全国高等中医药院校中药学类专业双语规划教材
Bilingual Planned Textbooks for Chinese Materia Medica Majors in TCM Colleges and Universities

中药学
Chinese Materia Medica

（供中药学类专业使用）
(For Chinese Materia Medica Majors)

主　编　张一昕　叶耀辉

副主编　杨　敏　张　艳　林海燕　王雪敏

编　者　（以姓氏笔画为序）

王　茜（河北中医学院）　　　　王英豪（福建中医药大学）

王科军（滨州医学院）　　　　　王雪敏（河北中医学院）

王琳琳（辽宁中医药大学）　　　叶耀辉（江西中医药大学）

刘立萍（辽宁中医药大学）　　　杨　敏（成都中医药大学）

杨青山（安徽中医药大学）　　　李　丽（河北医科大学）

余　娜（湖南中医药大学）　　　张　艳（山东中医药大学）

张一昕（河北中医学院）　　　　沈　月（云南中医药大学）

林海燕（滨州医学院）　　　　　金素安（上海中医药大学）

周　鹏（天津中医药大学）　　　孟　洁（河北中医学院）

赵　彤（重庆医科大学）　　　　郝二伟（广西中医药大学）

胡晨霞（广州中医药大学）　　　柳海艳（北京中医药大学）

高　峰（陕西中医药大学）　　　管家齐（浙江中医药大学）

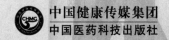

中国健康传媒集团
中国医药科技出版社

内 容 提 要

　　本教材是"全国高等中医药院校中药学类专业双语规划教材"之一。分为总论和各论两部分，系统地介绍了中药及中药学的概念、中药的起源和发展、中药的产地与采集、中药的炮制、中药的性能、中药的功效和临床应用等内容。本教材为书网融合教材，即纸质教材有机融合电子教材、教学配套资源（PPT、微课、视频、图片等）、题库系统、数字化教学服务（在线教学、在线作业、在线考试），使教学资源更加多样化、立体化。

　　本教材供全国高等中医药院校中药学、中药制药等中药学类专业及中医学、药学等相关专业使用，也可供从事中药研究、生产、销售工作的人员参考。

图书在版编目（CIP）数据

中药学：汉英对照 / 张一昕，叶耀辉主编 .—北京：中国医药科技出版社，2020. 8
全国高等中医药院校中药学类专业双语规划教材
ISBN 978-7-5214-1873-6

Ⅰ. ①中… 　Ⅱ. ①张…②叶… 　Ⅲ. ①中药学 – 双语教学 – 中医学院 – 教材 – 汉、英 　Ⅳ. ①R28

中国版本图书馆 CIP 数据核字（2020）第 097259 号

美术编辑　陈君杞
版式设计　辰轩文化

出版　**中国健康传媒集团** | 中国医药科技出版社
地址　北京市海淀区文慧园北路甲 22 号
邮编　100082
电话　发行：010-62227427　邮购：010-62236938
网址　www.cmstp.com
规格　889×1194 mm ¹⁄₁₆
印张　31
字数　877 千字
版次　2020 年 8 月第 1 版
印次　2020 年 8 月第 1 次印刷
印刷　三河市万龙印装有限公司
经销　全国各地新华书店
书号　ISBN 978-7-5214-1873-6
定价　98.00 元

获取新书信息、投稿、为图书纠错，请扫码联系我们。

近些年随着世界范围的中医药热潮的涌动，来中国学习中医药学的留学生逐年增多，走出国门的中医药学人才也在增加。为了适应中医药国际交流与合作的需要，加快中医药国际化进程，提高来中国留学生和国际班学生的教学质量，满足双语教学的需要和中医药对外交流需求，培养优秀的国际化中医药人才，进一步推动中医药国际化进程，根据教育部、国家中医药管理局、国家药品监督管理局等部门的有关精神，在本套教材建设指导委员会主任委员成都中医药大学彭成教授等专家的指导和顶层设计下，中国医药科技出版社组织全国 50 余所高等中医药院校及附属医疗机构约 420 名专家、教师精心编撰了全国高等中医药院校中药学类专业双语规划教材，该套教材即将付梓出版。

本套教材共计 23 门，主要供全国高等中医药院校中药学类专业教学使用。本套教材定位清晰、特色鲜明，主要体现在以下方面。

一、立足双语教学实际，培养复合应用型人才

本套教材以高校双语教学课程建设要求为依据，以满足国内医药院校开展留学生教学和双语教学的需求为目标，突出中医药文化特色鲜明、中医药专业术语规范的特点，注重培养中医药技能、反映中医药传承和现代研究成果，旨在优化教育质量，培养优秀的国际化中医药人才，推进中医药对外交流。

本套教材建设围绕目前中医药院校本科教育教学改革方向对教材体系进行科学规划、合理设计，坚持以培养创新型和复合型人才为宗旨，以社会需求为导向，以培养适应中药开发、利用、管理、服务等各个领域需求的高素质应用型人才为目标的教材建设思路与原则。

二、遵循教材编写规律，整体优化，紧跟学科发展步伐

本套教材的编写遵循"三基、五性、三特定"的教材编写规律；以"必需、够用"为度；坚持与时俱进，注意吸收新技术和新方法，适当拓展知识面，为学生后续发展奠定必要的基础。实验教材密切结合主干教材内容，体现理实一体，注重培养学生实践技能训练的同时，按照教育部相关精神，增加设计性实验部分，以现实问题作为驱动力来培养学生自主获取和应用新知识的能力，从而培养学生独立思考能力、实验设计能力、实践操作能力和可持续发展能力，满足培养应用型和复合型人才的要求。强调全套教材内容的整体优化，并注重不同教材内容的联系与衔接，避免遗漏和不必要的交叉重复。

三、对接职业资格考试，"教考""理实"密切融合

本套教材的内容和结构设计紧密对接国家执业中药师职业资格考试大纲要求，实现教学与考试、理论与实践的密切融合，并且在教材编写过程中，吸收具有丰富实践经验的企业人员参与教材的编写，确保教材的内容密切结合应用，更加体现高等教育的实践性和开放性，为学生参加考试和实践工作打下坚实基础。

四、创新教材呈现形式，书网融合，使教与学更便捷更轻松

全套教材为书网融合教材，即纸质教材与数字教材、配套教学资源、题库系统、数字化教学服务有机融合。通过"一书一码"的强关联，为读者提供全免费增值服务。按教材封底的提示激活教材后，读者可通过 PC、手机阅读电子教材和配套课程资源（PPT、微课、视频等），并可在线进行同步练习，实时收到答案反馈和解析。同时，读者也可以直接扫描书中二维码，阅读与教材内容关联的课程资源，从而丰富学习体验，使学习更便捷。教师可通过 PC 在线创建课程，与学生互动，开展在线课程内容定制、布置和批改作业、在线组织考试、讨论与答疑等教学活动，学生通过 PC、手机均可实现在线作业、在线考试，提升学习效率，使教与学更轻松。此外，平台尚有数据分析、教学诊断等功能，可为教学研究与管理提供技术和数据支撑。需要特殊说明的是，有些专业基础课程，例如《药理学》等 9 种教材，起源于西方医学，因篇幅所限，在本次双语教材建设中纸质教材以英语为主，仅将专业词汇对照了中文翻译，同时在中国医药科技出版社数字平台"医药大学堂"上配套了中文电子教材供学生学习参考。

编写出版本套高质量教材，得到了全国知名专家的精心指导和各有关院校领导与编者的大力支持，在此一并表示衷心感谢。希望广大师生在教学中积极使用本套教材和提出宝贵意见，以便修订完善，共同打造精品教材，为促进我国高等中医药院校中药学类专业教育教学改革和人才培养做出积极贡献。

数字化教材编委会

主　编　张一昕　叶耀辉

副主编　杨　敏　张　艳　林海燕　王雪敏　王　茜

编　者　（以姓氏笔画为序）

王　茜（河北中医学院）　　王英豪（福建中医药大学）

王科军（滨州医学院）　　　王雪敏（河北中医学院）

王琳琳（辽宁中医药大学）　叶耀辉（江西中医药大学）

刘立萍（辽宁中医药大学）　杨　敏（成都中医药大学）

杨青山（安徽中医药大学）　李　丽（河北医科大学）

余　娜（湖南中医药大学）　张　艳（山东中医药大学）

张一昕（河北中医学院）　　沈　月（云南中医药大学）

林海燕（滨州医学院）　　　金素安（上海中医药大学）

周　鹏（天津中医药大学）　孟　洁（河北中医学院）

赵　彤（重庆医科大学）　　郝二伟（广西中医药大学）

胡晨霞（广州中医药大学）　柳海艳（北京中医药大学）

高　峰（陕西中医药大学）　管家齐（浙江中医药大学）

中医药是中华民族的宝贵财富，为中华民族的繁衍昌盛做出了巨大贡献。中药学是研究中药的基本理论和临床应用的学科，是中医药各专业的基础学科之一，记录着我国人民发明和发展中医药学的智慧创造。随着我国综合国力的提高，中药在世界各国逐渐被接受，因此亟需培养高层次的中药学双语人才，以促进中医药的国际化进程。为深入贯彻落实教育部《关于加强高等学校本科教学工作提高教学质量的若干意见》和《国务院关于扶持和促进中医药事业发展的若干意见》等相关文件精神，更好地适应当前高等教育改革发展的需求，培养适应行业发展需要的创新型、复合型人才，推动中医药对外交流，全国17所中医药院校的专家学者立足双语教学实际，在继承传统的基础上，结合现代研究成果，共同编写了本教材。

本教材主要围绕"学生好学、教师好教、医药行业好用"的"三好"目标制定编写体例，对接职业资格考试，明确学习目标，突出中药学的基础性、适用性和创新性。教材分为总论和各论两部分，共26章。其中总论部分共计5章，系统介绍了中药及中药学的基本概念、中药的起源和发展、中药的产地与采集、中药的炮制、中药的性能、中药的应用，编写力求突出重点、简明扼要。各论部分根据《国家执业药师资格考试大纲》要求，收载常用中药407味，按照功效分为21章，针对需要掌握和大部分需要熟悉的药物，在正文介绍来源、产地、采集、炮制、质量标准、药性、功效、应用、用法用量、使用注意、现代研究等内容；针对需要了解和少部分需要熟悉的药物，在每章末集中以表格形式阐释。文末以中药名拼音为序设置索引，方便检索。

本教材为书网融合教材，即纸质教材有机融合电子教材、教学配套资源（PPT、微课、视频、图片等）、题库系统、数字化教学服务（在线教学、在线作业、在线考试），使教学资源更加多样化、立体化。本教材供全国高等中医药院校中药学、中药制药等中药学类专业及中医学、药学等相关专业使用，也可供从事中药研究、生产、销售工作的人员参考。

本教材在编写过程中得到了相关院校的大力支持，在此致以诚挚的谢意！尽管编写力臻完善，但难免存在疏漏或不足之处，敬请各位读者批评指正！

编　者
2020 年 4 月

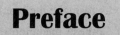

Preface

Chinese medicine is the precious wealth of the Chinese nation and has made great contributions to the prosperity of the Chinese nation. Chinese Materia Medica is the basic theory and clinical application of traditional Chinese medicine, is one of the basic disciplines of Chinese medicine, recording the people of our country to invent and develop the wisdom of traditional Chinese medicine. With the improvement of China's comprehensive national strength, traditional Chinese medicine has been gradually accepted all over the world. It is urgent to cultivate high-level bilingual talents of traditional Chinese medicine to promote the internationalization of traditional Chinese medicine.

In order to thoroughly implement the spirit of relevant documents such as *Ministry of Education's Opinions on Strengthening the Undergraduate Teaching and Improving the Teaching Quality of Colleges and Universities* and *State Council's Opinions on Supporting and Promoting the Development of Traditional Chinese Medicine*, better adapt to the needs of the current reform and development of higher education, cultivate innovative and compound talents to meet the needs of the industry development, and promote the development of traditional Chinese medicine. Based on the practice of bilingual teaching, experts and scholars from 17 colleges and universities of traditional Chinese medicine have jointly compiled this textbook on the basis of inheriting the tradition and combining the results of modern research.

This textbook mainly focuses on the "three convenient" goals of student convenient in learning, teacher convenient in teaching, and the pharmaceutical industry convenient in application. It integrates vocational qualification examination, defines learning objectives, and highlights the foundation, applicability and innovation of Chinese pharmacy. The textbook is divided into two parts: general introduction and each theory, totaling 26 chapters. There are five chapters in the general part, which systematically introduce the concept of traditional Chinese medicine and Chinese medicine, the origin and development of traditional Chinese medicine, the origin and collection of traditional Chinese medicine, the processing of traditional Chinese medicine, the performance of traditional Chinese medicine, the application of traditional Chinese medicine, and strive to highlight the core content and be concise. According to the requirements of the national qualification examination program for licensed pharmacists, 407 kinds of commonly used traditional Chinese medicines are collected in each part, which are divided into 21 chapters according to their efficacy. For the drugs that need to be mastered and those whose major contents need to be familiar with, the source, place of origin, collection, processing, quality standard, property, efficacy, application, usage and dosage, attention to use, chemical composition, pharmacological research and other contents are introduced in the text; for some drugs whose minor contents need to be familiar with and for the drugs that need to be understood are explained in tabular form at the end of each section. The index is set up according to the Pinyin of Chinese medicine names for convenient search.

This textbook is the book-network integration textbook, that is, the paper textbook organically integrates the electronic textbook, teaching supporting resources (PPT, micro-class, video, picture, etc.), question bank system, digital teaching services (online teaching, online homework, online examination), so as to make the teaching resources more diversified and three-dimensional. This book is for the use of Chinese medicine majors such as Chinese medicine, Chinese medicine pharmacy, etc., in colleges and universities of Chinese medicine in China, as well as related majors such as Chinese medicine and pharmacy, and also for the reference of personnel engaged in the research, production and sales of Chinese medicine.

The compilation of this textbook strives to be concise, easy to understand and easy to learn. In this process, it has been greatly supported by relevant colleges and universities. I sincerely thank you! Although the compilation is perfect, there are inevitably omissions or deficiencies and we are eagerly looking forward to your comments and corrects.

Editor
April, 2020

目录┊Contents

总 论
General introduction

各 论
Special discussion

总　论
General introduction

第一章 绪 言
Chapter 1 Introduction

 学习目标 | Learning goals

1. **掌握** 中药、中药学、临床中药学的含义。

2. **熟悉** 本草、中药材、中药饮片、中成药的含义；历代具有代表性的本草著作名称、作者及主要学术成就。

3. **了解** 中药学与临床中药学的区别；先辈对中药基本知识与中药学基础理论的认知过程；中药对人类防治疾病做出的重大贡献。

1. Master the meaning of Chinese medicinal, Chinese Materia Medica and Clinical Chinese Pharmacy.

2. Familiar with the meaning of materia medica, Chinese medicinal materials, Chinese medicinal pieces, and Chinese patent medicines; the titles, authors and major academic achievements of the representative works of the past dynasties.

3. Understand the difference between Chinese Materia Medica and Clinical Chinese Pharmacy, the cognitive process of the basic knowledge of Chinese medicinal and the basic theory of Chinese Materia Medica; the great contribution of Chinese medicinals to the prevention and treatment of human diseases.

我国幅员辽阔，地形复杂，气候条件多样，有着丰富的中药天然资源，主要包括植物资源、动物资源、矿物资源。古代本草文献所载的中药已超过 3000 种。20 世纪 90 年代全国中药资源普查资料表明，中药资源已达 12 807 种。数千年来，中国人民以这些资源作为防病治病的主要工具，为中华民族的繁衍和健康发挥了巨大的作用。

China has a vast territory, complex terrain, diverse climate conditions, and rich natural resources of traditional Chinese medicinals, mainly including plant resources, animal resources, and mineral resources. According to the ancient literature of materia medica, there are more than 3000 kinds of Chinese medicinals. The general survey of Chinese medicinal resources in 1990s showed there were 12 807 kinds of Chinese medicinals. For thousands of years, these resources have been used as the main tools for disease prevention and treatment, and played a huge role in the reproduction and health of the Chinese nation.

医药大学堂
WWW.YIYAODXT.COM

第一节 中药与中药学的基本概念
Section 1 General concepts of Chinese medicinal and Chinese Materia Medica

1. **中药** 是我国传统药物的总称,是在中医药理论指导下,用于预防、治疗、诊断疾病并具有康复与保健作用的物质,主要包括中药材、中药饮片和中成药等。

(1) Chinese medicine Chinese medicine is the general term of traditional Chinese medicinal materials. It is, under the guidance of the theory of traditional Chinese medicine (TCM), used to prevent, treat and diagnose diseases and has the function of rehabilitation and health care, mainly including Chinese medicinal materials, Chinese herbal pieces and Chinese patent medicine.

2. **中药学** 是研究中药的基本理论和中药的品种来源、药材鉴别、种植、采收、贮存、加工炮制、制剂、性能、功效、应用、药理、化学成分等一切与中药有关内容的一级学科,是"广义的中药学"。随着学科的不断发展,逐步分化为中药资源学、中药栽培学、中药鉴定学、中药炮制学、中药化学、中药药剂学、中药药理学、临床中药学和中成药学等分支学科。

(2) Chinese Materia Medica It is a first level discipline related to Chinese medicinals, which studies the basic theory, as well as the source of varieties, identification, planting, collection, storage, processing, preparation, property, efficacy, application, pharmacology, chemical composition of various Chinese medicines, also known as "generalized Chinese Materia Medica". With the continuous development of this discipline, it is gradually divided into Resourceology of Chinese Medicinals, Science of Chinese Medicinal Cultivation, Identification of Chinese Pharmacy, Science of Chinese Medicinal Processing, Chinese Medical Chemistry, Chinese Pharmaceutics, Chinese Pharmacology, Clinical Chinese Pharmacy, and Science of Chinese Patent Medicines.

3. **临床中药学** 是以中药的性能、功效、主治为核心,以临床安全、有效、合理用药为目的,研究中药基础理论和各药临床应用的二级学科,是"狭义的中药学"。临床中药学是衔接中医学和中药学、中医基础学科和临床各科之间的桥梁,是一门重要的专业基础课程。中药性能理论、功效理论、配伍理论、应用理论,以及影响临床效用的相关知识,均属于临床中药学的研究范畴。

(3) Clinical Chinese Pharmacy It is a secondary discipline, also known as "narrow sense Chinese Materia Medica", which studies the basic theory of Chinese medicinals and clinical application of each medicinal with the property, efficacy and main treatment as the core and clinical safe, effectiveness and rational medication as the purpose. Clinical Chinese Pharmacy is an important professional basic course, bridging TCM and Chinese Materia Medica, basic and clinical disciplines. The property theory, efficacy theory, combination theory, application theory of Chinese medicinals, as well as related knowledge affecting clinical effect, all belongs to the research category of Clinical Chinese Pharmacy.

4. **本草** 是中国古代所称的中药以及中药著作。中药的来源虽然有植物、动物、矿物以及某些生物制品,但以植物药为最多,故有"诸药以草为本"的说法。因而自古相沿把中药称为本草,将记载中药的有关著作也冠以本草之名。

(4) Materia medica It refers to the ancient Chinese medicinals and works on it. Although Chinese medicinals are from plants, animals, minerals and some chemical and biological products, most of them are plant medicine, so there is a saying that "all kinds of medicinals are based on herbs". Therefore,

Chinese medicinal has been called "Materia Medica" since ancient times, and relevant works are also named "Materia Medica".

5. **中药材** 是指未经精制加工或未制成成品的原生药材（生药）。一般指原植物、动物、矿物、除去非药用部位的商品药材，符合药品标准，具有天然药物属性，是生产中药饮片的原料。

(5) **Chinese medicinal materials** They refer to the crude medicine (crude drug) that has not been refined or processed. Generally, they refer to the original plants, animals, minerals, and commercial medicinal materials excluding non medicinal parts, which meet the drug standards and have the natural drug properties, and are the raw materials for the production of Chinese herbal pieces.

6. **中药饮片** 是在中医药理论指导下，根据中药炮制规范，将中药材进行加工炮制，制成的一定规格、可直接用于中医临床调配和制剂的中药。

(6) **Chinese herbal pieces** They refer to the medicinals which are processed into certain specifications and directly used in clinical deployment and preparation according to the processing standards of Chinese medicinals under the guidance of TCM theory.

7. **中成药** 是在中医药理论指导下，以中药饮片为原料，按规定的处方和标准制成的具有一定规格的剂型，是直接用于防治疾病的制剂。中成药具有特定的名称和剂型，在标签和说明书上注明批准文号、品名、规格、处方成分、功效和适应证、用法用量、禁忌、使用注意、生产批号、有效期等内容。

(7) **Chinese patent medicine** It is a kind of preparation with certain specifications and directly used in the prevention and treatment of diseases. It is made of Chinese herbal pieces according to the specified prescription and standard under the guidance of TCM theory. Chinese patent medicine has a specific name and dosage form, and the label and instruction indicate the approval number, product name, specification, prescription compositions, efficacy and indications, dosage and administration, contraindications, precautions, batch number, expiry date, etc.

第二节　中药知识的初步积累和中药学的发展

Section 2　Preliminary accumulation of Chinese medicinal knowledge and development of Chinese Materia Medica

PPT

一、中药知识的初步积累
1. Preliminary accumulation of Chinese medicinal knowledge

中药的发现与应用有着悠久的历史。早在原始社会，人们为了生存，通过长期的采集食用植物和狩猎活动，逐步观察和了解到有些植物、动物不仅可以充饥果腹，而且可以减缓病痛，或引起中毒，甚至危及生命，造成死亡。古人经过无数次有意识的反复试验和观察，逐步形成了早期的药物认知。《淮南子·修务训》中记述的"神农尝百草之滋味……一日而遇七十毒"的传说，生动而形象地概括了人类药物知识的萌芽是与寻求食物的生活实践密切相关的。

The discovery and application of Chinese medicinals has gone through a very long history. As early as in the primitive society, people undertook collecting of edible plants and hunting for survival. They gradually observed and understood that these plants and animals could satisfy hunger, some could relieve pains, and some could cause poisoning, even endanger life and cause death. After countless conscious repeated experiments and observations, the ancients gradually formed early drug knowledge. *Huái Nán Zǐ—Xiū Wù Xùn* records a legend that "Shennong tasted hundreds of herbs…and met 70 poisons in one day", which vividly illustrated the rudiments of medicinal knowledge and has a close connection to living practice of foraging for food.

人类早期主要以植物性食物充饥，因而最先发现的是植物药。在广泛的渔猎活动开展之后，又相继认识了某些动物药。进入原始社会后期，随着开矿、采石和冶炼的兴起，又相继发现并掌握了矿物药的加工和应用知识。在这一时期，我们的祖先还从野果与谷物自然发酵的启示中，逐步发现并掌握了酒的酿制技术。至殷商时期，酿酒业已十分兴盛，酒除了作为饮料之外，还具有祛寒邪、通血脉、行药势、作为溶媒等多方面的医疗作用，故古人将酒誉为"百药之长"。

The primitive human beings alleviated their hunger with vegetables, so vegetable medicines were first found. Some animal medicines were recognized after the development of fishing and hunting. In the late period of primitive society, along with the rise of mining, quarrying and smelting, processing and utilizing knowledge of mineral medicines were discovered and mastered. During this period, our ancestors gradually discovered and mastered the brewing technology of wine from the inspiration of natural fermentation of wild fruits and grains. In the Yin and Shang Dynasties, wine making industry was very prosperous. Besides being a drink, wine also had many medical functions, such as dispelling cold pathogen, dredging blood and channels, helping drugs function better, and acting as a solvent. Therefore, wine was regarded as the "parent of all medicines" in ancient times.

随着文字的创造和使用，药物知识也由口耳相传发展为文字记载。从现有文献可知，先秦时期认识的药物品种已十分可观。如《诗经》中用以比喻吟咏的植物和动物有 300 余种，其中大多为后世所常用。用以记述山川及物产的《山海经》，介绍了植物、动物、矿物药 120 余种，所言各物产地更加具体，还介绍了其医疗用途。20 世纪 70 年代初，长沙马王堆汉墓出土的《五十二病方》，虽并非药学专著，但留存医方 283 首，涉及药物已达 247 种之多，对药物的贮藏、炮制、制剂、用法、禁忌等均有记述。日渐丰富的药物知识为本草专著的产生奠定了基础。

With the creation and use of written words, medicinal knowledge has developed from oral to written records. It can be seen from the existing literature that the varieties of drugs recognized in the pre-Qin period are quite considerable. For example, in *Book of Songs* (*Shī Jīng*), there are more than 300 kinds of plants and animals, most of which are commonly used in later generations. There are more than 120 kinds of plant, animal and mineral medicine as well as their specific place of origins and their medical uses in *The Classic of Mountains and Seas* (*Shān Hǎi Jīng*), which mainly records mountains and rivers and their products. In the early 1970s, *Formulas for Fifty-two Diseases* (*Wǔ Shí Èr Bìng Fāng*) unearthed from Mawangdui Han tomb in Changsha was not a monograph on pharmacy, but there were 283 prescriptions in existence, involving 247 kinds of medicines, and there were records on the storage, processing, preparation, usage and contraindications of medicines. The growing knowledge of pharmacy has laid the foundation for the production of the monograph of Materia Medica.

二、中药学的发展
2. Development of Chinese Materia Medica

本草著作的出现，是中药学形成的重要标志。各个历史时期的主要本草著作是当时中药学发展的集中体现，其发展简况如下。

The emergence of the works of materia medica marked the formation of Chinese Materia Medica. The main works of Materia Medica in each historical period are the concentrated embodiment of the development of Chinese Materia Medica. Its development is as follows.

（一）秦汉时期（公元前 221~ 公元 220 年）

2.1 Qin and Han Dynasties (221B. C. ~220A. D.)

秦汉之际，本草学已初具规模，并有药学专著问世。成书于东汉末年的《神农本草经》（简称《本经》），是对汉以前药学知识的总结，代表了秦汉时期最高的药学成就，是我国现存最早的药学专著。全书分为"序录（总论）"和"药物（各论）"两部分，总论部分简要论述了四气、五味、有毒无毒、配伍法度、药物对剂型的选择以及产地、采收、加工、真伪等多方面内容，初步奠定了中药学理论的基础。各论部分载药 365 种，按照有毒无毒以及功效分为上、中、下三品。上品 120 种，功能滋补强壮，延年益寿，无毒或毒性很弱；中品 120 种，功能治病补虚，有毒或无毒；下品 125 种，功专治病攻邪，多具毒性，这是药物按功效分类的创始。每药项下，主要介绍性味、功效、主治等内容。其所载药效，大多朴实有验，如麻黄平喘、黄连治痢、人参补虚、茵陈退黄、半夏止呕等，至今亦为临床常用之品。该书为研究秦汉医药发展情况留下了宝贵的资料。其编写体例和内容，成为后世本草的范例和基础，为中药学的全面发展奠定了理论基石。

At the time of Qin and Han Dynasties, material medica had begun to take shape, and monographs on pharmacy appeared. *Shen Nong's Classic of the Materia Medica* (*Shén Nóng Běn Cǎo Jīng*), also called *Classic of Materia Medica* (*Běn Jīng*) for short, was compiled at the end of the Eastern Han Dynasty and is a summary of the pharmaceutical knowledge before the Han Dynasty, represents the highest pharmaceutical achievements of the Qin and Han Dynasties, and is the earliest existing pharmaceutical monograph in China. The book is divided into two parts: "Preface (general discussion)" and "Medicinals (specific discussion)". The first part briefly discusses four qi, five flavors, toxic and non-toxic, compatibility, drug selection of dosage forms, as well as the origin, collection, processing, authenticity and other aspects, which initially lays the foundation of the theory of Chinese Materia Medica. The second part contains 365 kinds of medicinals which is divided into three categories according to their toxicity and efficacy: top grade, medium grade, and low grade. 120 kinds of top grade medicinals with no or slight toxicity function as nourishing and improving health, prolonging life; 120 kinds of medium grade medicinals with or without toxicity function as treating disease and tonifying deficiency; 125 kinds of low grade medicinals with toxicity are special in treating disease and attacking pathogens. It is the beginning of drug classification according to function. Each item mainly introduces the property, nature, efficacy, and indications, most of which are plain and effective, such as *má huáng* (Ephedrae Herba) for relieving dyspnea, *huáng lián* (Coptidis Rhizoma) for dysentery, *rén shēn* (Ginseng Radix et Rhizoma) for tonifying deficiency, *yīn chén* (Artemisiae Scopariae Herba) for removing jaundice, and *bàn xià* (Pinelliae Rhizoma) for stopping vomiting, which are also commonly used in clinical practice. This book leaves valuable information for the study of Qin and Han medicine. Its writing style and content became the example and foundation of the future Materia Medica, and laid a theoretical foundation for the comprehensive development of Chinese Materia Medica.

（二）魏晋南北朝时期（公元 220~581 年）

2.2 Wei, Jin, Southern and Northern Dynasties (220~581 A. D.)

随着临床用药不断发展，医家应用的药物种类日渐增多，加之南北融合和与外国交往的扩大，本草学的内容更加丰富。此期本草著作有近百种之多，且形式多样，有综合性、炮制类、专科用药类、配伍宜忌、食物类，以及单味药专论、采药、药图等。对后世影响较大者除《吴普本草》《名医别录》、李当之《药录》及徐之才《药对》外，首推梁代陶弘景辑成的《本草经集注》（简称《集注》）。该书完成于公元500年左右，以《本经》为基础，又从《名医别录》中选取365种药物，加上陶氏自注而成，全书共7卷，载药730种。书中"序录"部分，首先回顾本草学发展概况，随后对《本经》序文13条逐一注释、发挥，补充了许多采收、鉴别、加工、炮制、制剂、配伍、合理配方取量方面的理论和操作原则，极大丰富了药学总论的内容。其增列的"诸病通用药"，实为病证用药索引，便于临床医生查询。各论部分首创按药物自然属性分类的方法，列玉石、草木、虫兽、果、菜、米谷及有名未用七类，各类中又结合三品分类排列药物顺序，每味药物项下不仅转录《本经》和《名医别录》的内容，并增加自注，以阐明作者的用药经验和见解。该书对魏晋以来300余年的药学成就进行了全面总结，奠定了我国大型骨干本草编写的雏形，标志着综合本草模式的初步确立。其编写体例和内容，一直为后世许多本草学家所沿袭习用。

Along with the continuous development of clinical medication, more and more kinds of medicines were used by doctors. With the integration of North and South and the expansion of sino foreign exchanges, the content of Materia Medica was more abundant. Nearly one hundred works on materia medica appeared at that time, and they are various in forms, comprehensive, processing, specialty medication, incompatible, food, and single drug monograph, drug collection, drug pictures, and so on. Among the works that have a great influence on later generations, except for *Wu Pu's Materia Medica* (*Wú Pǔ Běn Cǎo*), *Miscellaneous Records of Famous Physicians* (*Míng Yī Bié Lù*), Li Dang's *Materia Medica Records* (*Yào Lù*) and Xu Zhicai's *Medicinal Pairs* (*Yào Duì*), *Collective Commentaries on the Classic of Materia Medica* (*Běn Cǎo Jīng Jí Zhù*) compiled by Tao Hongjing in the Liang Dynasty is the most important one, which was completed around 500 A.D. based on the book of *Classic of Materia Medica* (*Běn Jīng*) and selected 365 kinds of medicinals from *Miscellaneous Records of Famous Physicians* (*Míng Yī Bié Lù*) with his own notes. It is composed of 7 volumes consisting 730 kinds of medicinals. General Discussion of the book reviews the development of Material Medica, and then annotates and develops the 13 items in the preface of the book one by one, adding a lot of theories and operation principles in the aspects of collection, identification, processing, preparation, compatibility and reasonable formula, so as to enrich the content of the general theory of pharmacy. The added "general medicines for all diseases" is actually the index of medicine used for syndromes, which is convenient for clinicians to query. Specific Discussion of book initiated the method of classification according to the natural attributes of medicinals, which was classified into seven categories: jade, plants, insects and animals, fruits, vegetables, grains and those having names but not used. In each category, the order of drugs was arranged in combination with the classification of three grades. It attaches notes to each article of *Classic of Materia Medica* (*Běn Jīng*) and *Miscellaneous Records of Famous Physicians* (*Míng Yī Bié Lù*) to reflect the author's experience and opinions on medication. The book comprehensively summarizes the pharmaceutical achievements of more than 300 years since the Wei and Jin Dynasties, and establishes the rudiment of the compilation of materia medica in China, marking the preliminary establishment of the writing pattern for comprehensive materia medica. Its writing style and content have been used by many herbalists in later generations.

南朝刘宋时期，雷敩总结了当时药物炮制的经验，撰成《雷公炮炙论》，该书系统地介绍了300种中药的炮制方法，提出药物经过炮制可以提高药效，降低毒性，便于贮存、调剂、制剂等。原书虽已散佚，但其内容多为后世本草书籍及有关著作所引述。该书是我国第一部炮制专著，标志着本草中又一新兴分支学科的出现，对后世中药炮制产生了极大的影响，书中记载的某些炮制方法至今仍有很大参考价值。

In the Liu Song Period of Southern Dynasty, Lei Yu summarized the experience of medicinal processing at that time and compiled *Master Lei's Discourse on Medicinal Processing* (*Léi Gōng Páo Zhì Lùn*). The book systematically introduced the processing methods of 300 kinds of Chinese medicinals, and proposed that the processed drugs could improve the efficacy, reduce the toxicity, and be convenient for storage, dispensing and preparation. Although the original book has been lost, most of its contents are quoted by the later works. This book is the first processing monograph in our country, marking the emergence of another new branch of materia medica, which has a great impact on the medicinal processing in later generations. Some processing methods recorded in the book still have great reference value.

（三）隋唐时期（公元 581~960 年）

2.3 Sui and Tang Dynasties (581-960 A.D.)

隋唐时期，尤其是盛唐之时，政权统一，经济文化日渐繁荣，交通不断发达，海外交往逐步扩大，医药学有了较大的发展。相继从海外输入的药材品种亦有所增加，本草内容更加丰富，各地使用的药物总数已达千种之多。此外，长期分裂、战乱等原因造成药物品种及名称混乱，加之《本草经集注》成书之际，正处于南北分裂时期，对北方药物情况缺乏了解，内容上存在一定的局限性，而且，在一百年来的传抄中出现了不少错误，因而有必要对本草做一次全面的整理和总结。

In the Sui and Tang Dynasties, especially in the heyday of the Tang Dynasty, with the unity of political power, the prosperity of economy and culture, the continuous development of transportation, and the gradual expansion of overseas exchanges, great progress had been made in medicine. The varieties of medicinal materials imported from overseas had also increased, and materia medica had become more abundant. The total number of medicines used in various regions reached as many as one thousand. In addition, medicinal varieties and names were confused due to the long-term division, war and other reasons, and *Collective Commentaries on the Classic of Materia Medica* (*Běn Cǎo Jīng Jí Zhù*) was compiled in north and south split period and there were some limitations in the content of this book due to lack of knowledge about medicinals in the north. Moreover, many errors appeared in the private copying in the past 100 years, so it was necessary to make a comprehensive summarization of the materia medica.

唐显庆四年（公元 659 年），由唐政府组织编纂、颁行，长孙无忌、李勣、苏敬等 23 人撰写的《新修本草》（又名《唐本草》），是我国历史上第一部官修本草，也是世界上最早公开颁布的药典性本草著作，比公元 1542 年欧洲颁布的《纽伦堡药典》要早 800 余年。全书共 54 卷，载药 850 种（一说为 844 种），分为玉石、草、木、兽禽、虫、鱼、果菜、米谷、有名未用九类。在编写过程中，唐政府通令全国各地选送当地道地药材，作为实物标本进行描绘，从而增加了绘制考究的药物图谱，并辅以文字说明，以介绍各药形态特征。这种图文对照的编写形式，开创了世界药学著作的先河，其内容丰富，取材精要，具有较高的学术水平和科学价值，反映了唐代本草学的辉煌成就，奠定了我国大型骨干本草编写的格局，对国内外医药学发展产生了巨大影响。该书以崭新的形式和内容广为流传，成为我国唐代及当时日本等医生的必修课本。

In the fourth year of Xianqing of Tang Dynasty (659 A.D.), *Newly Revised Materia Medica* (*Xīn Xīu Běn Cǎo*), also known as *Tang Materia Medica* (*Táng Běn Cǎo*), was compiled and promulgated by the government. It was written by 23 people, such as Zhangsun Wuji, Li Ji and Su Jing. It is the first official revised materia medica in history of China and the earliest published works of pharmacopeia in the world more than 800 years earlier than the European *Nuremberg Pharmacopoeia* in 1542 A.D. The treatise consists of 54 volumes, containing 850 medicinals (or 844), which was classified into nine categories: jade, grass, woods, animals, insects, fish, fruits and vegetables, grains and those having names but not used. In the process of compilation, the government ordered all parts of the country to select and send authentic medicinal materials as physical samples for description, thus increasing the preparation of a sophisticated medicinal map, supplemented by text description, to introduce the morphological characteristics of each medicinal. This kind of compilation form of contrast between pictures and texts created the forerunner of pharmaceutical works in the world. This book is rich in content, essential in materials and of high academic level and scientific value. It reflects the brilliant achievements of Materia Medica in Tang Dynasty, establishes the pattern of large-scale key materia medica compilation in China and has a great impact on the development of medicine at home and abroad. With its new form and content, it became a compulsory textbook for doctors in Tang Dynasty and Japan at that time.

唐开元年间（公元 713~741 年），陈藏器对《新修本草》进行了增补和辨误，著成《本草拾遗》。他广泛收集资料，不仅搜集了《唐本草》所遗漏的民间药物，而且辨识品类也极审慎，充实了本草学的内容，并根据药物功效提出药有宣、通、补、泻、轻、重、滑、涩、燥、湿十类，成为日后药物和方剂按功效分类的发端。

In the Kaiyuan period of the Tang Dynasty (713-741 A.D.), Chen Cangqi supplemented and identified *Newly Revised Materia Medica* (*Xīn Xiū Běn Cǎo*) and compiled *Supplement to the Materia Medica* (*Běn Cǎo Shí Yí*). He collected a wide range of data, not only collecting the folk drugs omitted in *Tang Materia Medica* (*Táng Běn Cǎo*), but also identifying the categories with great prudence, enriching the content of Material Medica. According to the medicinal efficacy, he put forward ten categories of medicinals: dispersing, dredging, tonifying, purgative, light, heavy, lubricant, astringent, dry and damp, which became the starting point of later medicinals and prescriptions classified by efficacy.

此外，由孟诜原著、张鼎增补的《食疗本草》，较全面地总结了唐代的食疗经验。李珣所辑《海药本草》，则为介绍外来药的专著。

In addition, *Materia Medica for Dietary Therapy* (*Shí Liáo Běn Cǎo*) written by Meng Shen, supplemented by Zhang Ding, comprehensively summarized the dietotherapy experience of Tang Dynasty. *Materia Medica from the [Southern] Seaboard Area* (*Hǎi Yào Běn Cǎo*) is a monograph introducing foreign medicinals.

（四）宋、金、元时期（公元 960~1368 年）
2.4 Song, Jin and Yuan Dynasties (960-1368 A.D.)

雕版印刷等技术的应用，为医药书籍的编纂和刊行提供了有利条件。宋代初年，依靠国家力量对药材的来源和品种进行了全面考订，相继刊行了多部官修本草。如 973~974 年刊行了《开宝本草》，书成之后，发现尚有遗漏，翌年又进行增订，名为《开宝重订本草》，1060 年刊行《嘉祐补注本草》，1061 年刊行《本草图经》（又称《图经本草》），附有 900 多幅药图，是我国现存最早的版刻本草图谱。当时《嘉祐补注本草》与《图经本草》各自刊行，使用不便，因而四川医者陈承将两书合并，并增加古今论说及个人见解，名为《重广补注神农本草图经》。

Development of economy, culture, science and technology, commerce and transportation, especially the application of engraving and printing technology, provided favorable conditions for the compilation and publication of medical books. In the early years of Song Dynasty, with the supporting of the government, the source and variety of medicinal materials were comprehensively examined and revised, and many official revised works of materia medica were published successively. For example, *Materia Medica of the Kaibao Era* (*Kāi Bǎo Běn Cǎo*) was published in 973-974, was renewed for the second time the following year, named *Revised Materia Medica of the Kaibao Era* (*Kāi Bǎo Chóng Dìng Běn Cǎo*), since some omissions were found in the book. In 1060, *Supplementary Annotations on Materia Medica of the Jiayou Era* (*Jiā Yòu Bǔ Zhù Běn Cǎo*) was published. In 1061, *Illustrated Classic of Materia Medica* (*Běn Cǎo Tú Jīng*, also known as *Tú Jīng Běn Cǎo* in Chinese) was published, with more than 900 medicinal pictures attached. It is the earliest version of Materia Medica with engraving illustrations in China. However, *Materia Medica of the Jiayou Era* and *Illustrated Classic of Materia Medica* were published separately, which made it inconvenient to use. Therefore, Chen Cheng, a doctor in Sichuan, combined the two books and added ancient and modern theories and personal opinions, which was titled *Revised Extensively Supplementary Annotation* of *Illustrated Classic of Materia Medica* (*Chóng Guǎng Bǔ Zhù Shén Nóng Běn Cǎo Tú Jīng*).

宋代最有代表性的大型综合本草，为四川名医唐慎微个人编纂的《经史证类备急本草》(简称《证类本草》)，书以《嘉祐补注本草》和《本草图经》为基础，整理了经史百家典籍中有关药学的资料，载药 1746 种（各种刊本的数字略有出入），附列单方 3000 余首。每味药物附有图谱，这种方药兼收，图文并重的编写体例，较前代本草又有所进步，使我国大型骨干本草编写格局臻于完备。该书对所收载的资料采用原文照录、注明出处的方法，使得宋以前许多已经亡佚的本草资料得以流传后世，具有很高的学术价值、实用价值和重要的文献价值。

The most representative large-scale comprehensive treatise on materia medica in the Song Dynasty is *Classified Materia Medica from Historical Classics for Emergency* (*Jīng Shǐ Zhèng Lèi Bèi Jí Běn Cǎo*, also known as *Zhèng Lèi Běn Cǎo* in Chinese) compiled by Tang Shenwei, a famous doctor in Sichuan. The treatise, based on the *Materia Medica of the Jiayou Era* and *Illustrated Classic of Materia Medica*, collates the materials related to pharmacy in hundreds of classics and historical books. It contains 1746 kinds of medicinals (the number of various publications varies slightly), and lists more than 3000 single prescriptions. Each medicinal has an attached illustration. This compilation pattern, which includes both prescriptions and medicinals, and lays equal stress on illustrations and text, is more advanced than the former ones of previous generations, making perfect the writing pattern of large-scale key treatise on materia medica in China. Since it records the original words and indicates the place of origin, many of the lost materials before the Song Dynasty can be handed down to later generations by the excerpt of this treatise, which not only has high academic value and practical value, but also has important document value.

金元时期的本草一般出自医家之手，药味不多，内容简要，具有明显的临床药学特征。如寇宗奭的《本草衍义》、张元素的《珍珠囊》、李东垣的《药类法象》和《用药心法》、王好古的《汤液本草》、朱丹溪的《本草衍义补遗》等。这些本草著作发展了升降浮沉、归经等药性理论，并使之系统化，进一步完善了中药性能的内容，而且根据中医理论，结合药物主治经验，总结各药功效，提高了本草的学术性、临床实用性和可读性。

The materia medica works of Jin and Yuan Dynasties were generally produced by doctors with fewer medicinals, brief contents, and obvious clinical pharmaceutical characteristics, such as *Extension of the Materia Medica* (*Běn Cǎo Yǎn Yì*) compiled by Kou Zongshi, *Pouch of Pearls* (*Zhēn Zhū Náng*) by Zhang Yuansu, *Medicinal Property and Action* (*Yào Lèi Fǎ Xiàng*) and *Teachings on Medication* (*Yòng Yào Xīn Fǎ*) by Li Dongyuan, *Materia Medica for Decoctions* (*Tāng Yè Běn Cǎo*) by Wang Haogu, and *Supplement to the Extension of the Materia Medica* (*Běn Cǎo Yǎn Yì Bǔ Yí*) by Zhu Danxi. These works developed and systematized the theories of medicinal properties, such as ascending, descending, floating and sinking, and meridian tropism. According to the theory of TCM, combined with the experience of main medicinal treatments, it summed up the efficacy of various medicinals, and improved the academic, clinical practicality and readability of materia medica.

元代忽思慧编著的《饮膳正要》是饮食疗法的专著，书中对养生避忌、妊娠食忌、高营养物的烹调法、营养疗法、食物卫生、食物中毒都有论述，介绍了许多回、蒙民族的食疗方法，至今仍有较高的参考价值。

Principles of Correct Diet (*Yǐn Shàn Zhèng Yào*) compiled by Hu Sihui is a monograph of dietotherapy, which discusses health contraindications, contraindications during, high nutrition cooking methods, nutrition therapy, food hygiene and food poisoning, and introduces many dietotherapy methods of Hui and Meng nationalities, which still have high reference value.

（五）明代（公元 1368~1644 年）
2.5　Ming Dynasty (1368-1644 A.D.)

随着医药学的发展，明代药学知识和技术进一步积累，沿用已久的《证类本草》已经不符合时代的要求。我国伟大的医药学家李时珍在《证类本草》的基础上，博采群书，经过走访调研，临床实践，实地考察，对古本草进行了系统全面的总结整理，补充修正。历时 27 年，三易其稿，终于在公元 1578 年完成了 200 多万字的本草巨著《本草纲目》。全书共 52 卷，载药 1892 种（新增 374 种），附方 11 000 余首，附图 1109 幅。序例中介绍历代诸家本草，全面总结明代以前的药性理论内容，保存了大量医药文献。该书按自然属性将药物分为水、火、土、金石、草、谷、菜、果、木、器服、虫、鳞、介、禽、兽、人共 16 部，62 类，每药标正名为纲，纲之下列目，纲目清晰，被认为是当时世界上最先进的分类法，为植物学分类奠定了基础。

With the development of medicine and pharmacy, the knowledge and technology of pharmacy were further accumulated in Ming Dynasty, and the long-standing *Zhèng Lèi Běn Cǎo* did not meet the requirements of the times. Li Shizhen, a great pharmacist in China, based on *Zhèng Lèi Běn Cǎo*, studied a lot of medical books, gathered materials, practiced personally, extensively investigated on the spot, systematically and comprehensively summarized and revised the ancient works on materia medica, and finally accomplished the monumental masterpiece *The Grand Compendium of Materia Medica* (*Běn Cǎo Gāng Mù*) in 1578 after 27 years and three times reversions. It has over two million Chinese characters, consisting of 52 volumes, with 1892 medicinals (374 newly-added), more than 11 000 formulas and 1109 attached pictures. The preface part introduces all kinds of Materia Medica in the past dynasties, summarizes the theory of medicinal property before the Ming Dynasty, and saves a lot of medical literature. The is divided into 16 sections and 62 categories according to the medicinal natural attributes: water, fire, earth, stone, grass, grain, vegetable, fruit, wood, clothing and tools, insect, fish, crustaceans, bird, animal and human. Every medicinal is compiled with its official name (*gang*), to which is attached many specific information (*mu*). With its clear *gang* and *mu*, it is considered the most advanced classification method in the world at that time, laying a foundation for botanical classification.

《本草纲目》中的每一味药都按释名、集解、修治、气味、主治、发明、附方等项分别叙述。详细地介绍了药物名称的由来和含义、产地、形态、真伪鉴别、采集、栽培、炮制方法、性味功能、主治特点。尤其是发明项下，主要介绍李时珍对药物观察、研究和实际应用的新发现、新经验，更加丰富了本草学的内容。该书集我国 16 世纪以前药学成就之大成，在训诂、语言文字、历史、地理、植物、动物、矿物、冶金、农学、气象等许多方面均有突出成就，其影响远超出了本草学的范围。自 1598 年刊行之后，很快风行全国，17 世纪初期流传到国外，先后被译为拉丁、日、法、德、英等 20 多种语言，在世界广泛流传，被国外学者誉为"16 世纪中国的百科全书"。2011 年，《本草纲目》作为世界物质文化遗产，与《黄帝内经》入选《世界记忆名录》。

Each material medica in *The Grand Compendium of Materia Medica* (*Běn Cǎo Gāng Mù*) is described separately with the following items: notes to the name, collection comprehensive explanations, rectification, odor, indications, invention and attached formulas, introducing in detail the origin and meaning of the name, place of origin, morphologic characteristics, identification of authenticity, collection, cultivation, processing, property and action, and indications. Especially the item of invention mainly introduces Li Shizhen's new discovery and experience in medicinal observation, research and practical application, which enriches the content of Material Medica. The treatise not only collects all the medicinal achievements of China before the 16th century and makes great achievements in the fields of exegesis, language, history, geography, plants, animals, minerals, metallurgy, agronomy, meteorology and so on. Its influence is far beyond the scope of Materia Medica. Since its publication in 1598, it has been popular all over the country and was spread abroad in the early 17th century. It has been translated into more than 20 languages, such as Latin, Japanese, French, German, and English. Widely spread in the world, it is known as the "Encyclopedia of China in the 16th century" by foreign scholars. In 2011, *The Grand Compendium of Materia Medica*, as a world material and cultural heritage, was selected into *The World Memory List* together with *The Yellow Emperor's Inner Classic* (*Huáng Dì Nèi Jīng*).

明代的专题本草也取得了瞩目成就。缪希雍的《炮炙大法》是明代影响最大的炮制专著。朱橚的《救荒本草》（1406 年）为食疗专著，收集了民间可供食用的 400 余种植物，丰富了植物学、本草学内容。李中立的《本草原始》对本草名实、性味、形态加以考证，绘图逼真，注重生药学的研究。兰茂编著的《滇南本草》是一部专门记载云南地区药物知识的地方本草。

The monographic texts of Ming Dynasty also made remarkable achievements. Miao Xiyong's *Great Processing Methods* (*Páo Zhì Dà Fǎ*) is the most influential monograph in Ming Dynasty; Zhu Su's *Materia Medica for Famine Relief* (*Jiù Huāng Běn Cǎo*) (1406) is a monograph on dietotherapy, which collects more than 400 kinds of folk edible plants and enriches the contents of Botany and Materia Medica; Li Zhongli's *Origins of the Materia Medica* (*Běn Cǎo Yuán Shǐ*) makes a textual research on the name, nature, flavor and form of Materia Medica with vivid drawings and stresses the study of pharmacognosy; Lan Mao's *Materia Medica of South Yunnan* (*Diān Nán Běn Cǎo*) is a local materia medica specially recording the knowledge of medicinals in Yunnan.

（六）清代（公元 1644~1911 年）
2.6 Qing Dynasty (1644-1911 A.D.)

在《本草纲目》的影响下，清代研究本草之风盛行，本草的数量达 400 种之多，代表作当推赵学敏的《本草纲目拾遗》（1765 年）。全书共 10 卷，载药 921 种，仅新增品种达 716 种之多，主要是民间药和外来药，同时收录了大量已散佚的方药书籍中的部分内容，极大地丰富了本草学的内容，具有重要的文献价值。它不仅拾《本草纲目》之遗漏，而且对《本草纲目》备而不详者加以补充修订，疏漏之处加以厘正。

Under the influence of *The Grand Compendium of Materia Medica* (*Běn Cǎo Gāng Mù*), the research on materia medica prevailed in Qing Dynasty and there were more than 400 kinds of treatises on it. Among them, *Supplement to the Grand Compendium of Materia Medica* (*Běn Cǎo Gāng Mù Shí Yí*) (in 1765) is a representative one. It contains 10 volumes and 921 medicinals, out of which 716 are newly-added, mainly folk and foreign medicinals. At the same time, it also collects contents of a large number of lost prescription books, which greatly enriches Material Medica and has important literature value. It not only picks up the omissions of *The Grand Compendium of Materia Medica*, but also supplements and revises the omissions and those without detailed information.

为配合临床需要，以临床实用为原则，撷取《本草纲目》精粹，旁引众家，兼抒己见，编撰成临床节要性本草，具有较高的质量，影响较大，如汪昂的《本草备要》、吴仪洛的《本草从新》、黄宫绣的《本草求真》等。另外，受考据和崇古思想的影响，清人辑复《神农本草经》等古典文献及阐释之风盛行，前者有孙星衍、顾观光等人的辑本，后者有《本草崇原》《本经逢原》《神农本草经百种录》《本经疏证》等，对学习研究《神农本草经》都有参考价值。

In order to meet the clinical needs, some essential treatises were compiled with high quality and great influence, which selected the essence of *The Grand Compendium of Materia Medica* and cited various authorities with clinical practice as principle, such as Wang Ang's *Essentials of Materia Medica* (*Běn Cǎo Bèi Yào*), Wu Yiluo's *Thoroughly Revised Materia Medica* (*Běn Cǎo Cóng Xīn*), and Huang Gongxiu's *Seeking Accuracy in the Materia Medica* (*Běn Cǎo Qiú Zhēn*). In addition, under the influence of textual research and the thought of worshiping the ancients, it was popular for the Qing people to collect and interpret classical documents such as *Shen Nong's Classic of the Materia Medica* (*Shén Nóng Běn Cǎo Jīng*). The former included editions by Sun Xingyan and Gu Guanguang, while the latter included *Reverence for the Origin of the Materia Medica* (*Běn Cǎo Chóng Yuán*), *Encountering the Sources of the Classic of Materia Medica* (*Běn Jīng Féng Yuán*), *A Hundred Records on Shen Nong's Classic of the Materia Medica* (*Shén Nóng Běn Cǎo Jīng Bǎi Zhǒng Lù*), and *Commentary on the Classic of Materia Medica* (*Běn Jīng Shū Zhèng*), which has great reference value for studying *Shen Nong's Classic of the Materia Medica*.

清代专题类本草门类齐全，其中不乏佳作，如张仲岩的《修事指南》，为炮制类专著；郑肖岩的《伪药条辨》，为优秀的辨药专书；吴其浚的《植物名实图考》，详记每种植物形态、产地、栽培、用途、药用部位、效用治验等内容，并附有插图，为研究药用植物提供了宝贵的文献资料。

In Qing Dynasty, there were all kinds of works on materia medica, including some excellent ones. For example, Zhang Zhongyan's *Guide to Preparation of Medicinals* (*Xiū Shì Zhǐ Nán*) is a monograph for processing; Zheng Xiaoyan's *Systematic Differentiation of Erroneous Medicinals* (*Wěi Yào Tiáo Biàn*) is an excellent monograph for differentiation of medicinals; Wu Qijun's *Illustrated Reference of Botanical Nomenclature* (*Zhí Wù Míng Shí Tú Kǎo*) details the form, origin, cultivation, use, medicinal parts, treating efficacy of each plant, with illustrations attached, and provides us with valuable literature and information for research on medicinal plants.

（七）民国时期（1912~1949年）

2.7 Period of the Republic of China (1912-1949A.D.)

民国时期我国医药学发展的特点是中西医药并存，中药辞书的产生和发展是这一时期中药学发展的一项重要成就，其中成就和影响最大的当推陈存仁主编的《中国药学大辞典》。全书约200万字，收录词目4300条，既广罗古籍，又博采新说，且附有标本图册，受到药界之推崇。虽有不少错讹，仍不失为近代第一部具有重要影响的大型药学辞书。

The development of Chinese medicine in the Republic of China is characterized by the coexistence of Chinese and Western medicine. The emergence and development of Chinese medicine dictionaries is an important achievement in the development of Chinese medicine in this period, among which the greatest achievement and influence is *Chinese Pharmacy Dictionary* (*Zhōng Guó Yào Xué Dà Cí Diǎn*) edited by Chen Cunren, Which is about 2 million words, including 4300 entries. It is not only a wide range of ancient books, but also a wide range of new ideas, with specimen atlas, which is highly praised by the pharmaceutical field. Although there are many mistakes, it is still the first large pharmaceutical dictionary with important influence in modern times.

随着中医学校的兴建，涌现了一批适应中医药教育需要的实用性强、内容简要、体例新颖的中药学讲义,如张山雷的《本草正义》、何廉臣的《实验药物学》、秦伯未的《药物学》、张锡纯的《药物讲义》等。这些讲义对各药功用主治的论述更加充实。其中,《本草正义》多是作者对药物疗效的新见解和临床经验,是理论结合实际的名著。

With the construction of schools of traditional Chinese medicine, a number of practical, simple and novel Chinese medicine handbooks have emerged, such as Zhang Shanlei's *Orthodox Interpretation of the Materia Medica* (*Běn Cǎo Zhèng Yì*), He Lianchen's *Experimental Pharmacology* (*Shí Yàn Yào Wù Xué*), Qin Bowei's *Pharmacology* (*Yào Wù Xué*), and Zhang Xichun's *Lecture Notes on Pharmacology* (*Yào Wù Jiǎng Yì*). These are more substantial in the discussion of the functions and indications of various medicinals, among which *Orthodox Interpretation of the Materia Medica* is about the author's new views and clinical experience on medicinal efficacy and is a famous work combining theory with practice.

民国时期,随着西方药学知识和化学、生物学、物理学等近代科学技术在我国的迅速传播和发展,初步建立了以中药为主要研究对象的药用动物学、药用植物学、生药学、中药鉴定学、中药药理学等新兴学科。在当时条件下,研究成果集中在中药的生药、药理、化学分析、有效成分提取及临床验证等方面,在一定程度上促进了中药学的发展。

During this period, with the rapid spread and development of Western pharmaceutical knowledge, Chemistry, Biology, Physics and other modern science and technology in China, new disciplines, such as Medicinal Zoology, Medicinal Botany, Pharmacognosy, Chinese Medicinal Identification and Chinese Pharmacology, were initially established, with Chinese medicinals as the main research object. At that time, its achievements focused on the crude drug, pharmacology, chemical analysis, effective component extraction and clinical verification of Chinese medicinals, and promoted the development of pharmacy to a certain extent.

(八)中华人民共和国成立以后

2.8　After the founding of the People's Republic of China

中华人民共和国成立以后,我国社会主义事业取得了伟大成就,政治稳定,经济繁荣,许多先进技术被引入医药学研究中,大大促进了中医药学的发展。

After the founding of the People's Republic of China, China's socialist cause has made great achievements with political stability and economic prosperity, and many advanced technology has been introduced into medicine, greatly promoting the development of traditional Chinese medicine.

在本草方面,陆续影印、重刊或校点评注了《神农本草经》《新修本草》(残卷)、《证类本草》《滇南本草》《本草品汇精要》《本草纲目》等数十种重要的古代本草专著。20世纪60年代以来,对亡佚本草的辑复也取得突出成绩,其中有些已正式出版发行,对本草学的研究、发展做出了较大贡献。

In the aspect of Materia Medica, dozens of important ancient materia medica monographs, such as *Shen Nong's Classic of the Materia Medica* (*Shén Nóng Běn Cǎo Jīn*), *Newly Revised Materia Medica* (*Xīn Xiū Běn Cǎo*) (remnant volume), *Materia Medica Arranged According to Pattern* (*Zhèng Lèi Běn Cǎo*), *Materia Medica of South Yunnan* (*Diān Nán Běn Cǎo*), *Essentials of Materia Medica Distinctions* (*Běn Cǎo Pǐn Huì Jīng Yào*) and *The Grand Compendium of Materia Medica* (*Běn Cǎo Gāng Mù*), have been photocopied, reprinted or commented. Since the 1960s, remarkable achievements have been made in the collection and recovery of lost Materia Medica, some of which have been officially released, making great contributions to the research and development of Material Medica.

20世纪70年代后期,中药新著不断问世,数以千计各具特色的中药著作,多角度、全方位地将本草学提高到崭新的水平。其中最能反映当代本草学术成就的,有各版《中华人民共和国药典》(简称《中国药典》)、《中药志》《全国中草药汇编》《中药大辞典》《原色中国本草图鉴》《中华本草》等。《中国药典》(一部)作为中药生产、供应、检验和使用的依据,以法典的形式确定了中药在当代医药卫生事业中的地位,也为中药材及中药制剂质量的提高、标准的确定,起到了巨大的促进作用,在一定程度上反映当代药学水平。《中药大辞典》是中华人民共和国成立以来最全面的巨型中药工具书之一。《全国中草药汇编》是对中华人民共和国成立20多年来中药研究和应用的一次大总结。《中华本草》几乎涵盖了当时中药学的全部内容,总结了我国两千多年来中药学成就,是一部反映20世纪中药学科发展水平的综合性本草巨著。

In the late 1970s, new works of Chinese medicinals were published continuously. Thousands of unique works of Chinese medicinals raised the level of Materia Medica to a new level from multiple and all-round perspectives. What best reflected the academic achievements of contemporary materia medica are *Pharmacopoeia of the people's Republic of China* (*Zhōng Huá Rén Mín Gòng Hé Guó Yào Diǎn*, *Chinese Pharmacopoeia* for short), *Records of Chinese Medicinals* (*Zhōng Yào Zhì*), *National Collection of Chinese Herbal Medicines* (*Quán Guó Zhōng Cǎo Yào Huì Biān*), *Encyclopedia of Chinese Medicinals* (*Zhōng Yà Dà Cí Diǎn*), *Yuanse Illustrated Chinese Materia Medica* (*Yuán Sè Zhōng Guó Běn Cǎo Tú Jiàn*), *Chinese Materia Medica* (*Zhōng Huá Běn Cǎo*). *Chinese Pharmacopoeia* (Volume I), as the basis for the production, supply, inspection and application of Chinese medicinals, has determined the position of Chinese medicine in the contemporary medical and health undertakings in the form of code, and has greatly promoted the quality improvement and standard determination of Chinese medicinal and its preparations, reflecting the level of contemporary pharmacy to a certain extent. *Encyclopedia of Chinese Medicinals* is one of the most comprehensive giant reference books of Chinese medicinals since the founding of the People's Republic of China. *National Collection of Chinese Herbal Medicines* is a grand summary of the research and application of Chinese herbal medicine over the past 20 years since the founding of the People's Republic of China. *Chinese Materia Medica* covers almost all the contents of modern Chinese pharmacy. It summarizes the achievements of Chinese medicine in more than 2000 years in China and is a great comprehensive work reflecting the development level of Chinese pharmacy in the 20th century.

中华人民共和国成立以来,政府先后4次组织各方面人员进行全国性的中药资源普查,基本摸清了天然药物的种类、产区分布、生态环境、野生资源、蕴藏量、收购量和社会需要量等情况。在资源调查的基础上,编著出版了全国性中药志及一大批药用植物志、药用动物志及地区性中药志,蒙、藏、维、傣、苗、彝等少数民族药也得到科学整理。

Since the founding of the People's Republic of China, the government has organized four nationwide surveys of Chinese medicinal resources, basically made out the types of natural medicinals, distribution of production areas, ecological environment, wild resources, reserves, acquisitions and social needs. On the basis of resource investigation, the national Chinese medicinal records, a large number of medical plant records, medical animal records and regional Chinese medicinal records have been compiled and published. Mongolian, Tibetan, Uygur, Dai, Miao, Yi and other ethnic medicine have also been scientifically sorted out.

随着现代自然科学的迅速发展及中药事业自身发展的需要,中药现代研究在深度和广度上都取得了瞩目成就,中药鉴定学、中药化学、中药药理学、中药炮制学、中药药剂学等分支学科都取得了很大发展。

With the rapid development of modern natural science and the needs of the development of Chinese medicinals, the modern medicinal research has made remarkable achievements in depth and breadth, and the branches as Chinese Medicinal Identification, Chinese Medicinal Chemistry, Chinese Pharmacology, Chinese Medicinal Processing, and Chinese Pharmaceutics have made great development.

当代中药教育事业的振兴，使中医中药由家传师授的培养方式转入国家高等教育的轨道，造就了一大批高质量的专业人才。自 1978 年恢复培养研究生制度后，全国不少高等院校及药学科研机构开始招收中药学硕士学位和博士学位研究生。我国的中药教育形成了从中专、大专、本科到硕士、博士研究生多层次培养的完整体系。为了适应中药教育的需要，各种中药教材也多次编写修订，质量不断提高。

The revitalization of contemporary Chinese medicine education has transferred the training mode from the family teacher to the national higher education, and created a large number of high-quality professionals. Since 1978, many universities and pharmaceutical research institutions began to recruit postgraduates with master's degree and doctor's degree. Chinese medicinal education has formed a complete multi-level training system from technical secondary school, college, undergraduate to master's and doctoral students. In order to meet the needs of Chinese medicinal education, all kinds of teaching materials have been compiled and revised for many times, and the quality has been continuously improved.

中医药学历史源远流长，内容浩博。经过数千年的实践检验，中医药的疗效有目共睹，在多次大型传染性疾病暴发之际发挥了重要的临床作用。吾辈当继承传统，守正创新，在已取得成绩的基础上，动员多学科力量，使中药学取得更大的成就，使安全有效、质量可控的优质中药早日走向世界，为世界人民的医疗保健做出更大的贡献。

Chinese medicine has a long history and a vast content. After thousands of years of practice, the curative effect of TCM is universally recognized, and it has played an important clinical role in the outbreak of many large infectious diseases. On the basis of achievements, we should inherit tradition, keep innovation, mobilize multi-disciplinary forces to make more achievements in the rich and colorful Chinese pharmacy, make the excellent Chinese medicinals with safe, effective and controllable quality go to the world as soon as possible, and make greater contributions to the health care of the people of the world.

（王 茜 张一昕）

题库

第二章 中药的产地和采集
Chapter 2 Place of origin and collection

 学习目标 | Learning goals

1. **熟悉** 道地药材的含义和重要的道地药材品种。
2. **了解** 中药的质量、疗效与中药的产地和采集的关系；各类药材的一般采收原则。

1. Familiar with the meaning and important varieties of genuine medicinal materials.
2. Understand the quality and efficacy of Chinese medicinals and the relationship between the origin and collection of Chinese medicinals; the general collection principles of all kinds of Chinese medicinals.

中药绝大部分来源于天然植物，其次是动物、矿物，尚有部分人工制品。中药的产地与采集是否适宜，直接影响中药的质量和疗效。早在《神农本草经》中即指出："阴干、曝干，采造时月，生熟，土地所出，真伪陈新，并各有法。"认为药物的品种、产地、采集、贮存与其加工炮制同样重要。《用药法象》则明确强调"凡诸草木昆虫，产之有地；根叶花实，采之有时。失其地则性味少异，失其时则性味不全。"历代医药家都十分重视中药的产地与采集，并在长期的实践中积累了丰富的经验和知识。研究药物的产地和采集规律，对于保证和提高药材的质量以及保护药源均有十分重要的意义。

The vast majority of Chinese medicinals originate from natural plants, followed by animals, minerals, and some artificial products. The place of origin and collection time directly affects the quality and efficacy. *Shen Nong's Classic of the Materia Medica* (*Shén Nóng Běn Cǎo Jīng*) says that "There are standards for drying in the shade or in the sun, collection time, raw and ripe, place of origin, authenticity and freshness". It is considered that the species, origin, collection and storage of drugs are as important as their processing. *Applying Chinese Medicinals with Natural Phenomena* (*Yòng Yào Fǎ Xiàng*) clearly emphasizes that "all plants and insects have their own places of origin and roots, leaves, flowers and fruits have their collection time. The efficacies will change if the places of origin and collection time change". Physicians of all ages have attached great importance to the origin and collection of Chinese medicinals, and have accumulated rich experience and knowledge in long-term practice. It is very important to study the producing area and collecting rule of medicine for ensuring and improving the medicinal quality and protecting the resources of Chinese medicinals.

第一节　中药的产地

Section 1　Place of origin

PPT

　　天然药材的生长或形成，都离不开一定的自然环境和条件。我国疆土辽阔，地形复杂，气候、日照、湿度、温差、土质等生态环境因地而异，甚至差别很大，因而天然中药材大多具有一定的地域性，且产地与其产量、质量具有密切的关系。对于这种现象，古人早有认识，如《本草经集注》提出："诸药所生，皆有境界。"《千金要方》指出："用药必依土地。"《本草蒙筌》强调："地产南北相殊，药力大小悬隔。"古代医药家经过长期使用、观察和比较，发现即使分布较广的药材，由于各地自然条件的不同，其质量优劣也不一样，因而自唐宋以来，逐渐形成了"道地药材"的概念。

The growth or production of natural medicinals are inseparable from certain natural environment and conditions. China has a vast territory and complex terrains. The climate, sunlight, humidity, temperature, soil texture and other ecological environments vary from place to place, even greatly. Therefore, most of the natural Chinese herbal medicines have certain regional characteristics, and the origin is closely related to its yield and quality. The ancients have known this phenomenon for a long time. As the *Collective Commentaries on the Classic of Materia Medica* (*Běn Cǎo Jīng Jí Zhù*) says, "all medicines have their own places of origin". *Important Formulas Worth a Thousand Gold Pieces* (*Qiān Jīn Yào Fāng*) points out that "medicine must be based on land". *Enlightening Primer of Materia Medica* (*Běn Cǎo Méng Quán*) emphasizes that "the products of the north and the south are different, and the size of the medicinal power is separated". After long-term use, observation and comparison, ancient pharmacists found that the quality of widely distributed medicinal materials was different due to different natural conditions. Therefore, since the Tang and Song Dynasties, the concept of "genuine regional medicinals" has gradually formed.

　　所谓"道地药材"，是指历史悠久，品种优良，疗效突出，具有明显地域性的药材。如四川的黄连、附子、川芎、川贝母，东北的人参、细辛、五味子，河南的山药、地黄、牛膝，甘肃的当归，山东的阿胶，宁夏的枸杞，广东的砂仁，江苏的薄荷，广西的肉桂，广东的陈皮等，都是著名的道地药材，深受广大医药家的赞誉。这些道地药材习惯上在药名之前冠以产地名表示，如宁枸杞、北细辛、辽五味、云茯苓等。确定道地药材的依据是多方面的，其中最关键的是临床疗效。道地药材的产区在实践中形成以后，并不是一成不变的。如三七原以广西为上，称为广三七或田七，云南后来居上，成为新的道地药材产区。

Genuine regional medicinals refer to the medicinal materials with a long history, high quality, outstanding curative effects and obvious regional characteristics, such as *huáng lián* (Coptidis Rhizoma), *fù zǐ* (Aconiti Lateralis Radix Praeparata), *chuān xiōng* (Chuanxiong Rhizoma), *chuān bèi mǔ* (Fritillariae Cirrhosae Bulbus) in Sichuan, *rén shēn* (Ginseng Radix et Rhizoma), *xì xīn* (Asari Radix et Rhizoma), *wǔ wèi zǐ* (Schisandrae Chinensis Fructus) in the northeast China, *shān yào* (Dioscoreae Rhizoma), *dì huáng* (Rehmanniae Radix), *niú xī* (Achyranthis Bidentatae Radix) in Henan, *dāng guī* (Angelicae Sinensis Radix) in Gansu, *ē jiāo* (Corii Asini Colla) in Shandong, *gǒu qǐ* (Lycii Fructus) in Ningxia, *shā rén* (Amomi Fructus) in Guangdong, *bò he* (Menthae Herba) in Jiangsu, *ròu guì* (Cinnamomi Cortex) in Guangxi, *chén pí* (Citri Reticulatae Pericarpium) in Guangdong, all of which are famous genuine medicinals and are highly praised by the majority of medical experts. These genuine medicinal materials are customarily named with place before their names, such as *níng gǒu qǐ*, *běi xì xīn*, *liáo wǔ wèi*, *yún fú líng*, and so on. Many factors can decide the genuine regional medicinals but the clinical efficacy is the most important one. The production areas of genuine medicinals are not unchangeable after they are formed in practice. For example, *sān qī* (Notoginseng Radix et Rhizoma) in Guangxi was originally the best, known as *guǎng sān qī* or *tián qī*, and Yunnan came from behind to become a new production area of genuine medicinal materials.

实践证明，重视道地药材的开发和使用，对于确保品种来源正确、疗效安全可靠，起着十分重要的作用。然而，随着中医药事业不断发展，药材需求量日益增加，道地药材已无法满足临床用药和康复保健的需要。因而在积极扩大道地药材生产的同时，深入研究道地药材的生态环境，创造特定的生产条件，科学规范地进行植物药异地引种及药用动物人工驯养，发展优质药材生产，开拓新的药材资源，是当今乃至今后的一项十分艰巨的任务。

Practice has shown that paying attention to the development and application of genuine regional medicinals plays an important role in ensuring the correct sources and safe and reliable curative effect. However, with the continuous development of TCM and the increasing consumption of medicinals, genuine regional medicinals has been unable to meet the needs of clinical medication, rehabilitation and health care. Therefore, as well as actively expanding the production of genuine medicinals, it is a very arduous task to study their ecological environment, create specific production conditions, scientifically and normatively introduce herbs from other places, domesticate medicinal animals, develop the production of high-quality medicinal materials, and open up new medicinal resources.

第二节　中药的采集
Section 2　Collection

PPT

中药的采收时间和方法与中药的质量和疗效有密切关系，正如《千金要方》云："早则药势未成，晚则盛势已歇。"《千金翼方》进一步强调："不依时采取，与朽木无殊，虚费人工，卒无裨益。"因动、植物在其生长发育的不同阶段，所含有效成分不同，药效也有较大的差异。故适时而合理的采收，不仅可以保证药材质量，还能增加产量，有利于保护药材资源。一般而言，中药材的采集应在有效成分含量最高的时候进行，通常以入药部位的成熟程度为依据。

The harvest time and method are closely related to the quality and efficacy of Chinese medicinals. As the saying goes in *Important Formulas Worth a Thousand Gold Pieces* (*Qiān Jīn Yào Fāng*), "collected early, the medicinal efficacy will not be the best while the best efficacy cannot be achieved if collected late". *Supplement to Important Formulas Worth a Thousand Gold Pieces* (*Qiān Jīn Yì Fāng*) also stresses that "if they are not collected on time, they make no difference from the rotten wood, which will waste manpower and be of no benefit". In their different growing stages, their active ingredients are in plants and animals are different, so their efficacy is also different. Therefore, timely and reasonable collecting can not only ensure the quality of medicinals, but also increase the output, and is conducive to the protection of medicinal resources. Generally speaking, the collection should be carried out when the content of active ingredients is the highest, usually based on the maturity of the medicinal parts.

一、植物类药材的采集
1. Collection of botanical medicinals

1. **全草类** 多在植株充分生长、枝叶茂盛的花前期或初见花时采收。此时是植物生长最旺盛的时期，茎叶中的有效成分往往含量最高，不仅质量好，而且产量高。若不用根，则割取地上部分，如青蒿、薄荷、益母草、广藿香等；若需带根入药，则连根拔起，如车前草、蒲公英、紫花地丁等。有的需要幼嫩全草或带叶花梢，如茵陈、夏枯草等，则需适时采收。

(1) Entire plant Most are collected in the early stage of flowering when the plants are fully grown and the branches and leaves are luxuriant. It is the most vigorous period of plant growth, and the content of effective components in stems and leaves is often the highest, with high quality and the yield. The parts above the ground are cut for medicinal use if the roots are not used, such as *qīng hāo* (Artemisiae Annuae Herba), *bò he* (Menthae Herba), *yì mǔ cǎo* (Leonuri Herba) and *guǎng huò xiāng* (Pogostemonis Herba). If the roots are also used, the whole plants are rooted up, such as *chē qián cǎo* (Plantaginis Herba), *pú gōng yīng* (Taraxaci Herba) and *zǐ huā dì dīng* (Violae Herba). Some should have their tender sprouts, or tips with its leaves and flowers collected timely, such as *yīn chén* (Artemisiae Scopariae Herba) and *xià kū cǎo* (Prunellae Spica).

2. **叶类** 多在花蕾将放或花正盛开时采收。此时叶片茂盛，有效成分含量高，药力雄厚，应及时采集，如大青叶、枇杷叶、荷叶等。少数药材如桑叶，需在深秋或初冬经霜后采集，习称"霜桑叶"或"冬桑叶"。

(2) Leaf They are usually collected when the flower is still in bud or in full bloom. At this time, the leaves are luxuriant, the contents of active ingredients are the highest, and the quality is the best, such as *dà qīng yè* (Isatidis Folium), *pí pá yè* (Eriobotryae Folium) and *hé yè* (Nelumbinis Folium). A few herbs should be collected after frost at late autumn or early winter, such as *sāng yè* (Mori Folium), also named *shuāng* (frost) *sāng yè* or *dōng* (winter) *sāng yè*.

3. **花类** 多采收未开放的花蕾或初开的花朵，以免香味散失、花瓣散落而影响质量，如金银花、菊花等。由于花蕾大多次第形成和开放，所以应分批次及时采摘。红花则要在花冠由黄转为橙红时采收；蒲黄等以花粉入药者，应在花朵完全开放后采收。

(3) Flower They are always collected when the flowers are still in bud or in the early stage of bloom so as not to lose the fragrance and petals, such as *jīn yín huā* (Lonicerae Japonicae Flos) and *jú huā* (Chrysanthemi Flos). Since the buds form and bloom in sequence, the collection should be timely and in batches. The best collection time for *hóng huā* (Carthami Flos) is when its corolla turns from yellow to arrange, while *pú huáng* (Typhae Pollen) with pollen as the medicinal, should be collected in its full bloom.

4. **果实或种子类** 多在果实成熟时或将至成熟时采收，如瓜蒌、枸杞、山楂等。少数需在果实未成熟时采集果皮或果实，如青皮、枳实、乌梅等。以种子入药者，大多在果实完全成熟后采集，如银杏、莲子等。有些既用全草又用种子入药者，可在种子成熟后割取全草，将种子打下后分别晒干贮存，如车前子、苏子等。对于果实成熟后，其果壳开裂而易致种子散失者，如牵牛子、小茴香、豆蔻等，应见熟即收。

(4) Fruit or seed The best collection time for those with fruits as the medicinal art is usually when the fruits are ripe or approaching maturity, such as *guā lóu* (Trichosanthis Fructus), *gǒu qǐ* (Lycii Fructus), and *shān zhā* (Crataegi Fructus). A few need to collect the peel or fruit when the fruit is immature, such as *qīng pí* (Citri Reticulatae Viride Pericarpium), *zhǐ shí* (Aurantii Immaturus Fructus) and *wū méi* (Mume Fructus). Those with seeds as the medicinal part are usually collected after the fruits are fully mature, such as *yín xìng* (Ginkgo Semen) and *lián zǐ* (Nelumbinis Semen). For those with both whole plants and seeds as the medicinal parts, the whole plants may be cut after the seeds are mature, and the seeds should be dried and stored, such as *chē qián zǐ* (Plantaginis Semen) and *sū zǐ* (Perillae Fructus). For those whose shell is cracked and the seeds are subject to abscission in time of their maturity, the seeds should be collected as soon as they become ripe, such as *qiān niú zǐ* (Pharbitidis Semen), *xiǎo huí xiāng* (Foeniculi Fructus) and *dòu kòu* (Amomi Rotundus Fructus).

5. **根和根茎类**　一般以春初或秋末，即阴历二、八月采收为佳。古人认为"（初春）津润始萌，未充枝叶，势力淳浓""至秋枝叶干枯，津润归流于下"，同时还强调"春宁宜早，秋宁宜晚"。早春时节（阴历二月），植物根茎处于休眠状态，新芽未萌，营养物质未被茎叶消耗；深秋（阴历八月）以后，多数植物地上部分停止生长，精微物质贮于地下之根或根茎，故有效成分含量高。此时采收该类药材，不仅质量优，而且产量高，如天麻、大黄、葛根等。也有少数例外者，如半夏、延胡索等宜在夏季采挖。

(5) Root and rootstock　Generally, it is better to collect in late autumn or early spring, that is, the eighth month or the second month of the lunar year. The ancients believed that in the early spring, the roots and rootstocks of plants are still in dormant state and the new buds do not sprout, so the nutrition substances have not been consumed by the stems and leaves; while in the late autumn, the overground parts of most plants stop growing and the nutrients substances will be stored in the roots or rootstocks, so the contents of active ingredients are high. The medicinals collected at these times are excellent in quality and high in yield, such as *tiān má* (Gastrodiae Rhizoma), *dà huáng* (Rhei Radix et Rhizoma) and *gé gēn* (Puerariae Lobatae Radix). However, there are a few exceptions, such as *bàn xià* (Pinelliae Rhizoma) and *yán hú suǒ* (Corydalis Rhizoma), which should be collected in summer.

6. **树皮和根皮类**　一般在清明至夏至（即春、夏时节）间剥取。此时植物生长旺盛，树皮中贮存和运输的营养物质丰富，其药材质量较佳；而且因树木枝干内浆汁多，形成层细胞分裂迅速，其皮易于剥离，如黄柏、厚朴、杜仲等。但以树皮入药的肉桂，则宜在10月剥皮，此时油多容易剥取。另有些根皮以秋后采集为佳，此时植物养分多贮于根部，如牡丹皮、地骨皮、桑白皮等。树皮类药材大多来源于乔木，其生长期长，成材缓慢，应尽量避免伐树取皮，或环剥树皮造成树木枯死的掠夺式方法，最好每次纵剥1/3的树皮，以保护药源。

(6) Bark and root cortice　They are usually peeled from Qingming to summer solstice (i.e., spring and summer). At this time, the plants grow vigorously, the barks are rich in nutrients stored and transported, and the quality of the medicinal materials is better; moreover, the barks are easy to peel off since the serous fluid is plentiful in the stems and branches and the cambium cells divide rapidly, such as *huáng bó* (Phellodendri Chinensis Cortex), *hòu pò* (Magnoliae Officinalis Cortex) and *dù zhòng* (Eucommiae Cortex). An exception is ròu guì (Cinnamomi Cortex), which should be peeled in October when the rich oil makes it easy to peel. As for the root cortices, the best collection time is late autumn when the nutrients are mostly stored in the roots, such as *mǔ dān pí* (Moutan Cortex), *dì gǔ pí* (Lycii Cortex) and *sāng bái pí* (Mori Cortex). Most medicinals of this type come from arbors which have a long growth period and slow growth, so felling bark or girdling bark should be avoided to cause tree dead. It is advisable to peel 1/3 of bark vertically each time to protect the medicinal resource.

二、动物类药材的采集
2. Collection of animal medicinals

动物类药材因品种不同而采收时间各异，以保证药效、容易获得和利于保护资源为原则。如桑螵蛸应在3月中旬收集，过时则虫卵孵化；鹿茸应在清明后45~50天锯取头茬茸，过时则角化；制取阿胶的驴皮，应于冬至后剥取，其皮厚而质优；小昆虫类应在数量多的活动期捕获。

Different kinds of animal medicinal materials have different collecting time. The principle is to ensure the medical efficacy, to obtain easily and to protect resources. For example, *sāng piāo xiāo* (Mantidis Oötheca) should be collected in the middle of March, for after this time the ovums will hatch; *lù róng* (Cervi Cornu Pantotrichum) should be collected 45 to 50 days after the Qingming, for after this time it will be keratinized; donkey hide for *ē jiāo* (Corii Asini Colla) should be collected after the winter solstice, for the hide is thick with high quality; insects should be caught when they are in active period in large quantity.

三、矿物类药材的采集
3. Collection of mineral medicinals

矿物类药材一般全年皆可采集，不拘时间。
Mineral medicinals can be collected all year round, regardless of time.

（叶耀辉）

题库

第三章　中药的炮制
Chapter 3　Processing of Chinese medicinals

学习目标 | Learning goals

1. **掌握**　中药炮制的目的。
2. **熟悉**　水飞、炒、炙、煅、煨、淬、焯等主要炮制方法的含义。
3. **了解**　炮制的含义和分类方法。

1. Master the purpose of processing Chinese medicinals.
2. Familiar with the meaning of main processing methods, such as grinding with water, stir-frying, stir-frying with liquid adjuvant, calcining, roasting, quenching, blanching, etc.
3. Understand the meaning and classification of processing.

中药炮制，古时又称"炮炙""修事""修治"，是指药物在使用前或制成各种剂型前，根据中医药理论，依照药材自身性质以及调剂、制剂和临床应用的不同要求，对中药所采取的必要的加工处理方法。它是我国制备中药饮片的一门传统制药技术。中药材大多是生药，其中不少药物必须经过一定的加工炮制处理，才符合临床用药需求。炮制方法有多种，炮制得当对保障药效、安全用药、便于制剂和调剂都有十分重要的意义。

微课

In ancient times, the processing of Chinese medicinals, also known as "*Paozhi*" "*Xiu shi*", and "*Xiu zhi*", refers to the necessary processing methods for Chinese medicinals before the application or preparation of various dosage forms, based on the traditional Chinese medical theories, according to the nature of the medicinals as well as the different requirements of prescription, preparation and clinical application. It is a traditional pharmaceutical technology to deal with Chinese medicinals. Since most of the Chinese medicines are raw, many of them must be processed to meet the requirements of clinical medication. There are many processing methods according to different medicinal properties and treatment requirements. Whether the processing is appropriate or not is of great significance to ensure the efficacy, medication safety, and medicinal preparation.

第一节　炮制目的
Section 1　Purposes of medicinal processing

PPT

中药的炮制方法较多，辅料各异。对于不同的药物，炮制目的不尽一致；在炮制某一具体药物时，常有几方面的目的。总体来说，炮制目的可以归纳为以下几方面。

There are many processing methods, different adjuvants of Chinese medicinals. For different medicinals, the purpose of processing is not the same; when processing a specific drug, there are often several purposes. In general, the purpose of processing can be summarized as follows.

一、降低或消除药物的毒性或副作用，保证用药安全
1. To reduce or eliminate the toxicity or side effects to ensure medication safety

一些具有毒性或明显副作用的药物，不经炮制而直接生用，即使在常用的有效剂量内，也容易产生毒性反应和副作用。如经过特殊的炮制处理，可以明显降低甚至消除某些毒性和副作用，确保临床用药安全。如川乌、附子、半夏、马钱子等生用内服易于中毒，炮制后能降低其毒性。巴豆有剧毒，泻下峻烈，去油用霜，可降低毒性；乳香、没药含刺激性挥发油，生品内服可引起呕吐和食欲减退，经炒制去油，可减缓其副作用。

Some Chinese medicinals with toxicity or obvious side effects, if used without processing, will result in toxic reactions and side effects even in the commonly used effective doses. Special processing can significantly reduce or even eliminate some side effects and ensure the safety of clinical medication. For example, *chuān wū* (Aconiti Radix), *fù zǐ* (Aconiti Lateralis Radix Praeparata), *bàn xià* (Pinelliae Rhizoma) and *mǎ qián zǐ* (Strychni Semen) are poisonous by oral administration, but their toxicity can be reduced after being processed. *Bā dòu* (Crotonis Fructus) is highly toxic and purge violently, but the toxicity may be reduced if it is used after its oil is removed and it is frosted. *Rǔ xiāng* (Olibanum) and *mò yào* (Myrrha) contain irritant volatile oil, which can cause vomiting and loss of appetite when taken orally. After frying, the side effects can be reduced.

二、增强药物作用，提高临床疗效
2. To enhance medicinal actions and increase clinical effects

在中药炮制时，常加入一些辅料，辅料的种类较多，其具体作用虽然不同，但主要是为了增强药物的作用，提高临床疗效。如蜜炙桑叶、百部能增强润肺止咳的作用；酒炒川芎、当归能增强温通活血的作用。不加辅料的炮制方法也能增强药物的作用。如决明子、莱菔子炒制，可使其表面爆裂，利于有效成分溶出而增强作用；麦芽炒焦，能增强消食作用。

In the processing of Chinese medicinals, some adjuvants are often added, which are of many kinds. Although their specific functions are different, they are mainly to enhance the medicinal actions and improve the clinical efficacy. For example, honey-fried *sāng yè* (Mori Folium) and *bǎi bù* (Stemonae Radix) can promote the effect of moistening lung and relieving cough; wine-fried *chuān xiōng* (Chuanxiong Rhizoma) and *dāng guī* (Angelicae Sinensis Radix) can promote the effect of warming channels and activating blood circulation. Other processing methods without auxiliary materials can also enhance the effect of drugs. For example, *jué míng zǐ* (Cassiae Semen) and *lái fú zǐ* (Raphani Semen) will crack after being dry-fried, which is conducive to the dissolution of effective ingredients and enhance the effect; *mài yá* (Hordei Germinatus Fructus) dry-fried until scorched will function better in promoting digestion.

三、改变药物性能和功效，使其更适应病情的需要
3. To change the nature and efficacy of medicinals to meet the requirements of diseases

某些药物通过炮制可以改变药性和功效，扩大临床应用范围。如生地黄性寒，功能清热凉血，适用于血热证，经蒸制为熟地黄后，药性偏温，以补血见长，适用于血虚证；何首乌生用能泻下通便，制熟后则失去泻下作用而专补肝肾。

Some medicinals can be processed to change their properties and efficacy, and expand the scope of clinical application. For example, *shēng dì huáng* (Rehmanniae Radix) is cold in nature, and is effective for clearing heat to cool blood, which is suitable for the syndrome of blood heat. After being steamed, it becomes *shú dì huáng* (Rehmanniae Radix Praeparata), which is slightly warm and applicable for blood deficiency. *Hé shǒu wū* (Polygoni Multiflori Radix) can be used to purge in raw form, but after being processed, it will lose its purgative effect and specially tonify liver and kidney.

四、改变药物性状，便于贮存和制剂
4. To change the properties and forms of medicinals to facilitate storage and preparation

大多数药材必须经过干燥处理，才有利于贮存。如马齿苋柔嫩多汁，必须入沸水焯后才能干燥；桑螵蛸必须蒸制以杀死虫卵或蚜虫，否则可因虫卵孵化而失效。将植物药切制成一定规格的片、丝、块、段等，有利于药效成分煎出，便于制剂；多数矿物药需经过煅、淬等处理，使之酥脆，便于煎煮或制剂。

Most of the medicinal materials must be dried to facilitate storage. For example, being delicate and juicy, *mǎ chǐ xiàn* (Portulacae Herba) must be soaked in boiling water before drying. *Sāng piāo xiāo* (Mantidis Oötheca) must be steamed to kill the ovum or aphids, otherwise it will lose effect due to the hatching of ovum. The botanical medicinals are cut into slices, sections, shreds or segments of certain specifications, which is conducive to the decocting of the effective ingredients and the preparation. Most mineral medicinals need to be calcined and quenched to make them easy to be ground into powder and be easily decocted or prepared.

五、提高药材纯净度，保证药材质量和称量准确
5. To improve the medicinal purity to guarantee the quality and the weighing accuracy

中药在采收、运输和贮存过程中，往往残留一些非药用部分或混有泥沙、霉变品等，既影响药材质量，又造成用量不准确，因此必须进行修制或特殊处理，使药物洁净。如茯苓去净泥土、枳壳去瓤、枇杷叶刷去毛以及动物类药去头、足、翅等。

In collection, transportation and storage, some non-medicinal parts, sediment and moldy products may be mixed in medicinal materials, which affects the medicinal quality and causes inaccurate dosage. Therefore, medicinals must be handled specially to achieve the pureness. The earth in *fú líng* (Poria) must be washed away; the pulp of *zhǐ qiào* (Aurantii Fructus) removed; the hair on *pí pa yè* (Eriobotryae

Folium) brushed off; the heads, feet and wings of animals removed.

六、矫味矫臭，便于服用
6. To get rid of unpleasant tastes and smells to make it easier to take

有些药材尤其是动物药、树脂类药等具有特殊的气味，服用后易引起恶心、呕吐等不良反应，经过炮制能矫正药材的异味，便于患者服用。如酒制乌梢蛇，醋制乳香、没药，醋炒五灵脂等。

Some medicinal materials, especially animal medicine and resins, have special smell, which may lead to adverse reactions such as nausea and vomiting after taking. Processing may get rid of the unpleasant smells and make it convenient for patients to take, such as wine-fried *wū shāo shé* (Zaocys), vinegar-prepared *rǔ xiāng* (Olibanum) and *mò yào* (Myrrha), and vinegar-fried *wǔ líng zhī* (Trogopterori Faeces).

第二节　炮制方法
Section 2　Methods of medicinal processing

中药炮制是历代逐步发展和充实起来的，其内容丰富，方法多样。根据现代的实际应用情况，炮制方法一般分为修治、水制、火制、水火共制及其他制法五大类。

The processing of Chinese medicinals is gradually developed and enriched in the past dynasties, with rich contents and various methods. According to the modern practical application, the processing methods are generally divided into five categories: common processing, water processing, fire processing, water and fire processing.

一、修治
1. Purifying, grinding and cutting

包括纯净、粉碎、切制药材三道工序。

It consists of three procedures: purifying, grinding and cutting.

1. **纯净药材**　采用挑、筛、簸、刷、刮、挖、撞等方法，除去药材中的杂质和非药用部分，使药材纯净。如拣去辛夷花的枝、叶，簸去薏苡仁的杂质，刷除枇杷叶背面的绒毛，刮去肉桂的粗皮，撞去白蒺藜的硬刺等。

(1) **Purifying**　It is the method of removing impurities and non medicinal parts in the medicinal materials by means of selecting, sieving, winnowing, brushing, scraping, digging and striking, so as to make the medicinal materials pure, such as picking *yì yǐ rén* (Coicis Semen), brushing off the fluff on the back of *pí pa yè* (Eriobotryae Folium), scraping off the coarse bark of *ròu guì* (Cinnamomi Cortex), and striking away the hard thorn of *bái jí lí* (Tribuli Fructus).

2. **粉碎药材**　采用捣、碾、研、磨、镑、锉等方法，使药材达到一定粉碎度，便于调配、制剂或服用。如牡蛎捣碎、川贝母研粉、角类药镑片或锉粉等。

(2) Grinding　It is the method of grinding medicinal materials into pieces by pounding, grinding, flaking, filing and other techniques to make it easier for further processing, preparation or administration, such as the pounding of *mǔ lì* (Ostreae Concha), the grinding of *chuān bèi mǔ* (Fritillariae Cirrhosae Bulbus), and the filing or flaking of horn medicine.

3. **切制药材**　采用切、铡的方法用刀具将药材切为一定规格的片、段、丝、块等，便于调配、制剂或贮存，利于有效成分煎出，提高煎药质量。如天麻切薄片、泽泻切厚片、黄芪切斜片、甘草切圆片、桑白皮切丝、茯苓切块、白茅根切段等。

(3) Cutting　It is the method of cutting the medicinal materials into slices, segments, sections or shreds of certain specifications for the convenience for further processing, preparation and storage, which is conducive to the decocting of effective ingredients, and improves the quality of decocting medicine, such as *tiān má* (Gastrodiae Rhizoma) cut into thin slices, *zé xiè* (Alismatis Rhizoma) into thick slices, *huáng qí* (Astragali Radix) into oblique slices, *gān cǎo* (Glycyrrhizae Radix et Rhizoma) into round slice, *sāng bái pí* (Mori Cortex) into shreds, *fú líng* (Poria) into sections, and *bái máo gēn* (Imperatae Rhizoma) into segments.

二、水制
2. Water processing

水制是以较低温度的水或其他液体辅料处理药物的多种方法的总称。常用的有漂洗、浸泡、闷润、喷洒、水飞等。主要目的是清洁药物、软化药物、除去杂质、便于切制、降低毒性及调整药性等。如芦根洗去泥土杂质、海藻漂去盐分、胆巴水浸泡附子、泡润槟榔、盖润大黄等。其中，水飞是将不溶于水的矿物类或贝壳类药材置于水中，反复研磨，制取极细粉末的加工方法。目的是制取极细而纯净的粉末，并防止加工时药粉飞扬。如水飞朱砂、水飞炉甘石等。

It is a general term for a variety of methods of processing medicinal materials with water at a lower temperature or other liquid adjuvant. Commonly used are rinsing and washing, soaking, moistening, spraying, and powder-refining with water, etc. The main purpose is to clean or soften drugs, to remove impurities, to be cut easily, to reduce toxicity and adjust medicinal properties, such as washing off the dirt and impurities of *lú gēn* (Phragmitis Rhizoma), rinsing the salt on *hǎi zǎo* (Sargassum), soaking *fù zǐ* (Aconiti Lateralis Radix Praeparata) in brine, soaking to moisten *bīng láng* (Arecae Semen), sealing to moisten *dà huáng* (Rhei Radix et Rhizoma). Powder-refining with water is a processing method of making extremely fine powder by repeatedly grinding the insoluble mineral or shell medicine in water. The purpose is to produce fine and pure powder and prevent the powder flying during processing, such as powder-refining *zhū shā* (Cinnabaris) and *lú gān shí* (Calamina) with water.

三、火制
3. Fire processing

火制是将药物经火加热处理的方法，目的是改变药性、提高疗效、消除或降低药物的毒性和烈性，并使坚硬的药材变得松脆，便于制剂和服用。常用的方法有炒、煅、煨等。

It is the method to process medicinal materials by heating the medicine by fire, with the purpose of changing the medicinal properties, improving the curative effect, eliminating or reducing the toxicity and intensity of the medicine, and making the hard medicinals become crunchy, convenient for preparation and taking. Common methods are stir-frying, calcining, roasting, etc.

1. 炒　是指将药物置锅中加热，不断翻动，炒至一定"火候"的方法。炒法分为清炒和加辅料炒两类。清炒是将药物置锅内，不加辅料直接翻炒，如炒牛蒡子、焦白术、焦山楂、艾叶炭等。根据加热程度不同，又有炒黄、炒焦和炒炭之分。用文火将药物表面炒至微黄，称为炒黄；用武火将药物炒至表面焦黄（褐），内部颜色加深并有焦香气，称为炒焦；将药物炒至表面焦黑，内部焦黄，但保留原有气味（存性），称为炒炭。加辅料炒是将药物与固体辅料拌炒，如砂烫龟甲、蛤粉炒阿胶、土炒白术、麸炒枳壳等。根据所加辅料砂、土、米、麸、蛤粉、滑石粉等的不同又有不同的炒法。

(1) Stir-frying　It is a method to heat the medicinals in the pot and stir it continuously until it reaches a certain degree. It falls into two categories: plain-frying and stir-frying with auxiliary materials. Plain-frying is to place the medicine in the pot and stir directly without any adjuvants, such as *chǎo niú bàng zǐ* (Arctii Fructus fried), *jiāo bái zhú* (Atractylodis Macrocephalae Rhizoma Praepareta), *jiāo shān zhā* (Crataegi Fructus Praepareta), and *ài yè tàn* (Artemisiae Argyi Folium Carbonisatum). It is subdivided into stir-frying to yellow, stir-frying to brown and stir-frying to scorch. Frying to yellow means frying the surface of the medicinals with mild fire until it is slightly yellow; frying to brown means frying the medicinals with strong fire until it is burnt yellow (brown) on the surface with deepening interior color and original smell; frying to scorch means frying the medicinals with strong fire until it is burnt black on the surface with burnt yellow interior color and originals smell (retain the original drug property). Stir-frying with auxiliary materials is mixing and stirring the medicinal materials and the solid adjuvants, such as sand, earth, wheat bran, clam powder, talcum powder and so on, such as scalding *guī jiǎ* (Testudinis Carapax et Plastrum) with sand, frying *ē jiāo* (Corii Asini Colla) with clam powder, frying *bái zhú* (Atractylodis Macrocephalae Rhizoma) with earth, and frying *zhǐ qiào* (Aurantii Fructus) with bran. The methods vary with different adjuvants.

2. 煅　是指用猛火直接或间接煅烧药材的方法。其中，将坚硬的矿物或甲骨类药材直接煅烧，煅至红透为度的方法，又称明煅，如煅牡蛎、煅石膏等；将质地轻松的药物置于耐高温的容器中密闭煅烧，至容器底部红透为度的方法，又称焖煅，如血余炭、棕榈炭。

(2) Calcining　It refers to the direct or indirect calcination of medicinal materials with high fire. The solid mineral or oracle bone medicine is directly calcined to the degree of red penetration, known as direct calcining, such as *duàn mǔ lì* (Ostreae Concha Praeparatum), and *duàn shí gāo* (Gypsum Fibrosum Praeparatum). The medicine with light texture is placed in a high-temperature container and sealed for calcination until the bottom of the container is totally red, which is called sealed calcining, such as *xuè yú tàn* (Crinis Carbonisatus) and *zōng lǚ tàn* (Trachycarpi Petiolus Carbonisatus).

3. 煨　是指将药材用湿面粉或湿草纸包裹置于火灰中，或用吸油纸与药物隔层分开加热的方法。如煨葛根、煨木香、煨肉豆蔻等。

(3) Roasting　It is the method of wrapping the medicinal materials with wet flour or wet paper in the hot ashes, or heating them separately with oil absorption paper and drug compartment, such as *wēi* (roasted) *gé gēn* (Puerariae Lobatae Radix), *wēi mù xiāng* (Aucklandiae Radix), and *wēi ròu dòu kòu* (Myristicae Semen).

四、水火共制
4. Water and fire processing

水火共制既要用水又要用火，有些药物还必须加入其他辅料进行炮制。其目的是改变药物性能、增强药效、降低或消除药物的毒性和副作用。常用的方法有煮、炙、淬、婵、蒸等。

This processing method needs both water and fire, and some medicinals must be processed with other auxiliary materials. The purpose is to change medicinal properties, enhance the therapeutic efficacy, reduce or eliminate toxicity and side effects. The commonly used methods are decocting, liquid-frying, quenching, and blanching steaming.

1. 煮　是指用水或其他液体辅料与药物置锅中同煮的方法。如醋煮芫花、姜矾煮半夏等。

(1) Decocting　It is the method of boiling medicinal materials with water or other liquid adjuvants together in a pot, such as *yuán huā* (Genkwa Flos) decocted in vinegar, *bàn xià* (Pinelliae Rhizoma) decocted with *shēng jiāng* (Zingiberis Recens Rhizoma) and *míng fán* (Alumen).

2. 炙　是指将药物与液体辅料共置锅中加热拌炒，使液体辅料逐渐渗入药物内部或附着于药物表面，以改变药性、增强疗效或降低毒性和副作用的方法。常用的液体辅料有蜜、酒、醋、姜汁、盐水等。如蜜炙百部、桑叶可增强润肺止咳作用；酒炙川芎、丹参可增强活血作用；醋炙柴胡、香附可增强疏肝解郁作用；姜炙半夏、竹茹可增强止呕作用；盐炙杜仲、补骨脂可引药入肾，并增强补肾作用；酒炙常山可减轻催吐作用。

(2) Liquid-frying　It is a processing method of heating and stir-frying medicinal materials and liquid adjuvants together in a pot, so that the adjuvants gradually permeate into the drug or attach to the surface for the purpose to change the medicinal properties, enhance the curative effect or reduce the toxic and side effects. Commonly used liquid adjuvants are honey, wine, vinegar, ginger juice, salt water, etc. For example, honey-fried *bǎi bù* (Stemonae Radix) and *sāng yè* (Mori Folium) can enhance the effect of moistening lung and relieving cough; wine-fried *chuān xiōng* (Chuanxiong Rhizoma) and *dān shēn* (Salviae Miltiorrhizae Radix et Rhizoma) can enhance the effect of promoting blood circulation; vinegar-fried *chái hú* (Bupleuri Radix) and *xiāng fù* (Cyperi Rhizoma) can enhance the effect of soothing liver and relieving depression; ginger juice-fried *bànxià* (Pinellia ternata) and *zhúrú* (Caulis Bambusae in Taenia) can enhance the effect of anti-nausea; salt-fried *dù zhòng* (Eucommiae Cortex) and *bǔ gǔ zhī* (Psoraleae Fructus) can lead drugs into the kidney and enhance the effect of tonifying kidney; wine-fried *cháng shān* (Dichroae Radix) can reduce the effect of vomiting.

3. 淬　是指将药物煅烧红后迅速投入冷水或液体辅料中，使之受冷而松脆的方法。如醋淬自然铜、醋淬磁石等。

(3) Quenching　It is the method of rapidly putting medicinal materials calcined red into cold water or liquid adjuvants to make it cold and crisp, such as vinegar-quenched *zì rán tóng* (Pyritum), and vinegar-quenched *cí shí* (Magnetitum).

4. 焯　是指将药物投入沸水中短暂潦过，迅速捞出的方法。如焯杏仁、焯马齿苋等。

(4) Blanching　It is the method of putting the medicinal materials into boiling water for a short time and quickly getting it out, such as blanched *xìng rén* (Armeniacae Amarum Semen) and blanched *mǎ chǐ xiàn* (Portulacae Herba).

5. 蒸　是指用水蒸气或附加成分将药物蒸熟的方法。如清蒸桑螵蛸、酒蒸山茱萸等。

(5) Steaming　It is the method of heating the medicinal materials with steam or other adjuvants, such as steamed *sāng piāo xiāo* (Mantidis Oötheca) and wine-steamed *shān zhū yú* (Corni Fructus).

五、其他制法
5. Other processing methods

其他制法是指上述四类炮制方法以外的特殊制法。主要有制霜、发芽、发酵等。

It refers to some special processing methods other than the above four processing methods. The commonly used methods are crystallizing, sprouting and fermenting.

1. **制霜** 是指将药材炮制加工成松散粉末或析出细小结晶的方法。包括去油制霜法、煎煮制霜法、升华制霜法和渗析制霜法。如巴豆霜、鹿角霜、砒霜、西瓜霜等。

(1) Crystallizing It is the methods of processing some medicinal materials into dispersible powder or separating out fine crystals, including crystallizing by removing fat, by decocting, by sublimating or by dialyzing, such as *bā dòu shuāng* (Crotonis Pulveratum Semen), *lù jiǎo shuāng* (Cervi Cornu Degelatinatum), *pī shuāng* (Arsenolite), and *xī guā shuāng* (Mirabilitum Praeparatum).

2. **发芽** 是指将具有发芽能力的种子类药材用水浸泡，并在一定的湿度和温度条件下，促使其萌发幼芽的方法。如谷芽、麦芽等。

(2) Sprouting It is the method of soaking the medicinal seeds with germinating ability in water and promoting their germination at a certain humidity and temperature, such as *gǔ yá* (Setariae Germinatus Fructus) and *mài yá* (Hordei Germinatus Fructus).

3. **发酵** 是指将药材与辅料拌和，保持一定的温度和湿度，利用霉菌和酶的催化分解作用，使药物发泡、生衣的方法。如神曲、淡豆豉等。

(3) Fermenting It is the method of mixing medicinal materials and adjuvants at a certain temperature and humidity and making them foaming and bacteria and algae parasitizing under the catalytic decomposition of mold and enzyme, such as *shén qū* (Medicata Fermentata Massa) and *dàn dòu chǐ* (Sojae Semen Praeparatum).

（叶耀辉）

题库

第四章 中药的性能

Chapter 4 Properties and actions of Chinese medicinals

 学习目标 | Learning goals

1. **掌握** 中药性能的含义；四气、五味、升降浮沉、归经的含义，确定的依据，所表示药物的作用及其对临床的指导意义；毒性的含义及使用有毒药物的注意事项。

2. **熟悉** 中药治病的基本作用；影响升降浮沉的因素；引起中药中毒的原因。

1. Master the definitions of properties and actions of Chinese medicinals; the meaning of four qi, five flavors, ascending-descending-floating-sinking, and meridian tropism; the precise basis, the functions of the medicinal and its clinical guiding significance; the meaning of toxicity and precautions for the application of toxic drugs.

2. Familiar with the basic role of Chinese medicine in treating diseases; the factors affecting the ascending, descending, floating and sinking; and the causes of Chinese medicinal poisoning.

中医学认为，疾病的发生和发展都是由于致病因素作用于人体，导致脏腑、经络功能异常，气血阴阳偏盛偏衰。中药治病的基本作用，不外去除病因，扶正固本，恢复脏腑功能的协调，纠正阴阳气血的偏盛偏衰，使之在最大程度上恢复到阴平阳秘的正常状态。

According to traditional Chinese medicine, the occurrence and development of diseases are due to pathogenic factors acting on the human body, resulting in disfunctions of *zang-fu* organs and meridians, and excess or deficiency of yin and yang of qi and blood. The basic function of Chinese medicinals in treating diseases is to eliminate the pathogens, reinforce healthy qi, restore the coordination of *zang-fu* function, rectify the excess or deficiency of yin and yang, and reestablish the balance in body to the greatest extent.

中药之所以能发挥上述作用，达到治愈疾病、恢复健康的目的，是因为药物自身具有的偏性。如《医原》说："药未有不偏者也，以偏救偏，故名曰药。"《神农本草经百种录》进一步指出："凡药之用，或取其气，或取其味，或取其色，或取其形……各以其偏胜而即资之疗疾，故能补偏救弊，调和脏腑。"所谓偏性，就是药物具有的各种特性和作用，即中药的性能。利用中药的偏性纠正机体疾病状态下阴阳的偏盛偏衰，是中药治病的一般原理。

The reason why Chinese medicine can play the above-mentioned role and achieve the goal of curing diseases and restoring health is that medicinals have their own preferences (properties and functions). Therefore, *Bases of Medicine* (*Yī Yuán*) says, "medicine has its preference, but the preference can be used to save preference of various abnormalities, so it is called medicine". *A Hundred Records on Shen Nong's Classic of the Materia Medica (Shén Nóng Běn Cǎo Jīng Bǎi Zhǒng Lù)* further points out that, "where a medicinal is used, its qi, its flavor, its color, or its shape shall be taken…It is the preference that cures a disease, that is, it can remedy the defects and rectify errors so as to reconcile *zang-fu* organs". The preferences refer to the various characteristics and functions of drugs, that is, the medicinal properties and actions. It is the general principle of Chinese medicinals to correct abnormal exuberance or debilitation of yin or yang under the condition of disease.

中药性能是在中医理论指导下，通过分析、归纳许多中药作用于机体的表现而形成的。对于一种具体的中药，描述其作用特性的性能越多，其个性特点就越鲜明，人们对该药利弊的认识就越清晰，临床用药时就越能按照中医药理论的要求准确选用，以扬长避短。中药性能是对中药作用的基本性质和特征的高度概括，是中药药性理论的核心及认识和使用中药的重要依据。其涵盖的内容比较丰富，本章重点介绍四气、五味、升降浮沉、归经、毒性等。

The medicinal properties and actions is formed through the analysis and induction under the guidance of the theory of TCM. For a specific Chinese medicine, the more performance described its function characteristics, and the more distinctive its personality characteristics, the more accurately people is able to select Chinese medicine in accordance with the requirements of chinese medicine theory. The properties and actions of Chinese medicinals refers to the highly generalization of the basic properties and characteristics of Chinese medicine, and is the core of the theory of Chinese materia medica and the important basis for understanding and applying medicinals, which covers a relatively rich content. This chapter focuses on four qi, five flavors, ascending-descending-floating-sinking, meridian tropism, toxicity, etc.

中药的性能和性状是两个不同的概念。中药性能是以服药后的人体为观察对象，根据机体用药反应，通过逻辑推理，对药物作用进行的概括和抽象；药物性状是以药物本身为观察对象，通过人的感觉器官直接感知的各种天然物理特征，如药材的形状、颜色、气味、滋味、质地等。

The property and characteristics of Chinese medicinals are two different concepts. The property is a generalization and abstraction of the function of a medicinal by logical reasoning based on the medication reaction of the body. The medicinal characteristics are all kinds of natural physical features directly perceived by human sensory organs, such as the shape, color, odor, taste, texture and so on.

第一节 四气

Section 1　Four qi

PPT

四气，是指寒、热、温、凉四种药性。它主要反映药物对人体阴阳盛衰、寒热变化方面的影响，是说明药物作用性质的重要理论之一，是中药性能的重要组成部分。

Four qi refers to the four medicinal natures, including cold, hot, warm and cool, which mainly reflects the influence of medicine on the exuberance or decline of yin and yang, cold and heat changes of human body, and is one of the important theories to explain the nature of medicinal action and an important part of medicinal properties.

药性分寒温，不晚于西汉时期。自《神农本草经》提出药"有寒热温凉四气"后，一直被后世袭用。宋代寇宗奭为了避免与药物的香臭之气相混淆，主张将"四气"称为"四性"。两种称谓的含义相同，而四气的称谓沿用已久，习称至今。

The time when medicinal nature fell into cold and warm was no later than the Western Han Dynasty. Since *Shen Nong's Classic of the Materia Medica* (*Shén Nóng Běn Cǎo Jīng*) put forward the medicine four qi, cold, hot, warm and cool, it has been used by later generations. Kou Zongshi of Song Dynasty advocated four natures instead of four qi to avoid being confused with the smell of medicine. The two kinds of appellation have the same meaning, while four qi has been used for a long time, and it has been used so far.

在寒、热、温、凉四性中，寒与凉、温与热分别是同一类药性，仅是程度上的差异，"凉次于寒""温次于热"。若进一步区分其程度，则又有"大热""大寒""微温""微凉"等描述。此外，还有一些平性药，是指寒热偏性不明显，药性平和、作用缓和的一类药。实际上也有偏温偏凉的不同，称其性平是相对而言，仍未超出四性的范围。四性从本质而言，实际上是寒、热二性。

In the four natures, cold and cool, warm and hot are different in intensity with the same nature; "cool is inferior to cold" "warm is inferior to hot". For further subdivision, some medicinals are marked as extremely hot, extremely cold, slightly warm and slightly cool. In addition, some Chinese medicinals are of neutral nature, whose medicinal preferences for cold or hot are inconspicuous, neutral in nature and mild in effect, even though actually they are also slightly warm or cool. It's relative to call it neutral, still not beyond the scope of the four natures. Therefore, in essence, the four natures are cold and hot.

药物的寒凉、温热是通过药物作用于人体所产生的不同效应总结出来的，与所治疾病的寒热性质相对而言。能够减轻或消除寒证的药物，其药性属于寒性或凉性，其清热之力较强者为大寒或寒性，清热之力较弱者为微寒或凉性。如石膏、知母能够治疗高热、汗出、口渴、脉洪数等温热病气分热证，因而这两种药物属于寒性。反之，能够减轻或消除热证的药物，其药性属于温性或热性。其祛寒之力强者为大热或热性，力稍次者为温性，力再次者为微温。如附子、干姜对于脘腹冷痛、四肢厥冷、脉微欲绝等寒证具有温里散寒作用，表明这两种药物具有热性。

The determination of the medicinal nature, cold, cool, warm or hot, is summed up from the different effects of the drug on the human body, which is relative to the cold and hot properties of the disease. The medicinals that can alleviate or eliminate cold syndrome belong to cold or cool nature. Those with stronger heat clearing force are of great cold or cold nature, and the drugs with weaker heat clearing force are of slight cold or cold in nature. For example, *shí gāo* (Gypsum Fibrosum) and *zhī mǔ* (Anemarrhenae Rhizoma) can treat the heat syndrome in qi aspect of some warm febrile diseases, such as high fever, sweating, thirst, surging and rapid pulse, so they are cold in nature. On the contrary, the medicinals which can reduce or eliminate the heat syndrome belong to the warm or hot nature. Those with strong force of dispelling cold are of great hot or hot in nature, those less strong are warm, and then slightly warm. For example, *fù zǐ* (Aconiti Lateralis Radix Praeparata) and *gān jiāng* (Zingiberis Rhizoma) have the effect of warming interior and dissipating cold on some cold syndromes such as abdominal cold pain, reversal cold of limbs, and faint pulse, which shows the two medicinals are hot in nature.

一般而言，寒凉药具有清热泻火、凉血解毒等作用；温热药则具有温里散寒、补火助阳、温经通络等作用。明确了四气的性质及其作用，就能以四气为依据指导临床用药。

Generally speaking, cold and cold medicinals have the functions of clearing heat and purging fire, cooling blood and removing toxin, while warm and hot medicinals have the functions of warming interior and dissipating cold, tonifying fire and assist yang, warming channels and dredging collaterals.

Understanding the nature and actions of the four qi can guide clinical medication.

1. **辨证用药** 是指在中医药理论指导下，辨明疾病的阴阳盛衰和寒热性质，有针对性地遣用寒性或热性药。《神农本草经》提出"疗寒以热药，疗热以寒药"，《素问》谓"寒者热之，热者寒之"，明确指出了药性寒热与治则的关系。阴寒证选用温热药，阳热证选用寒凉药，这是临床用药的一般原则，反之可能对患者造成不良影响，故王叔和明确提出"桂枝下咽，阳盛则毙；承气入胃，阴盛以亡"。

(1) Medication on syndrome differentiation Under the guidance of TCM theory, we should distinguish the exuberance or decline of yin and yang, cold or heat in nature, and dispatch the cold or heat drugs specially. *Shen Nong's Classic of the Materia Medica* (*Shén Nóng Běn Cǎo Jīng*) puts forward "treating cold diseases with hot medicinals while hot diseases with cold medicinals". *Basic Questions* (*Sù Wèn*) says "treating cold with heat, and treating heat with cold", clearly pointing out the relationship between the four qi and the treatment principle. It is the general principle of clinical medication that yin cold syndrome uses warm medicine and yang heat syndrome uses cold medicine. Or, it may cause adverse effects on the patients, so Wang Shuhe clearly warned "taking *guì zhī* (Cinnamomi Ramulus), the patient with yang exuberance may die; taking *Chéng Qì Tāng* (Purgative Decoction), the patient with yin exuberance may die".

2. **寒热并用** 临床实际中，疾病的表现往往复杂多样，单纯的寒证或热证比较少见，而表寒里热、上热下寒、寒热中阻等是疾病常见的表现形式。在治疗时当寒药与热药并用，使寒热并除，即《医碥》所谓："因其人寒热之邪夹杂于内，不得不用寒热夹杂之剂，古人每多如此。"《伤寒论》中半夏泻心汤、生姜泻心汤等就是寒温并用的典范。对于寒热错杂、阴阳格拒的病证，又当采用反佐之法治之，即张介宾"以热治寒，而寒拒热，则反佐以寒药而入之；以寒治热，而热拒寒，则反佐以热药而入之"之谓也。

(2) Use cold and hot together In clinical practice, the manifestations of diseases are often complex and diverse, and the simple cold syndrome or heat syndrome is relatively rare, while the more common ones are the mixed cold and heat syndromes such as exterior cold and interior heat, upper heat and lower cold, middle obstruction of cold-heat complex. In the treatment, cold and hot medicinals should be used together to remove cold and heat. It is said in *Danger Zone of Medicine* (*Yī Biān*) that "because of the pathogenic cold and heat mixed together, we have to use the mixture of cold and hot medicinals, and that's what the ancients did". Good examples of cold and warm combination are *Bàn Xià Xiè Xīn Tāng* (Pinellia Heart-Draining Decoction) and *Shēng Jiāng Xiè Xīn Tāng* (Fresh Ginger Heart-Draining Decoction) in *Treatise on Cold Damage* (*Shāng Hán Lùn*). For syndromes of cold-heat complex, and repelling of cold and heat, using corrigent is the treating method. That's just what Zhang Jie-bin said "treat cold with heat, and cold repels heat, and cold medicinals should be added; treat heat with cold, and heat repels cold, and hot medicinals should be added".

第二节　五味

Section 2　Five flavors

五味最早主要指烹饪、饮食调味，如《吕氏春秋》曰："调和之事，必以酸苦甘辛咸，先后多少。"将五味与药物结合起来，最早见于《黄帝内经》《神农本草经》，如《素问·脏气法时论》曰："辛散、酸收、甘缓、苦坚、咸软。"《神农本草经》曰："药有酸、咸、甘、苦、辛五味。"为中药五味的形成奠定了基础。经后世历代医家的补充完善，逐步形成了说明药物性质与作用的主要理论。

The five flavors originally refer to cooking and food seasoning. For example, *Mister Lv's Spring and Autumn Annals* (*Lǚ Shì Chūn Qiū*) says, "seasoning in cooking must depend on the order and quantity of sour, bitter, sweet, acrid and salty". The combination of five flavors and medicine was first seen in *The Yellow Emperor's Inner Classic* (*Huáng Dì Nèi Jīng*) and *Shen Nong's Classic of the Materia Medica* (*Shén Nóng Běn Cǎo Jīng*). *Basic Questions—Method of Internal Qi* (*Sù Wèn—Zàng Qì Fǎ Shí Lùn*) mentions "acrid means dispersing, sour absorbing, sweet moderating, bitter drying and salty softening". *Shen Nong's Classic of the Materia Medica* (*Shén Nóng Běn Cǎo Jīng*) says "Chinese medicinals have five flavors, sour, salty, sweet, bitter and acrid". Thus, it laid a foundation for the formation of five flavors of Chinese medicine. With the supplement and improvement of the doctors in the later generations, the main theories about the properties and functions of medicinals have been gradually formed.

所谓五味，是指药物有酸、苦、甘、辛、咸五种基本的味。药物或食物的滋味实际上不止五味，还有淡味或涩味。但由于长期以来将涩附于酸，淡附于甘，以合五行配属关系，故仍习称五味。

The five flavors refer to the five basic tastes of medicine: sour, bitter, sweet, acrid (pungent) and salty. The taste of medicine or food actually has actually more than five tastes, and there is also a bland or astringent taste. Although there are actually more than five kinds, it is still commonly known as "five flavors" because of its long-term attachment of astringency to sour and light attachment to sweetness in order to integrate the five elements.

五味最初用以表示通过口尝直接感知的真实滋味，如黄连味苦、生姜味辛、山楂味酸等。随着用药知识的积累，古人在长期的医疗实践中发现，不同滋味的药物作用于人体，会产生不同的功效，逐步发现各种药味与某些作用之间的相关性，如辛味、甘味、酸味分别具有发散、补虚、收涩等作用特点，因此以五味为纲，对各种作用的药物进行归类，从而总结归纳形成了早期的五味理论。随着临床实践的不断深入，药物品种增多，药物功用拓展，有的药物具有某种滋味，却并无早期五味理论中相应的作用特点，如山楂虽有真实的酸味，却并无收敛固涩的功效；而有的药物具有某种作用特点，又没有相应的味，如麻黄虽有较强的发散作用，但其滋味却无明显的辛味。因此就采用了以功效类推定味的方法，从而产生了抽象之味，即具有补益作用的定为甘味，具有发散作用的定为辛味等。由此可见，中药性能中的味，已经不仅是药物滋味的真实反映，更重要的是在功效基础之上，对药物实际效用的总结，对临床用药具有更直接的指导意义。

The determination of five flavors is initially used to express the real taste directly perceived through the mouth, such as the bitter taste of *huáng lián* (Coptidis Rhizoma), the pungent taste of *shēng jiāng* (Zingiberis Recens Rhizoma), the sour taste of *shān zhā* (Crataegi Fructus), etc. With the accumulation of drug knowledge, the ancients found in long-term medical practice that different tastes of drugs will have different functional effects when they act on the human body, and gradually found the correlation between various tastes and some effects, such as tastes of pungent, sweet, sour respectively corresponding to actions of dispersing, tonifying deficiency, astringency. Based on the five flavors, the medicinals with various functions are classified, and then the early five flavors theory came into being. With the deepening of clinical practice, the number of drug varieties and the expansion of functions, some drugs have a certain taste, but there is no corresponding feature in the early tasteless theory, such as *shān zhā* (Crataegi

Fructus). Although it has a real sour taste, it has no absorbing and astringent effect. Some drugs have the same characteristics of action, but no corresponding taste. For example, *má huáng* (Ephedrae Herba) has strong divergent effect, but no obvious pungent taste. Therefore, the method of using efficacy to infer flavors is adopted, which produces abstract flavors. Those with tonic effect are defined as sweet, and those with divergent effect are defined as acrid, etc. It can be seen that the flavor in the property of Chinese medicinals is not only the true reflection of the taste, but also the summary of the actual medicinal effect based on the establishment of efficacy, which has a more direct guiding significance for clinical medication.

1. 辛味 能散、能行，具有发散、行气、行血等作用。一般用治外感表证、气滞证、血瘀证，如生姜发散风寒、薄荷发散风热，分别用治风寒和风热表证；木香、陈皮行气调中，用治脾胃气滞证；川芎、红花活血化瘀，用治瘀血阻滞病证等。

(1) Acrid Acrid flavor can disperse and move, with the efficacy of dispersing, moving qi and activating blood. Acrid medicinals are generally used for exterior syndromes, syndromes of qi stagnation, syndromes of blood stasis, such as *shēng jiāng* (Zingiberis Recens Rhizoma) can disperse wind-cold, and *bò he* (Menthae Herba) can disperse wind-heat, respectively; *mù xiāng* (Aucklandiae Radix) and *chén pí* (Citri Reticulatae Pericarpium) can regulate qi to regulate the spleen; *chuān xiōng* (Chuanxiong Rhizoma) and *hóng huā* (Carthami Flos) can activate blood and remove blood stasis to treat syndromes of blood stasis.

2. 甘味 能补、能和、能缓，具有补益、和中、调和药性和缓急止痛的作用。一般用治虚证、脾胃不和、脘腹、四肢挛急疼痛、调和药性及中毒解救等方面。如人参补气、熟地黄能补血滋阴、饴糖能缓急止痛、甘草能调和药性，并解药食中毒等。

(2) Sweet Sweet flavor can nourish, harmonize and moderate, with the efficacy of tonifying, harmonizing the middle, moderating property of medicinals, moderating emergency and stopping pains. Sweet medicinals are often used in treatment of deficiency syndromes, spleen-stomach disharmony, spasm and pain in abdomen and limbs, medicinal moderation, moderating toxic, and so on. For example, *rén shēn* (Ginseng Radix et Rhizoma) can reinforce qi, *shú dì huáng* (Rehmanniae Radix Praeparata) can tonify blood and nourish yin, *yí táng* (Saccharum Granorum) can relieve spasm and pain, *gān cǎo* (Glycyrrhizae Radix et Rhizoma) can moderate medicinal nature and remove toxicity.

3. 苦味 能泄、能燥、能坚，"泄"的含义有三：一是清泄，即清热泻火，主要用治火热病证，如栀子、黄芩清热泻火等；二是降泄，主要用于肺胃气逆证，如苦杏仁降泄肺气、枇杷叶降泄肺胃之气等；三是通泄，即泻下，主要用于便秘，如大黄、芒硝泻下通便等。"燥"即燥湿，主要用于湿证。根据其药性寒温之不同，又有苦温燥湿和苦寒燥湿之分，前者多用于寒湿证，如苍术、厚朴等；后者多用于湿热证，如龙胆、黄连等。"坚"即坚阴，又称泻火存阴。通过清热泻火以保护阴液，用于治疗阴虚火旺证，如黄柏、知母等。

(3) Bitter Bitter flavor can purge, dry and firm. Purgation includes three aspects: firstly, clearing, referring to clearing heat and purging fire, mainly used for fire-heat syndromes, such as *zhī zǐ* (Gardeniae Fructus) and *huáng qín* (Scutellariae Radix); secondly, lowering, mainly used for the syndrome of lung and stomach qi counterflow, such as *kǔ xìng rén* (Armeniacae Amarum Semen) descending lung qi, and *pí pá yè* (Eriobotryae Folium) descending qi of lung and stomach; thirdly, discharging, mainly used for constipation, such as *dà huáng* (Rhei Radix et Rhizoma) and *máng xiāo* (Natrii Sulfas) discharging stool. Drying refers to drying dampness, mainly used for damp syndromes, including cold-damp syndrome and damp-heat syndrome according to different medicinal nature, the former mainly for cold-damp syndromes, such as *cāng zhú* (Atractylodis Rhizoma) and *hòu pò* (Magnoliae Officinalis Cortex); the latter mainly for damp-heat syndromes, such as *lóng dǎn* (Gentianae Radix et Rhizoma) and *huáng lián* (Coptidis Rhizoma). Firming, also known as purging fire and holding yin, which protects yin fluid through clearing heat and purging fire, mainly used for syndrome of yin deficiency and effulgent fire, such as *huáng bó* (Phellodendri Chinensis Cortex) and *zhī mǔ* (Anemarrhenae Rhizoma).

4. 酸（涩）味　能收、能涩，有收敛、固涩作用，具体表现为固表止汗、敛肺止咳、固精缩尿、涩肠止泻、固崩止血等功效。一般用治自汗盗汗、久咳虚喘、久泻久痢、遗精滑精、遗尿尿频、崩带不止等滑脱不禁的病证。如乌梅敛肺止咳、山茱萸敛汗涩精、五味子固表止汗等。此外，部分酸味药具有生津作用，可用治津亏口渴等，如乌梅、五味子等。

(4) Sour (astringent)　Sour (astringent) flavor can absorb and astringing, manifested in the functions of consolidating exterior and stopping sweating, astringing lung and relieving cough, securing essence and reducing urination, astringing intestines and checking diarrhea, stopping metrorrhagia and bleeding. Sour medicinals are often utilized to treat the syndrome of spontaneous sweating and night sweat, chronic cough deficiency-type dyspnea, chronic diarrhea and dysentery, seminal emission and involuntary emission, enuresis and frequent urination, metrorrhagia, etc., such as *wū méi* (Mume Fructus) astringing lung and relieving cough, *shān zhū yú* (Corni Fructus) arresting sweat and astringing intestines, and *wǔ wèi zǐ* (Schisandrae Chinensis Fructus) strengthening exterior and stopping sweating. In addition, some of the sour medicinals have the effect of promoting fluid production, and can be used to treat fluid consumption and thirst, such as *wū méi* (Mume Fructus) and *wǔ wèi zǐ* (Schisandrae Chinensis Fructus).

5. 咸味　能下、能软，有泻下、软坚散结作用。一般用治大便秘结以及痰核、瘿瘤、癥瘕痞块等。如芒硝软坚泻下、牡蛎软坚散结等。

(5) Salty　Salty flavor can purge and soften, functioning as relieving constipation and softening hardness and dissipating mass. Generally salty medicinals are used for constipation, phlegm nodule, goiter and tumor, and abdominal mass, such as *máng xiāo* (Natrii Sulfas) softening and purging, *mǔ lì* (Ostreae Concha) softening hardness and dissipating mass.

6. 淡味　能渗、能利，有渗湿、利水作用。一般用治水肿、小便不利之证。如茯苓、猪苓、薏苡仁等。

(6) Bland　Bland flavor can percolate dampness and promote urination. Bland medicinals are often used for edema and poor urination, such as *fú líng* (Poria), *zhū líng* (Polyporus) and *yì yǐ rén* (Coicis Semen).

每种药物都同时具有性和味，两者分别从不同角度说明药物的作用，因此必须将两者综合起来，才能准确地认识药物的作用及特点。一般而言，气味相同者，作用相近。如辛温的药物多具有发散风寒的作用，甘温的药物多具有补气或助阳的作用。气味不同，则作用有别。其中，气同味异者，如麻黄、杏仁、大枣、乌梅、肉苁蓉同属温性但五味不同，则麻黄辛温发汗解表、杏仁苦温降气止咳、大枣甘温补脾益气、乌梅酸温敛肺涩肠、肉苁蓉咸温补肾助阳；味同气异者，如桂枝、薄荷、附子、石膏均为辛味但四气不同，则桂枝辛温解表散寒、薄荷辛凉疏散风热、附子辛热补火助阳、石膏辛寒清热泻火。至于一药兼有数味，则往往作用更广，如当归味辛甘性温，甘能补血、辛能活血行气、温能祛寒，故有补血、活血、行气止痛、温经散寒等作用，可用治血虚、血瘀、血寒等病证。一般临床用药既用其性，又用其味，但有时在复方配伍用药时，可能出现或用其气，或用其味的不同情况。如升麻辛甘微寒，与葛根同用治麻疹不透时，则取其味辛以解表透疹；若与石膏同用治胃火牙痛时，则取其寒性以清热降火。由此可见，药物的气味所表示的药物作用以及气味配合的关系是比较复杂的。因此，既要熟悉四气五味的一般规律，又要掌握每一药物气味的特殊治疗作用以及气味配合的规律，这样才能更好地掌握药性，指导临床用药。

Each medicinal has both nature and flavor at the same time. They explain the role of drugs from different perspectives. Therefore, both of them must be integrated in order to accurately understand the functions and characteristics of medicinals. Generally speaking, those with the same flavors demonstrate similar functions. For example, pungent-warm medicine has the effect of dispersing wind and cold, and sweet-warm medicine has the effect of invigorating qi or assisting yang. Those with different flavors demonstrate different functions. Some medicinals are of the same natures but different flavors. For example, *má huáng* (Ephedrae Herba), *xìng rén* (Armeniacae Amarum Semen), *dà zǎo* (Jujubae Fructus), *wū méi* (Mume Fructus) and *ròu cōng róng* (Cistanches Herba) are all warm in nature but different in flavors, so *má huáng*, acrid and warm, can induce sweating and release exterior; *kǔ xìng rén*, bitter and warm, can descend qi and relieving cough; *dà zǎo*, sweet and warm, can tonify spleen and replenishing qi; *wū méi*, sour and warm, can astringe lung and intestines; *ròu cōng róng*, salty and warm, can tonify kidney and assist yang. Some medicinals are of the same flavors but different natures. For example, *guì zhī* (Cinnamomi Ramulus), *bò he* (Menthae Herba), *fù zǐ* (Aconiti Lateralis Radix Praeparata) and *shí gāo* (Gypsum Fibrosum) are all acrid but different in nature, so *guì zhī*, acrid and warm, can release exterior and dissipate cold; *bò he*, acrid and cool, can disperse wind and dissipate cold; *fù zǐ*, acrid and hot, can tonify fire and assist yang; *shí gāo*, acrid and cold, can clear heat and purge fire. As for one medicinal with several flavors, it often has a wider effect. For example, *dāng guī* (Angelicae Sinensis Radix) is acrid, sweet and warm, while sweet nature is to replenish blood, acrid to activate blood and move qi, warm to dispel cold, so *dāng guī* has the functions of replenishing blood, activating blood circulation, move qi to relieve pain, warming channels and dispersing cold, and can be used to treat blood deficiency, blood stasis and blood cold. The general clinical medication is to use both its nature and its flavor, but sometimes when the compound is used in combination, either nature or flavor may be adopted in different situations. For example, *shēng má* (Cimicifugae Rhizoma) is acrid, sweet and slightly cold, but its acrid nature is adopted to release exterior and promote eruption when used with *gé gēn* (Puerariae Lobatae Radix) to treat inadequate measles eruption; and its cold nature is adopted to clear heat and descend fire when used with *shí gāo* (Gypsum Fibrosum) to treat toothache due to stomach fire. It shows that the relationship between the functions of medicinals, demonstrated by its flavors and qi, and combination of the flavors and qi is complex. Therefore, it is necessary to be familiar with the general law of four qi and five flavors, as well as the special therapeutic effect and the coordination, so as to better grasp the medicinal properties and guide clinical medication.

第三节　升降浮沉

Section 3　Ascending, descending, floating and sinking

PPT

升降浮沉为古代升降出入理论在中药学中的具体应用，用以反映药物作用的趋向性，是说明药物作用性质的概念之一。

Ascending, descending, floating and sinking is the specific application of ancient upward-downward and outward-inward theory in Chinese medicine, which is used to reflect the tendency of medicinal action, and is one of the concepts to explain the nature of medicinal actions.

《素问·至真要大论》指出"升降出入，无器不有"，把升降出入作为自然界一切事物的基本运动形式。气机升降出入是人体生命活动的基础。若气机升降出入发生障碍，机体便处于疾病状态，产生不同的病势趋向，常表现为向上（如呕吐、咳喘）、向下（如脱肛、泄泻、崩漏）、向外（如自汗、盗汗）、向内（如表证未解而入里）等。中药能够针对病情，改善或消除这些病证，相对而言也就分别具有向下、向上、向内、向外的作用趋向。

It is pointed out in *Basic Questions—On the Supreme Truth (Sù Wèn · Zhì Zhēn Yào Dà Lùn)* that "ascending, descending, exiting and entering exist in everything", which takes the four tendencies as the basic movement of all things in nature. Ascending, descending, exiting and entering is the basis of human life activities. If there is an obstacle in the qi movement, the body will be in a state of disease, resulting in different disease inclination, which often manifests as ascending (vomiting, coughing and asthma), descending (prolapse, diarrhea, metrorrhagia), exiting (self perspiration, night perspiration), entering (inward penetration of exterior syndrome), etc. Chinese medicinals can improve or eliminate these syndromes according to the condition of the disease, which has the function trend of downward, upward, inward and outward respectively.

升是上升，表示作用趋向于上；降是下降，表示作用趋向于下；浮表示发散，作用趋向于外；沉表示收敛闭藏，作用趋向于内。升降浮沉之中，升与降、浮与沉是相对立的，升与浮、沉与降既有区别又有联系，升与浮、沉与降常相提并论。按阴阳属性区分，则升浮属阳，沉降属阴。从药物作用而言，升浮药作用趋向多上升向外，具有升阳、发表、祛风散寒、开窍、涌吐等作用；而沉降药作用趋向多下行向内，具有泻下、清热、利水、重镇安神、潜阳息风、平喘止咳、降逆止呕、收敛固涩等作用。大多数中药具有升浮或沉降之性，但有的药物升降浮沉的特性不明显，如川楝子、土荆皮等。也有少数药物具有升浮与沉降的双重性，如川芎既上行头目，又下行血海；麻黄既发汗解表，又利水消肿等。

Ascending is to demonstrate the uprising trend, while descending is to express the downward action. Floating means dispersing and acts outside, however sinking is collecting and hiding with action inside. In the trend of actions, ascending and descending, floating and sinking are opposite, while ascending and floating, descending and sinking are different but related, so they are often comparable. In yin and yang theory, ascending and floating belong to yang, descending and sinking to yin. From the aspect of actions, medicinals with ascending and floating trends are mainly to be upward and outward and have the functions of elevating yang, relieving exterior, expelling wind, dissipating cold, opening orifice and vomiting, while medicinals with descending and sinking trends are mainly to be downward and inward and have the functions of purging, clearing heat, promoting urination, tranquilizing mind with heavy sedatives, subduing yang, extinguishing wind, relieving dyspnea and cough, descending counterflow of qi, relieving vomiting, astringing and arresting discharge. Generally speaking, most of the Chinese medicinals have the characteristics of ascending-floating or descending-sinking, but some are not obvious, such as *chuān liàn zǐ* (Toosendan Fructus) and *tǔ jīng pí* (Pseudolaricis Cortex). There are a few medicinals with the dual characteristics of ascending-floating or descending-sinking, such as *chuān xiōng* (Chuanxiong Rhizoma) moving upward to head and eyes as well as downward to *Xuehai*, and *má huáng* (Ephedrae Herba) inducing sweating to releasing exterior as well as promoting urination and alleviating edema.

药物升降浮沉趋向，即是药物本身固有的，也受炮制、配伍等诸多因素的影响，诚如《本草纲目》所言："升降在物，亦在人。"影响药物升降浮沉的因素主要有以下几方面。

The tendency of ascending, descending, floating and sinking is inherent, and at the same time influenced by many factors such as processing and compatibility. As *The Grand Compendium of Materia Medica* (*Běn Cǎo Gāng Mù*) says, "ascending and descending exist naturally but also artificially".The main factors affecting ascending, descending, floating and sinking of medicinals are as follows.

1. **性味**　中药的性味是升降浮沉性能的内在依据。一般而言，药性升浮者，大多具有辛甘之味和温热之性，如麻黄、升麻、黄芪等；药性沉降者，大多具有苦酸咸涩之味和寒凉之性，如大黄、芒硝、乌梅等。故《本草纲目》云："酸咸无升，辛甘无降，寒无浮，热无沉。"

(1) Property　The property of Chinese medicinal is the internal basis of ascending, descending, floating and sinking. Generally speaking, most of medicinals with ascending and floating trends are acrid and sweet in flavor, warm and hot in nature, such as *má huáng* (Ephedrae Herba), *shēng má* (Cimicifugae Rhizoma), and *huáng qí* (Astragali Radix). Most of those with descending and sinking trends are bitter, sour, salty and astringent in flavor, cold and cool in nature, such as *dà huáng* (Rhei Radix et Rhizoma), *máng xiāo* (Natrii Sulfas) and *wū méi* (Mume Fructus). Therefore, *The Grand Compendium of Materia Medica* (*Běn Cǎo Gāng Mù*) says, "medicinals with sour and salty flavors have no ascending trend, acrid and sweet no descending, cold no floating, and hot no sinking".

2. **质地**　前人重视药物升降浮沉与药物质地轻重的关系。汪昂《本草备要》药性总义云："凡药轻虚者浮而升；重实者沉而降。"一般而言，花、叶、皮、枝等质轻的药物大多升浮，如苏叶、菊花、桑枝等；而种子、果实、矿物、贝壳等质重者大多是沉降药，如苏子、枳实、赭石等。然而，前人也认识到，上述关系并非绝对，如旋覆花功能降气、消痰、止呕，药性沉降而不升浮；苍耳子散风寒、通鼻窍、祛风湿，药性升浮而不沉降，故有"诸花皆升，旋覆独降；诸子皆降，苍耳独升"之说。

(2) Quality　Previous researchers paid attention to the relationship between the ascending-descending-floating-sinking and the quality of medicinals. Wang Ang said in *Essentials of Materia Medica* (*Běn Cǎo Bèi Yào*), "all medicines that are light and empty tend to ascend and float; those that are heavy and solid tend to descend and sink". Generally speaking, the medicinals with light quality such as flowers, leaves, barks and branches are mostly ascending and floating, such as *sū yè* (Perillae Folium), *jú huā* (Chrysanthemi Flos), and *sāng zhī* (Mori Ramulus), while those with heavy quality such as seeds, fruits, minerals, and shells are mostly descending and sinking, such as *sū zǐ* (Perillae Fructus), *zhǐ shí* (Aurantii Immaturus Fructus) and *zhě shí* (Haematitum). However, the predecessors also realized that the above relationship is not absolute. For example, *xuán fù huā* (Inulae Flos) functions to reduce qi, eliminate phlegm, and relieve vomiting, but its property is descending and sinking without ascending and floating; *cāng ěr zǐ* (Xanthii Fructus) can disperse wind-cold, unblock stuffy nose, and dispel wind dampness, but its property is ascending and floating without descending and sinking, so there is a saying that "all flowers are ascending except *xuán fù* which descending, while all seeds are descending except *cāng ěr* which ascending".

3. **炮制**　其对药物升降浮沉趋向的影响较复杂，其中炮制辅料的影响最为明显。李时珍指出："升者引之以咸寒，则沉而直达下焦，沉者引之以酒，则浮而上至巅顶。"一般而言，酒制则升，姜炒则散，醋炒收敛，盐炒下行。如大黄属于沉降药，功能泻热通便，经酒炒后则清上焦火热，可用治目赤咽肿、牙龈肿痛。

(3) Processing　The influence of processing on the four tendencies of medicinals is complex, but the influence of processing adjuvants is the most obvious. Li Shizhen pointed out: "those who ascend are added with salty and cold adjuvants will sink to the lower-energizer, while those who sink are added with wine will float to the top." Generally speaking, wine-processed medicinals will ascend, ginger-fried medicinals will disperse, vinegar-fried will astringe, salt-fried will descend. For example, *dà huáng* (Rhei Radix et Rhizoma) belongs to descending and sinking medicinals, and can relieve heat and defecate. After being stir fried with wine, it will clear fire-heat of upper-energizer and can be used to treat red eye, swelling throat, swelling and pain of gingival.

4. 配伍　中药的配伍影响其升降浮沉的性能。在复方配伍中，将少量升浮药与较多沉降药同用，其升浮之性会受到制约，该复方总的作用趋向以沉降为主；反之，少量沉降药与较多升浮药配伍，其沉降之性会受到抑制。如麻黄与大量石膏同用，其升浮发汗之力受到制约，可治疗肺热咳喘证；大黄与防风、白芷、荆芥等同用，其沉降之性受到制约，可治疗上焦风热证。

(4) Combination　The combination of Chinese medicinals affects its properties of ascending, descending, floating and sinking. In the combination of compound formula, when a small amount of ascending and floating medicine is used together with a large number of descending and sinking medicine, its ascending and floating property will be restricted, and the general function of the compound tends to be mainly descending and sinking; on the contrary, when a small amount of descending and sinking medicine is combined with a large number of ascending and floating medicine, its descending and sinking property will be restrained. For example, when *má huáng* (Ephedrae Herba) is used together with a large number of *shí gāo* (Gypsum Fibrosum), its function of ascending and sweating is restricted, which can be used to treat the syndrome of lung heat, cough and asthma; When *dà huáng* (Rhei Radix et Rhizoma) is used together with *fáng fēng* (Saposhnikoviae Radix), *bái zhǐ* (Angelicae Dahuricae Radix) and *jīng jiè* (Schizonepetae Herba), its function of descending and sinking is restricted, which can be used to treat upper-energizer wind-heat syndrome.

掌握药物升降浮沉的性能，可以更好地指导临床用药，以纠正机体功能的失调，使之恢复正常，或因势利导，有助于祛邪外出。具体而言，病变部位在上在表者，宜升浮不宜沉降，如外感风热应选用薄荷、菊花等以疏散表邪；病变部位在下在里者，宜沉降不宜升浮，如热结便秘者应选用大黄、芒硝等以泻热通便。病势上逆者，宜降不宜升，如肝阳上亢之头晕目眩，应选用赭石、石决明等以平肝潜阳；病势下陷者，宜升不宜降，如气虚下陷之久泻、脱肛，应用黄芪、升麻等以益气升阳。

Mastering the ascending-descending-floating-sinking properties of medicinals can better guide clinical medication, retrieve the imbalance of body function, take it back to normal, or guide according to the circumstances, and help expel pathogens out. In particular, those with the lesion in the upper part or on the surface should be ascended and floated rather than descended and sunk. For example, external-contraction wind-heat should use *bò he* (Menthae Herba) and *jú huā* (Chrysanthemi Flos) to disperse exterior pathogen. Those with the lesion in the lower part or inside should be descended and sunk rather than ascended and floated. For example, constipation due to heat accumulation should use *dà huáng* (Rhei Radix et Rhizoma) and *máng xiāo* (Natrii Sulfas) to purge heat and relaxing bowels. For those with adverse rising, the descending medicinal is advisable, such as dizziness due to ascendant hyperactivity of liver yang, which should use *zhě shí* (Haematitum) and *shí jué míng* (Haliotidis Concha) to pacify liver and subdue yang; for those with sinking tendency, the ascending medicinal is advisable, such as chronic diarrhea and anorectal prolapse due to qi sinking, which should use *huáng qí* (Astragali Radix) and *shēng má* (Cimicifugae Rhizoma) to replenish qi and elevate yang.

第四节　归经

Section 4　Meridian tropism

归经是药物作用的定位概念，即表示药物作用部位。归是作用的归属，经是脏腑经络的概称。所谓归经，是指药物对于机体某部位的选择性作用，即中药对某些脏腑经络的病变起着主要或特殊的治疗作用。药物的归经不同，其治疗作用也不同。归经阐明了药物治病的适用范围，说明了药效所在，包含了药物作用定位的内容，是阐明药物作用机理，指导临床用药的性能理论之一。

Meridian tropism is the concept of the location of medicinal action, that is, the site of a medicinal act. Tropism is the attribution of function, and the meridian is the general term of *zang-fu* organs, channels, collaterals and their subordinates. Meridian tropism refers to the selective effect of medicinals on a certain part of the body, that is, Chinese medicinals play a major or special therapeutic role in the pathological changes of some organs or meridians. The therapeutic effect is different with different meridian tropism. Meridian tropism points out the scope of application of medicinal treatment, explains the efficacy, contains the content of medicinal action orientation, and is one of the performance theories to clarify the mechanism of medicinal action and guide clinical medication.

前人在用药实践中观察到，一种药物往往主要对某一经或某几经产生明显的作用，而对其他经的作用较小，甚至没有作用。同属性寒清热的药物，有的偏于清肺热，有的偏于清胃热，有的偏于清心热或清肝热；同属补药，也有补脾、补肾、补肝、补肺的不同。反映了药物在机体产生效应的部位各有侧重。将这些认识加以归纳，使之系统化，便形成了归经理论。

It has been observed in the practice of medication that a medicinal often has an obvious effect on a certain meridian or several meridians, but has little or no effect on other meridians. Some medicinals with the same property of cold and heat-clearing are partial to clearing the lung heat, partial to clearing the stomach heat, partial to clearing the heart heat or clearing the liver heat; even tonic have differences in tonifying the spleen, kidney, liver and lung, which reflects that there are different emphases in the parts of the body where the medicinals have effects. These understandings are summed up and systematized to form the theory of meridian tropism.

归经是在中医基本理论指导下，以脏腑经络学说为基础，以药物所治疗的具体病证为依据，经过长期临床实践总结出来的用药理论。经络能沟通人体内外表里，所以一旦机体发生疾病，体表病变可以通过经络影响到内在脏腑；反之，内在脏腑病变也可以反映到体表。由于发病所在脏腑及经络循行部位不同，临床上所表现的症状则各不相同。能够治疗特定脏腑、经络疾病就决定了该药的归经所在。如心经病变多见心悸失眠，酸枣仁、朱砂能治疗心悸失眠，因而归心经；杏仁、苏子能够治疗喘咳胸闷，因而归肺经；白芍、钩藤能治疗胁痛、抽搐，因而归肝经。许多中药可以治疗多脏腑、经络疾病，因而归数经。如麻黄既治外感风寒及咳喘病证，又能治疗水肿，因而归肺、膀胱经。

Guided by the basic theory of TCM, based on the theory of *zang-fu* organs, meridians and collaterals, and based on the specific diseases and syndromes, meridian tropism is a medication theory summarized through long-term clinical practice. Meridians and collaterals can communicate the interior of the body with the exterior, so once the body has diseases, the lesions on the body surface can affect the internal organs through meridians and collaterals; otherwise, the lesions on the internal organs can also be reflected on the body surface. Due to the different location of *zang-fu* organs and meridians, the clinical symptoms are different. The Chinese medicinals which can treat the diseases of specific organs and meridians determines the meridian tropism of the medicinal. For example, palpitation and insomnia are often seen in the pathological changes of heart meridian. *Suān zǎo rén* (Ziziphi Spinosae Semen) and *zhū shā* (Cinnabaris) can treat palpitation and insomnia, entering heart meridian. In the same way, *xìng rén* (Armeniacae Amarum Semen) and *sū zǐ* (Perillae Fructus) can treat asthma, cough and chest distress, entering lung meridian; *bái sháo* (Paeoniae Alba Radix) and *gōu téng* (Uncariae Cum Uncis Ramulus) can treat hypochondriac pain and convulsion, entering liver meridian. Many medicinals can treat the diseases of multiple organs and meridians, so one medicinal may enter several meridians. For example, *má huáng* (Ephedrae Herba) can treat not only the syndrome of exterior-contraction wind-cold and cough and asthma, but also edema, so it enters lung and bladder meridians.

掌握药物的归经，就认识了该药作用部位的个性专长，可以增强用药的准确性，提高临床疗效。根据疾病的临床表现，通过辨证，明确病变所在脏腑经络部位，按照归经理论来选择适当药物进行治疗。如治疗心悸失眠，选择归心经的药物；治疗咳嗽气喘，选择归肺经的药物。

Mastering the meridian tropism of medicinals makes it easy to know the individual specialty of the action site of the medicinal, which can enhance the accuracy of medication and improve the clinical efficacy. According to the clinical manifestations of the disease, through syndrome differentiation, the location of the lesions in *zang-fu* organs and meridians should be determined, and the appropriate medicinal should be selected for treatment according to the meridian tropism. For example, in the treatment of palpitation and insomnia, select the medicinal that enters the heart meridian; in the treatment of cough and asthma, select the medicinal that enters the lung meridian.

掌握药物的归经，便于临床根据脏腑经络关系配伍用药。脏腑经络在生理上相互联系，在病理上相互影响，因此，在临床用药时并不单纯选用某一经的药物，而是根据脏腑经络之间的关系，予以合理的配伍，以提高临床疗效。如肝阳上亢往往由于肾阴不足，临证治疗时常以平肝潜阳药与滋补肾阴药同用，使肝有所涵而亢阳自潜。咳喘虽不离于肺，但亦常与脾虚、肾虚或肝火有关，若以健脾、补肾或清肝火之药与归肺经的补肺、清肺、化痰、止咳平喘药同用，能明显提高疗效。若拘泥于见肝治肝、见肺治肺的单纯分经用药，其效果必受影响。正如徐灵胎所说："不知经络而用药，其失也泛，必无捷效；执经络而用药，其失也泥，反能致害。"

Mastering the meridian tropism of medicinals makes it convenient for clinical combination according to the relationship between organs and meridians. The *zang-fu* organs and meridians are interrelated in physiology and influence each other in pathology. Therefore, the medicinal of a certain meridian is not simply used in clinical medication, but is reasonably combined according to the relationship between *zang-fu* organs and meridians, so as to improve the clinical efficacy. For example, ascendant hyperactivity of liver yang is often due to the deficiency of kidney yin. The clinical treatment often uses medicinals of pacifying liver and subduing yang and medicinals of nourishing kidney yin together, so that the liver is nourished and yang hyperactivity is subdued. Although cough and asthma are not separated from the lung, they are often related to spleen deficiency, kidney deficiency or liver fire. If the medicinals of invigorating spleen, tonifying kidney or clearing liver fire are used together with the medicinals of invigorating lung, clearing lung, resolving phlegm and relieving cough and asthma, the curative effect can be significantly improved. Sticking to the treatment of liver or lung, the effect will be affected. As Xu Lingtai said, "if the doctor does not know how to use medicine through the meridians and collaterals, there must be a lot of faults, which will not have a rapid and significant effect; if the doctor is too constrained to use medicine through the meridians and collaterals, there will be many faults, which will cause harm to the patients".

在运用归经理论指导药物临床应用时，还必须与四气五味、升降浮沉结合起来，才能做到准确用药。如同归肺经的药物，由于有四气的不同，其治疗作用也异。如紫苏温散肺经风寒、薄荷凉散肺经风热、干姜性热温肺化饮、黄芩性寒清肺泻火。同归肺经的药物，由于五味的不同，作用亦殊。如乌梅酸以收涩、敛肺止咳，麻黄辛以发表、宣肺平喘，党参甘以补虚、补肺益气，陈皮苦以下气、止咳化痰，蛤蚧咸以补肾、益肺平喘。同归肺经的药物，因其升降浮沉之性不同，作用迥异。如桔梗、麻黄药性升浮，故能开宣肺气以平喘咳；杏仁、苏子药性沉降，故能降肺止咳平喘。四气五味、升降浮沉、归经同是药性理论的重要组成部分，在应用时必须结合起来，全面分析，才能准确地指导临床用药。

When using the theory of meridian tropism to guide the clinical medication, it must be combined with qi, flavors, ascending, descending, floating and sinking to achieve accurate medication. Take medicinals of lung meridian for instance. They are different in therapeutic effects because of the difference of four qi. For example, *zǐ sū* (Perillae Folium) is warm in nature for dissipating wind-cold of lung meridian, *bò he* (Menthae Herba) is cool for dissipating wind-heat of lung meridian, *gān jiāng* (Zingiberis Rhizoma) is hot for warming lung and resolving fluid retention, *huáng qín* (Scutellariae Radix) is cold for clear lung and draining fire. They have different therapeutic effects because they have different flavors. For example, *wū méi* (Mume Fructus) is sour for astringing, astringing lung and relieving cough, *má huáng* (Ephedrae Herba) is acrid for releasing exterior, ventilating lung and relieving dyspnea, *dǎng shēn* (Codonopsis Radix) is sweet for tonifying deficiency, tonifying lung and replenishing qi, *chén pí* (Citri Reticulatae Pericarpium) is bitter for lowering qi, relieving cough and resolving phlegm, *gé jiè* (Gecko) is salty for tonifying kidney, replenishing lung and relieving dyspnea. They are also different in therapeutic effects because of the difference of ascending, descending, floating and sinking. For example, *jié gěng* (Platycodonis Radix) and *má huáng* (Ephedrae Herba) are ascending and floating for dispersing lung qi, relieving cough and dyspnea, *xìng rén* (Armeniacae Amarum Semen) and *sū zǐ* (Perillae Fructus) are descending and sinking for descending lung and relieving cough and dyspnea. Four qi, five flavors, ascending, descending, floating and sinking, and meridian tropism are the important parts of the medicinal property and should be combined in application for overall analysis to guide clinical medication accurately.

第五节 毒性

PPT

Section 5　Toxicity

毒性是用以反映药物安全程度的性能。毒性和副作用不同，毒性是指药物对机体产生的不良影响和损害性，它对人体的危害较大，甚至危及生命；副作用是指在常用治疗剂量下出现的与治疗需要无关的不适反应，一般比较轻微，对机体危害不大，停药后可自行消失。为了确保安全合理用药，必须认识中药的毒性，了解毒性发生的原因，掌握中药中毒的解救方法和预防措施。

Toxicity is used to reflect the extent of medicinal safety. Toxic reactions are different from side effects. Toxic reactions refer to the adverse effects and damages of drugs on the body. They do great harm to the human body and even endanger life. Side effects refer to the discomfort reactions that have nothing to do with the need of treatment under the commonly used treatment dose. They are generally mild and do little harm to the body, and they can disappear automatically after the drug is stopped. In order to ensure the safety and rational use of drugs, one must understand the toxicity of Chinese medicinals, understand the causes of toxicity, and master the rescue methods and preventive measures of Chinese medicinal poisoning.

西汉以前 "毒药" 是一切药物的总称。《周礼·天官》云："医师掌医之政令，聚毒药以供医事。"《素问·脏气法时论》云："毒药攻邪，五谷为养，五果为助。"对此，丹波元简《药治通义》指出："毒药二字，古多连称，见《素问》及《周官》，即总括药饵之词。"古代的毒药概念，一方面反映了药、食分离在认识上的进步，另一方面也反映出当时对药物的治疗作用和毒性及副作用还不能很好地把握，故笼统称为 "毒药"。

Before the Western Han Dynasty, *dú* (poison) *yào* (herbs) was the general term of all drugs. *The Zhou Rituals—Cheongwan* (*Zhōu Lǐ—Tiān Guān*) says that "the doctor is in charge of medical law, gathering poisons for medical service". *Basic Questions—On Zang Qi Comforting to Seasons* (*Sù Wèn—Zàng Qì Fǎ Shí Lùn*) points out "all medicine is to remove pathogens that invade the body which needs the nourishment of gains and all kinds of fruits to help". In this regard, Danboyuan Jian said in *General Meaning of Medicaiton* (*Yào Zhì Tōng Yì*) that "the two characters, *dú yào*, is often put together in ancient times, seen in *Basic Questions* and *The Zhou Rituals*, and is a generalization of drugs". The ancient concept of *dú yào*, on the one hand, reflected the progress in the understanding of the separation of drugs and food, on the other hand, also reflected at that time, the therapeutic effect and side effects of drugs were not well mastered, so *dú yào* is a general term.

东汉时期，《本经》提出了 "有毒、无毒" 的区分，并谓："若用毒药疗病，起如黍粟，病去即止，不去倍之，不去十之，取去为度。"《内经》七篇大论中，亦有大毒、常毒、小毒等论述。从毒药连称到有毒、无毒的区分，反映了人们对毒性认识的进步。东汉以后的本草著作对有毒药物都标出其毒性。

In the Eastern Han Dynasty, *Classic of Materia Medica* (*Běn Jīng*) put forward the distinction of "toxic and non-toxic", and said "when you use poison to treat the disease, use the medicine as big as millet at the beginning, and stop medication if the symptoms vanish. If not, the dosage of the medicine should be doubled. If the disease has not been removed, it should be treated with ten times the amount of medicine, taking the complete removal of the disease as the limit". In the seven major treatises of *The Inner Classic* (*Nèi Jīng*), there are also treatises on big poison, regular poison and small poison. From the serial name of poison and herbs to the distinction of toxic and non-toxic, it reflects the progress of people's understanding of toxicity. After the Eastern Han Dynasty, all the works of Materia Medica marked the toxicity of toxic medicinals.

前人以偏性的强弱来解释有毒、无毒及毒性大小。有毒药物的治疗剂量与中毒剂量比较接近或相当，因而治疗用药时安全度小，易引起中毒反应。无毒药物安全度较大，但并非绝对不会引起毒性反应。人参、知母、柴胡等皆有中毒反应的报道，这与剂量过大或服用时间过长等有密切关系。

Previous scholars used the strength of bias to explain the toxic, nontoxic and toxic level. The therapeutic dose of toxic drugs is close to or equal to the medium toxic dose, which results in low medicinal safety and makes it easy to cause toxic reaction. The safety of nontoxic drugs is relatively high, but it does not mean it will never cause toxic reactions. *Rén shēn* (Ginseng Radix et Rhizoma), *zhī mǔ* (Anemarrhenae Rhizoma) and *chái hú* (Bupleuri Radix) have been reported to have toxic reactions, which are closely related to the excessive dosage or taking time.

毒性反应是临床用药时应当尽量避免的，本教材中的有毒药物，沿用历代本草的记载，分别标注为"有大毒""有毒""有小毒"。由于毒性反应的产生与药物贮存、加工炮制、配伍、剂型、给药途径、用量、使用时间以及患者的体质、年龄、证候性质等都有密切关系，使用有毒药物时，应从上述各个环节进行控制，避免中毒发生。

Toxic reactions should be avoided as far as possible in clinical medication. The toxic medicinals in this textbook, following the records of all previous generations of Chinese materia medica, are respectively marked as "extremely toxic" "toxic" and "slightly toxic". The toxic reactions are closely related to storage, processing, combination, dosage form, route of administration, dose, length of use, as well as the constitution, age and syndrome of patients. Therefore, every factors mentioned above should be controlled to avoid poisoning when toxic medicinals are used.

有毒药物偏性强，根据以偏纠偏、以毒攻毒的原则，在保证用药安全的前提下，使用某些有毒药物治疗某些疾病。如用雄黄治疗疔疮恶肿，水银治疗疥癣、梅毒，砒霜治疗白血病等，古今积累了大量经验，应当积极加以利用，让有毒中药更好地为临床服务。

Toxic medicinals have a strong preference, and can be used to treat some diseases one the premise of ensuring the medicinal safety according to the principle of rectifying deviation with deviation and attacking poison with poison. For example, *xióng huáng* (Realgar) is used to treat furuncles and swelling, *shuǐ yín* (Hydrargyrum) treats scabies and syphilis, *pī shuāng* (Arsenolite) treats leukemia. A great deal of experience has been accumulated in ancient and modern times, which should be actively used to better serve the clinical application of toxic medicinals.

古代文献中有关药物毒性的记载大多是正确的，但由于历史条件和个人经验与认识的局限性，其中也有一些错误之处。如《本经》认为丹砂无毒，且列为上品药之首；《本草纲目》认为马钱子无毒等。应当借鉴古代用药经验和现代药理毒理学及临床研究成果，全面客观地认识中药的毒性。

Most records about toxicity of Chinese medicinals in ancient literature are correct, but there are also some mistakes due to the limitations of historical conditions and personal experience and cognition. For example, *dān shā* (Cinnabaris) was considered nontoxic and was regarded as the best medicinal in *Classic of Materia Medica* (*Běn Jīng*); *mǎ qián zǐ* (Strychni Semen) in *The Grand Compendium of Materia Medica* (*Běn Cǎo Gāng Mù*) is also considered nontoxic. We should learn from the experience of ancient medication and modern pharmacology, toxicology and clinical research results, and comprehensively and objectively understand the toxicity of Chinese medicinals.

需要注意的是，古人对药物毒性的认识大多是从急性中毒反应的观察中总结出来的，对于亚急性毒性、亚慢性毒性、慢性毒性和特殊毒性（如致癌、致突变、致畸、成瘾），由于历史条件的限制，未能进行系统、深入的观察和总结。目前这方面的研究虽然已经取得了一些成效，但还需要做大量、深入的工作。

It should be noted that the ancients' understanding of toxicity was mostly summed up from the observation of acute toxic reaction. For sub-acute toxicity, sub-chronic toxicity, chronic toxicity and special toxicity such as carcinogenesis, mutagenesis, teratogenesis, addiction, etc., due to the limitations of historical conditions, they failed to carry out systematic and in-depth observation and summary. At present, although some achievements have been made in this field, a lot of work still remains to be done.

（张一昕）

第五章 中药的应用
Chapter 5 Application of Chinese medicinals

 学习目标｜ Learning goals

1. 掌握 中药"七情"的含义及对临床用药的指导意义；配伍禁忌、妊娠禁忌；确定中药剂量的依据。

2. 熟悉 中药配伍的目的；中药剂量与药效的关系；中药的煎法（先煎、后下、包煎、另煎、烊化等）及服法。

3. 了解 证候禁忌；饮食禁忌；中药剂量的含义。

1. Master the meaning of *qi qing* (seven compatibilities) of Chinese medicinals and its guiding significance for clinical medication, prohibited combination, contraindications during pregnancy, and the basis for determining the dosage of Chinese medicinals.

2. Familiar with the purpose of compatibility; the relationship between dosage and efficacy of Chinese medicinals; the decocting methods of Chinese medicine (including different requirements of decocting first, decocting later, wrap-boiling, decocting separately, melting) and methods of administration.

3. Understand the contraindications of syndrome medication, dietary incompatibility and the meaning of dosage of Chinese medicinal.

第一节 配伍
Section 1 Combination

PPT

配伍是指根据病情需要和药性特点，按照一定原则有选择地将两味或两味以上的药物配合应用。

Combination refers to the selective combination of two or more than two medicinals for clinical application, according to the needs of the disease and the characteristics of medicinal properties.

中药之所以要配伍应用，是因为单味中药在一定用量下，其作用强度有限，对病势沉重者常嫌药力不济；单味药虽有多种功效，但对于复杂多变的病情往往不能全面照顾；有的药物还具有毒性和副作用，单味应用不安全。如果根据病情和药物的需要，并按照一定的原则，将药物配合使用，可增强药力，全面照顾病情，减轻或消除药物的毒性和副作用，使临床用药更安全、更有效。

The reason that Chinese medicinals are combined in application is that under a certain dosage, a single medicinal has limited potency and is not powerful for severe cases; it may have multiple effects, but is often unable to cover the complicated and multivariate conditions; some medicinals have toxicity or side effects, and would not be safe if used alone. According to the requirements of the disease and medicinals, and in accordance with certain principles, the medicinals can be used together to enhance the medicinal power, take full care of the disease, reduce or eliminate the toxic and side effects, and make clinical medication safer and more effective.

前人把单味药的应用及药物之间的配伍关系概括为七种情况，称为药物的"七情"。七情的提法首见于《神农本草经》，其序例云："药……有单行者，有相须者，有相使者，有相恶者，有相畏者，有相杀者，有相反者。凡此七情，和合视之。"中药的七情，就是药物相互作用、相互影响的配伍关系，现将七情内容分述于下。

The application of single medicinal and the combination between medicinals was summarized into seven compatibilities, called *qi qing*, which first appeared in *Shen Nong's Classic of the Materia Medica (Shén Nóng Běn Cǎo Jīng)*. Its preface says "medicinals… have various relations, single application, mutual reinforcement, mutual assistance, mutual inhibition, mutual restraint, mutual suppression, and mutual antagonism. There are seven compatibilities in medication, which should be combined according to different conditions". *Qi qing* of Chinese medicinals is the combination of medicinal interaction and mutual influence. The content of *qi qing* is described below.

1. 单行 一般认为，单行就是单味药治病。病情单纯或病势较轻，单用一味针对性较强的药物即能获得疗效。如清金散单用一味黄芩治疗轻度肺热咯血，现代单用鹤草芽驱除绦虫等。此外，某些药物单味重用，乃取其功专力宏，以应急用。如《十药神书》中独参汤，即单用一味人参补气救脱。

(1) Single application It is generally believed that single application is using one medicinal alone. It is applied in treatment of simple syndrome or diseases for which one appropriate medicinal can have desired effect. For example, in *Qīng Jīn Sǎn* (Lung-Heat-Clearing Powder), *huáng qín* (Scutellariae Radix) is used alone to treat mild hemoptysis due to lung heat; in modern time *hè cǎo yá* (Agrimoniae Herba et Gemma) is used alone to expel tapeworm. In addition, some medicinals can be used alone in a heavy dose for their specific and powerful effect, so they should be used in response to urgent needs. For example, *Dú Shēn Tāng* (Pure Gingseng Decoction) in *Divine Book of Ten Medicinal Formulas (Shí Yào Shén Shū)*, *rén shēn* (Ginseng Radix et Rhizoma) is used to tonify qi and save from collapse.

《神农本草经》在提出中药七情时，虽未作具体说明，但推敲其"凡此七情，和合视之"等文字，单行应当是指各药单独取效，互不影响临床效应的两味药之间的配伍关系。实际上，在临床用药时这样的情况是广泛存在的。两味药可能同为病情所需，但此两药之间可能不具有增减疗效或毒性的特殊关系。这种认识应该更符合《神农本草经》中"单行"的原意。

In *Shen Nong's Classic of the Materia Medica (Shén Nóng Běn Cǎo Jīng)*, *qi qing* is not specifically explained, but "there are seven compatibilities in medication, which should be combined according to different conditions" and other words indicates that single application refers to the compatibility relationship between two medicinals that each medicinal takes effect independently and does not affect each other's clinical effect. In fact, such a situation is widespread in clinical medication. Both medicinals may be necessary for the disease, but there may be no special relationship between them in terms of increasing or decreasing efficacy or toxicity. This should be more in line with the original meaning of "single application" in *Shen Nong's Classic of the Materia Medica*.

2. **相须** 就是将性能功效类似的药物合用，以增强原有药物功效的配伍关系。如麻黄与桂枝配伍，能明显增强发汗解表、祛风散寒的治疗效果；大黄与芒硝配伍，能明显增强泻下通便的治疗效果；半夏与陈皮配伍，能明显增强燥湿化痰的治疗效果。

(2) Mutual reinforcement It is the combination of medicinals with similar property and efficacy which can significantly reinforce each other's therapeutic effects. For example, the combination of *má huáng* (Ephedrae Herba) and *guì zhī* (Ramulus Cinnamomi) can significantly reinforce the effect of promoting sweating, releasing exterior, expelling wind and dispersing cold; *dà huáng* (Rhei Radix et Rhizoma) combined with *máng xiāo* (Natrii Sulfas) can markedly enhance the effect of relieving constipation by purgation; *bàn xià* (Pinelliae Rhizoma) combined with *chén pí* (Citri Reticulatae Pericarpium) can markedly reinforce the effect of drying dampness and resolving phlegm.

3. **相使** 就是将性能功效有某些共性，或性能功效虽不相同但治疗目的一致的药物配合应用，且以一种药物为主，其他药物为辅，辅药可以提高主药疗效的配伍关系。如治疗气虚水肿，以黄芪补气利水为主药，辅以茯苓健脾利湿，两药合用，茯苓能增强黄芪补气利水的治疗效果；又如，治疗湿热泻痢，腹痛里急，以黄连清热燥湿、解毒止痢为主药，辅以木香行气止痛，两药合用，可增强黄连清热燥湿、行气止痛的治疗效果。

(3) Mutual assistance It is the combination of medicinals with commonness in property and efficacy, or those with different property and efficacy but the same treatment purpose, while one medicinal takes on the major role and others an assistant which can improves the effect of the major medicinal. For example, in the treatment of qi deficiency and edema, *huáng qí* (Astragali Radix) is used as the major medicinal, with *fú líng* (Poria) as the assistant which can invigorate spleen and promoting urination, while *fú líng* helps *huáng qí* to reinforce the medicinal efficacies of supplementing qi and promoting urination; in the treatment of diarrhea and dysentery due to damp heat and abdominal pain and urgency, *huáng lián* (Coptidis Rhizoma) is used as the major medicinal with *mù xiāng* (Aucklandiae Radix) as the assistant which can move qi and relieve pain, while *mù xiāng* helps *huáng lián* to reinforce its medicinal efficacies of clearing heat, drying dampness, resolving toxin and stopping dysentery.

4. **相畏** 就是一种药物的毒性或副作用，能被另一种药物减轻或消除的配伍关系。如生半夏和生南星的毒性能被生姜减轻或消除，所以说生半夏和生南星畏生姜。

(4) Mutual restraint It is the combination of medicinals in which the toxicity or side effects of one medicinal can be reduced or eliminated by the other. For example, the toxicity of *shēng bàn xià* (Pinelliae Rhizoma) and *shēng nán xīng* (Arisaematis Rhizoma) can be reduced or eliminated by *shēng jiāng* (Zingiberis Recens Rhizoma). In other words, *shēng bàn xià* and *shēng nán xīng* are restrained by *shēng jiāng*.

5. **相杀** 就是一种药物能够降低或消除另一种药物的毒性或副作用的配伍关系。如生姜可以减轻或消除生半夏、生南星的毒性。所以说生姜杀生半夏、生南星的毒。由此可见，相畏和相杀实际上是同一配伍关系的两种提法。

(5) Mutual suppression It is the combination of medicinals in which one medicinal may reduce or eliminate the toxicity or side effects of the other medicinal. For example, *shēng jiāng* may reduce or eliminate the toxicity or side effects of *shēng bàn xià* and *shēng nán xīng*. In other words, *shēng jiāng* suppresses the toxicity of *shēng bàn xià* and *shēng nán xīng*. It can be seen that mutual restraint and mutual suppression are actually two formulations of the same compatibility relationship.

6. **相恶** 就是两药合用，一种药物能使另一种药物的功效降低甚至丧失的配伍关系。如人参恶莱菔子，莱菔子能削弱人参的补气作用；生姜恶黄芩，黄芩能削弱生姜的温胃和温肺作用。

(6) Mutual inhibition It is the combination of two medicinals in which one may reduce or even eliminate the medicinal efficacies of the other. For example, *rén shēn* (Ginseng Radix et Rhizoma) is inhibited by *lái fú zǐ* (Raphani Semen), as the latter can reduce the former's effect of tonifying qi; *shēng jiāng* (Zingiberis Recens Rhizoma) is inhibited by *huáng qín* (Scutellariae Radix), as the latter can reduce the former's effect of warming stomach and lung.

7. 相反　就是两药合用，能产生或增强毒性或副作用的配伍关系。详见本章第二节"用药禁忌"。

(7) Mutual antagonism　It is the combination of two medicinals which may generate or reinforce their toxicity or side effects. For details, see "Medication contraindications" in this chapter.

上述中药配伍中，相须、相使配伍能提高疗效；相畏、相杀配伍可使有害效应削弱或消除，有利于临床安全用药，都是临床用药时应充分利用的配伍形式。相恶配伍会使疗效降低或丧失；相反配伍会增强或产生新的毒性和副作用，故相恶、相反配伍都是临床用药时应尽量避免的配伍形式。

In the above combinations of Chinese medicinals, mutual reinforcement and mutual assistance can improve the curative effect; mutual restraint and mutual suppression can weaken or eliminate the harmful effect, which is conducive to the safety of clinical medication. They are all the compatibility forms that should be fully used in clinical medication. Mutual inhibition will reduce or lose the therapeutic effect; mutual antagonism will enhance the side effects or produce new side effects, therefore, the two combinations should be avoided in clinical medication.

基于上述可知，从单味药到配伍应用，是通过很长的实践与认识过程逐渐积累和丰富起来的。药物的配伍应用是中医用药的主要形式，七情是中药应用的基本形式。药物按一定法度加以组合，并确定一定的分量比例，制成适当的剂型，即是方剂。方剂是药物配伍的发展，君臣佐使的配伍应用是中药配伍的高级形式。

Based on the above, it can be seen that either single medicinal or combination is gradually accumulated and enriched through a long process of practice and understanding. The combination is the main form of Chinese medicinals, and *qi qing* (seven kinds of compatibility) is the basic form of Chinese medicinal application. Medicinals are combined according to a certain rules and a certain proportion of components to make an appropriate dosage form, that is, formula. Formula is the development of medicinal combination, and the compatibility application of sovereign, minister, assistant and guiding medicinals is the advanced form of Chinese medicinal combination.

第二节　用药禁忌

Section 2　Medication contraindications

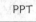

为了保证疗效和安全用药，必须注意用药禁忌。中药的用药禁忌主要包括配伍禁忌、证候禁忌、妊娠禁忌和饮食禁忌四个方面。

Much attention must be paid to the medication contraindications in order to ensure the efficacy and safety of medication. The medication contraindications of Chinese medicinals mainly include prohibited combinations, syndrome medication contraindication, contraindication during pregnancy and dietary

51

微课

incompatibility.

一、配伍禁忌
1. Prohibited combination

配伍禁忌是指某些药物合用会产生或增加毒性和副作用，或降低和破坏药效，应尽量避免，即《神农本草经》所谓："勿用相恶、相反者。"历代关于配伍禁忌的认识不完全一致，目前医药界公认的配伍禁忌，为金元时期《儒门事亲》概括的"十八反"和明代《医经小学》概括的"十九畏"。

Prohibited combination refers to that some medicinals may produce or increase toxicity or side effects, or reduce and destroy the efficacy and should be avoided to be combined with other medicinals, that is what *Shen Nong's Classic of the Materia Medica* (*Shén Nóng Běn Cǎo Jīng*) says that medicinals in mutual inhibition and mutual antagonism cannot be used. The understanding of medication contraindications in the past dynasties is not completely consistent. At present, the medication contraindications recognize by the pharmaceutical field is Eighteen Antagonisms summarized in *Confucians' Duties to Their Parents* (*Rú Mén Shì Qīn*) in the Jin and Yuan Dynasties and Nineteen Incompatibilities summarized in the *Primary Study of the Medical Classics* (*Yī Jīng Xiǎo Xué*) in the Ming Dynasty.

1. "十八反"　即乌头反贝母、瓜蒌、半夏、白及、白蔹；甘草反甘遂、大戟、海藻、芫花；藜芦反人参、丹参、玄参、沙参、苦参、细辛、芍药。

(1) Eighteen Antagonisms　*wū tóu* (Aconiti Radix) with *bèi mǔ* (Fritillaria Bulbus), *guā lóu* (Trichosanthis Fructus), *bàn xià* (Pinelliae Rhizoma), *bái jí* (Bletillae Rhizoma) and *bái liǎn* (Ampelopsis Radix); *gān cǎo* (Glycyrrhizae Radix et Rhizoma) with *gān suí* (Kansui Radix), *dà jǐ* (Cirsii Japonici Herba), *hǎi zǎo* (Sargassum) and *yuán huā* (Genkwa Flos); *lí lú* (Veratri Nigri Radix et Rhizoma) with *rén shēn* (Ginseng Radix et Rhizoma), *dān shēn* (Salviae Miltiorrhizae Radix et Rhizoma), *xuán shēn* (Scrophulariae Radix), *shā shēn* (Adenophorae seu Glehniae Radix), *ku shen* (Sophora flavescens), *xì xīn* (Asari Radix et Rhizoma) and *sháo yào* (Paeoniae Radix).

2. "十九畏"　即硫黄畏朴硝，狼毒畏密陀僧，巴豆畏牵牛，丁香畏郁金，川乌、草乌畏犀角，牙硝畏三棱，官桂畏赤石脂，人参畏五灵脂。

(2) Nineteen Incompatibilities　*liú huáng* (Sulphur) with *pò xiāo* (Mirabilitum), *láng dú* (Euphorbiae Fischerianae Radix) with *mì tuó sēng* (Lithargyrum), *bā dòu* (Crotonis Fructus) with *qiān niú* (Pharbitidis Semen), *dīng xiāng* (Caryophylli Flos) with *yù jīn* (Curcumae Radix), *chuān wū* (Aconiti Radix) and *cǎo wū* (Aconiti Kusnezoffii Radix) with *xī jiǎo* (Rhinocerotis Cornu), *yá xiāo* (Natrii Sulfas) with *sān léng* (Sparganii Rhizoma), *guān guì* (Cinnamomi Cortex) with *chì shí zhī* (Halloysitum Rubrum), *rén shēn* (Ginseng Radix et Rhizoma) with *wǔ líng zhī* (Trogopterori Faeces).

十八反、十九畏作为中药配伍禁忌，有其历史渊源，在《中国药典》中也有体现，因此应将十八反、十九畏作为用药禁忌来遵循。但是，应该看到，古今文献中，也有应用十八反、十九畏配伍用药的记载。因此，对十八反、十九畏的配伍应采取审慎的态度，若无充分根据和用药经验，一般不宜使用，以免发生意外。

Eighteen Antagonisms and Nineteen Incompatibilities, as the incompatibility of Chinese medicinals, have their historical origins and are also reflected in *Chinese Pharmacopoeia*. Therefore, Eighteen Antagonisms and Nineteen Incompatibilities should be followed as prohibited combinations. However,

医药大学堂
WWW.YIYAODXT.COM

it should be noted that in ancient and modern literature, there are also records of the application of the medicinals of Eighteen Antagonisms and Nineteen Incompatibilities. Therefore, medicinal combination of Eighteen Antagonisms and Nineteen Incompatibilities should used with a prudent attitude, and should not be utilized without full evidence and practical experience to avoid accidents.

二、证候禁忌
2. Syndrome medication contraindication

证候禁忌是指某种或某类病证不宜使用某种或某类药物。由于药物皆有偏性，或寒或热，或补或泻……用之得当，可以以其偏性纠正疾病的病理偏向；使用不当，其偏性又会反助病势，加重病情或造成新的病理偏向。因此，凡药不对证，药物功效不为病情所需，有可能导致病情加重，原则上都属于证候禁忌范围。如表虚自汗、阴虚盗汗者，忌用具有发汗作用的药物，以免加重出汗；里寒证忌用具有清热作用的药物，以免寒凉伤阳；里热证忌用具有温里作用的药物，以免助火伤阴；脾胃虚寒便溏者，忌用具有泻下作用的药物，以免损伤脾胃，加重病情；阴虚津伤者，忌用具有燥湿、化湿作用的药物，以免耗伤津液；妇女月经过多及出血无瘀滞者，忌用破血逐瘀药，以免加重出血；邪实而正不虚者，忌用补虚药，以免误补益疾；痰湿内阻者，忌用补血滋阴之品，以免滋腻助湿；表邪未解者，忌用收敛止汗药；湿热泻痢者，忌用收涩止泻药等。证候禁忌是用药禁忌中涉及最广的内容，几乎见于各类和各种药物。详见各论中每味药物的"使用注意"部分。

Syndrome medication contraindication refers to a certain disease or a certain type of syndromes should avoid application of some kinds of medicinals. Each medicinal has its bias: cold or hot, tonifying or purging. If used properly, the bias can be used to correct the deviation of pathological changes of a disease; if not, its bias will aggravate the disease or cause new pathological bias. Therefore, if the medicinal does not fit for the syndrome and the efficacy is not required by the disease, it may lead to aggravation of the disease, which in principle belongs to the scope of syndrome medication contraindications. For example, those who suffer from the spontaneous sweating due to interior deficiency and night sweating due to yin deficiency should not use medicinals with perspiration effect to avoid aggravating perspiration. Interior cold syndrome should avoid heat-clearing medicinals for fear of impairing yang. Interior hear syndrome should not use interior-warming medicinals for fear of assisting fire to impair yin. Those with loose stool due to deficiency of spleen and stomach should not use purgative medicinals to avoid damage to spleen and stomach and aggravation of the disease. Those with yin deficiency and fluid injury should not use dampness-drying and dampness-resolving medicinals to avoid body fluid consumption. Women with excessive menstruation and bleeding without stasis should not use medicinals for breaking and expelling blood stasis to avoid aggravating bleeding. Those with excess of pathogenic qi and sufficiency of healthy qi should not use tonifying medicinals to avoid aggravating the disease by mistakenly tonifying. Those with internal obstruction of phlegm-dampness should not use blood-tonifying and yin-nourishing medicinals to avoid nourishing sliminess and aggravating dampness. Those with exterior pathogens unresolved should not use astringent antiperspirant; those with diarrhea due to damp-heat should not use astringent antiperspirant, etc. Syndrome contraindication is the most extensive content in medication contraindications, almost all kinds of medicinals involved. For details, refer to "Precautions section" of each medicinal in specific discussions.

三、妊娠禁忌
3. Contraindication during pregnancy

妊娠禁忌是指妇女妊娠期间，除为了中断妊娠外，慎用或禁用某些药物。一般而言，凡能引起堕胎或损害胎元的药物，均应作为妊娠禁忌的药物。根据药物对于胎元损害程度的不同，一般可分为慎用与禁用两类。慎用的药物包括通经祛瘀、行气破滞及辛热滑利之品，如桃仁、红花、牛膝、大黄、枳实、附子、肉桂、干姜、木通、冬葵子、瞿麦等；禁用的药物包括毒性较强或药性猛烈的药物，如巴豆、牵牛、大戟、商陆、麝香、三棱、莪术、水蛭、斑蝥、雄黄、砒霜等。凡禁用的药物绝对不能使用，慎用的药物可以根据病情的需要斟酌使用。

Contraindication during pregnancy refers to the medicinals forbidden during pregnancy, except for interruption of pregnancy or induction of labor. Generally speaking, any medicinals that can cause abortion or damage the original qi of fetus should be regarded as the contraindication during pregnancy. According to the damage degree to original qi of fetus, the contraindicated medicinals can be divided into two categories: cautious use and forbidden use. The medicinals used with caution include those for dredging channels and dispelling stasis, moving qi and removing stagnation, and lubricant ones with pungent and heat, such as *táo rén* (Persicae Semen), *hóng huā* (Carthami Flos), *niú xī* (Achyranthis Bidentatae Radix), *dà huáng* (Rhei Radix et Rhizoma), *zhǐ shí* (Aurantii Immaturus Fructus), *fù zǐ* (Aconiti Lateralis Radix Praeparata), *ròu guì* (Cinnamomi Cortex), *gān jiāng* (Zingiberis Rhizoma), *mù tōng* (Akebiae Caulis), *dōng kuí zǐ* (Malvae Fructus) and *qú mài* (Dianthi Herba); while the forbidden medicinals refer to those with strong toxicity or strong properties, such as *bā dòu* (Crotonis Fructus), *qiān niú* (Pharbitidis Semen), *dà jǐ* (Euphorbiae Pekinensis Radix), *shāng lù* (Phytolaccae Radix), *shè xiāng* (Moschus), *sān léng* (Sparganii Rhizoma), *é zhú* (Curcumae Rhizoma), *shuǐ zhì* (Hirudo), *bān máo* (Mylabris), *xióng huáng* (Realgar) and *pī shuāng* (Arsenolite). Any banned medicinals must not be used, while medicinals used with caution can be used according to the needs of the disease.

四、饮食禁忌
4. Dietary incompatibility

饮食禁忌是指服药期间禁忌进食某些食物，又称服药食忌，简称食忌，也就是俗称的"忌口"。一般在服药期间，应忌食生冷、油腻、腥膻、辛辣、不易消化以及有刺激性的食物，以免妨碍脾胃功能，影响药物吸收，使疗效降低。某些对治疗不利的食物也应忌口，如热性病，应忌食辛辣、油腻、煎炸食物；寒性病，应忌食生冷食物、清凉饮料等。还应避免食用某些与所服药物可能发生不良反应的食物。如服用使君子、土茯苓忌饮茶，服用薄荷忌食鳖肉，服用绵马贯众忌油，以及蜜反生葱、柿反蟹等。

Dietary incompatibility refers to the foods that are forbidden in the course of taking certain medicinals. Generally, uncooked and cold, greasy, fishy, spicy and hot, indigestible and irritant food are avoided so as not to hinder the function of spleen and stomach, affect the absorption and reduce the efficacy of medicinals.Some foods that are unfavorable for treatment should also be avoided. For example, spicy and hot, greasy, or fried food is forbidden in heat diseases, and cold diseases should avoid uncooked and cold food, cool beverages. It is also necessary to avoid certain foods that may have adverse reactions to the drugs taken. For example, *shǐ jūn zǐ* (Quisqualis Fructus) and *fú líng* (Poria)

should not taken with tea, *bò he* (Menthae Herba) with turtle meat, *mián mǎ guàn zhòng* (Dryopteridis Crassirhizomatis Rhizoma) with oil, honey with onions, and persimmon with crabs.

第三节　剂量
Section 3　Dosage

剂量，即药物的用量。本教材中每味药物标明的用量，除特别注明以外，都是指干燥后饮片，入汤剂内服的成人一日用量，入丸、散剂内服的一次用量。

Dosage is medication amount. Unless otherwise specified, the dosage of each medicinal in this textbook refers to the daily amount for adults taking in decoction after drying, or the dosage for once in pill or powder.

中药计量单位，古今有别。传统计量有重量（斤、两、钱、分、厘）、度量（寸、尺等）、容量（勺、合、升、斗等）、数量（片、条、枚、支、角、只）等多种方法。明清以来，我国普遍采用 16 进位制，即 1 市斤 = 16 两 = 160 钱。自 1979 年起我国对中药生药计量统一采用公制，即 1 公斤 = 1000g。为了处方和调剂计算方便，特别是古方剂量的换算，通常按规定以如下的近似值进行换算：1 市两（16 进位制）= 30 克；1 钱 = 3 克；1 分 = 0.3 克；1 厘 = 0.03 克。

The measurement unit of Chinese medicinal varies from ancient to modern times. Traditional measurement methods include weight (*jin, liang, qian, fen, li*), length (*chi, cun,* etc.), capacity (*shao, he, sheng, dou,* etc.), quantity (*pian, tiao, mei, zhi, jiao, zhi*). Since the Ming and Qing Dynasties, China has generally adopted the hexadecimal system, i.e., 1 kg=16 *liang*=160 *qian*. Since 1979, the metric system has been adopted for the measurement of crude Chinese medicine, i.e., 1kg=1000g. In order to facilitate the calculation of prescription and dispensing, especially the conversion of ancient prescription dose, the following approximate values are usually used for conversion according to the regulations: 1 *liang* (hex)=30g; 1 *qian*=3g; 1 *fen*=0.3g; 1 *li*=0.03g.

尽管大多数中药的安全剂量幅度较大，用量不如化学药品严格，但用量得当与否，也是直接影响药效发挥和临床效果的重要因素之一。药量过小，起不到治疗作用可贻误病情；药量过大，戕伤正气，也可引起不良后果，或造成不必要的浪费。同时，中药多为复方应用，其中主要药物的剂量变化，可以影响整个处方的功效，改变主治病证。因此，对于中药的使用剂量应采取科学、谨慎的态度。一般来说，确定中药的剂量，应考虑如下几方面因素。

Although most of the safe dosage of Chinese medicinals is large and not as strict as that of chemical drugs, whether the dosage is appropriate or not is also one of the important factors that directly affect the efficacy and clinical effect. Too small dosage will not play a therapeutic role and delay illness; too large dosage will hurt the healthy qi and may cause adverse consequences, or cause unnecessary waste. At the same time, Chinese medicine is mostly compound application. Among them, the dosage change of the major medicinals can affect the efficacy of the whole prescription and the main symptoms. Therefore, a scientific and cautious attitude should be paid to the Chinese medicinal dosage. Generally speaking, to determine the dosage of Chinese medicinals, the following factors should be considered.

一、药物因素
1. Factors of medicinals

应考虑药物毒性有无、作用强弱、气味浓淡、质地轻重和药品干鲜等因素与剂量的关系。一般而言，剧毒药或作用峻烈的药物，应严格控制剂量，开始时用量宜轻，逐渐加量，一旦病情好转，应立即减量或停服，防止过量或蓄积中毒。花、叶、皮枝等质轻及气味浓厚、作用较强的药物用量宜小，矿物、介壳类质重及气味淡薄、作用温和的药物用量宜大。鲜品药材含水分较多，用量宜大（一般为干品的4倍）。贵重药材如羚羊角、麝香、牛黄、鹿茸等，在保证药效的前提下应尽量减少用量。

In the aspect of medicinals, it is necessary to consider whether the toxicity, the effect, the smell, the texture and the dry or fresh are related to the dosage. Generally speaking, the dosage of highly toxic medicinal or those with severe effects should be strictly controlled. The dosage should be light at first and gradually increased. Once the condition improves, the dosage should be reduced or stopped immediately to prevent excessive or accumulated poisoning. Medicinals from flowers, leaves, bark or branches with light quality, strong flavors and strong actions are administered in a small dosage, while those from metals, stones or shells with heavy quality, slight flavors and mild actions are in a large dosage. The fresh medicinal materials should used in a large dosage since they contain more water (generally 4 times of the dry ones). Precious medicinals such as *líng yáng jiǎo* (Saigae Tataricae Cornu), *shè xiāng* (Moschus), *niú huáng* (Calculus Bovis) and *lù róng* (Cervi Cornu Pantotrichum) should be used as little as possible under the premise of ensuring the efficacy.

二、患者因素
2. Factors of patients

应考虑患者的年龄、体质、病情轻重与缓急、病程长短与剂量的关系。一般而言，成人及平素体质壮实的患者用量宜重；老年人、小儿、产后妇女及体质虚弱的患者，用量宜轻。一般5岁以下的小儿用成人药量的1/4；5岁以上的儿童按成人用量减半服用。病情轻、病势缓、病程长者用量宜小；病情重、病势急、病程短者用量宜大。

In the aspect of patients, it is necessary to consider the relationship between age, constitution, severity of illness, medical history, duration of disease and dosage. Generally speaking, the dosage for adults and normal healthy patients should be heavy; for the elderly, children, women, postpartum and weak patients, the dosage should be light. Generally, children under 5 years old use 1/4 of that for adults; children over 5 years old take half of the adult dosage. The dosage should be small for the patients with mild illness, slow illness and long course, and large for the patients with severe illness, acute illness and short course.

三、应用因素
3. Factors of application

应考虑剂型、配伍、用法、用药目的与剂量的关系。一般而言，单味药使用比复方中应用剂量要大；在复方配伍使用时，主药比辅药用量要大。同一药物在不同剂型中，其用量亦不尽同，一般入汤剂比入丸、散剂的用量要大。临床用药目的不同，其用量也不同。如槟榔，用于消积、行气、利水，常用量为6~15g；而用以驱绦虫时，则需用到60~120g。又如牵牛子，"少则动大便，多则下水"，同是泻下，用以通便导滞，用量宜轻；用以峻下逐水，则用量宜重。

In the aspect of application, the relationship between dosage form, compatibility, usage, purpose and dosage should be considered. Generally speaking, the dosage of single medicinal is higher than that of compound medicine, and the dosage of major medicinal is higher than that of auxiliary medicine in combination. In different forms, the dosage of the same medicianl is also different. Generally, the dosage of the decoction is larger than that of the pill or powder. The dosage varies with the purpose of clinical medication. For example, *bīng láng* (Arecae Semen) is usually 6-15g when used for resolving accumulation, moving qi and promoting urination, while 60-120g when used for expelling tapeworms; *qiān niú zǐ* (Pharbitidis Semen) "less will relax bowels if used less, or will expel water if used more". As a purgative, the dosage of *qiān niú zǐ* should be light if it is to relieve constipation and remove food stagnation, and the dosage should be heavy if it is to expel water by drastic purgation.

在确定药物剂量时，除应注意上述因素外，还应考虑季节、气候及居住环境等方面的因素，做到"因时制宜""因地制宜"。

When determining the dosage of medicinals, season, climate and living natural environment, in addition to the above-mentioned factors, should also be taken into account, so as to "adapt to the times" and "adapt to local conditions".

除了剧毒药、峻烈药、精制药及某些贵重药外，一般中药常用内服剂量为5~10g；部分药物常用量较大，为15~30g；新鲜药物常用量为30~60g。

Except highly toxic, drastic, refined and valuable medicinals, the commonly used Chinese medicinal for oral administration is about 5-10g; some are usually in large quantities, with a dosage of 15-30g; and fresh ones are commonly in 30-60g.

第四节　用法
Section 4　Administration

PPT

本教材所述中药的用法，主要是汤剂的煎煮方法及服用方法。

The administration of Chinese medicinals described in this textbook is mainly the decoction methods and taking methods.

一、汤剂煎煮法
1. Decocting methods

汤剂是临床应用中药最常用的剂型，煎药方法得当与否与疗效有密切的关系。汤剂的制作对煎具、用水、火候、煮法都有一定的要求。

Decoction is the most commonly used dosage form in clinical application of Chinese medicine.

Whether the decoction method is appropriate or not is closely related to the curative effect. The preparation of decoction has certain requirements for utensils, water, duration and degree, and boiling methods.

1. 煎药用具　以砂锅、瓦罐为好，不锈钢锅、搪瓷器皿次之。忌用铁、铜、铝锅，以免发生化学反应，影响疗效，甚至产生毒性和副作用。

(1) Decoction utensils　The best decocting utensils are casseroles and pots, followed by stainless steel pots and enamel pots. Do not use iron, copper, aluminum pot to avoid chemical reaction degrading the efficacy or even producing toxic and side effects.

2. 煎药用水　古时用长流水、井水、雨水、泉水、米泔水等煎煮。现多用自来水、井水、蒸馏水等，但总以水质洁净、新鲜为好。

(2) Water for decoction　In ancient times, it was decocted with long running water, well water, rainwater, spring water, rice swill, etc. At present, tap water, well water and distilled water are mostly used, but the water is required clean and fresh.

3. 加水量　按理论推算，加水量应为饮片吸水量、煎煮过程中蒸发水量及煎煮后所需药液量的总和，但实际操作时很难做到十分准确。通常根据饮片质地的疏密、吸水性能的强弱及煎煮所需时间的长短来估计加水量。第一煎用水量一般以将饮片适当加压后，液面高出药面 2~3cm 为宜，第二煎加水量为第一煎的 1/3~1/2。

(3) Capacity of water added　According to the theoretical calculation, the amount of water added should be the sum of the water absorption of the decoction pieces, the evaporation during the decocting and the amount of liquid needed after decocting, but it is difficult to add water accurately in the actual operation. Generally, the amount of water can only be estimated according to the density of texture, the strength of water absorption and the required time. The water consumption of the first decoction is 2-3cm higher than that of the medicine after the pieces are properly pressurized. The amount of water added in the second decoction was 1/3~1/2 of that in the first.

4. 煎前浸泡　煎煮前将中药饮片浸泡一定的时间，既有利于药物有效成分的溶出，又可缩短煎煮时间。一般用冷水浸泡 20~30 分钟即可。若以种子或果实为主者可浸泡 1 小时。夏天气温高，浸泡时间不宜过长，以免药液变质。

(4) Soaking before decoction　Soaking medicinal pieces before decocting for a certain time is not only beneficial to the dissolution of effective ingredients, but also can shorten the decocting time. Generally, it is better to soak in cold water for 20-30 minutes. For medicinals from seeds or fruits, 1 hour or so is advised. In summer, the temperature is high, and the soaking time should not be too long to avoid the deterioration of the liquid medicine.

5. 煎药火候　有文、武火之分。文火，即小火，是指使温度上升及水液蒸发缓慢的火候；武火，又称急火，是指使温度上升及水液蒸发迅速的火候。

(5) Duration and degree of decoction　There are mild fire and strong fire. Mild fire, that is, small fire, refers to the fire that causes the temperature to rise and the water to evaporate slowly; while strong fire, also known as rapid fire, refers to the fire that causes the temperature to rise and the water to evaporate rapidly.

6. 煎煮方法　一般药物煎煮时宜先用武火尽快使药液煮沸，后用文火继续煎煮，使药液保持沸腾状态，以免药汁溢出或过快熬干。解表药及其他含挥发性有效成分的药物，宜用武火煮沸，改用文火维持 10~15 分钟即可。有效成分不易煎出的矿物类、骨角类、贝壳类、甲壳类及滋补药物，宜文火久煎，使有效成分充分溶出。一般中药煎煮 2 次，两次煎液去渣滤净混合后，分 2~3

次服用。

(6) Decocting method　General medicinals can be decocted with strong fire at first to boil the liquid as soon as possible, and then continue to decocting with mild fire to keep the liquid boiling, so as to prevent the liquid medicine from overflowing or drying too fast. It is advisable to boil the exterior-releasing medicinals and those with volatile active ingredients with strong fire and maintain them for 10-15 minutes with mild fire. Medicinal from minerals, bone angles, shells, crustaceans and tonics whose effective ingredients are not easy to be decocted are generally decocted with mild fire for a long time to fully dissolve the effective ingredients. Common Chinese medicinals are decocted twice, and the decocted liquid is mixed with dregs removed and then taken 2-3 times.

某些药物因其质地不同，尚需特殊的煎煮方法，处方上需加以注明，归纳起来主要有以下几种。

Some of medicinals need to be decocted in a special way due to the different textures, which should be noted on the prescription. They can be summarized as follows.

（1）先煎　一些有效成分难溶于水的金石、矿物、介壳类药物，应打碎先煎，煮沸 20~30 分钟后，再下其他药物同煎，以使有效成分充分析出，如磁石、赭石、生石膏、龙骨、牡蛎、石决明、龟板、鳖甲等。附子、乌头等毒性较强的药物，宜先煎 45~60 分钟后再下他药，久煎可以降低毒性。

1) Decocting first　Some medicinals from stones, mineral and shells that are hard to dissolve in water should be smashed first and boiled for 20-30 minutes, and then fried with other medicinals, so as to fully separate the effective ingredients, such as *cí shí* (Magnetitum), *zhě shí* (Haematitum), *shēng shí gāo* (Gypsum Fibrosum), *lóng gǔ* (Draconis Os), *mǔ lì* (Ostreae Concha), *shí jué míng* (Haliotidis Concha), *guī bǎn* (Testudinis Plastrum) and *biē jiǎ* (Trionycis Carapax). In addition, *fù zǐ* (Aconiti Lateralis Radix Praeparata), *wú tóu* (Aconiti Radix) and other highly toxic medicinals should be decocted for 45-60 minutes before adding other drugs. Long decocting can reduce the toxicity.

（2）后下　一些气味芳香的药物，久煎其有效成分易于挥发而降低药效，须在其他药物煎好前 5~10 分钟放入同煎，如薄荷、木香、砂仁、豆蔻等。有些药物虽不属芳香药，但久煎也能破坏其有效成分，如钩藤、大黄、番泻叶等亦属后下之列。

2) Decocting later　Some aromatic medicinals should be added later for the effective ingredients tend to volatilize and the efficacy may be reduced if decocted for a long time. It should be put in 5-10 minutes before the decoction are almost done, such as *bò he* (Menthae Herba), *mù xiāng* (Aucklandiae Radix), *shā rén* (Amomi Fructus) and *dòu kòu* (Amomi Rotundus Fructus). Besides, some medicinals are not aromatic, long-term decocting can also damage the effective ingredients, such as *gōu téng* (Uncariae Cum Uncis Ramulus), *dà huáng* (Rhei Radix et Rhizoma), and *fān xiè yè* (Sennae Folium).

（3）包煎　一些黏性强、粉末状及带有绒毛的药物，宜先用纱布袋装好，再与其他药物同煎，以防止药液混浊或刺激咽喉引起咳嗽，以及沉于锅底，加热时引起焦化或糊化，如蛤粉、滑石、旋覆花、车前子、蒲黄等。

3) Wrap-boiling　Some medicinals with strong viscosity, powder and floss should be wrapped in gauze first, and then decocted together with other medicinals to prevent the medicinal liquid from being turbid, stimulating the throat to cause cough, sinking at the bottom, or causing coking or burning when heated, such as clam powder, *huá shí* (Talcum), *xuán fù huā* (Inulae Flos), *chē qián zǐ* (Plantaginis Semen) and *pú huáng* (Typhae Pollen).

（4）另煎　又称另炖，某些贵重药材为了更好地煎出有效成分，应单独煎煮 2~3 小时。煎液可以另服，也可与其他煎液混合服用，如人参、西洋参等。

4) Decocting separately   It is also known as stewed separately. Some valuable medicinal materials should be decocted or stewed separately for 2-3 hours in order to better decoct the effective ingredients. The decoction can be taken separately or mixed with other decoction, such as *rén shēn* (Ginseng Radix et Rhizoma), and *xī yáng shēn* (Panacis Quinquefolii Radix).

（5）溶化   又称烊化，某些胶类药物及黏性大而易溶的药物，为避免入煎粘锅或黏附其他药物影响煎煮，可单用水或黄酒将此类药加热溶化后，用煎好的药液冲服；也可将此类药放入其他药物煎好的药液中加热烊化后服用，如阿胶、鹿角胶、龟板胶、鳖甲胶及饴糖等。

5) Dissolving   Also known as melting. Some glue-like medicinals or those with high viscosity and solubility should be melted first by water or rice wine in order to avoid sticking to the pot or dregs, and then taken orally with other decoction or put into other decoction and taken orally after heating and melting, such as *ē jiāo* (Corii Asini Colla), *lù jiāo jiāo* (Cervi Cornus Colla), *guī bǎn jiāo* (Testudinis Plastri Colla), *biē jiǎ jiāo* (Trionycis Carapacis Colla) and *yí táng* (Saccharum Granorum).

（6）泡服   又称焗服，某些有效成分易溶于水或久煎容易破坏药效的药物，可以用少量开水或复方中其他药物滚烫的煎出液趁热浸泡，加盖闷润，减少挥发，半小时后去渣即可服用，如藏红花、番泻叶、胖大海等。

6) Soaking   Effective ingredients of some medicinals are easy to dissolve in water or long-term decoction and tend to damage the efficacy of the medicinal. It is advisable to soak such medicinals in a small amount of boiling water or other boiling decoction of the compound, seal and moisten it to reducing volatilization, and take it after half an hour with dregs removed, such as *zàng hóng huā* (Croci Stigma), *fān xiè yè* (Sennae Folium) and *pàng dà hǎi* (Sterculiae Lychnophorae Semen).

（7）冲服   某些贵重药，用量较轻，为防止散失，常需要研成细末制成散剂，用温开水或复方中其他药物煎液冲服，如珍珠、鹿茸、蛤蚧等。某些药物，根据病情需要，为提高药效，也常研成散剂冲服，如用于止血的三七、白及；用于息风止痉的蜈蚣、全蝎；用于制酸止痛的乌贼骨、海蛤壳等。某些药物高温容易破坏药效或有效成分难溶于水，也只能制成散剂冲服，如雷丸、鹤草芽、琥珀等。此外，还有一些液体药物如竹沥汁、姜汁、藕汁等也须冲服。

7) Taking infused   Some valuable medicinals in light dosage are ground into fine powder and infused with a decoction or with boiled water for oral administration, such as *zhēn zhū* (Margarita), *lù róng* (Cervi Cornu Pantotrichum), and *gé jiè* (Gecko). Some medicinals, according to the needs of the disease and in order to improve the efficacy, are often ground into powder, such as *sān qī* (Notoginseng Radix et Rhizoma) and *bái jí* (Bletillae Rhizoma) for stopping bleeding, *wú gōng* (Scolopendra) and *quán xiē* (Scorpio) for extinguishing wind and stopping convulsions, *wū zéi gǔ* (Sepiae Endoconcha) and *hǎi gé qiào* (Meretricis Concha seu Cyclinae) for inhibit acid to stop pain. Some medicinals are easily damaged by high temperature or the effective ingredients are difficult to dissolve in water, they can only be prepared into powder, such *léi wán* (Omphalia), *hè cǎo yá* (Agrimoniae Herba et Gemma) and *hǔ pò* (Succinum). In addition, some liquid medicine should be infused in water, such as *zhú lì zhī* (Bambusae Succus), *jiāng zhī* (Rhizomatis Zingiberis Succus) and *ǒu zhī* (Nelumbinis Rhizomatis Succus).

（8）煎汤代水   某些药物与其他药物同煎易使煎液混浊，难于服用，宜先煎后取其上清液代水再煎煮其他药物，如灶心土等。此外，某些药物质轻、用量大、体积大、吸水量大，如玉米须、丝瓜络、金钱草等，也须煎汤代水用。

8) Decoction for water   Some medicinals, in order to prevent the decoction from being turbid and difficult to take, should be decocted first and then the top clear liquid is taken to decoct other medicinals

in stead of water, such as *zào xīn tǔ* (Flava Usta Terra). Some medicinals are light in quantity, large in volume and large in water absorption is also necessary to be decocted instead of water, such as *yù mǐ xū* (Maydis Stigma), *sī guā luò* (Luffae Fructus Retinervus) and *jīn qián cǎo* (Lysimachiae Herba).

二、服药法
2. Administration methods

1. **服药次数**　汤剂一般每日 1 剂，煎 2 次，分 2~3 次服。病情急重者，可每隔 4 小时左右服用 1 次，昼夜不停，使药力顿挫病势。病情缓轻者，亦可间日服或煎汤代茶饮。

(1) Times　The decoction is usually taken 1 dose per day, 2 times decocting, for 2-3 times taking separately. For the severe or acute diseases, the medicinal should be taken once every 4 hours or so, day and night, so as to stop the development of the disease as early as possible, while for mild conditions, usually once every other day or decoction as tea.

2. **服药时间**　应根据胃肠状况、病情需要及药物特性来确定。如攻下药及治疗胃肠道疾病的药物宜饭前服，消食药及对胃肠有刺激的药物宜饭后服。无论饭前服还是饭后服，服药与进食都应间隔 1 小时左右，以免影响药效的发挥与食物的消化。此外，为了使药物能充分发挥作用，有些药还应在特定的时间服用。如安神药宜在睡前 0.5~1 小时服，截疟药宜在疟疾发作前 4 小时服；驱虫药、峻下逐水药宜在清晨空腹时服；慢性病定时服；急性病则不拘时服。

(2) Time　The specific administration time should be determined according to the gastrointestinal conditions, the needs of the disease and the characteristics of the medicinal. For example, offensive purgative and medicinals for gastrointestinal diseases should be taken before meals, while digestive medicinals and those stimulating stomach and intestines should be taken after meals. Whether taken before or after meals, the interval between administration and meal should be about 1 hour, so as not to affect the efficacy and digestion of food. In addition, some medicinals should be taken at a specific time to bring the medicinal into full play. For example, the tranquilizer should be taken 0.5-1 hour before going to bed; the antimalarial should be taken 4 hours before the onset of malaria; the vermifugal medicinals and drastic hydragogue should be taken in the morning with an empty stomach; medicinals should be taken regularly for chronic diseases and the acute diseases at any time.

3. **服药温度**　宜温服。但解表药要趁热服，服后还须温覆盖好衣被，或进热粥，以助汗出；寒证用热药宜热服，热证用寒药宜冷服，以防格拒于外。如出现真热假寒当寒药温服，真寒假热者则当热药冷服。

(3) Temperature　Decoction are usually taken when they are warm, but the exterior-releasing medicinals should be taken hot and the patient should cover up after taking the medicine or eat hot porridge to promoting sweating. The medicinals for cold syndrome should be taken hot, and the medicine for heat syndrome should be taken cold to prevent expelling. In case of true heat with false cold, the medicinals of cold nature are taken warm, while for true cold with false heat, the medicinals of warm nature should be taken cold.

此外，危重患者宜少量频服；呕吐患者可以浓煎药汁，少量频服；对于神志不清或因其他原因不能口服时，可采用鼻饲给药法。在应用发汗、泻下、清热药时，若药力较强，要注意患者个体差异，一般得汗、泻下、热降即可停药，适可而止，不必尽剂，以免汗、下、清热太过，损伤人体正气。

In addition, patients with critical conditions should take a small amount of medication frequently;

vomiting patients can take thick decoction, a small amount of medication frequently; patients who can't take orally because of delirium or other reasons can use the nasal feeding method. In the application of sweating, purgative and antipyretic medicinals, if the drug power is strong, the individual differences of patients should be noted. Generally, the drug can be stopped without using up the medicinals after sweating, purging and fever reduced in order to avoid excessive sweating, purgative and heat-clearing which may damage the healthy qi of human body.

（张一昕）

各 论
Special discussion

第六章 解 表 药
Chapter 6　Exterior-releasing medicinals

 学习目标｜Learning goals

1. **掌握** 解表药在功效、主治、性能、配伍及使用注意方面的共性；麻黄、桂枝、紫苏叶、荆芥、防风、羌活、薄荷、桑叶、菊花、牛蒡子、蝉蜕、柴胡、葛根的性能、功效、应用以及特殊的用法用量和特殊的使用注意。

2. **熟悉** 解表药的分类；香薷、生姜、白芷、细辛、苍耳子、蔓荆子的功效、主治以及特殊的用法用量和特殊的使用注意。

3. **了解** 解表药、发散风寒药、发散风热药及相关解表功效术语的含义；藁本、辛夷、淡豆豉的功效以及特殊的用法用量和特殊的使用注意。

1. Master the commonness of exterior-releasing medicinals in efficacy, indications, property, compatibility and cautions; the property, efficacy, application, special usage and dosage and special precautions of *má huáng, guì zhī, zǐ sū yè, jīng jiè, fáng fēng, qiāng huó, bò he, sāng yè, jú huā, niú bàng zǐ, chán tuì, chái hú,* and *gé gēn.*

2. Familiar with the classifications of exterior-releasing medicinals; the efficacy, indications, special usage and dosage and special precautions of *xiāng rú, shēng jiāng, bái zhǐ, xì xīn, cāng ěr zǐ,* and *màn jīng zǐ.*

3. Understand the definitions of exterior-releasing medicinals, wind-cold-dispersing medicinals, wind-heat-dispersing medicinals and related terms of exterior-releasing medicine; the efficacy, special usage and dosage and special precautions of *gǎo běn, xīn yí,* and *dàn dòu chǐ.*

凡以发散表邪为主要功效，常用以治疗表证的药物，称为解表药，又称发表药。

Medicinals with the main efficacy of dispersing exterior pathogens and usually indicated for exterior syndromes are called exterior-releasing medicinals.

解表药多具有辛味，药性疏散，主入肺、膀胱经，善走肌表，使肌表之邪外散或随汗出而解。主治恶寒发热、头身疼痛，无汗或有汗不畅、脉浮之外感表证。部分药物还可用于麻疹、风疹、水肿、咳喘、风湿痹痛、疮疡初起等兼有表证者。

Exterior-releasing medicinals are usually acrid in flavor, have the efficacy to release and disperse, and act on the lung and bladder meridians. They tend to work on the superficies to promote sweating and to disperse exterior pathogens with sweating. They are indicated for exterior syndromes manifested as aversion to cold, fever, headache, body pain, no sweating or inhibited sweating, and floating pulse. Some herbs can also be used for measles, rubella, edema, cough and asthma, rheumatism arthralgia, initial stage of ulcers and sores concomitantly with exterior syndromes.

根据解表药的药性及功效主治差异，可分为发散风寒药及发散风热药两类，也称辛温解表药与辛凉解表药，分别用于风寒表证和风热表证。

According to the difference of properties, efficacy and indications, they can be divided into two categories: wind-cold-dispersing medicinals and divergent wind-heat-dispersing medicinals, also known as acrid-warm exterior-releasing medicinals and acrid-cool exterior-releasing medicinals, which are respectively used for wind-cold syndromes and wind-heat syndromes.

应用解表药时，必须针对外感风寒或风热的不同，选用长于发散风寒或发散风热的药物。对于虚人外感者，应随证配伍益气、助阳、养阴、补血等扶正之品。此外，还应根据四时气候变化的不同，恰当地配伍祛暑、化湿、润燥、散寒药。若温病初起，邪在卫分，除选用发散风热药外，应配伍清热解毒药。

When in use, exterior-releasing medicinals are required to be those dispersing wind-cold or releasing wind-heat according to the difference between exterior wind-cold and wind-heat. In case of weak people with external contraction, they are required to combined to respectively with medicinals of tonifying qi, reinforcing yang, nourishing yin or replenishing blood. In addition, according to climate variations in four seasons, exterior-releasing medicinals are required to combine with medicinals of dispelling summer-heat, resolving dampness, moistening dryness and dispersing cold. Fro early-stage warm diseases with pathogens entering defensive stage, wind-heat-dispersing medicinals are used in combination with heat-clearing and toxin-removing medicinals.

使用发汗力强的解表药时，要注意发汗适度，以免汗出过多耗损阳气和津液。对于自汗、盗汗、淋证、失血、久患疮疡的患者，应慎用或忌用。入汤剂不宜久煎，以免有效成分挥发而降低药效。

When using the medicinals that strongly promotes sweat, the dosage should be smaller for fear that excessive sweating damage yang qi and bold fluids. For the patients with self perspiration, night perspiration, drenching syndrome, blood loss and long-term sore, it should be used with caution or avoided. The soup should not be decocted for a long time, so as to avoid the volatilization of effective ingredients and reduce the efficacy.

第一节　发散风寒药

Section 1　Wind-cold-dispersing medicinals

PPT

本类药物性味多辛温，以发散风寒为主要功效。主治风寒表证，症见恶寒发热、无汗或汗出不畅、头身疼痛、鼻塞流涕、舌苔薄白、脉浮紧等。部分药物兼有止咳平喘、祛风湿、止痛、通鼻窍、利水等功效，还可用治咳喘、风湿痹痛、头痛、鼻渊、水肿等兼有风寒表证者。

Wind-cold-dispersing medicinals are usually acrid in flavor and warm in property, so their major efficacy is to disperse wind-cold. They are used to treat exterior syndromes of wind-cold type, manifested as aversion to cold with fever, no sweating or unsmooth sweating, headache and body pain, nasal congestion, nasal discharge, no thirst, a thin and white tongue coating, and a floating and tense pulse. Some wind-cold-dispersing medicinals also have the efficacies of stopping coughing, relieve dyspnea, expelling wind, eliminating dampness, relieving pain, relieving stuffy nose, and promoting urination. They can also treat those with wind cold syndrome as cough and asthma, rheumatic arthralgia, headache, sinusitis and edema.

麻黄 *Má huáng* (Ehpedrae Herba)
《神农本草经》
Shen Nong's Classic of the Materia Medica (*Shén Nóng Běn Cǎo Jīng*)

【来源 / Origin】

为麻黄科植物草麻黄 *Ephedra sinica* Stapf、中麻黄 *Ephedra intermedia* Schrenk et C.A.Mey. 或木贼麻黄 *Ephedra equisetina* Bge. 的干燥草质茎。主产于山西、河北、甘肃等地。秋季采收，切段，生用或蜜炙用。本品气微香，味涩、微苦。《中国药典》规定，含盐酸麻黄碱（$C_{10}H_{15}NO·HCl$）和盐酸伪麻黄碱（$C_{10}H_{15}NO·HCl$）的总量不得少于 0.80%。

Má huáng is the dry herbaceous stem of *Ephedra sinica* Stapf, *Ephedra intermedia* Schrenk et C.A.Mey. or *Ephedra equisetina* Bge., pertaining to Ephedraceae, mainly produced in Shanxi, Hebei, and Gansu Province. It is collected in autumn, cut into sections, raw or honey roasted. It is slightly fragrant, astringent and bitter. According to *Chinese Pharmacopoeia*, the total content of ephedrine hydrochloride ($C_{10}H_{15}NO·HCl$) and pseudoephedrine hydrochloride ($C_{10}H_{15}NO·HCl$) shall not be less than 0.80%.

【性味归经 / Medicinal properties】

辛、微苦，温。归肺、膀胱经。

Acrid, warm and lightly bitter; act on the lung and bladder meridians.

【主要功效 / Medicinal efficacies】

发汗解表，宣肺平喘，利水消肿。

Induce sweating to release the exterior; diffuse the lung and relieve panting; promote urination and relieve swelling.

【临床应用 / Clinical application】

1. 风寒表证 本品味辛发散，性温散寒，善宣肺气、开腠理，以外散侵袭肌表的风寒之邪，其发汗之力强，尤宜用于外感风寒，腠理闭塞之恶寒发热、头身疼痛、无汗的风寒表实证，常与桂枝相须为用，以增强发汗解表之力。

(1) Wind-cold exterior pattern *Má huáng* is pungent and warm with an action to disperse cold, ventilate lung qi and loosen striae and interstice so as to disperse the exterior wind-cold pathogen invaded. It has a strong action of inducing sweating and is suitable for external-contraction of wind-cold of exterior excess patterns manifested as blocked striae and interstice, aversion to cold with fever, headache and body pain with no sweating, and is usually combined with *guì zhī* (Cinnamomi Ramulus) for mutual reinforcement to induce sweating and release exterior.

2. 咳嗽气喘 本品辛散苦降，入肺经，外能发散风寒，内能宣降肺气，有良好的宣肺平喘之功，适用于风寒外束，肺失宣降的喘咳，常与杏仁、甘草同用。对寒痰停饮，咳嗽气喘，痰多清稀者，常配伍细辛、干姜、半夏等。肺热喘咳者，多与石膏、杏仁、甘草伍用。

(2) Coughing and panting *Má huáng* is pungent for dispersing and bitter for descending, acting in lung meridian. Since it can disperse wind cold externally, and ventilate and descend lung qi internally, it can relieve panting and stop coughing, so is suitable for cough and panting due to wind-cold fettering and congestion of the lung qi, in combination with *xìng rén* (Armeniacae Amarum Semen) and *gān cǎo* (Glycyrrhizae Radix et Rhizoma). For cold phlegm-rheum manifested as cough, panting, profuse, clear and diluted sputum, it is usually combined with *xì xīn* (Asari Radix et Rhizoma), *gān jiāng* (Zingiberis Rhizoma) and *bàn xià* (Pinelliae Rhizoma). For those with cough and panting due to lung heat, it is combined with *shí gāo* (Gypsum Fibrosum), *xìng rén* (Armeniacae Amarum Semen) and *gān cǎo* (Glycyrrhizae Radix et Rhizoma).

3. 风水浮肿 本品上宣肺气，发汗解表，下输膀胱，利尿消肿，故宜于风邪袭表，肺失宣降之水肿、小便不利兼有表证者，常与生姜、白术等同用。

(3) Wind edema *Má huáng* can diffuse and descend lung qi for inducing sweating and releasing exterior, and transport to the bladder for promoting urination and reducing edema, so it treats edema and difficult urination with the exterior syndrome due to wind pathogen attacking the exterior and congestion of the lung qi, in combination with *shēng jiāng* (Zingiberis Recens Rhizoma) and *bái zhú* (Atractylodis Macrocephalae Rhizoma).

此外，取麻黄散寒通滞之功，尚可用治风寒湿痹、阴疽痰核。

In addition, *má huáng* can dissipate cold and unblock stagnation to treat *bì* syndrome of wind-cold and dampness, dorsal furuncle and phlegm node.

【用法用量 / Usage and dosage】

煎服，2~10g。本品生用发汗解表，蜜炙用润肺止咳，多用于表证已解、气喘咳嗽者。

Decocted, 2-10g. To induce sweating to release the exterior, it is used in the raw form, and decocted with honey to relieve cough and panting, mostly used for cases with exterior syndromes released, panting and cough.

【使用注意 / Precaution】

表虚自汗、阴虚盗汗、肺肾虚喘者均当慎用，失眠及高血压患者亦应慎用，运动员禁用。

It should be used with caution for those with spontaneous sweating due to exterior deficiency, night sweat due to yin deficiency, and deficiency-type panting due to insufficiency of lung and kidney; and also for those with insomnia and hypertension. It is contraindicated for athletes.

【现代研究 / Modern research】

本品主要含麻黄碱、伪麻黄碱、甲基伪麻黄碱、麻黄次碱等生物碱，以及挥发油、黄酮、多糖、儿茶酚、鞣质及有机酸等。具有发汗、解热、平喘、镇咳、祛痰、利尿、抗炎、抗菌、抗过敏、升高血压、加快心率和一定的中枢兴奋作用。

Má huáng mainly contains alkaloids such as ephedrine, pseudoephedrine, methylpseudoephedrine, and ephedine, and also contains volatile oil, flavonoids, polysaccharides, catechol, tannin and organic acids. It has the efficacies of inducing sweating, clearing heat, relieving panting and cough, dispelling phlegm, promoting urination, anti-inflammation, anti-bacteria, anti-allergy, raising hypertension, accelerating heart rate and certain central excitation.

桂枝 *Guì zhī* (Cinnamomi Ramulus)
《名医别录》
Miscellaneous Records of Famous Physicians (Míng Yī Bié Lù)

【来源 / Origin】

为樟科植物肉桂 *Cinnamomum cassia* Presl 的干燥嫩枝。主产于广东、广西及云南。春、夏二季采收。切片，生用。本品有特异香气，味甜、微辛，皮部味较浓。《中国药典》规定，干燥药材含桂皮醛（C_9H_8O）不得少于 1.0%。

Guì zhī is the tender twig of *Cinnamomum cassia* Presl, pertaining to Lauraceae. It is mainly produced in Guangdong Province, Guangxi Zhuang Autonomous Region and Yunnan Province, collected in summer and autumn and cut into slices for use in the raw form. It has peculiar fragrance, and is sweet and slightly pungent in flavor. The smell in the surface is quite strong. According to *Chinese Pharmacopoeia*, the content of cinnamaldehyde (C_9H_8O) in dried medicinal materials should not be less than 1.0%.

【性味归经 / Medicinal properties 】

辛、甘，温。归心、肺、膀胱经。

Acrid, sweet and warm; act on the heart, lung and bladder meridians.

【主要功效 / Medicinal efficacies 】

发汗解肌，温通经脉，助阳化气，平冲降逆。

Induce sweating to release muscles; warm and unblock meridians; reinforce yang and promote qi transformation; lower down flow of reversed qi.

【临床应用 / Clinical application 】

1. 风寒表证　本品辛温散寒，发汗之力较麻黄温和，凡外感风寒，无论表实无汗、表虚有汗者，皆可配伍使用。前者常与麻黄相须为用，后者常与白芍配伍。

(1) Wind-cold exterior syndrome　*Guì zhī* is to dissipate cold with pungent-warm, and induce sweating more moderate than *má huáng*. It is indicated for exterior wind-cold whether for exterior excess without sweating or exterior deficiency with sweating, the former combined with *má huáng* while the latter with *bái sháo* (Paeoniae Alba Radix).

2. 寒凝血滞诸痛证　本品辛散温通，有温通经脉、散寒止痛之效。用治胸阳不振，心脉瘀阻，胸痹心痛者，常与枳实、薤白同用。用治中焦虚寒，脘腹冷痛，常与白芍、饴糖同用。用治妇女寒凝血滞，经闭，痛经，多与当归、吴茱萸同用。用治风寒湿痹，肩背肢节酸痛，每与附子同用。

(2) Pains induced by wind-cold-damp arthralgia　*Guì zhī* is to dredge channels with warm, dissipate cold and relieve pains. To treat heart obstruction, and chest impediment and heart pain due to hypofunction of chest yang, *guì zhī* is combined with *zhǐ shí* (Aurantii Immaturus Fructus) and *xiè bái* (Allii Macrostemi Bulbus); to treat cold pain in stomach and abdomen due to deficiency-cold in middle *jiao*, it is combined with *bái sháo* (Paeoniae Alba Radix) and *yí táng* (Saccharum Granorum); to treat pattern of cold congeal and blood stasis, amenorrhea and dysmenorrheal, it is combined with *dāng guī* (Angelicae Sinensis Radix) and *wú zhū yú* (Evodiae Fructus); to treat wind-cold-damp arthralgia, and shoulder and back pain, it is combined with *fù zǐ* (Aconiti Lateralis Radix Praeparata).

3. 心悸、痰饮、水肿　本品甘温，可助心、脾、肾三脏之阳气。用治心阳不足，心动悸，脉结代，常与甘草、人参等同用。用治脾阳不运，水湿内停之痰饮眩晕，常与茯苓、白术等同用。用治肾阳不足，膀胱气化不行之水肿、小便不利，常与茯苓、猪苓、泽泻等同用。

(3) Palpitation, phlegm-fluid retention, edema　*Guì zhī* is sweet and warm and can assist yang qi of heart, spleen and kidney. To treat heart-yang deficiency, palpitation, irregularly or regularly intermittent pulse, it is often combined with *gān cǎo* (Glycyrrhizae Radix et Rhizoma) and *rén shēn* (Ginseng Radix et Rhizoma); to treat phlegm-fluid retention and dizziness due to dysfunction of spleen yang in transportation, retention of water and dampness, it is combined with *fú líng* (Poria) and *bái zhú* (Atractylodis Macrocephalae Rhizoma); to treat edema and dysuria due to kidney-yang insufficiency, disturbance of qi transformation in bladder, it is often combined with *fú líng* (Poria), *zhū líng* (Polyporus)

and *zé xiè* (Alismatis Rhizoma).

4. 奔豚　本品甘温，能温心阳，降冲逆。对于心阳不足，不能下温肾水，以致下焦阴寒之气上逆发为奔豚者，常重用本品以助阳化气、平冲降逆。

(4) Up-rushing of qi (like a running piglet)　*Guì zhī* is sweet and warm and can warm the yang of heart, descend the adverse qi. For up-rushing qi of yin-cold in lower-energizer due to heart-yang insufficiency failing to warm kidney water, it is often used in large dosage to assist yang and transform qi, descend adverse-rising qi.

【用法用量 / Usage and dosage】
煎服，3~10g。
Decoction, 3-10g.

【使用注意 / Precaution】
凡外感热病、阴虚火旺及血热妄行之出血证均当忌用。孕妇及月经过多者慎用。

Guì zhī should be avoided for those with warm pathogens, yin deficiency with effulgent fire, or reckless movement of the blood due to heat in blood. Pregnant women and women with menorrhagia should be used with caution.

【现代研究 / Modern research】
本品主要含桂皮醛等挥发油，尚含酚类、有机酸、多糖、苷类、香豆精及鞣质等。具有解热、降温、抑菌、镇痛、健胃、缓解胃肠痉挛及利尿、强心、镇静、抗惊厥等作用。

Guì zhī mainly contains volatile oil and cinnamaldehyde. In addition, it also contains phenols, organic acids, polysaccharides, glycosides, coumarins and tannins. It has the functions of dispelling heat, relieving fever, bacteriostasis, relieving pain, invigorating the stomach, relieving gastrointestinal spasm, promoting urine, strengthening the heart, calming and resisting convulsions.

羌活　*Qiāng huó* (Notopterygii Rhizoma et Radix)
《神农本草经》
Shen Nong's Classic of the Materia Medica (Shén Nóng Běn Cǎo Jīng)

【来源 / Origin】
为伞形科植物羌活 *Notopterygium incisum* Ting ex H.T.Chang 或宽叶羌活 *Notopterygium franchetii* H.de Boiss. 的干燥根茎和根。主产于四川、甘肃、青海等地。春、秋二季采挖，切片，生用。本品气香，味微苦而辛。《中国药典》规定，含挥发油不得少于 1.4%（ml/g），含羌活醇（$C_{21}H_{22}O_5$）和异欧前胡素（$C_{16}H_{14}O_4$）的总量不得少于 0.40%。

Qiāng huó is the dry rhizome and root of *Notopterygium Incosum* Ting ex H.T.Chang or *Notopterygium franchetii* H.de Boiss., pertaining to Apiaceae, mainly produced in Sichuan, Gansu, and Qinghai Province, collected in spring and autumn, sliced and used in raw form. It is fragrant, slightly bitter and pungent. According to *Chinese Pharmacopoeia*, the content of volatile oil shall not be less than 1.4% (ml/g), and the total content of notopterol ($C_{21}H_{22}O_5$) and isoimperatorin ($C_{16}H_{14}O_4$) shall not be less than 0.40%.

【性味归经 / Medicinal properties】
辛、苦，温。归膀胱、肾经。
Acrid, bitter, warm; act on bladder and kidney meridians.

【主要功效 / Medicinal efficacies】
解表散寒，祛风除湿，止痛。

Release exterior and dissipate cold, dispel wind and dampness, relieve pain.

【临床应用 / Clinical application】

1. 风寒夹湿表证　本品辛温散寒，苦燥胜湿，气味雄烈，有较强的解表散寒作用，为治风寒表证的常用药。又因其长于胜湿、止痛，故对外感风寒夹湿之恶寒发热、肌表无汗、头痛项强、肢体酸痛者尤为适宜，常与防风、细辛、川芎等同用。

(1) External-contraction of wind-cold complicated by dampness　*Qiāng huó* is acrid warm and dispersing cold, bitter dry overcoming dampness, strong smell, and is a common medicinal for wind cold syndrome since it has a strong effect of releasing exterior and dispersing cold. It is also good at overcoming dampness and relieving pain, it can treat those with external-contraction wind-cold complicated by dampness, manifested as aversion to cold, fever, no sweat on fleshy exterior, headache, rigid neck, and severe aching pain of the body, in combination with *fáng fēng*, *xì xīn* (Asari Radix et Rhizoma) and *chuān xiōng* (Chuanxiong Rhizoma).

2. 风寒湿痹，肩背酸痛　本品辛散祛风，味苦燥湿，性温散寒，有较强的祛风散寒、胜湿止痛功效。其入足太阳膀胱经，以除头项肩背之痛见长，善治上半身风寒湿痹，肩背肢节疼痛，多与防风、姜黄、当归等同用。

(2) Wind-cold-damp impediment and pain in shoulders and back　*Qiāng huó* is acrid dispersing and dispelling wind, bitter, dry and damp, warm in nature and dispersing cold, and has a strong effect of dispelling wind, dispersing cold, overcoming dampness and relieving pain. It acts on Taiyang bladder meridian, removing the pain of head, neck, shoulder and back, so it can treat wind-cold-damp impediment of upper body manifested as joints pain in shoulders and back in combination with *fáng fēng*, *jiāng huáng* (Curcumae Longae Rhizoma) and *dāng guī* (Angelicae Sinensis Radix).

【用法用量 / Usage and dosage】

煎服，3~10g。

Decoction, 3-10g.

【使用注意 / Precaution】

阴血亏虚者慎用，脾胃虚弱者不宜服用。

It should be used with caution for those with yin-blood deficiency, and be avoided for those with weakness of spleen and stomach.

【现代研究 / Modern research】

本品主要含α-侧柏烯、α-蒎烯、β-蒎烯等挥发油成分，另含紫花前胡苷、羌活醇、异欧前胡素、花椒毒酚以及脂肪酸、糖类等。具有解热、抗炎、镇痛、抑菌、抗心律失常、抗心肌缺血等作用。

Qiāng huó mainly contains volatile oil components such as α-platyclonene, α-pinene, and β-pinene, and also contains nodakenin, notopterol, isoimperatorin, zanthol, fatty acids, sugars, etc. It has antipyretic, anti-inflammatory, analgesic, antibacterial, antiarrhythmic, anti myocardial ischemia and other effects.

荆芥　*Jīng jiè* (Schizonepetae Herba)
《神农本草经》
Shen Nong's Classic of the Materia Medica (Shén Nóng Běn Cǎo Jīng)

【来源 / Origin】

为唇形科植物荆芥 *Schizonepeta tenuifolia* Briq. 的干燥地上部分。主产于江苏、浙江、江西等地。夏、秋二季采割，切段，生用。本品气清香，味微涩辛凉。《中国药典》规定，含挥发油不得少于0.60%（ml/g），含胡薄荷酮（$C_{10}H_{16}O$）不得少于0.020%；饮片含挥发油不得少于0.30%（ml/g），胡薄荷酮不得少于0.020%。

Jīng jiè is the dry aboveground part of *Schizonepeta tenuifolia* Briq., pertaining to Labiatae, mainly produced in Jiangsu, Zhejiang, and Jiangxi Province, collected in summer and autumn, cut and used in the form of raw segments. It is fragrant and slightly astringent, acrid and cool. According to *Chinese Pharmacopoeia*, the content of volatile oil shall not be less than 0.60% (ml/g), the content of menthol ($C_{10}H_{16}O$) shall not be less than 0.020%; the content of volatile oil in decoction pieces shall not be less than 0.30% (ml/g), and that of menthol shall not be less than 0.020%.

【性味归经 / Medicinal properties 】

辛，微温。归肺、肝经。

Acrid, slightly warm; act on lung and liver meridians.

【主要功效 / Medicinal efficacies 】

解表散风，透疹，消疮。

Release exterior and dispelling wind, promote eruption, resolve sore, and stop bleeding when stir-fried to scorch.

【临床应用 / Clinical application 】

1. 外感表证 本品辛散气香，微温不烈，药性和缓，长于发表散风，为发散风寒药中药性最为平和之品。对于外感表证，无论风寒、风热均可选用。治风寒表证之恶寒发热、头痛无汗者，常与防风、羌活等同用；治风热表证之发热头痛者，每与薄荷、金银花等同用。

(1) External-contraction exterior syndrome *Jīng jiè* is acrid, dispersing, fragrant, slightly warm, and mild, suitable for relieving exterior and dispersing wind, and is the mildest in all the medicinals for relieving exterior and dispersing wind. It can be used for external-contraction exterior syndrome, whether wind-cold or wind-heat. For wind-cold exterior syndrome manifested as aversion to cold, fever, headache with no sweating, it is often used with *fáng fēng* (Saposhnikoviae Radix) and *qiāng huó* (Notopterygii Rhizoma et Radix); for wind-heat exterior syndrome with fever and headache, it is used with *bò he* (Menthae Herba) and *jīn yín huā* (Lonicerae Japonicae Flos).

2. 风疹瘙痒，麻疹不透 本品轻扬透散，能宣散疹毒，祛风止痒。用治风疹瘙痒，可与防风、白蒺藜等同用；用治麻疹初起、疹出不畅，多与蝉蜕、薄荷等同用。

(2) Itchy rubella and measles failing to erupt *Jīng jiè* is light, dispersing and promoting eruption, expelling toxin, dispel wind and stopping itching. For itchy rubella, it is used with *fáng fēng* (Saposhnikoviae Radix) and *bái jí lí* (Tribuli Fructus); for measles at the early stage or measles failing to erupt, it is often used with *chán tuì* (Cicadae Periostracum) and *bò he* (Menthae Herba).

3. 疮疡初起 本品既能祛风解表，又能消疮，故可用于疮疡初起兼有表证者。若偏风寒，可与羌活、川芎等同用；若偏风热，则与金银花、连翘等同用。

(3) Sores and ulcers in early stage *Jīng jiè* can dispel wind and release exterior as well as eliminating sores, so it can treat sores and ulcers in early stage with exterior syndrome. For those with wind-cold, it is used with *qiāng huó* (Notopterygii Rhizoma et Radix) and *chuān xiōng* (Chuanxiong Rhizoma); for those with wind-heat, it is used with *jīn yín huā* (Lonicerae Japonicae Flos) and *lián qiáo* (Forsythiae Fructus).

【用法用量 / Usage and dosage 】

煎服，5~10g。不宜久煎。

Decoction, 5-10g. Avoid long time decocting.

【现代研究 / Modern research】

本品主要含胡薄荷酮、薄荷酮、右旋柠檬烯等挥发油，尚含荆芥苷、荆芥醇及黄酮类化合物等。具有解热、抑菌、抗炎、镇痛、抗补体、止血等作用。

Jīng jiè mainly contains menthol, d-limonene and other volatile oil, and also schizonoside, schizonepeta alcohol and flavonoids. It has the functions of relieving heat, antibacterial, anti-inflammatory, relieving pain, anti-complement, and stanching bleeding.

防风 *Fáng fēng* (Saposhnikoviae Radix)
《神农本草经》
Shen Nong's Classic of the Materia Medica (Shén Nóng Běn Cǎo Jīng)

【来源 / Origin】

为伞形科植物防风 *Saposhnikovia divaricata*（Turcz.）Schischk. 的干燥根。主产于黑龙江、内蒙古、吉林等地。春、秋二季采挖，切厚片，生用。本品气特异，味微甘。《中国药典》规定，含升麻素苷（$C_{22}H_{28}O_{11}$）和 5-O-甲基维斯阿米醇苷（$C_{22}H_{28}O_{10}$）的总量不得少于 0.24%。

Fáng fēng is the dry root of *Saposhnikovia divaricata* (Turcz.) Schischk., pertaining to Apiaceae, mainly produced in Heilongjiang province, Inner Mongolia Antonomous Region, and Jilin Province, collected in spring and autumn, cut thick slices and used in raw form. It has a special odor and tastes slightly sweet. According to *Chinese Pharmacopoeia*, the total content of cimicin glycoside ($C_{22}H_{28}O_{11}$) and 5-O-methylvisamifoside ($C_{22}H_{28}O_{10}$) shall not be less than 0.24%.

【性味归经 / Medicinal properties】

辛、甘，微温。归膀胱、肝、脾经。

Acrid, sweet, and slightly warm; act on bladder, liver and spleen meridians.

【主要功效 / Medicinal efficacies】

祛风解表，胜湿止痛，止痉。

Expel wind, release exterior, overcome damp to relieve pain, and arrest convulsion.

【临床应用 / Clinical application】

1. 外感表证 本品辛温发散，微温不燥，长于祛风解表。不论外感风寒、风热、风湿表证均可配伍应用。治风寒表证，头痛身痛，恶风寒者，常与荆芥、羌活等同用。治风热表证，发热恶风，咽痛口渴者，多与薄荷、连翘等同用。治风寒夹湿表证，头痛如裹，身重肢痛者，可与羌活、川芎等同用。

(1) External-contraction exterior syndrome *Fáng fēng* is acrid warm dispersing, slightly warm and not dry, and is suitable for expelling wind and releasing exterior. It can be used in combination to treat external-contraction exterior syndrome due to wind-cold, wind-heat or wind-dampness. For wind-cold exterior syndrome with headache, body pain, and aversion to wind-cold, it is often used with *jīng jiè* (Schizonepetae Herba) and *qiāng huó* (Notopterygii Rhizoma et Radix); for wind-heat exterior syndrome with fever, aversion to wind, sore throat and thirst, it is often used with *bò he* (Menthae Herba) and *lián qiáo* (Forsythiae Fructus); for exterior syndrome of wind-cold complicated by dampness with headache, heavy body and limbs pain, it is used with *qiāng huó* (Notopterygii Rhizoma et Radix) and *chuān xiōng* (Chuanxiong Rhizoma).

2. 风湿痹痛 本品辛散温通，能祛风散寒，胜湿止痛，为祛风湿、止痹痛的常用药。用治风寒湿痹，肢节疼痛，筋脉挛急者，常与羌活、独活等同用。

(2) Wind-dampness and pains of impediment *Fáng fēng* is acrid dispersing and warm dredging, and can expel wind, disperse cold, overcome damp to relieve pain, so it is commonly used for expel wind-dampness and stop pains due to impediment. For those with wind-cold-dampness impediment, pain of limbs and joints, and muscular spasm, it is often used with *qiāng huó* (Notopterygii Rhizoma et Radix) and *dú huó* (Angelicae Pubescentis Radix).

3. 风疹瘙痒 本品能祛风止痒，且药性较为平和，风寒、风热所致的瘾疹瘙痒均可选用。若偏于风寒，可与麻黄、白芷等同用；若偏于风热，常与薄荷、蝉蜕等同用；若偏于湿热，可与土茯苓、白鲜皮等同用。

(3) Itching rubella *Fáng fēng* can expel wind and relieve itching, and is mild in property and can be used to treat itching rubella due to wind-cold or wind-heat. For those with wind-cold, it is used with *má huáng* (Ephedrae Herba) and *bái zhǐ* (Angelicae Dahuricae Radix); for those with wind-heat, it is used with *bò he* (Menthae Herba) and *chán tuì* (Cicadae Periostracum); for those with dampness-cold, it is used with *tǔ fú líng* (Smilacis Glabrae Rhizoma) and *bái xiān pí* (Dictamni Cortex).

4. 破伤风 本品既能辛散外风，又能息内风以止痉。用治破伤风，四肢抽搐，项背强急，角弓反张者，常与天麻、天南星等同用。

(4) Tetanus *Fáng fēng* is acrid and can disperse external wind as well as extinguish wind and stop convulsions. For tetanus with convulsion of four limbs, spasm of nape and back, and opisthotonos, it is used with *tiān má* (Gastrodiae Rhizoma) and *tiān nán xīng* (Arisaematis Rhizoma).

【用法用量 / Usage and dosage】

煎服，5~10g。

Decoction, 5-10g.

【现代研究 / Modern research】

本品主要含 5-O- 甲基维斯阿米醇苷、防风色酮醇、升麻素苷等，尚含香柑内脂、酸性多糖、挥发油等。具有解热、抗炎、镇静、镇痛、抗惊厥、抗过敏等作用。

Fáng fēng mainly contains 5-*O*-methylvisamifosicle, fangfengchromol, cimicin glycoside, and also contains citrus internal fat, acid polysaccharide, volatile oil, etc. It has antipyretic, anti-inflammatory, sedative, analgesic, anticonvulsant and antiallergic effects.

紫苏叶 *Zǐ sū yè* (Perillae Folium)
《名医别录》
Miscellaneous Records of Famous Physicians (*Míng Yī Bié Lù*)

【来源 / Origin】

为唇形科植物紫苏 *Perilla frutescens*（L.）Britt. 的干燥叶（或带嫩枝）。主产于江苏、浙江、河北。夏季采收，切碎，生用。本品气清香，味微辛。《中国药典》规定，含挥发油不得少于0.40%（ml/g）；饮片不得少于 0.20%（ml/g）。

Zǐ sū yè is the dry leaf (or with tender twig) of *Perilla frutescens* (L.)Britt., pertaining to Labiatae, mainly produced in Jiangsu, Zhejiang and Hebei Province, and collected in summer, cup up and used in the raw form. It has faint scent and slightly acrid. According to *Chinese Pharmacopoeia*, the volatile oil content shall not be less than 0.40% (ml/g) and that of decoction pieces shall not be less than 0.20% (ml/g).

【性味归经 / Medicinal properties】

辛，温。归肺、脾经。

Acrid and warm; act on the lung and spleen meridians.

【主要功效 / Medicinal efficacies】

解表散寒，行气和胃。

Release exterior and disperse cold, move qi and harmonize stomach.

【临床应用 / Clinical application】

1. 风寒表证　本品辛温发散之性缓和，发汗解表之力亦不如麻黄、桂枝。轻证可单用，重证须与其他发散风寒药同用。因其外能解表宣肺，内能理脾胃之气，略兼化痰止咳之功，故善治风寒表证兼有肺脾气滞，胸脘满闷，恶心呕逆或咳嗽痰多者。治疗胸脘满闷，恶心呕逆，常与香附、陈皮同用；治疗咳嗽痰多，常与苦杏仁、半夏等同用。

(1) Wind-cold exterior syndrome　*Zǐ sū yè* has mild in nature of acrid warm and dispersing, and its perspiration is not as powerful as *má huáng* and *guì zhī*. It can used single for light syndrome, but for severe diseases, it should be used with other wind-cold-dispersing medicinals. Releasing exterior and ventilating lung, regulating the qi of the spleen and stomach, as well as resolving phlegm and relieving cough, *zǐ sū yè* is suitable for wind-cold-exterior syndrome with stagnation of lung and spleen qi, chest fullness, nausea and vomiting, or coughing with phlegm. To treat chest fullness, nausea and vomiting, it is often used with *xiāng fù* (Cyperi Rhizoma) and *chén pí* (Citri Reticulatae Pericarpium), to treat coughing with phlegm, it is often used with *kǔ xìng rén* (Armeniacae Amarum Semen) and *bàn xià* (Pinelliae Rhizoma).

2. 脾胃气滞，腹胀呕吐　本品味辛能行，入中焦脾胃经，能行气以宽中除胀、和胃止呕，兼有理气安胎之功。治脾胃气滞，脘腹胀满，恶心呕吐者，可与陈皮、厚朴等同用。治妊娠胎气上逆，恶心呕吐，胎动不安者，可与砂仁、陈皮等同用。治七情郁结，痰凝气滞之梅核气，常与半夏、厚朴、茯苓等同用。

(2) Stagnation of spleen and stomach qi, abdomina fullness and vomiting　*Zǐ sū yè* is acrid and can moving qi. It enters middle-energizer of spleen and stomach meridians and can promote qi flow to soothe the middle-energizer and ease distension, harmonize stomach and stop vomiting, and it also has some effect on regulating qi to prevent abortion. For those with stagnation of spleen and stomach qi, abdominal fullness and distention, nausea and vomiting, it can be combined with *chén pí* (Citri Reticulatae Pericarpium) and *hòu pò* (Magnoliae Officinalis Cortex); for those with fetus-qi flowing upward, nausea and vomiting, and excessive fetal movement, it is combined with *shā rén* (Amomi Fructus) and *chén pí*; for those with plum-stone qi (globus hystericus) due to stagnation of seven emotions, phlegm coagulation and qi stagnation, it is used with *bàn xià*, *hòu pò* and *fú líng* (Poria).

此外，本品能解鱼蟹毒，治疗鱼蟹中毒，腹痛吐泻者，可单用或与生姜、藿香、陈皮等药同煎服。

In addition, *zǐ sū yè* can detoxify fish and crab, so for those with fish and crab poisoning, abdominal pain and diarrhea, it can be used alone or decocted with *shēng jiāng*, *huò xiāng*, and *chén pí*.

【用法用量 / Usage and dosage】

煎服，5~10g。不宜久煎。

Decoction, 5-10g. Avoid long-time decocting.

【现代研究 / Modern research】

本品主要含紫苏醛、紫苏酮、左旋柠檬烯等挥发油。具有解热、促进消化液分泌、增强胃肠蠕动、减少支气管分泌、缓解支气管痉挛、抑菌等作用。

Zǐ sū yè mainly contains perillaldehyde, perilla ketone, l-limonene and other volatile oil. It has the functions of releasing fever, promoting secretion of digestive fluid, enhancing gastrointestinal peristalsis, reducing secretion of bronchus, relieving bronchospasm and bacteriostasis.

生姜 *Shēng jiāng* (Zingiberis Rhizoma Recens)
《名医别录》
Miscellaneous Records of Famous Physicians (Míng Yī Bié Lù)

【来源 / Origin】

为姜科植物姜 *Zingiber officinale* Rosc. 的新鲜根茎。主产于四川、贵州、湖北等地。秋、冬二季采挖，切厚片，生用。本品气香特异，味辛辣，以质嫩者佳。《中国药典》规定，含6-姜辣素（$C_{17}H_{26}O_4$）不得少于0.050%，8-姜酚（$C_{19}H_{30}O_4$）与10-姜酚（$C_{21}H_{34}O_4$）总量不得少于0.040%；饮片含6-姜辣素不得少于0.050%。

Shēng jiāng is the fresh rhizome of *Zingiber officinale* Rosc., pertaining to Zingiberaceae, mainly produced in Sichuan, Guizhou, Hubei and other places, collected in autumn and winter, cut thick slices and used in the raw form. It is spicy with a special fragrance and better when tender. According to *Chinese Pharmacopoeia*, the content of 6-gingerol ($C_{17}H_{26}O_4$) shall not be less than 0.050%; the total content of 8-gingerol ($C_{19}H_{30}O_4$) and 10-gingerol ($C_{21}H_{34}O_4$) shall not be less than 0.040%. The content of 6-gingerol in decoction pieces shall not be less than 0.050%.

【性味归经 / Medicinal properties】

辛，微温。归肺、脾、胃经。

Acrid, slightly warm; act on lung, spleen and stomach meridians.

【主要功效 / Medicinal efficacies】

解表散寒，温中止呕，化痰止咳，解鱼蟹毒。

Release exterior and dissipate cold, warm the middle and arrest vomiting, dissolve phlegm and relieve cough, remove toxins of fish and crab.

【临床应用 / Clinical application】

1. 风寒表证 本品辛温，有发汗解表散寒之功，但作用较弱，故适用于风寒表证的轻证，可单味服用或与红糖、葱白煎服。对于风寒表证较重者，多配入辛温解表剂中作辅助用药，以增强发汗解表之力。

(1) Wind-cold exterior syndrome *Shēng jiāng* can release exterior and dissipate cold with acrid-warm, but the function is mild, so it is suitable for wind-cold exterior syndrome, decocted alone or along with brown sugar and *cōng bái* (Allii Fistulosi Bulbus). For severe cases, acrid-warm exterior-releasing medicinal is often used as adjuvant to enhance the function of promoting sweating and release exterior.

2. 胃寒呕吐 本品长于温胃散寒，降逆止呕，因其善能止呕，故有"呕家圣药"之称，随证配伍可治疗多种呕吐。因其善能温胃，故尤宜于胃寒呕吐，可单味煎服或捣汁服。若治痰饮呕吐，常与半夏同用；若治胃热呕吐，常与黄连、竹茹等同用。

(2) Vomiting due to stomach cold *Shēng jiāng* is better to warm stomach, dissipate cold, descend counterflow of qi, and relieve vomiting. Due to its action of relieving vomiting, it's got the name "Medicine of vomit" and can be combined with other medicinals to treat various vomiting. Because it is good at warming the stomach, it is especially suitable for stomach cold and vomiting. It can be decocted alone or mashed juice. For vomiting due to phlegm-fluid retention, it is often used with *bàn xià* (Pinelliae Rhizoma); for vomiting due to stomach heat, it is often used with *huáng lián* (Coptidis Rhizoma) and *zhú rú* (Bambusae Caulis in Taenia).

3. 寒痰咳嗽 本品辛散性温，入肺经，有温肺散寒止咳之功。对肺寒咳嗽，无论有无外感风寒，有痰无痰皆可选用。治风寒犯肺，咳嗽痰多，恶寒头痛者，每与麻黄、苦杏仁同用；治外无表邪而痰多者，可与陈皮、半夏等同用。

(3) Cold-phlegm cough *Shēng jiāng* is acrid dispersing and warm in nature, acting on lung meridian with the function of warming lung, dissipating cold and arresting cough. For lung-cold cough, it can be used whether there is external-contraction wind-cold or phlegm. For those with wind-cold invading lung, cough with more phlegm, aversion to cold and headache, it is often used with *má huáng* (Ephedrae Herba) and *kǔ xìng rén* (Armeniacae Amarum Semen); for those with more phlegm without external pathogen, it is used with *chén pí* (Citri Reticulatae Pericarpium) and *bàn xià* (Pinelliae Rhizoma).

4. 鱼蟹中毒 本品能解鱼蟹毒及半夏、天南星之毒，主要用于鱼蟹等食物中毒及生半夏、生天南星等药物中毒，可用生姜汁冲服或煎汤内服。

(4) Intoxication by eating fish or crab *Shēng jiāng* is used to resolve the toxins of fish, crab, *bàn xià* and *tiān nán xīng* (Arisaematis Rhizoma) by drinking infused *shēng jiāng* juice or decoction.

【 用法用量 / Usage and dosage 】

煎服，3~10g，或捣汁服。

Decoction or pounded juice, 3-10g.

【 使用注意 / Precaution 】

热盛及阴虚内热者忌服。

Those with exuberant heat or suffering from yin deficiency with internal heat should avoid it.

【 现代研究 / Modern research 】

本品主要含姜醇、α- 姜烯、β- 水芹烯等挥发油，尚含辣味成分姜辣素等。具有解热、镇吐、促进消化液分泌、保护胃黏膜、抗溃疡、保肝、利胆、镇痛、抗炎、抗菌等作用。

Shēng jiāng mainly contains zingiberol, α-gingerene, β-carvone and other volatile oil, and also contains gingerol and so on. It has the functions of releasing heat, relieving vomiting, promoting secretion of digestive fluid, protecting gastric mucosa and liver, promoting the function of gallbladder, and relieving pain, and also it has anti-ulcer, anti-inflammatory and antibacterial effect.

白芷　*Bái zhǐ* (Angelicae Dahuricae Radix)
《神农本草经》
Shen Nong's Classic of the Materia Medica (Shén Nóng Běn Cǎo Jīng)

【 来源 / Origin 】

为伞形科植物白芷 *Angelica dahurica*（Fisch.ex Hoffm.）Benth.et Hook.f. 或杭白芷 *Angelica dahurica*（Fisch.ex Hoffm.）Benth.et Hook.f.var. formosana（Boiss.）Shan et Yuan 的干燥根。主产于浙江、四川、河南等地。夏、秋间采挖，切厚片，生用。《中国药典》规定，含欧前胡素（$C_{16}H_{14}O_4$）不得少于 0.080%。

Bái zhǐ is the dry root of *Angelica dahurica* (Fisch.ex Hoffm.) Benth.et Hook. f. or *Angelica dahurica* (Fisch.ex Hoffm.) Benth.et Hook.f.var.formosana (Boiss.) Shan et Yuan, pertaining to Umbelliferae, mainly produced in Zhejiang, Sichuan, and Henan Province, collected in summer and autumn, cut thick slices and used in raw form. According to *Chinese Pharmacopoeia*, the content of imperatorin ($C_{16}H_{14}O_4$) in dried medicinal materials should not be less than 0.080%.

【 性味归经 / Medicinal properties 】

辛，温。归胃、大肠、肺经。

Acrid and warm; act on stomach, large intestine and lung meridians.

【主要功效 / Medicinal efficacies】

解表散寒，祛风止痛，宣通鼻窍，燥湿止带，消肿排脓。

Release exterior and dissipate cold, dispel wind and relieve pain, diffuse and unblock the nasal orifices, dry dampness and arrest vaginal discharge, resolve swelling and expel pus.

【临床应用 / Clinical application】

1. 风寒表证　本品辛温发散，能外散风寒以解表，但作用温和，因其兼有较好的止痛和通鼻窍之功，故宜于风寒表证之头痛、鼻塞流涕者，常与防风、羌活、细辛等同用。

(1) **Wind-cold exterior syndrome** *Bái zhǐ* is acrid, warm and dispersing, and can dissipate wind-cold to release the exterior but mild. It is effective in relieving pain and unblocking the nasal orifices, so can treat wind-cold exterior syndrome manifested as headache, nasal obstruction and discharge in combination with *fáng fēng*, *qiāng huó* and *xì xīn* (Asari Radix et Rhizoma).

2. 头痛，眉棱骨痛，牙痛，风湿痹痛　本品辛温升散，芳香上达，长于止痛，善入足阳明胃经，治疗头面诸疾。用治阳明头痛，眉棱骨痛，头风痛，属外感风寒者，可单用，或与防风、细辛、川芎等同用；属外感风热者，可与薄荷、蔓荆子、菊花配伍。用治牙痛，属风冷者，多与细辛、全蝎、川芎等同用；属风火者，可与石膏、黄连等同用。用治风寒湿痹，关节疼痛，可与羌活、独活等同用。

(2) **Headache, pain in supra-orbital bone, toothache, and wind-damp impediment pain** *Bái zhǐ* is acrid, warm, descending and dissipating, fragrant upward, and is good at relieving pain and entering foot Yangming meridian for head diseases. It can be used alone to treat Yangming headache due to external-contraction of wind-cold, pain in supra-orbital bone or head-wind pain or in combination with *fáng fēng*, *xì xīn* and *chuān xiōng*; for external-contraction of wind-heat, it is combined with *bò he* (Menthae Herba), *màn jīng zǐ* (Viticis Fructus) and *jú huā* (Chrysanthemi Flos); for toothache due to wind-cold, combined with *xì xīn*, *quán xiē* (Scorpio) and *chuān xiōng*; for toothache due to wind-fire, combined with *shí gāo* (Gypsum Fibrosum) and *huáng lián* (Coptidis Rhizoma); for wind-cold-damp impediment and joints pain, it is often used with *qiāng huó* and *dú huó* (Angelicae Pubescentis Radix).

3. 鼻衄，鼻渊，鼻塞流涕　本品辛香温通，入肺经，可宣肺气，通鼻窍，止疼痛。用治鼻衄，鼻渊，鼻塞不通，浊涕不止，前额疼痛，常与细辛、苍耳子、辛夷等同用。

(3) **Allergic rhinitis, sinusitis, stuffy nose with discharge** *Bái zhǐ* is acrid, fragrant, warm and dredging, entering lung meridian to ventilate lung qi, unblock nasal orifices and relieve pain. It treats allergic rhinitis, sinusitis, nasal obstruction, excessive thick nasal discharge, and forehead pain in combination with *xì xīn*, *cāng ěr zǐ* (Xanthii Fructus) and *xīn yí* (Magnoliae Flos).

4. 带下　本品温燥气香，善除阳明经湿邪而燥湿止带。若治寒湿带下，常与鹿角霜、白术、山药等同用。若治湿热带下，宜与车前子、黄柏等同用。

(4) **Leukorrhea** *Bái zhǐ* is warm, dry and fragrant, and good at removing dampness pathogen of Yangming meridians to dry dampness and arrest vaginal discharge. It treats cold-dampness leucorrhea in combination with *lù jiǎo shuāng* (Cervi Cornu Degelatinatum), *bái zhú* (Atractylodis Macrocephalae Rhizoma) and *shān yào* (Dioscoreae Rhizoma); for cold-heat leucorrhea, it is used with *chē qián zǐ* (Plantaginis Semen) and *huáng bó* (Phellodendri Chinensis Cortex).

5. 疮疡肿痛　本品能消肿排脓，止痛。用治疮疡初起，红肿热痛者，多与金银花、连翘等同用；治脓成难溃者，可与人参、黄芪、当归等同用。

(5) Sores and ulcers with swelling and pain *Bái zhǐ* has the effect of resolving swelling, expelling pus, and relieving pain. For sores and ulcers in early stage manifested as reddish swelling with hot pain, it is used in combination with *jīn yín huā* (Lonicerae Japonicae Flos) and *lián qiáo* (Forsythiae Fructus); for pus failing to erupt, it is used with *rén shēn* (Ginseng Radix et Rhizoma), *huáng qí* (Astragali Radix) and *dāng guī* (Angelicae Sinensis Radix).

【用法用量 / Usage and dosage】

煎服，3~10g。外用适量。

Decoction, 3-10g. Appropriate amount for external use.

【使用注意 / Precaution】

阴虚血热者忌服。

It should be avoided for those with yin deficiency and blood heat.

【现代研究 / Modern research】

本品主要含欧前胡素、异欧前胡素、别欧前胡素等香豆素类成分和挥发油等。具有解热、抗炎、镇痛、解痉、抑菌、抗癌等作用。

Bái zhǐ mainly contains coumarins such as imperatorin, isoimperatorin, alloimperatorin and volatile oil. It has antipyretic, anti-inflammatory, analgesic, antispasmodic, bacteriostatic, anticancer and other functions.

细辛 *Xì xīn* (Asari Radix et Rhizoma)
《神农本草经》
Shen Nong's Classic of the Materia Medica (Shén Nóng Běn Cǎo Jīng)

【来源 / Origin】

为马兜铃科植物北细辛 *Asarum heterotropoides* Fr.Schmidt var. *mandshuricum*（Maxim.）Kitag.、汉城细辛 *Asarum sieboldii* Miq. var. *seoulense* Nakai 或华细辛 *Asarum sieboldii* Miq. 的干燥根和根茎。前二种习称"辽细辛"，主产于辽宁、吉林、黑龙江；后一种习称"华细辛"，主产于陕西。夏季或初秋采挖，切段，生用。《中国药典》规定，含马兜铃酸Ⅰ（$C_{17}H_{11}NO_7$）不得过 0.001%，含挥发油不得少于 2.0%（ml/g），含细辛脂素（$C_{20}H_{18}O_6$）不得少于 0.050%。

Xì xīn is the dry root and rhizome of *Asarum heterotropoides* Fr.Schmidt var. *mandshuricum* (Maxim.) Kitag., *Asarum sieboldii* Miq. var. *seoulense* Nakai or *Asarum sieboldii* Miq., pertaining to Aristolochiaceae. The first two are known as *liáo xì xīn*, mainly produced in Liaoning, Jilin and Heilongjiang. The latter is known as *huá xì xīn*, mainly produced in Shaanxi. It is collected in summer or early autumn, cut slices and used in raw form. According to *Chinese Pharmacopoeia*, the content of aristolochic acid Ⅰ ($C_{17}H_{11}NO_7$) shall not exceed 0.001%, the content of volatile oil shall not be less than 2.0% (ml/g), and the content of asaronin ($C_{20}H_{18}O_6$) shall not be less than 0.050%.

【性味归经 / Medicinal properties】

辛，温。归心、肺、肾经。

Acrid and warm; act on heart, lung and kidney meridians.

【主要功效 / Medicinal efficacies】

解表散寒，祛风止痛，通窍，温肺化饮。

Release exterior and dissipate cold, expel wind and relieve pain, unblock the orifices, warm the lung and dissolve fluid retention.

【临床应用 / Clinical application】

1. 风寒表证 本品辛温发散，解表散寒，祛风止痛。用治风寒表证，恶寒发热，鼻塞流涕且头身疼痛较甚者，常与羌活、防风、白芷等同用。本品既入肺经散表寒，又入肾经除里寒，能达表入里，祛内外之寒。若治素体阳虚，外感风寒，恶寒发热、无汗、脉沉者，每与麻黄、附子同用。

(1) Wind-cold exterior syndrome *Xì xīn* is acrid, warm and dissipating, releasing exterior and dissipating cold, expelling wind and relieving pain. It treats wind-cold exterior syndrome manifested as aversion to cold, fever, stuffy nose with discharge, headache and body pain in combination with *qiāng huó*, *fáng fēng* and *bái zhǐ*. It enters lung meridian to dissipate external cold, as well as kidney to remove internal cold. For congenital yang deficiency and external-contraction wind-cold manifested as aversion to cold, fever, no sweat and deep pulse, it is often used with *má huáng* (Ephedrae Herba) and *fù zǐ* (Aconiti Lateralis Radix Praeparata).

2. 头痛，牙痛，风湿痹痛 本品止痛之力颇强，因其辛散温通，气香走窜而祛风散寒，故尤宜于多种寒痛证。若治少阴头痛，常配伍独活、川芎等。若治外感风邪之偏正头痛，常与白芷、川芎、羌活等同用。若治风冷牙痛，可单用，或与高良姜、冰片等同用。若治风寒湿痹，腰膝冷痛，可与独活、桑寄生、防风等同用。

(2) Headache, toothache, and wind-dampness impediment pain *Xì xīn* is high effective in relieving pain due to its acrid dissipating and warm dredging, fragrant qi moving around to expel wind and dissipate cold, so it is especially effective on cold pains. For Shaoyin headache, it is combined with *dú huó* (Angelicae Pubescentis Radix) and *chuān xiōng* (Chuanxiong Rhizoma); for external contraction of wind pathogen manifested as migraine or headache, it is combined with *bái zhǐ* (Angelicae Dahuricae Radix), *chuān xiōng* (Chuanxiong Rhizoma) and *qiāng huó* (Notopterygii Rhizoma et Radix); for toothache due to wind cold, it is used alone or combined with *gāo liáng jiāng* (Alpiniae Officinarum Rhizoma) and *bīng piàn* (Borneolum Syntheticum); for wind-cold-dampness impediment, cold pain in lower back and knees, it is used with *dú huó* (Angelicae Pubescentis Radix), *sāng jì shēng* (Taxilli Herba) and *fáng fēng* (Saposhnikoviae Radix).

3. 鼻鼽，鼻渊，鼻塞流涕 本品辛温升散，芳香透窍，能散风寒，宣通鼻窍。常用治鼻鼽、鼻渊等鼻科疾病之鼻塞、流涕、头痛，为治鼻鼽、鼻渊之良药，每与白芷、苍耳子、辛夷等同用。

(3) Allergic rhinitis, sinusitis, stuffy nose with discharge *Xì xīn* is acrid, warm, descending and dissipating, opening orifices with aromatics, dispersing wind-cold, and unblocking nasal orifice. It is often used to treat nasal diseases such as allergic rhinitis and sinusitis with stuffy nose, nasal discharge and headache with good effect, in combination with *bái zhǐ* (Angelicae Dahuricae Radix), *cāng ěr zǐ* (Xanthii Fructus) and *xīn yí* (Magnoliae Flos).

4. 寒痰咳喘 本品辛散温燥，入肺经，既能发散风寒，又能温肺化饮。若治外感风寒，水饮内停之恶寒发热、无汗、咳喘、痰多清稀者，可与麻黄、桂枝、干姜等配伍。若治寒痰停饮，咳嗽胸满，气逆喘急者，可与茯苓、干姜、五味子等同用。

(4) Cold phlegm and cough *Xì xīn* is acrid dissipating and warm drying, entering lung meridian to disperse wind-cold as well as warm lung and resolving fluid retention. For external contraction wind-cold and fluid retention manifested as aversion to cold, fever, no sweat, cough and dyspnea, and profuse diluted sputum, it is often combined with *má huáng* (Ephedrae Herba), *guì zhī* (Cinnamomi Ramulus) and *gān jiāng* (Zingiberis Rhizoma); for cold phlegm, fluid retention, cough, fullness in chest, qi counterflow and dyspnea, it is in combination with *fú líng* (Poria), *gān jiāng* (Zingiberis Rhizoma) and *wǔ wèi zǐ* (Schisandrae Chinensis Fructus).

【用法用量 / Usage and dosage】

煎服，1~3g。散剂每次服 0.5~1g。外用适量。

Decoction, 1-3g; powder, 0.5-1g; a proper amount for external use.

【使用注意 / Precaution】

气虚多汗、阴虚阳亢头痛、阴虚燥咳或肺热咳嗽者忌用。不宜与藜芦同用。

It should be contraindicated for those with profuse sweat due to qi deficiency, headache due to yin deficiency with yang hyperactivity, dry cough due to yin deficiency or lung-heat cough. It should not used with *lí lú* (Veratri Nigri Radix et Rhizoma).

【现代研究 / Modern research】

本品主要含挥发油，主要为细辛醚、甲基丁香酚、黄樟醚、α- 蒎烯、莰烯、香叶烯、柠檬烯等，尚含细辛脂素和痕量的马兜铃酸 I。具有解热、镇静、镇痛、抗炎、表面麻醉和浸润麻醉作用。此外，还有强心、扩血管、增加心肌收缩力、松弛支气管平滑肌等作用。

Xì xīn mainly contains volatile oil, mainly asarone, methyl eugenol, safrole, α-pinene, camphene, geralene, and limonene, and also contains asaronin and trace aristolochic acid I. It has the functions of antipyretic, sedative, analgesic, anti-inflammatory, superficial and infiltrative anesthesia. In addition, it can also strengthen the heart, expand blood vessels, increase myocardial contractility and relax the smooth muscle of bronchus.

第二节　发散风热药

Section 2　Wind-heat-dispersing medicinals

本类药物性味多辛凉，以发散风热为主要作用。主治风热表证及温病初起，症见发热、微恶风寒、头痛、口干、微渴，或有汗、舌边尖红赤、脉浮数等。部分药物兼有清头目、利咽喉、透疹、止痒、止咳等功效，还可用治目赤肿痛、咽喉肿痛、麻疹不透、风疹瘙痒和风热咳嗽等。

Wind-heat-dispersing medicinals are usually acrid in flavor and cool in property, so their major efficacy is to disperse wind-heat. They are used to treat wind-heat exterior syndrome and warm diseases at the early stage manifested as fever, a little aversion to wind-cold, headache, dry mouth, slight thirst, or sweating, red tongue edge and tip, and floating and rapid pulse. Some of the medicinals have the functions of clearing head and eyes, soothing throat, promoting eruption, relieving itching and cough, and can be used to treat red swelling pain of the eyes, sore and swollen throat, measles without adequate eruption, pruritus of rubella and wind-heat cough.

薄荷　*Bò he* (Menthae Haplocalycis Herba)
《新修本草》
Newly Revised Materia Medica (Xīn Xīu Běn Cǎo)

【来源 / Origin】

为唇形科植物薄荷 *Mentha haplocalyx* Briq. 的干燥地上部分。主产于江苏、浙江、湖南等地。夏、秋二季采割，晒干或阴干，切段，生用。本品揉搓后有特殊清凉香气，味辛凉。《中国药典》

规定，含挥发油不得少于 0.80%（ml/g），含薄荷脑（$C_{10}H_{20}O$）不得少于 0.20%；饮片含挥发油不得少于 0.40%（ml/g）。

Bò he is the dry aboveground part of *Mentha haplocalyx* Briq., pertaining to Labiatae, mainly produced in Jiangsu, Zhejiang, and Hunan Province, collected in summer and autumn, dried in the sun or in the shade, cut into sections, and used in raw form. After kneading, it has a special cool fragrance. It is acrid and cool in property. According to *Chinese Pharmacopoeia*, the content of volatile oil shall not be less than 0.80% (ml/g), menthol ($C_{10}H_{20}O$) no less than 0.20%, and the volatile oil in decotion pieces no less than 0.40% (ml/g).

【性味归经 / Medicinal properties】

辛，凉。归肺、肝经。

Acrid and cool. Act on lung and liver meridians.

【主要功效 / Medicinal efficacies】

疏散风热，清利头目，利咽，透疹，疏肝行气。

Scatter and dissipate wind-heat, clear head and eyes, soothe throat, promote eruption, soothe liver and move qi.

【临床应用 / Clinical application】

1. 风热表证，温病初起　本品辛凉发散，入肺达表，善于外散肌表的风热之邪，为发散风热药中发汗作用较强者。用治风热表证及温病初起之发热、微恶风寒、头痛等症，常与金银花、连翘等同用。

(1) Wind-heat exterior syndrome and warm diseases at the early stage　*Bò he* is acrid cool and dissipating, entering lung meridian to the exterior, good at wind-heat pathogen in the fleshly exterior, and has a strong effect among the wind-heat-dispersing medicinals. It treats wind-heat exterior syndrome and warm diseases at the early stage manifested as fever, a little aversion to wind-cold, and headache in combination with *jīn yín huā* (Lonicerae Japonicae Flos) and *lián qiáo* (Forsythiae Fructus).

2. 风热头痛，目赤多泪　本品轻清芳香，辛凉通窍，能疏散肝经风热而清利头目。用治风热上攻，头痛眩晕，目赤多泪，多与桑叶、菊花、蔓荆子等配伍。

(2) Wind-heat headache and red eye with profuse tears　*Bò he* is light, clear, frangrant, acrid, cool, dredging orifices, and can soothe and dissipate wind-heat of liver meridian to clear head and eyes. It treats up-attacking of wind-heat, headache, dizziness, and red eye with profuse tears in combination with *sāng yè* (Mori Folium), *jú huā* (Chrysanthemi Flos) and *màn jīng zǐ* (Viticis Fructus).

3. 咽喉肿痛　本品清轻凉散，又能利咽。用治风热壅盛，咽喉肿痛，常与牛蒡子、蝉蜕、桔梗等同用。

(3) Sort throat and pain　*Bò he* is light, clear, cool and dissipating and can soothe throat. It treats exuberance of wind-heat and sore throat in combination with *niú bàng zǐ* (Arctii Fructus), *chán tuì* (Cicadae Periostracum) and *jié gěng* (Platycodonis Radix).

4. 麻疹不透，风疹瘙痒　本品质轻宣散，有疏散风热、宣毒透疹、祛风止痒之功，用治风热束表，麻疹不透，常配伍蝉蜕、牛蒡子等。用治风疹瘙痒，可与荆芥、防风等同用。

(4) Measles failing to erupt, itching rubella　*Bò he* is light and dissipating, and has the functions of soothing and dissipating wind-heat, expelling toxin, promoting eruption, dispelling wind and stopping itching. It treats wind-heat fettering exterior and measles failing to erupt in combination with *chán tuì* (Cicadae Periostracum) and *niú bàng zǐ* (Arctii Fructus); for itching rubella, it is used with *jīng jiè* (Schizonepetae Herba) and *fáng fēng* (Saposhnikoviae Radix).

5. 肝郁气滞证　本品辛散入肝经，能疏散肝气之郁滞。用治肝气郁滞，胸胁胀痛，月经不调等，常与柴胡、香附等同用。

(5) Syndrome of liver depression and qi stagnation　*Bò he* is acrid dissipating and entering liver meridian, and has the function of soothing liver qi. It treats liver qi depression and stagnation, fullness and pain in chest and hypochondrium, and irregular menstruation in combination with *chái hú* (Bupleuri Radix) and *xiāng fù* (Cyperi Rhizoma).

【用法用量 / Usage and dosage】
煎服，3~6g，后下。薄荷叶长于发汗解表，薄荷梗偏于行气和中。

Decoction, 3-6g. It should be decocted later. *Bò he* leaf is effective in inducing sweating to release exterior while *bò he* stem is effective in moving qi and harmonizing the middle.

【使用注意 / Precaution】
体虚多汗者不宜使用。

It is not advisable for those with excessive sweating due to weak body.

【现代研究 / Modern research】
本品主要含挥发油，其主要成分为薄荷脑、薄荷酮、异薄荷酮、胡薄荷酮、柠檬烯等。具有发汗、解热、抗病毒、抗菌、抗炎、镇痛、抗氧化、利胆、促进透皮吸收作用。

Bò he mainly contains volatile oil, and its main components are menthol, menthone, isomenthol, I-pulegone , limonene, etc. It has the functions of sweating, antipyretic, antiviral, antibacterial, anti-inflammatory, analgesic, anti-oxidation, cholagogue, and transdermal absorption.

牛蒡子　*Niú bàng zǐ* (Arctii Fructus)
《名医别录》
Miscellaneous Records of Famous Physicians (Míng Yī Bié Lù)

【来源 / Origin】
为菊科植物牛蒡 *Arctium lappa* L. 的干燥成熟果实。主产于东北及浙江等地。秋季采收，打下果实，晒干，生用或炒用。本品气微，味苦后微辛而稍麻舌。《中国药典》规定，含牛蒡苷（$C_{27}H_{34}O_{11}$）不得少于5.0%。

Niú bàng zǐ is the dry and mature fruit of *Arctium lappa* L., pertaining to Asteraceae, mainly produced in northeast China and Zhejiang Province, collected in autumn, dried in the sun, and used in raw form or stir-fried. It has a slightly flavor and tastes slightly bitter, acrid and numb. According to *Chinese Pharmacopoeia*, the content of arctiin ($C_{27}H_{34}O_{11}$) should not be less than 5.0%.

【性味归经 / Medicinal properties】
辛、苦，寒。归肺、胃经。

Acrid, bitter and cool; act on lung and stomach meridians.

【主要功效 / Medicinal efficacies】
疏散风热，宣肺透疹，解毒利咽。

Scatter and dissipate wind-heat, diffuse lung and promote eruption, resolve toxin and relieve sore-throat.

【临床应用 / Clinical application】
1. 风热表证，温病初起　本品辛散苦泄，寒能清热，升散之中具有清降之性，虽发散之力不及薄荷，但长于解毒利咽，兼能宣肺祛痰，故常用于风热感冒，或温病初起之发热、咽喉肿痛或咳嗽痰多者，前者常与薄荷、金银花、桔梗等同用；后者多配伍桑叶、前胡、桔梗等。

(1) Wind-heat exterior syndrome and warm diseases at the early stage　*Niú bàng zǐ* is acrid dispersing and bitter discharging, cold in nature for clearing heat, ascending and dispersing with function of discharging and descending, less powerful than *bò he* but better at removing toxin and relieving sore throat, as well as ventilating lung and expelling phlegm. It treats common cold due to wind-heat or warm diseases at the early stage, manifested as fever, sore throat, or cough with profuse phlegm, the former in combination with *bò he*, *jīn yín huā* (Lonicerae Japonicae Flos) and *jié gěng* (Platycodonis Radix), while the latter with *sāng yè* (Mori Folium), *qián hú* (Peucedani Radix) and *jié gěng*.

2. 麻疹不透，风疹瘙痒　本品味辛透散，苦寒清热，既可入肺达表，宣散肌表风热；又可内清热毒，促使疹毒透发。用治风热外束，热毒内盛所致的麻疹不透或透而复隐，可与荆芥、薄荷同用。

(2) Measles failing to erupt, itching rubella　*Niú bàng zǐ* is acrid dispersing, bitter cold and clearing heat. It can reach the lung to the exterior to dissipate wind-heat of the fleshy surface as well as clear external heat toxin to promote eruption of measles. For measles failing to erupt or hiding again caused by wind-heat fettering externally and heat toxin exuberance inside, it can be used in combination with *jīng jiè* (Schizonepetae Herba) and *bò he*.

3. 热毒壅盛证　本品苦寒清降，有清热解毒、消肿利咽之效。用治热毒壅盛之咽喉肿痛、疮痈肿毒、痄腮、丹毒等，常与板蓝根、黄芩、黄连等同用。因其性偏滑利，兼滑肠通便，故上述病证兼有大便秘结者尤为适宜。

(3) Syndrome of heat-toxin exuberance　*Niú bàng zǐ* is bitter, cold, clearing and descending, and has the function of clearing heat and removing toxin, eliminate swelling and promote pharynx. For heat-toxin exuberance manifested as swollen and painful throat, ulcer and carbuncles, mumps, and erysipelas, it is often used with *bǎn lán gēn* (Isatidis Radix), *huáng qín* (Scutellariae Radix) and *huáng lián* (Coptidis Rhizoma). Because of the action of lubricating, and smoothing intestines defecate, it is especially suitable for the above-mentioned diseases with constipation.

【用法用量 / Usage and dosage】
煎服，6~12g。炒用可使其苦寒及滑肠之性略减。

Decoction, 6-12g. After being stir-fried, its properties of bitter and cold and its efficacy to smooth intestine will be slightly reduced.

【使用注意 / Precaution】
气虚便溏者慎用。

It should be used with caution for those with loose stool due to qi deficiency.

【现代研究 / Modern research】
本品主要含牛蒡子苷、牛蒡醇、硬脂酸、棕榈酸、胡薄荷酮等，尚含脂肪油、维生素 A、维生素 B$_1$ 及生物碱等。具有解热、镇静、镇痛、抗病毒、抗菌、降血糖、抗肿瘤等作用。

Niú bàng zǐ mainly contains arctiin, arctiol, stearic acid, palmitic acid, and menthol, and also contains fat oil, vitamin A, vitamin B$_1$ and alkaloids, etc. It has antipyretic, sedative, analgesic, antiviral, antibacterial, hypoglycemic, and antitumor functions.

蝉蜕　*Chán tuì* (Cicadae Periostracum)
《神农本草经》
Shen Nong's Classic of the Materia Medica (Shén Nóng Běn Cǎo Jīng)

【来源 / Origin】
为蝉科昆虫黑蚱 *Cryptotympana pustulata* Fabricius 的若虫羽化时脱落的皮壳。主产于山东、河北、河南等地。夏、秋二季收集，晒干，生用。本品气微，味淡。

Chán tuì is slough shed by the nymph of *Cryptotympana pustulata* Fabricius, pertaining to Cicadidae, mainly produced in Shandong, Hebei, and Henan Province, collected in summer and autumn, dried in the sun, and used in raw form. It has a slight flavor and tastes bland.

【性味归经 / Medicinal properties】

甘，寒。归肺、肝经。

Sweet and cold; act on lung and liver meridians.

【主要功效 / Medicinal efficacies】

疏散风热，利咽，透疹，明目退翳，解痉。

Scatter and dissipate wind-heat, relieve sore throat, promote eruption of papules, improve acuity of vision and remove nebula, and relieve convulsions.

【临床应用 / Clinical application】

1. 风热表证，温病初起，咽痛音哑　本品甘寒清热，轻浮宣散，能疏散肺经风热以祛邪解表。用治风热表证或温病初起，发热头痛者，可与薄荷、牛蒡子、前胡等同用。因其尤长于疏散肺经风热以宣肺利咽、开音疗哑，故尤宜于风热表证或温病初起之声音嘶哑、咽喉痒痛者，常与薄荷、牛蒡子、胖大海等同用。

(1) Wind-heat exterior syndrome, warm diseases at the early stage, sore throat and hoarse voice　*Chán tuì* is sweet, cold and clearing heat, light floating and dissipating. It has the functions of scattering and dissipating wind-heat of lung meridian to remove pathogens and release exterior. For wind-heat exterior syndrome or warm disease at the early stage with fever and headache, it is often used with *bò he, niú bàng zǐ* and *qián hú* (Peucedani Radix). Since it is especially effective in dissipating wind-heat of lung meridian to ventilate lung, relieve sore throat, and opening voice for hoarseness, it treats wind-heat exterior syndrome, warm diseases at the early stage, sore throat and hoarse voice, in combination with *bò he, niú bàng zǐ* and *pàng dà hǎi* (Sterculiae Lychnophorae Semen).

2. 麻疹不透，风疹瘙痒　本品轻宣透散，具有透疹、止痒之功。用治风热外束，麻疹不透，常与荆芥、牛蒡子、升麻等配伍。用治风疹瘙痒，可与荆芥、防风等同用。

(2) Measles failing to erupt and itching rubella　*Chán tuì* is light ventilating, eliminating and dissipating. It has the functions of promoting eruption and relieving itching. For wind-heat fettering externally and measles failing to erupt, it is often used with *jīng jiè* (Schizonepetae Herba), *niú bàng zǐ* and *shēng má* (Cimicifugae Rhizoma); for itching rubella, it is used with *jīng jiè* and *fáng fēng* (Saposhnikoviae Radix).

3. 目赤翳障　本品甘寒清热，入肝经，善能疏散肝经风热以明目退翳。用治风热上攻或肝火上炎之目赤肿痛、翳膜遮睛，常与菊花、决明子等同用。

(3) Red eyes and nebula　*Chán tuì* is clearing heat with sweet cold and entering liver meridian, and has the functions of scattering and dissipiating wind-heat of liver meridian to improve acuity of vision and remove nebula. For redness, swelling and pain of eyes, and nebula due to up-attacking of wind-heat or up-flaming of liver fire, it is often used with *jú huā* (Chrysanthemi Flos) and *jué míng zǐ* (Cassiae Semen).

4. 小儿惊风，破伤风　本品甘寒，既能疏散肝经风热，又可凉肝息风止痉。若治小儿急惊风，可与钩藤、僵蚕等同用。若治小儿慢惊风，可与全蝎、天麻等配伍。若治破伤风，可与僵蚕、全蝎、天南星等同用。

(4) Infantile convulsions and tetanus　*Chán tuì* is sweet and cold, dissipating wind-heat of liver meridian as well as cool liver, extinguishing wind and relieving convulsions. It treats acute infantile convulsions in combination with *gōu téng* (Uncariae Cum Uncis Ramulus) and *jiāng cán* (Batryticatus Bombyx); For chronic infantile convulsions, it is used with *quán xiē* (Scorpio) and *tiān má* (Gastrodiae Rhizoma); for tetanus, it is used with *jiāng cán*, *quán xiē* and *tiān nán xīng* (Arisaematis Rhizoma).

【用法用量 / Usage and dosage 】

煎服，3~6g。

Decoction, 3-6g.

【使用注意 / Precaution 】

孕妇慎用。

It should be used with caution for pregnant women.

【现代研究 / Modern research 】

本品主要含甲壳质、壳聚糖，尚含异黄蝶呤、蛋白质、氨基酸、有机酸、微量元素等。具有解热、镇静、抗惊厥、抗炎、镇咳祛痰、平喘止痉、抗过敏、免疫调节、增强子宫平滑肌收缩等作用。

Chán tuì mainly contains chitin, chitosan, isoxanthin, protein, amino acid, organic acid, trace elements, etc. It has the functions of antipyretic, sedative, anticonvulsant, anti-inflammatory, antitussive and expectorant, antiasthmatic and antispasmodic, antiallergic, immunomodulatory, and enhancing the contraction of uterine smooth muscle.

桑叶 *Sāng yè* (Mori Folium)
《神农本草经》
Shen Nong's Classic of the Materia Medica (Shén Nóng Běn Cǎo Jīng)

【来源 / Origin 】

为桑科乔木植物桑 *Morus alba* L. 的干燥叶。我国各地大多有野生或栽培。初霜后采收，晒干，生用或蜜炙用。本品气微，味淡、微苦涩。《中国药典》规定，含芦丁（$C_{27}H_{30}O_{16}$）不得少于0.10%。

Sāng yè is the dry leaf of *Morus alba* L., pertaining to Moraceae. There are wild or cultivated in most parts of China. It is collected after the first frost, dried in the sun, and used raw or honey-fried. It has a slight flavor and tastes bland with a little bitterness. According to *Chinese Pharmacopoeia*, the content of rutin ($C_{27}H_{30}O_{16}$) shall not be less than 0.10%.

【性味归经 / Medicinal properties 】

甘、苦，寒。归肺、肝经。

Sweet, bitter and cold; act on lung and liver meridians.

【主要功效 / Medicinal efficacies 】

疏散风热，清肺润燥，清肝明目。

Dispel wind-heat, clear lung, moisten dryness, pacify liver to improve vision.

【临床应用 / Clinical application 】

1. 风热表证，温病初起　本品甘寒质轻，轻清疏散，疏散风热作用较为缓和。因其兼能清肺热、润肺燥而止咳，故适宜于风热表证及温病初起之发热、微恶风寒、咽痒、咳嗽者，常与菊花、杏仁、桔梗等同用。

(1) Wind-heat exterior syndrome and warm diseases at the early stage　*Sāng yè* is sweet cold and light, scattering and dissipating wind-heat with moderate effect. It can clear lung heat as well as moistening lung dryness to stop cough, so is suitable for wind-heat exterior syndrome and warm diseases at the early stage manifested as fever, slight aversion to wind cold, itching throat and cough in combination with *jú huā* (Chrysanthemi Flos), *xìng rén* (Armeniacae Amarum Semen) and *jié gěng* (Platycodonis Radix).

2. 肺热咳嗽，燥热咳嗽 本品苦寒清泄肺热，甘寒凉润肺燥，对于肺热或燥热伤肺，咳嗽痰少，色黄而黏稠，或干咳无痰等皆可配伍使用。轻者可配伍杏仁、沙参、浙贝母等；重者常与石膏、麦冬等同用。

(2) Cough due to lung heat and cough due to dryness-heat *Sāng yè* is clearing lung heat with bitter cold, and moistening lung dryness with sweet cold. It treats lung heat or dryness-heat damaging lung, manifested as cough, scanty and sticky sputum of yellow color, or dry cough with no sputum. For the mild case, it is in combination with *xìng rén* (Armeniacae Amarum Semen), *shā shēn* (Adenophorae seu Glehniae Radix) and *zhè bèi mǔ* (Fritillariae Thunbergii Bulbus); for severe case, it is used with *shí gāo* (Gypsum Fibrosum) and *mài dōng* (Ophiopogonis Radix).

3. 头晕头痛，目赤昏花 本品既能疏散风热，又苦寒入肝，能清肝明目。用治风热上攻或肝火上炎之目赤肿痛、羞明多泪，常与菊花、决明子等同用。若治肝肾精血不足之眼目昏花、视物模糊，须配伍黑芝麻、枸杞子等同用。

(3) Dizziness, headache, red eyes and blurred vision *Sāng yè* is dissipating wind-heat as well as bitter cold entering liver to clear liver and improve vision. It treats up-attacking of wind-heat or up-flaming of liver fire, manifested as red eyes with astringent pain, photophobia and excessive tears, in combination with *jú huā* (Chrysanthemi Flos) and *jué míng zǐ* (Cassiae Semen). For essence and blood deficiency of liver and kidney, and blurred vision, it should be combined with *hēi zhī ma* (Sesami Nigrum Semen) and *gǒu qǐ zǐ* (Lycii Fructus).

【用法用量 / Usage and dosage】

煎服，5~10g。蜜炙用增强润肺止咳作用。

Decoction, 5-10g. The honey-fried can enhance the effect of moistening lung and relieving cough.

【现代研究 / Modern research】

本品主要含芦丁、槲皮素、异槲皮素、桑苷、牛膝甾酮、脱皮甾酮、桑叶多糖等。具有抗炎、抑菌、降血糖、降血脂、降血压、抗凝血、延缓衰老等作用。

Sāng yè mainly contains rutin, quercetin, isoquercetin, sangin, achyranthes bidentata sterone, desquasterone, mulberry leaf polysaccharide, etc. It has anti-inflammatory, bacteriostatic, reducing blood sugar, blood fat and blood pressure, anticoagulant, anti-aging functions.

菊花 *Jú huā* (Chrysanthemi Flos)
《神农本草经》
Shen Nong's Classic of the Materia Medica (Shén Nóng Běn Cǎo Jīng)

【来源 / Origin】

为菊科植物菊 *Chrysanthemum morifolium* Ramat. 的干燥头状花序。主产于浙江、安徽、河南等省。9~11月花盛开时分批采收，阴干或焙干，或熏、蒸后晒干，生用。药材按产地和加工方法的不同，分为"亳菊""滁菊""贡菊""杭菊""怀菊"。本品气清香，味甘、微苦。《中国药典》规定，含绿原酸（$C_{16}H_{18}O_9$）不得少于0.20%，含木犀草苷（$C_{21}H_{20}O_{11}$）不得少于0.080%，含3,5-*O*-二咖啡酰基奎宁酸（$C_{25}H_{24}O_{12}$）不得少于0.70%。

Jú huā is the capitulum of *Chrysanthemum morifolium* Ramat., pertaining to Asteraceae, mainly produced in Zhejiang, Anwei, and Henan Province, collected from September to November when it is in full bloom, dried in the shade or baked, or dried in the sun after being fumed or steamed, and used in raw form. According to different producing areas and processing methods, *jú huā* can be classified into *bó jú*, *chú jú*, *gòng jú*, *háng jú*, and *huái jú*. It has a fragrance, and tastes sweet and slightly bitter. According to *Chinese Pharmacopoeia*, the content of chlorogenic acid ($C_{16}H_{18}O_9$), luteolin ($C_{21}H_{20}O_{11}$) and 3, 5-*O*-dicaffeoylquinic acid ($C_{25}H_{24}O_{12}$) should not be less than 0.20%, 0.080% and 0.70% respectively.

【性味归经 / Medicinal properties 】

甘、苦，微寒。归肺、肝经。

Sweet, bitter and slightly cold; act on lung and liver meridians.

【主要功效 / Medicinal efficacies 】

疏散风热，平肝明目，清热解毒。

Dispel wind-heat, pacify liver to improve vision, clear heat and resolve toxins.

【临床应用 / Clinical application 】

1. **风热表证，温病初起**　本品疏散达表，微寒清热，功能疏散肺经风热，但发散表邪之力和缓。用治风热表证，或温病初起，发热、头痛、咳嗽等症，常与桑叶、薄荷、连翘等同用。

(1) **Wind-heat exterior syndrome, and warm diseases at the early stage**　*Jú huā* is dispersing external pathogen, and clearing heat with slightly cold. It has the functions of dissipating wind-heat of lung meridian and moderately exterior pathogens. For wind-heat exterior syndrome or warm diseases at the early stage, manifested as fever, headache and cough, it is often used with *sāng yè* (Mori Folium), *bò he* (Menthae Herba) and *lián qiáo* (Forsythiae Fructus).

2. **肝阳上亢证**　本品苦寒入肝经，能清泄肝热、平降肝阳。用治肝阳上亢，头痛眩晕，每与石决明、钩藤等同用。若治肝火上攻，眩晕头痛及肝经热盛、热极动风者，常与羚羊角、钩藤等同用。

(2) **Hyperactivity of liver yang**　*Jú huā* is bitter and cold entering liver meridian, and has the functions of clearing liver heat, and pacifying liver yang. For hyperactivity of liver yang with headache and dizziness, it is often combined with *shí jué míng* (Haliotidis Concha) and *gōu téng* (Uncariae Cum Uncis Ramulus). For up-attacking of liver fire with dizziness and headache, and heat exuberance of liver meridian and syndrome of extreme heat generating wind, it is used with *líng yáng jiǎo* (Saigae Tataricae Cornu) and *gōu téng* (Uncariae Cum Uncis Ramulus).

3. **目赤肿痛，眼目昏花**　本品既能疏散肝经风热，又能清泄肝经实热，兼能益阴，有明目之功，且清肝明目之效甚佳。常用治肝经风热或肝火上攻所致的目赤肿痛，羞明流泪，前者多与蝉蜕、僵蚕等同用；后者多与夏枯草、决明子等同用。若治肝肾精血不足，眼目昏花，视物不清，常配伍枸杞子、山茱萸、熟地黄等。

(3) **Redness, swelling and pain of eyes, and blurred vision**　*Jú huā* can not only disperse wind-heat of liver meridian but also clear excess heat, and replenish yin, with the function of clearing liver and improving vision. It treats red and swollen eyes with pain due to wind-heat of liver meridian or up-attacking of liver fire, manifested as photophobia and tearing, in combination with *chán tuì* (Cicadae Periostracum) and *jiāng cán* (Batryticatus Bombyx) for the former, and *xià kū cǎo* (Prunellae Spica) and *jué míng zǐ* (Cassiae Semen) for the latter. For essence and blood deficiency of liver and kidney with blurred vision, it is often combined with *gǒu qǐ zǐ* (Lycii Fructus), *shān zhū yú* (Corni Fructus) and *shú dì huáng* (Rehmanniae Radix Praeparata).

4. **疮痈肿毒**　本品有清热解毒之功。用治疮痈肿毒，可与金银花、甘草同用。因其清热解毒之力和缓，故临床应用较少。

(4) Sore, carbuncle and abscess *Jú huā* has the functions of clearing heat and resolving toxins. It treats sore, carbuncle and abscess in combination with *jīn yín huā* (Lonicerae Japonicae Flos) and *gān cǎo* (Glycyrrhizae Radix et Rhizoma). But the function is so mild that it is less used in clinic.

【用法用量 / Usage and dosage】

煎服，5~10g。

Decoction, 5-10g.

【现代研究 / Modern research】

本品主要含挥发油、绿原酸、3,5-*O*-二咖啡酰基奎宁酸、木犀草苷、维生素 A、黄酮素。具有抗炎、抑菌、抗病毒、降压、降血脂、免疫调节、抗肿瘤、扩张冠脉、增加冠脉血流量等作用。

Jú huā mainly contains volatile oil, chlorogenic acid, 3, 5-*O*-dicaffeoylquinic acid, luteolin, vitamin A and flavonoid. It has the functions of anti-inflammatory, bacteriostatic, antiviral, antihypertensive, hypolipidemic, immunomodulatory, anti-tumor, expanding coronary artery and increasing coronary blood flow.

柴胡　*Chái hú* (Bupleuri Radix)
《神农本草经》
Shen Nong's Classic of the Materia Medica (Shén Nóng Běn Cǎo Jīng)

【来源 / Origin】

为伞形科植物柴胡 *Bupleurum chinense* DC. 或狭叶柴胡 *Bupleurum scorzonerifolium* Willd. 的干燥根。前者主产于河北、河南、辽宁等地，习称"北柴胡"；后者主产于湖北、四川、安徽等地，习称"南柴胡"。春、秋二季采挖，干燥，切段，生用或醋炙用。本品气微香，味微苦。《中国药典》规定，含柴胡皂苷 a（$C_{42}H_{68}O_{13}$）和柴胡皂苷 d（$C_{42}H_{68}O_{13}$）的总量不少于 0.30%。

Chái hú is the dry root of *Bupleurum chinense* DC. or *Bupleurum scorzonerifolium* Wild., pertaining to Umbelliferae. The former is mainly produced in Hebei, Henan, and Liaoning Province, commonly called *běi chái hú*; the latter is mainly produced in Hubei, Sichuan, and Anhui Province, commonly called *nán chái hú*. It is collected in spring and autumn, dried, sliced, and used for raw or vinegar-fried. *Chái hú* is slightly fragrant and bitter. According to *Chinese Pharmacopoeia*, the total content of saikosaponin a ($C_{42}H_{68}O_{13}$) and saikosaponin d ($C_{42}H_{68}O_{13}$) should not be less than 0.30%.

【性味归经 / Medicinal properties】

辛、苦，微寒。归肝、胆、肺经。

Acrid, bitter and slightly cold; act on liver, gallbladder and lung meridians.

【主要功效 / Medicinal efficacies】

疏散退热，疏肝解郁，升举阳气。

Dissipate and relieve fever, soothe liver and relieve depression, and raise yang qi.

【临床应用 / Clinical application】

1. 表证发热，少阳证 本品辛散疏泄，微寒退热，能祛邪解表，尤长于退热。对于表证发热，风寒、风热皆宜。若治风寒表证，恶寒发热、头身疼痛，可与羌活、防风等配伍。若治风热表证，发热、头痛，常与菊花、薄荷等同用。此外，本品又善入少阳，疏散少阳半表半里之邪，为治少阳证之要药。用治伤寒邪在少阳，寒热往来、胸胁苦满、口苦咽干、目眩，常与黄芩同用。

(1) Exterior syndrome with fever, lesser yang syndrome *Chái hú* is dispersing with acrid and reducing heat with slightly cold. It has the functions of expelling pathogens and releasing exterior, especially removing fever. It treats exterior syndrome with fever regardless of wind-cold or wind-heat. For wind-cold exterior syndrome with aversion to cold, fever, headache and body pain, it can be combined with *qiāng huó* (Notopterygii Rhizoma et Radix) and *fáng fēng* (Saposhnikoviae Radix). For wind-heat exterior syndrome with fever and headache, it is used with *jú huā* (Chrysanthemi Flos) and *bò he* (Menthae Herba). In addition, *Chái hú* tends to enter Shaoyang to eliminate pathogen in the half-exterior and half interior, and it is an important medicinal for lesser yang syndrome. For cold pathogen in Shaoyang, manifested as alternating chills and fever, fullness and discomfort in chest and hypochondrium, bitter taste in the mouth, dry throat, and dizzy vision, it is combined with *huáng qín* (Scutellariae Radix).

2. 肝郁气滞证 本品辛行苦泄，善能疏肝解郁。常用治肝郁气滞所致的胸胁或少腹胀痛、情志抑郁、月经失调、痛经等，每与香附、川芎、白芍等同用。

(2) Liver depression and qi stagnation *Chái hú* is acrid moving and bitter discharging, and can soothe liver and relieve depression. It treats distending pain in chest, hypochondrium, lassitude, depression, menstrual disorders and dysmenorrheal induced by liver depression and qi stagnation in combination with *xiāng fù* (Cyperi Rhizoma), *chuān xiōng* (Chuanxiong Rhizoma) and *bái sháo* (Paeoniae Alba Radix).

3. 中气下陷证 本品入于脾胃，能升举其清阳之气。用治中气不足，气虚下陷所致的脘腹重坠作胀，食少倦怠，久泻脱肛，胃、子宫、肾等脏器下垂，常与人参、黄芪、升麻等同用。

(3) Syndrome of sinking of middle qi *Chái hú* can ascend clear yang qi of spleen and stomach. For bearing down and distention of abdomen, poor appetite and tiredness, lasing diarrhea leading to rectum prolapse, and prolapse of stomach, uterus and kidney, it is often in combination with *rén shēn* (Ginseng Radix et Rhizoma), *huáng qí* (Astragali Radix) and *shēng má* (Cimicifugae Rhizoma).

【用法用量 / Usage and dosage】

煎服，3~10g。疏散退热宜生用，疏肝解郁宜醋炙，升举阳气可生用或酒炙。

Decoction, 3-10g. It is used raw to disperse and relieve fever, fried with vinegar to soothe liver and relieve depression, and used raw or fried with wine to ascend yang qi.

【使用注意 / Precaution】

阴虚阳亢、肝风内动、阴虚火旺及气机上逆者忌用或慎用。

It should be contraindicated or cautious for those with yin deficiency and yang hyperactivity, internal stirring of liver wind, vigorous fire due to yin deficiency, and upward reversal of qi.

【现代研究 / Modern research】

本品主要含柴胡皂苷 a、柴胡皂苷 b、柴胡皂苷 d、柴胡皂苷 f 及柴胡皂苷元 E、柴胡皂苷元 F、柴胡皂苷元 G 等，尚含挥发油、多糖、植物甾醇和黄酮类等。具有解热、镇静、镇痛、镇咳、抗炎、降血脂、保肝、利胆、兴奋肠平滑肌、抑制胃酸分泌、抗溃疡、抗肿瘤、调节免疫等作用。

Chái hú mainly contains saikosaponin a, b, d, f and saikosapogenin E, F, G, and also volatile oil, polysaccharide, phytosterol and flavonoids. It has the functions of antipyretic, sedative, analgesic, antitussive, anti-inflammatory, hypolipidemic, hepatoprotective, cholagogic, stimulating intestinal smooth muscle, inhibiting gastric acid secretion, anti ulcer, anti-tumor, and regulating immunity.

葛根　*Gé gēn* (Puerariae Lobatae Radix)
《神农本草经》
Shen Nong's Classic of the Materia Medica (Shén Nóng Běn Cǎo Jīng)

【来源 / Origin】

为豆科植物野葛 *Pueraria lobata*（Willd.）Ohwi 的干燥根。主产于湖南、河南、广东等地。秋、冬二季采挖，切厚片或小块，干燥，生用或煨用。本品气微，味微甜。《中国药典》规定，含葛根素（$C_{21}H_{20}O_9$）不得少于 2.4%。

Gé gēn is the dry root of the legume *Pueraria lobata* (Willd.) Ohwi, pertaining to Leguminosae, mainly produced in Hunan, Henan, and Guangdong Province, collected in autumn and winter, cut into thick slices or small pieces, dried and used raw or simmered. It has a slight flavor and a slight sweet taste. According to *Chinese Pharmacopoeia*, the content of Puerarin ($C_{21}H_{20}O_9$) should not be less than 2.4%.

【性味归经 / Medicinal properties】

甘、辛，凉。归脾、胃、肺经。

Sweet, acrid and cool; act on spleen, stomach and lung meridians.

【主要功效 / Medicinal efficacies】

解肌退热，生津止渴，透疹，升阳止泻，通经活络，解酒毒。

Release flesh and relieve fever, promote fluid production to quench thirst, promote eruption, ascending yang and arrest diarrhea, dredge channels and activate collaterals, and resolve alcoholism.

【临床应用 / Clinical application】

1. 表证发热，项背强痛　本品辛凉升散，有解肌退热之功，凡是外感表证发热，无论风寒、风热，均可选用。用治风热表证，发热，头痛等，多与薄荷、菊花等同用。若治外感风寒，邪郁化热，发热重，恶寒轻，头痛无汗，目痛鼻干，口微渴，苔薄黄等，常与柴胡、黄芩等同用。本品既能发散表邪以退热，又善于缓解外邪郁阻、经气不利、筋脉失养所致的颈背强痛，故适宜于外感表证兼有项背强痛者，常与麻黄、桂枝等同用。

(1) Exterior syndrome with fever, rigid and painful neck and back　*Gé gēn* is ascending and dispersing with acrid cool, and has the functions of releasing flesh and relieving fever. It can be used for high fever of exterior syndromes due to external contraction either by wind-cold or wind-heat. For wind-heat exterior syndrome with fever and headache, it is used with *bò he* (Menthae Herba) and *jú huā* (Chrysanthemi Flos). For external contraction by wind-cold, pathogen accumulation transforming into heat with high fever, mild aversion to cold, headache, absence of sweating, eye pain and dry nose, slight thirst, and thin yellow fur, it is often used with *chái hú* (Bupleuri Radix) and *huáng qín* (Scutellariae Radix). *Gé gēn* can both disperse exterior pathogen to relieve fever and relieve the rigid and painful neck and back induced by external pathogen stagnation, disturbance of meridian qi, tendon and vessel malnutrition, so it is suitable for external-contraction exterior syndromes accompanied by rigid and painful neck and back in combination with *má huáng* (Ephedrae Herba) and *guì zhī* (Cinnamomi Ramulus).

2. 热病口渴，消渴　本品甘凉，能清泄胃热，生津止渴。用治热病津伤口渴，常与天花粉、知母等同用。若治内热消渴，口渴多饮，体瘦乏力，气阴不足者，可与黄芪、麦冬等配伍。

(2) Thirst due to warm diseases and diabetes　*Gé gēn* is sweet and cool, and has the functions of clearing stomach heat, promoting the fluid production and quenching thirst. It treats fluid consumption and thirst in combination with *tiān huā fěn* (Trichosanthis Radix) and *zhī mǔ* (Anemarrhenae Rhizoma).

For diabetes due to internal heat, manifested as thirst, excessive drinking, emaciation, lassitude, as well as deficiency of qi and yin, it is combined with *huáng qí* (Astragali Radix) and *mài dōng* (Ophiopogonis Radix)

3. 麻疹不透 本品有发表散邪，解肌退热，透发麻疹之功。用治麻疹初起，表邪外束，疹出不畅，常与升麻、薄荷、牛蒡子等同用。

(3) Measles failing to erupt *Gé gēn* has the actions of releasing exterior and expelling external pathogens, releasing flesh and relieving fever, and promoting the eruption of measles. It treats measles at the early stage, exterior pathogens fettering and measles without adequate eruption in combination with *shēng má* (Cimicifugae Rhizoma), *bò he* (Menthae Herba) and *niú bàng zǐ* (Arctii Fructus).

4. 脾虚泄泻 本品有升发清阳，鼓舞脾胃清阳之气上升而奏止泻痢之效。治疗脾虚泄泻，常与人参、白术、木香等同用。若治湿热泻痢，当与黄芩、黄连等同用。

(4) Diarrhea due to spleen deficiency *Gé gēn* has the functions of ascending and dispersing clear yang qi, promoting the clear qi of spleen and stomach to flow upward so as to stop diarrhea. It treats diarrhea due to spleen deficiency in combination with *rén shēn* (Ginseng Radix et Rhizoma), *bái zhú* (Atractylodis Macrocephalae Rhizoma) and *mù xiāng* (Aucklandiae Radix). It treats diarrhea due to dampness-heat in combination with *huáng qín* (Scutellariae Radix) and *huáng lián* (Coptidis Rhizoma).

5. 中风偏瘫，胸痹心痛，眩晕头痛 本品具有通经活络之功。用治中风偏瘫，胸痹心痛，眩晕头痛，可与三七、丹参、川芎等同用。

(5) Apoplectic hemiplegia, heart pain due to chest impediment, dizziness and headache *Gé gēn* has the functions of dredging channels and activating collaterals. It treats apoplectic hemiplegia, heart pain due to chest impediment, dizziness and headache in combination with *sān qī* (Notoginseng Radix et Rhizoma), *dān shēn* (Salviae Miltiorrhizae Radix et Rhizoma) and *chuān xiōng* (Chuanxiong Rhizoma).

6. 酒毒伤中 本品尚能解酒毒。用治酒毒伤中，恶心呕吐，脘腹痞满，可与紫苏叶、陈皮、枳椇子等同用。

(6) Alcoholic intoxication damaging the middle *Gé gēn* can resolve alcoholic toxin. It treats alcoholic intoxication damaging the middle manifested as nausea, vomiting, abdominal stuffiness and fullness in combination with *zǐ sū yè* (Perillae Folium), *chén pí* (Citri Reticulatae Pericarpium) and *zhī jǔ zǐ* (Hoveniae Semen).

【用法用量 / Usage and dosage】

煎服，10~15g。解肌退热、透疹、生津宜生用，升阳止泻宜煨用。

Decoction, 10-15g. It should be used raw for releasing flesh, relieving fever, and promoting eruption and fluid production, while used roasted for ascending yang and arrest diarrhea.

【现代研究 / Modern research】

本品主要含黄酮类成分葛根素、大豆苷、大豆素-4,7 二葡萄糖苷、葛根素 –7– 木糖苷等。具有解热、镇痛、抗炎、扩张冠状动脉、抗心肌缺血、改善心功能、改善脑循环、降血压、降血脂、抑制血小板聚集、抗肿瘤等作用。

Gé gēn mainly contains flavonoids: puerarin, daidzein, daidzein-4,7 diglucoside, and puerarin-7-xyloside. It has the functions of antipyretic, analgesic, anti-inflammatory, dilating coronary artery, anti myocardial ischemia, improving heart function, improving cerebral circulation, lowering blood pressure and blood lipid, inhibiting platelet aggregation, and anti-tumor.

升麻 *Shēng má* (Cimicifugae Rhizoma)
《神农本草经》
Shen Nong's Classic of the Materia Medica (Shén Nóng Běn Cǎo Jīng)

【来源 / Origin】

为毛茛科植物大三叶升麻 *Cimicifuga heracleifolia* Kom.、兴安升麻 *Cimicifuga dahurica*（Turcz.）Maxim. 或升麻 *Cimicifuga foetida* L. 的干燥根茎。主产于辽宁、吉林、黑龙江等地。秋季采挖，晒干，切片，生用或蜜炙用。本品气微，味微苦而涩。《中国药典》规定，含异阿魏酸（$C_{10}H_{10}O_4$）不得少于 0.10%。

Shēng má is the dry rhizome of *Cimicifuga heracleifolia* Kom., *Cimicifuga dahurica* (Turcz.) Maxim. or *Cimicifuga foetida* L., pertaining to Ranunculaceae, mainly produced in Liaoning, Jilin, and Heilongjiang Province, collected in autumn, dried, sliced, and used raw or honey-fried. *Shēng má* has a slight flavor, tastes slightly bitter and astringent. According to *Chinese Pharmacopoeia*, the content of isoferulic acid ($C_{10}H_{10}O_4$) should not be less than 0.10%.

【性味归经 / Medicinal properties】

辛、微甘，微寒。归肺、脾、胃、大肠经。

Acrid, slightly sweet and slightly cold; act on lung, spleen, stomach, and large intestine.

【主要功效 / Medicinal efficacies】

发表透疹，清热解毒，升举阳气。

Release exterior to promote eruption, clear heat and resolve toxin, and elevate yang qi.

【临床应用 / Clinical application】

1. 风热表证，温病初起　本品辛凉发散，有发表退热之功。用治风热表证或温病初起，发热、头痛等，可与薄荷、菊花等同用。若治风寒表证，发热、恶寒、头痛者，当与麻黄、白芷等配伍。

(1) **Wind-heat exterior syndrome, warm diseases at the early stage** *Shēng má* can disperse with acrid cool and has the function of releasing exterior and relieving fever. It treats wind-heat exterior syndrome, warm diseases at the early stage with fever and headache in combination with *bò he* (Menthae Herba) and *jú huā* (Chrysanthemi Flos). It treats wind-cold exterior syndrome manifested as fever, aversion to cold and headache, in combination with *má huáng* (Ephedrae Herba) and *bái zhǐ* (Angelicae Dahuricae Radix).

2. 麻疹不透　本品辛散发表，有透发麻疹之效。用治麻疹初起，透发不畅，常与葛根、白芍、甘草等同用。

(2) **Measles failing to erupt** *Shēng má* is acrid dispersing and releasing exterior with the function of promoting eruption of measles. It treats measles difficult to erupt at the early stage in combination with *gé gēn* (Puerariae Lobatae Radix), *bái sháo* (Paeoniae Alba Radix) and *gān cǎo* (Glycyrrhizae Radix et Rhizoma).

3. 热毒证　本品具有清热解毒之功，可用治多种热毒证。因其善解阳明热毒，故多用治胃火亢盛，牙龈肿痛、口舌生疮、咽肿喉痛等，常与黄连、石膏、丹皮等同用。若治风热疫毒上攻之大头瘟，头面红肿，咽喉肿痛者，常与黄芩、黄连、板蓝根等同用。若治疖腮肿痛，可与黄连、连翘、牛蒡子等同用。

(3) **Heat toxin syndrome** *Shēng má* is bitter and cool, and has the function of clearing heat and resolving toxins. It can be used to treat many kinds of heat toxin syndromes. Because it is effective

to clear heat toxin of Yangming meridians, it is often used to treat intense stomach fire manifested as swelling and pain of gums, aphtha and tongue sores, and sore throat in combination with *huáng lián* (Coptidis Rhizoma), *shí gāo* (Gypsum Fibrosum) and *dān pí* (Moutan Cortex). For swollen-head infection induced by up-attacking of wind-heat and epidemic toxin, manifested as redness and swelling of head, and swelling and pain in throat, it is in combination with *huáng qín* (Scutellariae Radix), *huáng lián* (Coptidis Rhizoma) and *bǎn lán gēn* (Isatidis Radix). For mumps, it is combined with *huáng lián* (Coptidis Rhizoma), *lián qiáo* (Forsythiae Fructus) and *niú bàng zǐ* (Arctii Fructus).

4. 中气下陷证　本品药性升浮，入脾胃经，能升举脾胃清阳之气，且升提之力强于柴胡。用治中气下陷所致的久泻脱肛，胃、子宫、肾等脏器下垂，常配伍黄芪、人参、柴胡等。

(4) Sinking of middle qi　*Shēng má* is ascending and floating in nature, entering stomach merdian to raise clear yang qi of spleen and stomach more powerfully than *chái hú* (Bupleuri Radix). It treats anorectal prolapse due to lasting diarrhea and prolapse of stomach, uterus and kidney, in combination with *huáng qí* (Astragali Radix), *rén shēn* (Ginseng Radix et Rhizoma) and *chái hú* (Bupleuri Radix).

【用法用量 / Usage and dosage】

煎服，3~10g。发表透疹、清热解毒宜生用，升阳举陷宜炙用。

Decoction, 3-10g. It should be used raw for releasing exterior and promoting eruption while be fried for elevating yang and raising the drooping.

【使用注意 / Precaution】

阴虚阳浮，气逆不降以及麻疹已透者忌用。

It should be contraindicated for those with yin deficiency with yang floating, qi counterflow without descending, and measles having erupted.

【现代研究 / Modern research】

本品主要含异阿魏酸、升麻碱 A~E、水杨酸、咖啡酸、升麻苦味素、升麻醇、升麻醇木糖苷、北升麻醇、升麻素、皂苷等。具有解热、抗炎、镇痛、抗菌、抗过敏、减慢心律、降低血压、抑制肠管和子宫平滑肌痉挛等作用。

Shēng má mainly contains isoferulic acid, cimicine A, B, C, D, E, salicylic acid, caffeic acid, and cimicifugin, cimicifugol, cimicifugol xyloside, north cimicifugol, cimicifugin, saponin, etc. It has the functions of antipyretic, anti-inflammatory, analgesic, antibacterial, antiallergic, slowing down the heart rate, lowering blood pressure, inhibiting the spasm of intestine and uterine smooth muscle.

其他解表药功用介绍见表 6-1。

The efficacies of other exterior-releasing medicinals are shown in table 6-1.

表 6-1　其他解表药功用介绍

分类	药物	药性	功效	应用	用法用量
发散风寒药	香薷	辛，微温。归肺、胃经	发汗解表，化湿和中，利水消肿	暑湿表证，水肿，小便不利	煎服，3~10g
	藁本	辛，温。归膀胱经	祛风，散寒，除湿，止痛	风寒表证，巅顶疼痛，风寒痹痛	煎服，3~10g
	荆芥炭	辛、涩，微温。归肺、肝经	收敛止血	便血，崩漏，产后血晕	煎服，5~10g
	荆芥穗	辛，微温。归肺、肝经	解表散风，透疹，消疮	感冒，头痛，麻疹，风疹，疮疡初起	煎服，5~10g

续表

分类	药物	药性	功效	应用	用法用量
发散风寒药	辛夷	辛，温。归肺、胃经	散风寒，通鼻窍	风寒头痛，鼻渊鼻鼽，鼻塞流涕	煎服，3~9g，包煎
	苍耳子	辛、苦，温；有毒。归肺经	散风寒，通鼻窍，祛风湿	风寒头痛，鼻渊鼻鼽，鼻塞流涕，风疹瘙痒	煎服，3~10g
发散风热药	蔓荆子	辛、苦，微寒。归膀胱、肝、胃经	疏散风热，清利头目	风热表证，头昏头痛，目赤多泪，牙龈肿痛，目暗不明，头晕目眩	煎服，5~10g
	淡豆豉	苦、辛，凉。归肺、胃经	解表，除烦，宣发郁热	感冒之寒热头痛，烦躁胸闷，虚烦不眠	煎服，6~12g

（张一昕　王茜　李丽）

题库

医药大学堂
WWW.YIYAODXT.COM

第七章 清 热 药
Chapter 7　Heat-clearing medicinals

 学习目标┆ Learning goals

　　1. 掌握　清热药在性能、功效、主治、配伍及使用注意方面的共性；石膏、知母、栀子、夏枯草、黄芩、黄连、黄柏、金银花、连翘、板蓝根、鱼腥草、蒲公英、射干、白头翁、地黄、玄参、牡丹皮、赤芍、青蒿、地骨皮的性能、功效、应用以及特殊的用法用量和特殊的使用注意。

　　2. 熟悉　清热药的分类；天花粉、淡竹叶、决明子、龙胆、苦参、大青叶、土茯苓、大血藤、山豆根、青黛、白花蛇舌草、白薇的功效、主治以及特殊的用法用量和特殊的使用注意。

　　3. 了解　清热药、清热泻火药、清热燥湿药、清热解毒药、清热凉血药、清虚热药及相关功效术语的含义；芦根、淡竹叶、竹叶、谷精草、密蒙花、青葙子、秦皮、白鲜皮、败酱草、野菊花、半边莲、马齿苋、穿心莲、紫花地丁、金荞麦、鸦胆子、垂盆草、马勃、木蝴蝶、半枝莲、水牛角、胡黄连、银柴胡的功效以及特殊的用法用量和特殊的使用注意。

　　1. Master the commonness of heat-clearing medicinals in efficacy, indications, property, compatibility and cautions; as well as the property, efficacy, application, special usage and dosage and special precautions of *shí gāo, zhī mǔ, zhī zǐ, xià kū cǎo, huáng qín, huáng lián, huáng bó, jīn yín huā, lián qiáo, bǎn lán gēn, yú xīng cǎo, pú gōng yīng, shè gān, bái tóu wēng, dì huáng, xuán shēn, mǔ dān pí, chì sháo, qīng hāo* and *dì gǔ pí*.

　　2. Familiar with the classifications of heat-clearing medicinals; and the efficacy, indications, special usage, dosage and special precautions of *tiān huā fěn, dàn zhú yè, jué míng zǐ, lóng dǎn, kǔ shēn, dà qīng yè, tǔ fú líng, dà xuè téng, shān dòu gēn, qīng dài, bái huā shé shé cǎo* and *bái wēi*.

　　3. Understand the definitions of heat-clearing medicinals, heat-clearing and fire-draining medicinals, heat-clearing and damp-drying medicinals, heat-clearing and detoxicating medicinals, heat-clearing and blood-cooling medicinals, deficiency-heat-clearing medicinals and related efficacy terms; and the efficacy, special usage and dosage and special precautions of *lú gēn, zhú yè, gǔ jīng cǎo, mì méng huā, qīng xiāng zǐ, qín pí, bái xiān pí, bài jiàng cǎo, yě jú huā, xióng dǎn, bàn biān lián, mǎ chǐ xiàn, chuān xīn lián, zǐ huā dì dīng, jīn qiáo mài, yā dǎn zǐ, chuí pén cǎo, mǎ bó, mù hú dié, bàn zhī lián, zǐ cǎo, shuǐ niú jiǎo, hú huáng lián* and *yín chái hú*.

凡以清泄里热为主要功效，常用于治疗里热证的药物，称为清热药。

Medicinals with the main function of clearing interior heat are called heat-clearing medicinals, which are usually used to treat interior heat syndrome.

清热药药性皆为寒凉，长于清泄里热，然其功效特点各有所长，具体来说，有清热泻火、清热燥湿、清热解毒、清热凉血及清虚热之区别。主治各种里热证，常见的有温热病气分证、温热病营血分证、脏腑热证、湿热诸证、痈肿疮毒以及虚热证等。部分药物还可用于外感表证、风湿痹证、水肿等兼有里热者。

Heat-clearing medicinals are usually cold and cool in nature and often used to clear interior heat. Specifically, their functions can be differentiated into clearing heat and draining fire, clearing heat and drying damp, clearing heat and detoxicating, clearing heat and cooling blood, as well as clearing deficient heat. They are indicated to treat various commonly encountered interior heat syndromes, such as qi aspect syndrome in warm-heat disease, blood aspect syndrome in warm-heat disease, heat syndrome of the viscera, damp-heat syndromes, carbuncle, swelling, sore and toxin, as well as deficient heat syndrome. Some medicinals are also applied to treat syndromes with interior heat, such as exogenous exterior syndrome, wind-damp *bì* syndrome and edema.

根据清热药的药性及功效主治差异，可分为清热泻火药、清热燥湿药、清热解毒药、清热凉血药和清虚热药五类。

According to their differences in property, efficacy and indication, heat-clearing medicinals can be classified into heat-clearing and fire-draining medicinals, heat-clearing and damp-drying medicinals, heat-clearing and detoxicating medicinals, heat-clearing and blood-cooling medicinals as well as deficiency-heat-clearing medicinals.

应用清热药时，必须针对热邪所在的部位、阶段及虚实不同，有针对性地选用不同的清热药进行治疗。同时应根据火热邪气的致病特点进行配伍，如火热易耗气伤阴、动血生风、易生肿疡等，应随证配伍益气养阴、生津润燥、凉血止血、息风止痉和解毒消肿药。若里热证兼有表证，应配伍相应的解表药以表里同治，或先解表后治里。里热兼有胃肠积滞者，应配伍泻下药。

When using heat-clearing medicinals, doctors must select different heat-clearing medicinals according to the locations and levels of pathogenic heat, and also the excessive or deficient nature of pathogens. Besides, proper compatibility should be made based on the characteristics of pathogenic fire-heat. For example, fire-heat tends to consume qi and damage yin, cause bleeding and produce wind, and give rise to swelling and sores. Therefore, medicinals with functions of reinforcing qi and nourishing yin, generating yin fluid and moistening dryness, cooling blood and stanching bleeding, extinguishing wind to arrest convulsion, as well as detoxicating and relieving swelling should be combined according to different syndromes. As for interior heat syndrome accompanied by exterior syndrome, proper exterior-releasing medicinals should be combined to treat the interior and exterior simultaneously, or to release the exterior first and then treat the interior; in case of interior heat with stagnation in the stomach and intestines, purgative medicinals should be combined.

清热药药性寒凉，易伤脾胃，脾胃虚弱、食少便溏者应慎用。在使用本类药时，亦须避免过用导致不良反应，如寒凉伤阳、苦寒败胃、苦燥伤阴、甘寒助湿等。

Heat-clearing medicinals are cold and cool in nature, and they are likely to impair spleen and stomach. So it should be used with caution for those with qi deficiency in stomach and spleen, manifested as poor appetite and loose stool.

第七章　清热药┊ Chapter 7　Heat-clearing medicinals

第一节　清热泻火药

Section 1　Heat-clearing and fire-draining medicinals

PPT

本类药物性味多苦寒或甘寒，以清泄温热病气分实热和脏腑实热为主要功效。主治温热病气分证，症见高热、汗出、烦渴甚至神昏谵语、脉洪大有力等。因作用部位不同，又分别能清肺、胃、心、肝等脏腑实热，适用于各脏腑的实热证。

These medicinals are mostly bitter-cold and sweet-cold, so their main efficacy is to clear excess heat in the qi level of warm-heat disease and viscera. They are mainly used to treat qi level syndrome in warm-heat disease, manifested as high fever, sweating, dysphoria and thirst, or even loss of consciousness and delirium speech, large and powerful pulse. They can also clear excess heat in the viscera, such as excess heat in the lung, stomach, heart and liver, etc.

石膏　*shí gāo* (Gypsum Fibrosum)
《神农本草经》
Shen Nong's Classic of the Materia Medica (Shén Nóng Běn Cǎo Jīng)

【来源 / Origin】

为含水硫酸钙纤维状结晶聚合体的矿石。主产于湖北、甘肃、四川等地。随时可采挖。生用或煅用。本品无臭，味淡。《中国药典》规定，含水硫酸钙（CaSO$_4$·2H$_2$O）含量不得少于95.0%。

Shí gāo pertains to anhydrite of sulfates, mainly containing hydrous calcium sulfate. It is mainly produced in Hubei, Gansu and Sichuan Province in China. It can be collected at any time. It is used in the raw form and ground into powder or calcined. It has a slight flavor and tastes bland. According to *Chinese Pharmacopoeia*, the content of hydrous calcium sulfate (CaSO$_4$·2H$_2$O) should be no less than 95.0%.

【性味归经 / Medicinal properties】

甘、辛，大寒。归肺、胃经。

Acrid, sweet and extremely cold; act on the lung and stomach meridians.

【主要功效 / Medicinal efficacies】

生用：清热泻火，除烦止渴；煅用：收湿、生肌、敛疮、止血。

Raw *shí gāo*: clear heat and drain fire, relieve vexation and thirst; calcined *shí gāo*: eliminate damp, engender flesh, close sore, stanch bleeding.

【临床应用 / Clinical application】

1. 温热病气分证　本品辛甘大寒，寒能清热泻火，甘寒除烦止渴，辛以解肌退热，为清泻肺胃气分实热之要药。适用于温热病邪在气分，高热、汗出、烦渴、脉洪大等，常与知母相须为用。

(1) **Qi level in warm-heat diseases** *Shí gāo* is acrid with effect of releasing the muscles and reducing fever, sweet and cold for relieving vexation and thirst, and its cold nature functions to clear heat and reduce fire. It is the most powerful medicinal to clear excess heat in the qi level of the lung and

stomach. It clears excess heat in the qi level in warm-heat diseases manifested as high fever, sweating, dysphoria, thirst, and surging pulse, in combination with *zhī mǔ* (Anemarrhenae Rhizoma) for mutual reinforcement.

2. 肺热喘咳　本品性寒入肺经，善清肺经实热，适用于邪热壅肺之咳逆喘促，常配伍麻黄、杏仁等。若治痰热咳嗽，多与浙贝母、瓜蒌、黄芩等同用。

(2) Cough and dyspnea due to lung heat　*Shí gāo* is cold and acts on the lung meridian. It is good at clearing excess heat in the lung meridian, and is suitable to treat cough and dyspnea due to lung heat in combination with *má huáng* (Ephedrae Herba) and *xìng rén* (Armeniacae Amarum Semen). To treat cough caused by coexistence of phlegm and heat, it is often combined with *zhè bèi mǔ* (Fritillariae Thunbergii Bulbus), *guā lóu* (Trichosanthis Fructus) and *huáng qín* (Scutellariae Radix).

3. 胃火牙痛，头痛　本品入胃经，又善清泻胃火。用治胃火亢盛的牙龈肿痛、头痛、咽肿口疮、口臭等，常与黄连、升麻等配伍。用治胃热消渴，常与生地、知母、麦冬等同用。

(3) Toothache and headache due to stomach fire　It acts on the stomach meridian and is effective in clearing stomach fire. To treat swollen and painful gums, headache, swollen throat and oral ulcer and fetid smell in the mouth, it is often combined with *huáng lián* (Coptidis Rhizoma) and *shēng má* (Cimicifugae Rhizoma). To treat *xiao kě* caused by consumption of body fluid due to up-steaming of stomach fire, it is often combined with *shēng dì* (Rehmanniae Radix), *zhī mǔ* (Anemarrhenae Rhizoma) and *mài dōng* (Ophiopogonis Radix).

4. 溃疡不敛，湿疹瘙痒，水火烫伤，外伤出血　本品煅后研末外用，有收湿、敛疮、生肌、止血之功，用治溃疡不敛，常与红粉配用。用治湿疹、湿疮，可配伍枯矾外用。用治水火烫伤，可与青黛配用。用治外伤出血，可单用研末外撒。

(4) Unhealing ulcer, eczema and itching, burn due to hot liquid or fire, and traumatic bleeding　Calcined *shí gāo* can be ground into powder for external application with functions of eliminating damp, engendering flesh, closing sore and stanching bleeding. To treat unhealing ulcer, it is often combined with *hóng fěn* (Oxydum Rubrum Hydrargyri). To treat eczema and itching, it can be combined with *kū fán* (Dehydratum Alumen) for external application. To treat burn due to hot liquid or fire, it can be used with *qīng dài* (Indigo Naturalis). It is ground into powder for external application to treat traumatic bleeding.

【用法用量 / Usage and dosage】

煎服，15~60g，宜打碎先煎；内服宜生用；外用多煅后研末。

Decoction, 15-60g. It should be broken and decocted first. The raw form is suitable for oral taking, while for external application, it can be calcined before grinding into powder.

【使用注意 / Precaution】

脾胃虚寒及阴虚内热者忌用。

It should be contraindicated for those suffering deficiency-cold of spleen and stomach and yin deficiency with internal heat.

【现代研究 / Modern research】

本品主要含含水硫酸钙，尚含有机物、硫化物及钛、铝、硅、铜等。具有解热、抗炎、抗病毒、降血糖、增强免疫、抑制神经应激能力、降低骨骼肌兴奋性、降低毛细血管通透性及促进骨缺损愈合等作用。

Shí gāo mainly contains hydrous calcium sulfate. It also contains organic substance, sulphide, titanium, aluminum, silicon and copper. It has the functions of relieving fever, antagonizing inflammation, antagonizing virus, lowering blood sugar, enhancing immunity, inhibiting the ability of nervous stress, reducing the excitability of skeletal muscle, lowering permeability of capillaries and strengthening the healing of bone defects.

知母　*Zhī mǔ* (Anemarrhenae Rhizoma)
《神农本草经》
Shen Nong's Classic of the Materia Medica (Shén Nóng Běn Cǎo Jīng)

【来源 / Origin】

为百合科植物知母 *Anemarrhena asphodeloides* Bge. 的根茎。主产于河北、山西等地。春、秋二季采挖。切段，生用或盐水炙用。本品味微甘、略苦，嚼之带黏性。《中国药典》规定，芒果苷（$C_{19}H_{18}O_{11}$）、知母皂苷 B Ⅱ（$C_{45}H_{76}O_{19}$）的含量分别不得少于 0.70% 和 3.0%。

Zhī mǔ is the rhizome of *Anemarrhena asphodeloides* Bge., pertaining to Liniaceae, mainly produced in Hebei and Shanxi Province in China. It is collected in spring and autumn, sliced, used raw or stir-fried with salt solution. It has a slight flavor, tastes slightly sweet and bitter, and is sticky in property. According to *Chinese Pharmacopoeia*, the content of mangiferin ($C_{19}H_{18}O_{11}$) and anemarsaponin B Ⅱ ($C_{45}H_{76}O_{19}$) should be no less than 0.70% and 3.0% respectively.

【性味归经 / Medicinal properties】

苦、甘，寒。归肺、胃、肾经。

Bitter, sweet and cold; act on the lung, stomach and kidney meridians.

【主要功效 / Medicinal efficacies】

清热泻火，滋阴润燥。

Clear heat and drain fire, nourish yin and moisten the dryness.

【临床应用 / Clinical application】

1. 温热病气分证　本品苦寒清热泻火，其清泻气分实热之功与石膏相似，且甘寒质润，又可滋阴润燥。善治温热病气分热盛，高热、烦渴、汗出，脉洪大者，常与石膏相须为用。

(1) Warm diseases with excess heat in the qi aspect　*Zhī mǔ* is bitter and cold for clearing heat and draining fire. Its efficacy of clearing excess heat in qi level is similar to that of *shí gāo* (Gypsum Fibrosum). It is sweet and cold with moistening nature, so it can also nourish yin and moisten the dryness. It is good at treating warm disease with excess heat in the qi level, manifested as high fever, thirst and dysphoria, sweating, large and powerful pulse in combination with *shí gāo* (Gypsum Fibrosum) for mutual reinforcement.

2. 肺热咳嗽，阴虚燥咳　本品苦甘而性寒，入肺经。既能清泻肺热，又能滋肺阴、润肺燥。用治肺热咳嗽，咳痰黄稠，常配伍黄芩、桑白皮等。用治阴虚燥咳、干咳少痰或无痰，常与川贝母、麦冬等同用。

(2) Cough due to lung heat, dry cough due to yin-deficiency　It is bitter and sweet with cold in nature and acts on the lung meridian. It can not only clear lung heat, but also nourish lung-yin and moisten dryness of the lung. To treat cough due to lung heat with yellow and thick sputum, it is often combined with *huáng qín* (Scutellariae Radix) and *sāng bái pí* (Mori Cortex). To treat cough due to deficiency of yin, it is often used with *chuān bèi mǔ* and *mài dōng*.

3. 胃热口渴，消渴　本品苦寒，能清泻胃火，甘寒又能滋养胃阴、生津止渴。用治胃热津伤、口渴，常与石膏、熟地黄、麦冬等同用。用治阴虚内热，消渴，津伤口渴或消渴引饮者，常配伍天花粉、葛根等同用。

(3) Thirst due to stomach heat, consumptive thirst It is bitter and cold with effect of clearing stomach fire. It is sweet and cold with action of nourishing and moistening stomach yin, as well as generating fluid to relieve thirst. To treat thirst caused by damage of fluid due to stomach heat, it is often combined with *shí gāo* (Gypsum Fibrosum), *shú dì huáng* (Rehmanniae Radix Praeparata) and *mài dōng* (Ophiopogonis Radix). To treat thirst due to damage of fluids or consumptive thirst caused by yin deficiency and internal heat, it is often combined with *tiān huā fěn* (Trichosanthis Radix) and *gé gēn* (Puerariae Lobatae Radix).

4. 骨蒸潮热　本品入肾经，能滋肾阴，退虚热。用治肾阴不足，阴虚火旺，骨蒸潮热，盗汗遗精等，常配伍熟地黄、黄柏等。

(4) Steaming bone and tidal fever It acts on the kidney meridian to nourish kidney yin and eliminate deficient heat. To treat steaming bone and tidal fever, night sweat and spermatorrhea due to exuberant fire caused by shortage of kidney yin, it is often combined with *shú dì huáng* (Rehmanniae Radix Praeparata) and *huáng bó* (Phellodendri Chinensis Cortex).

5. 阴虚肠燥便秘　本品能滋阴润燥以通便。用治阴虚肠燥便秘，常与生地黄、玄参、麦冬等同用。

(5) Constipation due to intestinal dryness caused by yin deficiency *Zhī mǔ* can nourish yin and moisten intestine to promote defecation. To treat constipation due to intestinal dryness caused by yin deficiency, it is often combined with *sheng dì huáng* (Rehmanniae Radix), *xuán shēn* (Scrophulariae Radix) and *mài dōng* (Ophiopogonis Radix).

【用法用量 / Usage and dosage 】

煎服，6~12g。

Decoction, 6-12g.

【使用注意 / Precaution 】

脾虚便溏者忌用。

It should be contraindicated for those suffering loose stool due to spleen deficiency.

【现代研究 / Modern research 】

本品主要含知母皂苷、薯蓣皂苷、芒果苷、异芒果苷等，尚含黄酮类、多糖类、生物碱类、有机酸等。具有解热、抗炎、抗病原微生物、免疫调节、降血糖、利胆、抗血小板聚集、抗肿瘤等作用。

It mainly contains anemarsaponin, dioscin, mangiferin and isomangiferin. It also contains flavonoids, polysaccharide, alkaloids and organic acids. It has functions of relieving fever, antagonizing inflammation, antagonizing pathogenic microorganism, immunoregulation, reducing blood sugar, promoting the action of gallbladder, anti-platelet aggregation and antitumor.

天花粉　*Tiān huā fěn* (Trichosanthis Radix)
《神农本草经》
Shen Nong's Classic of the Materia Medica (Shén Nóng Běn Cǎo Jīng)

【来源 / Origin 】

为葫芦科植物栝楼 *Trichosanthes kirilowii* Maxim 或双边栝楼 *T. rosthornii* Harms 的干燥根。主产于河南、山东、江苏等地。秋、冬二季采挖。切片，生用。本品无臭，味微苦。

Tiān huā fěn is the dried root of *Trichosanthes kirilowii* Maxim or *T. rosthornii* Harms, pertaining to Cucurbitaceae. It is mainly produced in Henan, Shandong and Jiangsu Province in China, collected in autumn and winter, cut into slices, used raw. It has a slight flavor and tastes slightly bitter.

【性味归经 / Medicinal properties 】

甘、微苦，微寒。归肺、胃经。

Sweet, slightly bitter and slightly cold; act on the lung and stomach meridians.

【主要功效 / Medicinal efficacies 】

清热泻火，生津止渴，消肿排脓。

Clear heat and drain fire, produce fluid to quench thirst, relieve swelling and expel pus.

【临床应用 / Clinical application 】

1. 热病烦渴　本品甘苦微寒，清泻气分实热之力较弱，但长于生津止渴，故治温热病气分热盛，津伤口渴者，常与石膏、知母等同用。若治表热证而见口渴者，可配伍发散风热药。

(1) **Irritation and thirst in febrile disease**　It is sweet, bitter and slightly cold with mild effect of clearing excess heat in qi level. But it is good at generating fluid to quench thirst. To treat thirst caused by exuberant heat in qi level of warm disease, it is often combined with *shí gāo* (Gypsum Fibrosum) and *zhī mǔ* (Anemarrhenae Rhizoma). To treat thirst accompanied by exterior heat syndrome, it can be combined with wind-heat-expelling medicinals.

2. 内热消渴　本品能清泻胃热，生津止渴。用治胃热伤津口渴，多与石膏、芦根等同用。治阴虚内热，消渴多饮，常配伍葛根、知母、五味子等。

(2) **Consumptive thirst due to internal heat**　It can reduce stomach heat, produce fluid to quench thirst. To treat thirst caused by damage of fluid due to stomach heat, it is often combined with *shí gāo* (Gypsum Fibrosum) and *lú gēn* (Phragmitis Rhizoma). To treat *xiāo kě* due to yin deficiency generating internal heat, it is often combined with *gé gēn* (Puerariae Lobatae Radix), *zhī mǔ* (Anemarrhenae Rhizoma) and *wǔ wèi zǐ* (Schisandrae Chinensis Fructus).

3. 肺热燥咳　本品入肺经，能清肺热，润肺燥。用治肺热咳嗽，咳痰黄稠，可与黄芩、浙贝母等同用。用治燥热伤肺，干咳无痰或痰少而黏者，常与沙参、麦冬等同用。

(3) **Dry cough due to lung heat**　It acts on the lung meridian to clear lung heat and moisten dryness of the lung. To treat cough, yellow and thick sputum due to lung heat, it is often combined with *huáng qín* (Scutellariae Radix) and *zhè bèi mǔ* (Fritillariae Thunbergii Bulbus). To treat dry cough without sputum or with little and sticky sputum due to impairment of lung by dry-heat, it is often combined with *shā shēn* (Adenophorae seu Glehniae Radix) and *mài dōng* (Ophiopogonis Radix).

4. 疮疡肿毒　本品苦寒，有清热解毒、消肿排脓之效。用治热毒炽盛，疮痈初起，红肿热痛，或脓成未溃者，常与金银花、白芷、穿山甲等同用。

(4) **Sores and ulcers, swelling and toxin**　*Tiān huā fěn* is bitter and cold with effect of clearing heat and relieving toxin, relieving swelling and expelling pus. It treats sores and ulcers in the early stage with red, swollen and heat-painful skin by preventing the formation of pus or expelling pus to relieve sores, in combination with *jīn yín huā* (Lonicerae Japonicae Flos), *bái zhǐ* (Angelicae Dahuricae Radix) and *chuān shān jiǎ* (Manitis Squama).

【用法用量 / Usage and dosage 】

煎服，10~15g。外用适量。

Decoction, 10-15g. An appropriate amount for external application.

【使用注意 / Precaution 】

孕妇慎用。不宜与川乌、制川乌、草乌、制草乌、附子同用。

It should be used with caution for pregnant women. It should not be used together with *chuān wū*

(Aconiti Radix), *zhì chuān wū* (Aconiti Radix Praeparata), *cǎo wū* (Aconiti Kusnezoffii Radix), *zhì cǎo wū* (Aconiti Kusnezoffii Radix Praeparata) and *fù zǐ* (Aconiti Lateralis Radix Praeparata).

【现代研究 / Modern research】

本品主要含天花粉蛋白、α-羟甲基丝氨酸、L-天冬氨酸、核糖、阿拉伯糖、泻根醇酸、植物凝集素等。具有降血糖、抗菌、抗病毒、增强免疫、抗肿瘤、抗早孕及引产等作用。

Tiān huā fěn mainly contains trichosanthin, α-hydroxymethylserine, L-aspartic acid, ribose, arabinose, bryonolic acid and phytoagglutinins. It has functions of reducing blood sugar, antibacterial, antivirus, improving the immune function of organism, antitumor, anti early pregnancy and inducing labor.

栀子 *Zhī zǐ* (Gardeniae Fructus)
《神农本草经》
Shen Nong's Classic of the Materia Medica (Shén Nóng Běn Cǎo Jīng)

【来源 / Origin】

为茜草科植物栀子 *Gardenia jasminoides* Ellis 的成熟果实。主产于长江以南各地。9~11 月采收。生用或炒焦用。本品气微，味微酸而苦。《中国药典》规定，含栀子苷（$C_{17}H_{24}O_{10}$）不得少于1.8%；饮片不得少于 1.5%。

Zhī zǐ is the ripe fruit of *Gardenia jasminoides* Ellis, pertaining to Rubiaceae. It is mainly produced in the south areas of the Yangtze River and is collected from September to November, used raw or stir-fried to scorch. It has a slight flavor, and tastes slightly sour and bitter. According to *Chinese Pharmacopoeia*, the content of geniposide ($C_{17}H_{24}O_{10}$) should be no less than 1.8%, and decoction no less than 1.5%.

【性味归经 / Medicinal properties】

苦，寒。归心、肝、肺、胃、三焦经。

Bitter and cold; act on the heart, liver, lung, stomach and triple energizer meridians.

【主要功效 / Medicinal efficacies】

泻火除烦，清热利湿，凉血解毒；外用消肿止痛。

Drain fire and relieve vexation, clear heat and drain damp, cool the blood and resolve toxin, relieve swelling and pain for external application.

【临床应用 / Clinical application】

1. 热病心烦　本品苦寒清泄之力较强，善于清心火而除烦，为治热病心烦、躁扰不宁之要药，常与淡豆豉同用。用治热病火毒炽盛，高热烦躁，神昏谵语，常与黄芩、黄连等同用。

(1) Vexation in warm disease　It is bitter and cold with strong effect of clearing and draining. It is good at clearing heart fire to relieve vexation. Which serves as an essential medicinal to treat dysphoria and restlessness caused by warm disease, and is often combined with *dàn dòu chǐ* (Sojae Semen Praeparatum). To treat high fever, vexation, loss of consciousness and delirium speech caused by exuberant fire toxin of warm disease, it is often combined with *huáng qín* (Scutellariae Radix) and *huáng lián* (Coptidis Rhizoma).

2. 心、肝、胃热证　本品能清泻三焦之火，但以心、肝、胃经为主，故常用于心、肝、胃热诸证。用治热扰心神，心胸烦闷，燥热不宁，甚至狂言乱语，常配伍黄连、连翘等。用治肝热上炎，目赤肿痛，烦躁易怒，常配伍龙胆草、大黄等。用治胃火上炎，口舌生疮，或咽喉、牙龈肿痛者，可与黄连、石膏等同用。

(2) Heat syndrome of the heart, liver and stomach　*Zhī zǐ* can clear fire of triple energizer, which mainly centers on the the heart, liver and stomach meridians. So it is usually used to treat various morbid conditions caused by heat syndrome of the heart, liver and stomach. To treat vexation, tight chest, restlessness or even manic raving due to heat disturbing the mind, it is often combined with *huáng lián* (Coptidis Rhizoma) and *lián qiáo* (Forsythiae Fructus). To treat reddish, painful and swollen eyes, irritation and dysphoria due to upward flaming of liver heat, it is often combined with *lóng dǎn cǎo* (Gentianae Radix et Rhizoma) and *dà huáng* (Rhei Radix et Rhizoma). To treat sores in the mouth and tongue, or swollen throat, swollen and painful gum caused by upward flaming of stomach fire, it is often used with *huáng lián* (Coptidis Rhizoma) and *shí gāo* (Gypsum Fibrosum).

3. 湿热黄疸，热淋涩痛 本品苦寒沉降，通利三焦，能导湿热从小便而出，具有清利湿热、退黄通淋之功。用治湿热黄疸，常配伍茵陈、青蒿、大黄等。用治热淋涩痛或血淋，常与车前子、木通等同用。

(3) Jaundice due to damp-heat, strangury with difficult and painful urination It is bitter and cold with sinking and descending effect. It can remove damp-heat through urination to clear damp-heat in the triple energizer. So it has efficacies of clearing heat and draining damp, as well as removing jaundice and treating stranguria. To treat jaundice due to damp-heat, it is often combined with *yīn chén* (Artemisiae Scopariae Herba), *qīng hāo* (Artemisiae Annuae Herba) and *dà huáng* (Rhei Radix et Rhizoma). To treat heat strangury with astringent pain or blood strangury, it is used with *chē qián zǐ* (Plantaginis Semen) and *mù tōng* (Akebiae Caulis).

4. 血热出血 本品入血分，既能清血分之热，又有止血之功。用治血热妄行所致的多种出血，如吐血、咯血、衄血、尿血等，常与白茅根、生地黄、侧柏叶等同用。

(4) Bleeding due to blood heat It acts on blood level. It can not only clear heat in blood aspect, but also stop bleeding. To treat various hemorrhages, such as hematemesis, hemoptysis, epistaxis and hematuria caused by blood heat, it is often combined with *bái máo gēn* (Imperatae Rhizoma), *shēng dì huáng* (Rehmanniae Radix) and *cè bǎi yè* (Platycladi Cacumen).

5. 热毒疮疡 本品苦寒，有清热泻火、凉血解毒之功。用治热毒疮疡，红肿热痛，常与金银花、连翘、大黄等同用。

(5) Sores and ulcers due to heat toxin It is bitter and cold with effect of clearing heat and draining fire, cooling blood and removing toxin. To treat sores and ulcers due to heat toxin with symptoms of red, swelling, heat and pain, it is often combined with *jīn yín huā* (Lonicerae Japonicae Flos), *lián qiáo* (Forsythiae Fructus) and *dà huáng* (Rhei Radix et Rhizoma).

6. 扭挫伤痛 本品外用能消肿止痛，用治扭挫伤痛，可用生栀子粉与黄酒调糊外敷。

(6) Sprain and contusion *Zhī zǐ* has efficacy of relieving swelling and pain for external use. Its powder can be mixed with yellow wine into paste to treat sprain and contusion.

【用法用量 / Usage and dosage】
煎服，6~10g。外用生品适量，研末调敷。本品炒焦长于止血，多用于血热出血。

Decoction, 6-10g. The amount of raw powder should be proper for external application. The *zhī zǐ* stir-fried to scorch is superior in stop bleeding, and is mostly used in bleeding caused by blood heat.

【使用注意 / Precaution】
脾虚便溏者忌用。

It should be contraindicated in those suffering loose stool due to spleen deficiency.

【现代研究 / Modern research】
本品主要含栀子苷（京尼平苷）、去羟栀子苷、藏红花素、藏红花酸、栀子素、绿原酸以及有机酸、挥发油、多糖、胆碱、多种微量元素等。具有解热、抗炎、镇静、镇痛、保肝、利胆、抗菌、抗内毒素、抗胰腺炎、抗病毒等作用。

Zhī zǐ mainly contains geniposide, gardenoside, crocin, potassium, gardenin, chlorogenic acid and organic acid, volatile oil, polysaccharide, choline and various trace elements. It has the functions of relieving fever, antagonizing inflammation, tranquilizing, relieving pain, protecting liver, promoting gallbladder function, inhibiting bacteria, antiendotoxin, and enhancing pancreatic secretion and antivirus.

夏枯草　*Xià kū cǎo* (Prunellae Spica)
《神农本草经》
Shen Nong's Classic of the Materia Medica (Shén Nóng Běn Cǎo Jīng)

【来源 / Origin】

为唇形科植物夏枯草 *Prunella vulgaris* L. 的果穗。我国各地均产。夏季采收。生用。本品气微清香，味淡。《中国药典》规定，迷迭香酸（$C_{18}H_{16}O_8$）含量不得少于 0.20%。

Xià kū cǎo is the spike of *Prunella vulgaris* L., pertaining to Labiatae, and is produced in all parts of China. It is collected in summer, and used raw. *Xià kū cǎo* has a light flavor, tastes bland. According to *Chinese Pharmacopoeia*, the content of rosmarinicacid ($C_{18}H_{16}O_8$) should be no less than 0.20%.

【性味归经 / Medicinal properties】

苦、辛，寒。归肝、胆经。

Bitter, acrid and cold; act on the liver and gallbladder meridians.

【主要功效 / Medicinal efficacies】

清肝泻火，明目，散结消肿。

Clear liver heat and drain fire, improve vision, dissipate masses and subside swelling.

【临床应用 / Clinical application】

1. 目赤肿痛，头痛眩晕　本品苦寒清降，入肝经，善于清热泻火，清肝明目。用治肝火上炎，目赤肿痛，常与菊花、决明子等同用。用治肝阴不足，目珠疼痛，至夜尤甚者，当与枸杞子、当归、熟地黄等同用。用治肝火上炎或肝阳上亢之头痛眩晕者，应与石决明、钩藤等同用。

(1) Red eyes with swelling and pain, headache and dizziness　*Xià kū cǎo* is bitter and cold for clearing and descending and acts on liver meridian. It is suitable to clear heat and reduce fire, as well as clear liver fire to improve vision. To treat reddish, swollen and painful eyes due to upward flaming of liver fire, it is often combined with *jú huā* (Chrysanthemi Flos) and *jué míng zǐ* (Cassiae Semen). To treat eyeball pain and even worsened at night due to liver yin deficiency, it is often combined with *gǒu qǐ zǐ* (Lycii Fructus), *dāng guī* (Angelicae Sinensis Radix) and *shú dì huáng* (Rehmanniae Radix Praeparata). To treat headache and dizziness due to upward flaming of liver fire or hyperactivity of liver yang, it should be used with *shí jué míng* (Haliotidis Concha) and *gōu téng* (Uncariae Cum Uncis Ramulus).

2. 瘰疬，瘿瘤、乳痈、乳癖　本品辛能散结，苦寒泄热，具有清肝泻火、散结消肿之效。用治肝郁化火，痰火郁结之瘰疬，常与浙贝母、玄参等同用。用治瘿瘤，常与昆布、玄参等同用。用治乳痈、乳癖、乳房胀痛，常配伍金银花、蒲公英、浙贝母等。

(2) Scrofula, goiter, mastitis and mammary hyperplasia　It is acrid for dissipating masses and bitter and cold for reducing fire. Thus, it has efficacies of clearing liver heat and draining liver fire, dissipating masses and resolving swelling. To treat scrofula caused by liver constraint transforming into fire and accumulation of phlegm and fire, it is often combined with *zhè bèi mǔ* (Fritillariae Thunbergii Bulbus) and *xuán shēn* (Scrophulariae Radix). It is often combined with *kūn bù* (Laminariae Thallus)

and *xuán shēn* (Scrophulariae Radix) to treat goiter. For mastitis, mammary hyperplasia and mammary distension and pain, it is usually used with *jīn yín huā* (Lonicerae Japonicae Flos), *pú gōng yīng* (Taraxaci Herba) and *zhè bèi mǔ* (Fritillariae Thunbergii Bulbus).

【用法用量 / Usage and dosage】
煎服，9~15g。
Decoction, 9-15g.

【使用注意 / Precaution】
脾胃虚弱者慎用。
It should be used with caution for those suffering deficiency of spleen and stomach.

【现代研究 / Modern research】
本品主要含迷迭香酸、齐墩果酸、熊果酸、芦丁、木犀草素、矢车菊素、甾类、香豆素类、挥发油等。具有抗病原微生物、抗病毒、降血压、抗炎、降血糖、抗肿瘤等作用。

Xià kū cǎo mainly contains rosmarinicacid, uosolic acid, rutinum, luteolin, cyanidin, steroids, coumarins and volatile oil. It has functions of antipathogenic microorganism, antivirus, lowering blood pressure, antagonizing inflammation, lowering blood sugar and antitumor.

决明子　*Jué míng zǐ* (Cassiae Semen)
《神农本草经》
Shen Nong's Classic of the Materia Medica (Shén Nóng Běn Cǎo Jīng)

【来源 / Origin】
为豆科植物决明 *Cassia obtusifolia* L.、小决明 *Cassia. tora* L. 的成熟种子。我国各地均有栽种。秋季采收。生用或炒用。本品气微，味微苦。《中国药典》规定，大黄酚（$C_{15}H_{10}O_4$）和橙黄决明素（$C_{17}H_{14}O_7$）的含量分别不得少于 0.20% 和 0.080%。

Jué míng zǐ is the mature seed of *Cassia obtusifolia* L. or *Cassia. tora* L., pertaining to Leguminosae, mainly produced in all parts of China. It is collected in autumn, used raw or stir-fried. It has a slight flavor and tastes slightly bitter. According to *Chinese Pharmacopoeia*, the content of chrysophanol ($C_{15}H_{10}O_4$) and aurantio-obtusin ($C_{17}H_{14}O_7$) should be no less than 0.20% and 0.080% respectively.

【性味归经 / Medicinal properties】
甘、苦、咸，微寒。归肝、大肠经。
Sweet, bitter, salty and slightly cold; act on the liver and large intestine meridians.

【主要功效 / Medicinal efficacies】
清肝明目，润肠通便。
Clear liver heat and improve vision, moisten the intestines to promote defecation.

【临床应用 / Clinical application】
1. 目赤肿痛，视物昏花　本品苦寒泄热，甘咸益阴，主入肝经，既能清泄肝火，又能益肝阴，为明目佳品，虚实目疾，均可应用。用治肝火上炎，目赤涩痛，羞明多泪等，常配伍黄芩、赤芍、木贼等。用治风热上攻之目赤疼痛，常配伍菊花、桑叶等。若肝肾阴亏，视物昏花，目暗不明，常与山茱萸、枸杞子、熟地黄等配伍。

(1) Red eyes with swelling and pain, blurred vision　*Jué míng zǐ* is bitter and cold for reducing heat, sweet and salty for nourishing yin, and acts on the liver meridian. It can not only clear liver fire, but also nourish liver yin, which serves as an essential medicinal to improve vision. It can be used to treat disorders of the eyes without considering deficiency or excess type. To treat red and swelling eyes with pain, photophobia and profuse tears caused by upward flaming of liver fire, it is often used with *huáng qín* (Scutellariae Radix), *chì sháo* (Paeoniae Rubra Radix) and *mù zéi* (Equiseti Hiemalis Herba). To treat red eyes with pain due to wind-heat attacking the upper, it is often combined with *jú huā* (Chrysanthemi Flos) and *sāng yè* (Mori Folium). To treat blurred vision and dim vision caused by deficiency of liver-kidney yin, it is often combined with *shān zhū yú* (Corni Fructus), *gǒu qǐ zǐ* (Lycii Fructus) and *shú dì huáng* (Rehmanniae Radix Praeparata).

2. 头痛眩晕 本品既能清泄肝火，又能平抑肝阳，用治肝火上炎或肝阳上亢之头痛眩晕，常与夏枯草、菊花、钩藤等同用。

(2) Headache and dizziness *Jué míng zǐ* has efficacies of clearing liver fire and soothing liver yang. To treat headache and dizziness caused by upward flaming of liver fire or hyperactivity of liver yang, it is combined with *xià kū cǎo* (Prunellae Spica), *jú huā* (Chrysanthemi Flos) and *gōu téng* (Uncariae Cum Uncis Ramulus).

3. 肠燥便秘 本品味甘咸质润，入大肠经，能清热润肠通便，用治肠燥津亏，大便秘结，可与火麻仁、瓜蒌仁等同用。

(3) Constipation due to intestinal dryness It is sweet and salty with moistening nature and acts on the large intestine. It has efficacy of clearing heat and moistening the intestine to promote defecation. For constipation due to intestinal dryness and shortage of fluid, it is used with *huǒ má rén* (Cannabis Fructus) and *guā lóu rén* (Trichosanthis Semen).

【 用法用量 / Usage and dosage 】

煎服，9~15g。用于润肠通便，不宜久煎。

Decoction, 9-15g. For moistening the intestines to promote defecation, it is not allowed to be over-decocted.

【 使用注意 / Precaution 】

脾虚便溏者忌用。

It should be contraindicated in those suffering loose stool due to spleen deficiency.

【 现代研究 / Modern research 】

本品主要含大黄酚、黄素甲醚、大黄素、决明子素、芦荟大黄素、大黄酸等蒽醌类化合物，尚含脂肪酸、甾醇、糖类等。具有降血压、泻下、降血脂、抗动脉粥样硬化、抗血小板聚集、保肝、免疫调节作用。

Jué míng zǐ mainly contains anthraquinones, such as chrysophanol, flavin methyl ether, emodin, obtusifolin, aloeemodin, rhein. It also contains fatty acid, sterol and carbohydrate. It has the functions of lowering blood pressure, purgation, lowering blood fat, anti-arteriosclerosis, antiplatelet aggregation, protecting liver and regulating immune system.

第二节　清热燥湿药

Section 2　Heat-clearing and damp-drying medicinals

PPT

本类药物性味多苦寒，以清热燥湿为主要功效。主治湿热病证。湿热病证在临床上表现比较复杂，因湿热侵袭机体不同部位，故有多种临床表现。如湿温或暑湿之身热不扬，胸脘痞闷，小便短赤；脾胃湿热之脘腹胀满，恶心呕吐；大肠湿热之泄泻、痢疾；肝胆湿热之黄疸尿赤，胁肋疼痛，耳肿流脓；下焦湿热之带下色黄，热淋涩痛。若湿热流注关节，可见关节红肿热痛；若湿热浸淫肌肤，则见湿疹、湿疮等。本类药物常兼有清热泻火和清热解毒的功效，还可用治脏腑气分实热和疮痈肿痛等热毒证。

Heat-clearing and damp-drying medicinals are mostly bitter and cold. Their main efficacy is to clear heat and dry damp. They are mainly indicated to treat damp-heat syndromes. Clinically, damp-heat syndromes are complicated which present different clinical manifestations according to different locations of diseases. For example, the hiding fever, *pǐ* and fullness in the stomach cavity and chest, scanty and brown urine caused by damp-warm or summer-damp; distension and fullness of stomach cavity and abdomen, nausea and vomiting due to damp-heat in the stomach and spleen; diarrhea and dysentery caused by damp-heat in the large intestine; jaundice, brown urine, hypochondriac pain and swollen ears with pus due to damp-heat in the liver and gallbladder; yellowish vaginal discharge and dripping discharge of urine with astringent pain due to damp-heat in the lower energizer; red, swollen, heat and painful joints due to damp-heat accumulating in the joints; eczema and damp sores due to damp-heat accumulating in the skin. In addition, these medicinals can also clear heat, reduce fire and resolve toxins. They can also be used to treat heat-toxin syndrome, such as excess heat in the qi level of *zang-fu* organs, sores and carbuncles with swelling and pain due to heat toxin.

黄芩 *Huáng qín* (Scutellariae Radix)
《神农本草经》
Shen Nong's Classic of the Materia Medica (Shén Nóng Běn Cǎo Jīng)

【来源 / Origin】

为唇形科植物黄芩 *Scutellaria baicalensis* Georgi 的干燥根。主产于河北、山西、内蒙古等地。春、秋二季采挖。切段，生用或酒炒用。本品气微，味苦。《中国药典》规定，含黄芩苷（$C_{21}H_{18}O_{11}$）不得少于 9.0%。

Huáng qín is the root of *Scutellaria baicalensis* Georgi, pertaining to Labiatae. It is mainly produced in Hebei and Shanxi Province and the Inner Mongolia Autonomous Region. It is collected in spring and autumn, cut into segments and used raw or stir-fried with wine. This medicinal has a slight flavor and tastes bitter. According to *Chinese Pharmacopoeia*, the content of Baicalins ($C_{21}H_{18}O_{11}$) should be no less than 9.0%.

【性味归经 / Medicinal properties】

苦，寒。归肺、胆、脾、大肠、小肠经。

Bitter and cold; act on the lung, gallbladder, spleen, large intestine and small intestine meridians.

【主要功效 / Medicinal efficacies】

清热燥湿，泻火解毒，止血，安胎。

Clear heat and dry damp, reduce fire to remove toxin, stop bleeding, calm the fetus.

【临床应用 / Clinical application】

1. 湿温暑湿，湿热痞满，黄疸，泻痢 本品苦能燥湿，性寒清热，有较强的清热燥湿作用，能清多个脏腑的湿热，可广泛用于多种湿热证，尤长于清中、上焦湿热。用治湿温或暑湿，身热不扬，胸脘痞闷，恶心呕吐等，常配伍滑石、豆蔻等。用治湿热中阻，寒热互结之痞满呕吐，舌苔黄腻，常与黄连、半夏、干姜等同用。用治湿热黄疸，常与茵陈、栀子等同用。用治湿热泻痢，常与葛根、黄连等同用。用治湿热淋证，可与木通、淡竹叶等配伍。

(1) Damp-warm, summer-damp, stuffiness and fullness due to damp-heat, diarrhea and dysentery, jaundice *Huáng qín* is bitter for drying damp, cold in nature with effect of clearing heat. It has strong efficacy of clearing heat and drying damp and can clear damp-heat in various *zang-fu* organs, which can be used to treat various damp-heat syndromes, especially the damp-heat in the middle and upper energizer. To treat hiding fever, stuffiness and oppression in the chest and stomach cavity, nausea and vomiting due to damp-warm or summer-damp diseases, it is often combined with *huá shí* (Talcumand) and *dòu kòu* (Amomi Rotundus Fructus). To treat stuffiness, fullness, vomiting, yellowish and greasy coating caused by coexistence of cold and heat due to damp-heat obstructing the middle energizer, it is often combined with *huáng lián* (Coptidis Rhizoma), *bàn xià* (Pinelliae Rhizoma) and *gān jiāng* (Zingiberis Rhizoma). To treat jaundice caused by damp-heat, it can be combined with *yīn chén* (Artemisiae Scopariae Herba) and *zhī zǐ* (Gardeniae Fructus). To treat diarrhea and dysentery due to damp-heat, it is often combined with *gé gēn* (Puerariae Lobatae Radix) and *huáng lián* (Coptidis Rhizoma). To treat strangury due to damp-heat, it is often combined with *mù tōng* (Akebiae Caulis) and *dàn zhú yè* (Lophatheri Herba).

2. 肺热咳嗽 本品苦寒，长于清肺热，为治肺热咳嗽之要药。治肺热壅遏，咳嗽痰黄单用有效，或配伍瓜蒌仁、枳实、杏仁等。

(2) Cough due to lung heat It is bitter and cold and good at clearing lung heat, which serves as an essential medicinal to treat cough due to lung heat. To treat cough and yellowish sputum due to lung heat accumulation, it can be used singly, or combined with *guā lóu rén* (Trichosanthis Semen), *zhǐ shí* (Aurantii Immaturus Fructus) and *xìng rén* (Armeniacae Amarum Semen).

3. 热病烦渴，寒热往来 本品有清热泻火之功，温热病气分证亦常用之。若治外感热病，高热烦渴，尿赤便秘，常与栀子、大黄、薄荷等同用。本品又长于清半表半里之热，用治邪在少阳，寒热往来，常与柴胡配伍。

(3) Dysphoria and thirst due to warm disease, alternate attacks of chill and fever It has efficacy of clearing heat and draining fire, which is frequently used to treat qi level syndrome in warm-heat disease. To treat heat disease manifested as high fever, dysphoria, thirst, brown urine and constipation, it is often combined with *zhī zǐ* (Gardeniae Fructus), *dà huáng* (Rhei Radix et Rhizoma) and *bò he* (Menthae Herba). For Shaoyang syndrome with alternating attacks of chill and fever, it is combined with *chái hú* (Bupleuri Radix).

4. 痈肿疮毒，咽喉肿痛 本品有清热解毒、消肿止痛之功。用治痈肿疮毒、咽喉肿痛等热毒病证，常配伍黄连、山豆根、连翘等。

(4) Carbuncle, swelling, sore and toxin, swollen and painful throat It has efficacy of clearing heat and resolving toxin, removing swelling and relieving pain. To treat heat-toxin syndrome, such as carbuncle, swelling, sore and toxin, swollen and painful throat, it is usually combined with *huáng lián* (Coptidis Rhizoma), *shān dòu gēn* (Sophorae Tonkinensis Radix et Rhizoma) and *lián qiáo* (Forsythiae Fructus).

5. 血热出血 本品既清热凉血，又能止血。用治血热妄行之吐血、衄血、便血、尿血、崩漏等，常与生地黄、侧柏叶、地榆等同用。

(5) Hemorrhages due to blood heat *Huáng qín* can clear heat and cool blood, as well as stanch bleeding. To treat hematemesis, epistaxis, bloody stool, hematuria and uterine bleeding due to blood heat, it is often combined with *sheng dì huáng* (Rehmanniae Radix), *cè bǎi yè* (Platycladi Cacumen) and *dì yú*

(Sanguisorbae Radix)

6. 胎动不安　本品能清热安胎，用治妊娠热盛，胎动不安者，常与白术、当归等同用。

(6) Restless fetus　It has effect of clearing heat to calm the fetus. To treat restless fetus due to exuberant heat, it is combined with *bái zhú* (Atractylodis Macrocephalae Rhizoma) and *dāng guī* (Angelicae Sinensis Radix).

【用法用量 / Usage and dosage】

煎服，3~10g。清热多生用，安胎多炒用，清上焦热酒炙用，止血炒炭用。

Decoction, 3-10g. For clearing heat, the raw form is used; for restless fetus, it is often stir-baked; for clearing heat in the upper energizer, it is wine-baked; for stanching bleeding, it is stir-baked for charcoal.

【使用注意 / Precaution】

脾胃虚寒者忌用。

It should be contraindicated in those suffering loose stool due to spleen deficiency.

【现代研究 / Modern research】

本品主含黄芩苷、黄芩素、汉黄芩素、汉黄芩苷、黄芩新素等黄酮类成分。具有抑菌、抗病毒、解热、抗炎、抗过敏、保肝、利胆、降脂、抗血小板聚集、抗凝血、解痉、降血压、镇静、利尿等作用。

Huáng qín mainly contains flavonoid, such as baicalin, baicalein, wogonin, wogonoside and skullcapflavone. It has the functions of inhibiting bacteria, antivirus, relieving fever, antagonizing inflammation, antiallergic, protecting liver, promoting gallbladder function, lowering blood fat, antiplatelet aggregation, anticoagulant, antispasmodic, reducing blood pressure, tranquilizing and diuresis.

黄连　*Huáng lián* (Coptidis Rhizoma)
《神农本草经》
Shen Nong's Classic of the Materia Medica (Shén Nóng Běn Cǎo Jīng)

【来源 / Origin】

为毛茛科植物黄连 *Coptis chinensis* Franch.、三角叶黄连 *C. deltoidea C. Y. Cheng et* Hsiao 或云连 *C. teeta* Wall. 的干燥根茎。以上三种分别习称"味连""雅连""云连"。多系栽培。味连、雅连主产于四川、湖北，云连主产于云南。秋季采挖，切片，生用或清炒、姜汁炙、酒炙、吴茱萸水炙用。本品气微，味极苦。《中国药典》规定，味连中小檗碱（$C_{20}H_{17}NO_4$）、表小檗碱（$C_{20}H_{17}NO_4$）、黄连碱（$C_{19}H_{13}NO_4$）、巴马汀（$C_{21}H_{21}NO_4$）的含量分别不得少于 5.5%、0.80%、1.6%、1.5%。雅连含小檗碱不得少于 4.5%。云连含小檗碱不得少于 7.0%。味连饮片含小檗碱不得少于 5.0%，含表小檗碱、黄连碱、巴马汀的总量不得少于 3.0%。

Huáng lián is the rhizome of *Coptis chinensis* Franch., *C. deltoidea C. Y. Cheng et* Hsiao or *C. teeta* Wall., pertaining to Ranunculaceae, which are respectively called *wèi lián*, *yǎ lián* and *yún lián*. It is poly cultivated. *Wèi lián* and *yǎ lián* are mainly produced in Sichuan and Hubei Province in China, while *yún lián* is mainly produced in Yunnan Province. *Huáng lián* is collected in fall and cut into slices. It is used in the raw or plainly stir-fried, stir-fried with ginger juice, stir-fried with wine, or stir-fried with *wú zhū yú* solution. It has a slight flavor and tastes extremely bitter. According to *Chinese Pharmacopoeia*, the content of berberine ($C_{20}H_{17}NO_4$), epiberberine ($C_{20}H_{17}NO_4$), coptisine ($C_{19}H_{13}NO_4$), palmatine ($C_{21}H_{21}NO_4$) in *wèi lián* should be no less than 5.5%, 0.80%, 1.6%, 1.5% respectively. The content of berberine in *yǎ lián* should be no less than 4.5%. The content of berberine in *yún lián* should be no less than 7.0%. The content of berberine in the prepared slices of *wèi lián* should be no less than 5.0%, and the total content of epiberberine, coptisine, palmatine in the prepared slices of *wèi lián* should be no less than 3.0%.

【性味归经 / Medicinal properties】

苦，寒。归心、脾、胃、肝、胆、大肠经。

Bitter and cold; act on the heart, spleen, stomach, liver, gallbladder, and large intestine meridians.

【主要功效 / Medicinal efficacies】

清热燥湿，泻火解毒。

Clear heat and dry damp, reduce fire and remove toxin.

【临床应用 / Clinical application】

1. 湿热痞满，呕吐，泻痢　本品苦寒，清热燥湿之力胜于黄芩，因其主入中焦，故善清中焦湿热。用治湿热中阻，气机不畅，脘腹痞满，恶心呕吐，常与黄芩、半夏、干姜等同用。本品为治湿热泻痢之要药，若伴里急后重腹痛者，常与白芍、木香、槟榔等同用；若兼表证发热者，常配伍葛根、黄芩等；若治热毒痢疾，下痢脓血，常与白头翁、秦皮、黄柏等同用。

(1) Stuffiness and fullness due to damp-heat, vomiting, diarrhea and dysentery　*Huáng lián* is bitter and cold, which has stronger effect of clearing heat and drying damp than *huáng qín* (Scutellariae Radix). As it mainly acts on the middle energizer, it is especially effective in clearing damp-heat in the middle energizer. To treat stuffiness and fullness in the stomach cavity and abdomen, nausea and vomiting caused by unsmooth qi flow due to damp-heat obstructing the middle energizer, it is often combined with *huáng qín* (Scutellariae Radix), *bàn xià* (Pinelliae Rhizoma) and *gān jiāng* (Zingiberis Rhizoma). It is an essential medicinal to treat diarrhea and dysentery due to damp-heat, if accompanied by tenesmus and abdominal pain, it is usually combined with *bái sháo* (Paeoniae Alba Radix), *mù xiāng* (Aucklandiae Radix) and *bīng láng* (Arecae Semen); if accompanied by exterior syndrome with fever, it is often used together with *gé gēn* (Puerariae Lobatae Radix) and *huáng qín* (Scutellariae Radix); for treating dysentery with pus and blood due to heat-toxin, it is often combined with *bái tóu wēng* (Pulsatillae Radix), *qín pí* (Fraxini Cortex) and *huáng bó* (Phellodendri Chinensis Cortex).

2. 心火亢盛证　本品有较强的清热泻火作用，长于清心经实火。用治外感热病，心经热盛，壮热烦躁，甚至神昏谵语，常配伍连翘、牛黄等。用治心火亢盛，心烦不眠，常与朱砂、生甘草同用。用治心火亢盛，阴血耗伤之虚烦不眠、惊悸怔忡，常配伍阿胶、白芍等。治心火上炎，口舌生疮，心烦，或心热下移小肠之小便淋沥涩痛，多与栀子、竹叶等同用。

(2) Exuberance of heart-fire syndrome　It has strong effect of clearing heat and draining fire, and is good at clearing excess fire in the heart meridian. To treat high fever, vexation, even loss of consciousness, delirium speech due to exuberant heat in the heart meridian in warm disease, it is often combined with *lián qiáo* (Forsythiae Fructus) and *niú huáng* (Calculus Bovis). To treat dysphoria, insomnia caused by predominance of heart fire, it is often combined with *zhū shā* (Cinnabaris) and *shēng gān cǎo* (Glycyrrhizae Radix et Rhizoma). To treat deficient vexation, insomnia and palpitation caused by exuberant heat damaging yin blood, it is often combined with *ē jiāo* (Corii Asini Colla) and *bái sháo* (Paeoniae Alba Radix). To treat ulcer in the mouth and tongue, dysphoria due to upward flaming of heart fire, or dripping urine with astringent pain due to heart-heat transmitting down to small intestine, it is often combined with *zhī zǐ* (Gardeniae Fructus) and *zhú yè* (Lophatheri Herba).

3. 胃火炽盛证　本品亦有较强的清泄胃火功效。用治胃热呕吐，常与半夏、竹茹等同用。用治胃火上炎之牙龈肿痛，常与石膏、升麻、牡丹皮等同用。用治胃热炽盛，消谷善饥，消渴等，常配伍生地黄、麦冬、天花粉等。用治肝火犯胃之胁肋胀痛、呕吐吞酸，每与吴茱萸同用。

(3) Exuberance of stomach fire syndrome It also has strong effect of clearing stomach fire. To treat vomiting caused by stomach heat, it is combined with *bàn xià* (Pinelliae Rhizoma) and *zhú rú* (Bambusae Caulis in Taenia). For treating swollen and painful gum due to upward flaming of stomach fire, it is often used with *shí gāo* (Gypsum Fibrosum), *shēng má* (Cimicifugae Rhizoma) and *mǔ dān pí* (Moutan Cortex). To treat swift digestion and rapid hungering, *xiāo kě* caused by exuberant stomach fire, it is often in combination with *dì huáng* (Rehmanniae Radix), *mài dōng* (Ophiopogonis Radix) and *tiān huā fěn* (Trichosanthis Radix). To treat hypochondriac distension and pain, vomiting and acid regurgitation due to liver fire invading stomach, it is often combined with *wú zhū yú* (Evodiae Fructus).

4. 痈肿疔疮，目赤肿痛 本品清解热毒之功胜于黄芩、黄柏，是皮肤疮痈等外科及五官科热毒证的常用药。用治热毒内盛，痈肿疔疮，常配伍金银花、黄芩、连翘等药，亦可配伍当归、黄柏、姜黄等制为软膏，局部外用。用治目赤肿痛，可以本品用人乳浸汁滴眼。

(4) Carbuncle, abscess, furuncle, sores, swollen and painful eyes Its effect of clearing heat and resolving toxin is stronger than that of *huáng qín* (Scutellariae Radix) and *huáng bó* (Phellodendri Chinensis Cortex). It is a commonly used medicinal to treat heat-toxin syndrome, such as sores and carbuncles of the skin and other diseases concerned with ophthalmology and otorhinolaryngology. To treat carbuncle, abscess, furuncle and sores due to exuberance of heat toxin, it is often combined with *jīn yín huā* (Lonicerae Japonicae Flos), *huáng qín* (Scutellariae Radix) and *lián qiáo* (Forsythiae Fructus). It can also be combined with *dāng guī* (Angelicae Sinensis Radix), *huáng bó* (Phellodendri Chinensis Cortex) and *jiāng huáng* (Curcumae Longae Rhizoma) to make into ointment for external application. For treating swollen and painful eyes, it can be soaked in human milk and drop the eyes.

5. 湿疹湿疮，耳道流脓 本品清热燥湿，泻火解毒，治湿疹、湿疮，可用本品制为软膏外敷。用治耳道疖肿，耳道流脓，可浸汁涂患处。

(5) Eczema, purulent discharge of auditory canal It clears heat and dries damp, reduces fire and resolves toxin. It can be made into ointment for external use to treat eczema. To treat furuncle and purulent discharge of auditory canal, the infusion can be used to afflicted area.

【用法用量 / Usage and dosage】

煎服，2~5g。外用适量。生用清热燥湿泻火力较强；炒用可缓其寒性；酒黄连善清上焦火热；姜黄连清胃和胃止呕；萸黄连舒肝和胃止呕。

Decoction, 2-5g. A proper amount is used externally. The raw form has stronger effect of clearing heat, drying damp and draining fire; the stir-fried form can weaken its cold nature; when stir-baked with wine, it is suitable to clearing heat and fire in the upper energizer; when stir-baked with ginger juice, it can harmonize the stomach to arrest vomiting by clearing stomach fire; when stir-baked with *wú zhū yú* (Evodiae Fructus) solution, it functions to harmonize the stomach to arrest vomiting by soothing the liver.

【使用注意 / Precaution】

脾胃虚寒者忌用。阴虚津伤者慎用。

It should be contraindicated in those suffering deficiency cold of spleen and stomach. It should be used with caution for patients with damage of fluid due to yin deficiency.

【现代研究 / Modern research】

本品主含小檗碱、黄连碱、甲基黄连碱、巴马汀、药根碱、表小檗碱等多种生物碱，以及阿魏酸、黄柏酮、黄柏内酯等成分。具有抑制病原微生物、抗炎、解热、镇静、抗腹泻、抗溃疡、利胆、降血糖、降血脂、抗氧化、抗肿瘤等作用。

Huáng lián mainly contains alkaloids, such as berberine, coptisine, worenine, palmatine, jatrorrhizine and epiberberine. It also contains ferulic acid, obacunone and baculactone. It has the functions of inhibiting pathogenic microorganisms, antagonizing inflammation, relieving fever, tranquilizing, antidiarrhea, antiulcer, promoting gallbladder function, lowering blood sugar, lowering blood fat, antioxidation and antitumor.

黄柏 *Huáng bó* (Phellodendri Chinensis Cortex)
《神农本草经》
Shen Nong's Classic of the Materia Medica (Shén Nóng Běn Cǎo Jīng)

【来源 / Origin】

为芸香科植物黄皮树 *Phellodendron chinense* Schneid. 的树皮，又称川黄柏。主产于四川、贵州等地。清明之后剥取树皮，切丝，生用或盐水炙、炒炭用。本品气微，味甚苦。《中国药典》规定，盐酸小檗碱含量不得少于 3.0%。

Huáng bó is the bark of *Phellodendron chinense* Schneid., pertaining to Rutaceae, which is also called *chuān huáng bó*. It is mainly produced in Sichuan and Guizhou Province in China. It is collected after Qingming, when the bark is peeled and cut into threads. It is used in the raw or stir-fried with salt-water, or stir-baked with charcoal. This medicinal has a slight flavor and tastes quite bitter. According to *Chinese Pharmacopoeia*, the content of berberine should be no less than 3.0%.

【性味归经 / Medicinal properties】

苦，寒。归肾、膀胱经。

Bitter and cold; act on the kidney and bladder meridians.

【主要功效 / Medicinal efficacies】

清热燥湿，泻火除蒸，解毒疗疮。

Clear heat and dry dampness, reduce fire and remove steaming fever, remove toxin and heal up sores.

【临床应用 / Clinical application】

1. 湿热泻痢，黄疸，带下阴痒，热淋涩痛，脚气痿躄 本品苦寒，亦有较强的清热燥湿作用，入肾和膀胱经，偏走下焦，善清下焦湿热。用治湿热痢疾，常与黄连、白头翁等同用。用治湿热黄疸，常与栀子同用。用治湿热下注，带下黄臭，阴肿阴痒，常与车前子、芡实等同用。用治湿热淋证，小便短赤涩痛，常配伍车前子、萆薢等。用治湿热下注，脚气肿痛，痿软无力，常与苍术、牛膝同用。

(1) Diarrhea and dysentery due to damp-heat, jaundice, pruritus vulvae, heat strangury with astringent pain, beriberi with crippling *wěi* *Huáng bó* is bitter and cold with stronger effect of clearing heat and drying damp. It acts on the kidney and bladder meridians, and is suitable to clear damp-heat in the lower energizer. To treat diarrhea and dysentery due to damp-heat, it is often used with *huáng lián* (Coptidis Rhizoma) and *bái tóu wēng* (Pulsatillae Radix). For jaundice caused by damp-heat, it is often used with *zhī zǐ* (Gardeniae Fructus). To treat yellowish and fetid vaginal discharge, swollen and itching vulva due to downward flow of damp-heat, it is combined with *chē qián zǐ* (Plantaginis Semen) and *qiàn shí* (Euryales Semen). To treat scanty and brown urine with astringent pain caused by heat strangury, it is combined with *chē qián zǐ* (Plantaginis Semen) and *bì xiè* (Dioscoreae Hypoglaucae Rhizoma). To treat beriberi with swelling and pain, flaccidity due to downward flow of damp-heat, it is combined with *cāng zhú* (Atractylodis Rhizoma) and *niú xī* (Achyranthis Bidentatae Radix).

2. 疮痈肿毒，湿疹湿疮 本品苦寒，既能清热燥湿，又能泻火解毒。用治热毒疮痈，红肿疼痛，常配伍黄芩、黄连、栀子等。用治湿疹、湿疮，可研末撒敷或煎汤浸洗。

(2) Sores, carbuncle, swelling, toxin and eczema It is bitter and cold with effect of clearing heat and drying damp, draining fire and removing toxin. To treat sores and carbuncle, swelling and pains due to heat toxin, it is combined with *huáng qín* (Scutellariae Radix), *huáng lián* (Coptidis Rhizoma) and *zhī zǐ* (Gardeniae Fructus). For eczema, it is ground into powder scattered to the afflicted area or decocted for soaking and washing.

3. 骨蒸潮热，盗汗，遗精 本品入肾经，长于泻相火，退虚热。用治肾阴不足，虚火上炎，骨蒸潮热，盗汗，遗精等，常与知母、地黄、山药等同用。

(3) Steaming bone fever, tidal fever, night sweating, seminal emission It acts on the kidney meridian, and good at purging away the ministerial fire and relieving deficient heat. To treat steaming bone, tidal fever, night sweating, seminal emission caused by upward flaming of deficient fire due to shortage of kidney yin, it is often used with *zhī mǔ* (Anemarrhenae Rhizoma), *dì huáng* (Rehmanniae Radix) and *shān yào* (Dioscoreae Rhizoma).

【用法用量 / Usage and dosage】

煎服，3~12g。外用适量。生用清热燥湿，泻火解毒力强；盐黄柏滋阴降火。

Decoction, 3-12g. A proper amount is used externally. The raw form has stronger effect of clearing heat and drying damp, draining fire and removing toxin; being stir-fried with salt-water, it can nourish yin and reduce fire.

【使用注意 / Precaution】

脾胃虚寒者忌用。

It should be contraindicated in those suffering deficiency cold of spleen and stomach.

【现代研究 / Modern research】

本品主要含小檗碱、木兰花碱、巴马汀、药根碱、黄柏碱等生物碱类成分。具有抑菌、抗病毒、解热、降压、利胆、抗溃疡、利尿、抗痛风、降血糖等作用。

Huáng bó mainly contains alkaloids, such as berberine, magnoflorine, palmatine, jatrorrhizine and phellodendrine. It has functions of inhibiting bacteria, antivirus, relieving fever, lowering blood pressure, promoting gallbladder function, antiulcer, diuresis, antigout and decreasing blood sugar.

龙胆　*Lóng dǎn* (Gentianae Radix et Rhizoma)
《神农本草经》
Shen Nong's Classic of the Materia Medica (Shén Nóng Běn Cǎo Jīng)

【来源 / Origin】

为龙胆科植物条叶龙胆 *Gentiana manshurica* Kitag.、三花龙胆 *G. triflora* pall. 或坚龙胆 *G. rigesceras* Franch. 的根及根茎。全国各地均产，以东北产量较大。秋季采挖，切段，生用。本品气微，味甚苦。《中国药典》规定，龙胆含龙胆苦苷（$C_{16}H_{20}O_9$）含量不得少于 3.0%，坚龙胆含龙胆苦苷不得少于 1.5%。

Lóng dǎn is the root and rhizome of *Gentiana manshurica* Kitag., *G. triflora* pall., or *G. rigesceras* Franch., pertaining to Gentianaceae. It is produced in almost all parts of China, and its output in northeast China is the highest. It is collected in fall, cut into segments and used raw. It has a slight flavor and tastes quite bitter. According to *Chinese Pharmacopoeia*, the content of gentiopicroside ($C_{16}H_{20}O_9$) in *lóng dǎn* should be no less than 3.0%, while that in *jiān lóng dǎn* should be no less than 1.5%.

【性味归经 / Medicinal properties】

苦，寒。归肝、胆经。

Bitter and cold; act on the liver and gallbladder meridians.

【主要功效 / Medicinal efficacies】

清热燥湿，泻肝胆火。

Clear heat and dry damp, drain liver and gallbladder fire.

【临床应用 / Clinical application】

1. **湿热黄疸，阴肿阴痒，带下，湿疹** 本品苦寒，清热燥湿力强，主入肝胆经，善清肝胆湿热和下焦湿热。用治湿热黄疸，常与茵陈、栀子等同用。用治湿热下注，带下黄臭、阴肿阴痒，或阴囊肿痛等，常与车前子、泽泻、木通等同用。用治湿疹瘙痒，常与苦参、黄柏、蛇床子等同用。

(1) **Jaundice due to damp-heat, swelling of vulvae with pruritus, leucorrhea and itching eczema** *Lóng dǎn* is bitter and cold with strong effect of clearing heat and drying damp. It acts on the liver and gallbladder meridians, and is suitable to clear damp-heat in the liver and gallbladder, as well as lower energizer. To treat jaundice due to damp-heat, it is often combined with *yīn chén* (Artemisiae Scopariae Herba) and *zhī zǐ* (Gardeniae Fructus). To treat yellowish and fetid vaginal discharge, swollen and itching vulva or swollen and painful scrotum due to downward flow of damp-heat, it is combined with *chē qián zǐ* (Plantaginis Semen), *zé xiè* (Alismatis Rhizoma) and *mù tōng* (Akebiae Caulis). To treat itching eczema, it is often combined with *kǔ shēn* (Sophorae Flavescentis Radix), *huáng bó* (Phellodendri Chinensis Cortex) and *shé chuáng zǐ* (Cnidii Fructus).

2. **肝火炽盛证** 本品苦寒清泄，善清肝胆实火。用治肝胆火盛，头痛目赤，耳鸣耳聋，胁痛，口苦等，常与栀子、黄芩等同用。若治肝经热盛，热极生风之高热惊风，手足抽搐，常与牛黄、钩藤、黄连等同用。

(2) **Syndrome of exuberant liver fire** It is bitter and cold with effect of clearing and draining, and is good at clearing excess fire of liver and gallbladder. To treat headache, red eyes, deafness, tinnitus, hypochondriac pain and bitter taste in the mouth due to exuberant liver and gallbladder fire, it is often used together with *zhī zǐ* (Gardeniae Fructus) and *huáng qín* (Scutellariae Radix). To treat high fever, convulsion, tetany caused by extreme heat in the liver channel producing wind, it is often combined with *niú huáng* (Calculus Bovis), *gōu téng* (Uncariae Cum Uncis Ramulus) and *huáng lián* (Coptidis Rhizoma).

【用法用量 / Usage and dosage】

煎服，3~6g。

Decoction, 3-6g.

【使用注意 / Precaution】

脾胃虚寒者忌用。阴虚津伤者慎用。

It should be contraindicated for those suffering deficiency cold of spleen and stomach. It should be used with caution for those suffering fluid consumption due to yin deficiency.

【现代研究 / Modern research】

本品主要含龙胆苦苷、当药苦苷、当药苷、苦龙胆酯苷、龙胆碱、龙胆黄碱等。具有抑菌、抗炎、解热、利胆、保肝、健胃、镇静、降压等作用。

Lóng dǎn mainly contains gentiopicroside, swertianolin, drug glucoside, amarogentin, gentianine, and gentioflavine. It has the functions of inhibiting bacteria, antagonizing inflammation, relieving fever, promoting gallbladder function, protecting the liver, strengthening the stomach, tranquilizing and lowering blood pressure.

苦参 *Kǔ shēn* (Sophorae Flavescentis Radix)
《神农本草经》
Shen Nong's Classic of the Materia Medica (*Shén Nóng Běn Cǎo Jīng*)

【来源 / Origin】

为豆科植物苦参 *Sophora flavescens* Ait. 的干燥根。我国各地均产。春、秋二季采挖，切片，生用。本品气微，味极苦。《中国药典》规定，含苦参碱（$C_{15}H_{24}N_2O$）和氧化苦参碱（$C_{15}H_{24}N_2O_2$）的总量不得少于 1.2%。

Kǔ shēn is the dried root of *Sophora flavescens* Ait., pertaining to Leguminosae. It is produced in almost all parts of China, collected in spring and autumn, cut into slices and used raw. It has a slight flavor and tastes extremely bitter. According to *Chinese Pharmacopoeia*, the total content of matrine ($C_{15}H_{24}N_2O$) and oxymatrine ($C_{15}H_{24}N_2O_2$) should be no less than 1.2%.

【性味归经 / Medicinal properties】

苦，寒。归心、肝、胃、大肠、膀胱经。

Bitter and cold; act on the heart, liver, stomach, large intestine and bladder meridians.

【主要功效 / Medicinal efficacies】

清热燥湿，杀虫止痒，利尿。

Clear heat and dry damp, kill worms and relieve itching, promote urination.

【临床应用 / Clinical application】

1. 湿热泻痢，黄疸，带下，阴肿阴痒 本品苦寒之性较强，既能清热燥湿，又能利尿，从而导湿热之邪外出，可用于多种湿热病证。用治湿热泻痢，常与白芍、木香等同用。用治湿热黄疸，可与龙胆、栀子等同用。用治湿热痔疮肿痛、便血，常与黄柏、冰片等同用。用治湿热带下，阴肿阴痒，常与黄柏、椿皮等同用。

(1) Diarrhea and dysentery due to damp-heat, jaundice, leucorrhea and swelling of vulvae with pruritus It is extremely bitter and rather cold in nature with effect of clearing heat and drying damp as well as promoting urination to remove damp-heat out of human body. It can be used to treat various damp-heat syndromes. To treat diarrhea and dysentery due to damp-heat, it is combined with *bái sháo* (Paeoniae Alba Radix) and *mù xiāng* (Aucklandiae Radix). To treat jaundice caused by damp-heat, it is used with *lóng dǎn* (Gentianae Radix et Rhizoma) and *zhī zǐ* (Gardeniae Fructus). To treat hemorrhoid with swelling and pain, hematofecia due to damp-heat, it is often combined with *huáng bó* (Phellodendri Chinensis Cortex) and *bīng piàn* (Borneolum Syntheticum). To treat leucorrhea, swelling of vulvae with pruritus caused by damp-heat, it is often used with *huáng bó* (Phellodendri Chinensis Cortex) and *chūn pí* (Ailanthi Cortex).

2. 湿疹湿疮，皮肤瘙痒，疥癣麻风 本品有清热燥湿，杀虫止痒之功。为治瘙痒性皮肤病之要药。用治湿疹、湿疮，可单用煎水外洗，或配伍黄柏、蛇床子煎水外洗。用治风疹瘙痒，可与防风、蝉蜕等同用。用治疥癣瘙痒，常与蛇床子、地肤子、黄柏等同用。治滴虫性阴道炎，可单用煎汤灌洗，或局部用栓剂。

(2) Eczema, itching skin, acariasis and leprosy It has efficacies of clearing heat and drying damp, killing worms and relieving itching, which serves as a vital medicinal to treat itching dermal diseases. To treat eczema, it can be decocted singly for external washing, or decocted with *huáng bó* (Phellodendri Chinensis Cortex) and *shé chuáng zǐ* (Cnidii Fructus) for external washing. To treat itching due to rubella, it can be used with *fáng fēng* (Saposhnikoviae Radix) and *chán tuì* (Cicadae Periostracum).

For itching due to acariasis, it is often used with *shé chuáng zǐ* (Cnidii Fructus), *dì fū zǐ* (Kochiae Fructus) and *huáng bó* (Phellodendri Chinensis Cortex). To treat trichomonal vaginitis, it can be decocted singly for vaginal douche, or administered with suppository in local parts.

3. 小便不利，灼热涩痛　本品苦寒沉降，能清膀胱湿热而利小便。用治湿热蕴结膀胱，小便不利，灼热涩痛，常与车前子、栀子等同用。

(3) Dysuria, difficulty and burning pain in micturition　It is bitter and cold for sinking and descending with effect of clearing damp-heat in bladder to promote urination. To treat dysuria, difficulty and burning pain in micturition due to damp-heat accumulating in bladder, it is often combined with *chē qián zǐ* (Plantaginis Semen) and *zhī zǐ* (Gardeniae Fructus).

【用法用量 / Usage and dosage】

煎服，4.5~9g。外用适量。

Decoction, 4.5-9g. A proper amount for external application.

【使用注意 / Precaution】

脾胃虚寒者忌用。阴虚津伤者慎用。反藜芦。

It should be contraindicated for those suffering deficiency cold of spleen and stomach. It should be used with caution for those suffering fluid consumption due to yin deficiency. It should not be used with *lí lú* (Veratri Nigri Radix et Rhizoma).

【现代研究 / Modern research】

本品主要含苦参碱、氧化苦参碱、槐果碱、异苦参碱、苦参素、槐定碱等生物碱，尚含苦参醇、新苦参醇、苦参酮、新苦参酮等黄酮类化合物。具有抑菌、解热、抗炎、抗心律失常、抗变态反应、抗心肌缺血、抗肿瘤、抗胃溃疡、镇静、升高白细胞等作用。

Kǔ shēn mainly contains alkaloids such as matrine, oxymatrine, sophocarpine, iosmatrine and sophoridine. It also contains flavonoids such as kurarinol, neo-kurarinol, kurarinon and norkurarinone. It has functions of inhibiting bacteria, antagonizing inflammation, relieving fever, antiarrhythmia, anti-allergy, anti-myocardial ischemia, antitumor, antigastric ulcer, tranquilizing and elevating white blood cells.

第三节　清热解毒药
Section 3　Heat-clearing and detoxicating medicinals

本类药物多性味苦寒，以清热解毒为主要功效，主治各种热毒病证，如疮痈疔疖、咽喉肿痛、丹毒、痄腮、痢疾、水火烫伤以及蛇虫咬伤、癌肿等。

Medicinals of this type are mostly bitter and cold with main efficacy of clearing heat and detoxicating. They are used to treat various heat-toxin patterns, such as carbuncle, furuncle, sores, deep-rooted boil, swollen throat, erysipelas, mumps, dysentery, burns and scalds, insect and snake bites as well as cancer swelling.

金银花　*Jīn yín huā* (Lonicerae Japonicae Flos)
《新修本草》
Newly Revised Materia Medica (Xīn Xīu Běn Cǎo)

【来源 / Origin】

为忍冬科植物忍冬 *Lonicera japonica* Thunb. 的干燥花蕾或带初开的花。主产于山东、河南。夏初花开放前采收，干燥，生用、炒用或制成露剂使用。本品气清香，味淡、微苦。《中国药典》规定，含绿原酸（$C_{16}H_{18}O_9$）不得少于 1.5%，木犀草苷（$C_{21}H_{20}O_{11}$）不得少于 0.050%。

Jīn yín huā is the dried bud or that with early blossoming flower of *Lonicera japonica* Thunb., pertaining to Caprifoliaceae. It is mainly produced in Shandong and Henan Province in China, collected in early summer before blossom, and then dried. It is used raw, stir-fried or processed as distillate. It has a delicate fragrance, and tastes bland and slightly bitter. According to *Chinese Pharmacopoeia*, the content of chlorogenic acid ($C_{16}H_{18}O_9$) should be no less than 1.5%, while that of luteoloside ($C_{21}H_{20}O_{11}$) should be no less than 0.050%.

【性味归经 / Medicinal properties】

甘，寒。归肺、心、胃经。

Sweet and cold; act on the lung, heart and stomach meridians.

【主要功效 / Medicinal efficacies】

清热解毒，疏散风热。

Clear heat and resolve toxins, dissipate wind-heat.

【临床应用 / Clinical application】

1. 疮痈疔疖　本品甘寒，清热解毒之力较佳，为治热毒疮痈疔疖之要药。用治疮痈初起，红肿热痛，常与穿山甲、白芷、皂角刺等同用。用治疔疮肿毒，坚硬根深者，常配伍野菊花、蒲公英等。用治肠痈腹痛，常与大血藤、薏苡仁等同用。用治肺痈咳吐脓血，常与鱼腥草、桔梗、芦根等同用。用治血热毒盛，丹毒红肿，多与大青叶、紫花地丁等同用。

(1) Ulcer, carbuncle and furuncle　It is sweet and cold with good effect of clearing heat and removing toxin, which serves as an essential medicinal to treat ulcer, carbuncle and furuncle due to heat-toxin. To treat ulcer and carbuncle in the early stage, manifested as red, swelling, heat and pain, it is often combined with *chuān shān jiǎ* (Manitis Squama), *bái zhǐ* (Angelicae Dahuricae Radix) and *zào jiǎo cì* (Gleditsiae Spina). To treat furuncle, ulcer, swelling and toxin, marked by hardness and deep root, it is combined with *yě jú huā* (Chrysanthemi Indici Flos) and *pú gōng yīng* (Taraxaci Herba). For abdominal pain due to intestinal abscess, it is often combined with *dà xuè téng* (Sargentodoxae Caulis) and *yì yǐ rén* (Coicis Semen). To treat lung abscess, manifested as cough with pus and blood, it is often combined with *yú xīng cǎo* (Houttuyniae Herba), *jié gěng* (Platycodonis Radix) and *lú gēn* (Phragmitis Rhizoma). To treat erysipelas due to blood heat and exuberant toxin, it is often combined with *dà qīng yè* (Isatidis Folium) and *zǐ huā dì dīng* (Violae Herba).

2. 风热表证，温病发热　本品甘寒质轻，芳香疏透，既能清热解毒，又能疏散风热，为治疗风热表证的常用药，也可用于温热病的各个阶段。用治风热表证或温病初起，邪在卫分，发热，微恶风寒，咽痛口渴者，常与连翘、薄荷、牛蒡子等同用。用治温病气分热盛，壮热烦渴者，可与石膏、知母等同用。用治温病热入营分，身热夜甚，神烦少寐，常与生地黄、玄参等同用。用治温病热入血分，高热神昏，斑疹吐衄，可与连翘、生地黄等同用。

(2) Wind-heat exterior syndrome, warm disease with fever　It is sweet and cold with fragrance and light property. Which has efficacies of clearing heat and resolving toxin, as well as dissipating wind-heat. It is considered as a commonly used medicinal to treat wind-heat exterior syndrome, and can be used in different stages of warm disease. To treat wind-heat exterior syndrome, or early stage of warm disease, pathogenic factors locating in defense aspect, manifested as fever, aversion to wind-cold, sore throat and thirst, it is often combined with *lián qiáo* (Forsythiae Fructus), *bò he* (Menthae Herba) and *niú bàng zǐ* (Arctii Fructus). To treat exuberant heat in the qi level of warm disease, manifested as high fever, vexation and thirst, it is often combined with *shí gāo* (Gypsum Fibrosum) and *zhī mǔ* (Anemarrhenae Rhizoma). To treat heat entering nutritive aspect in warm disease, manifested as fever worsened at night, spiritual vexation and insomnia, it is often combined with *shēng dì huáng* (Rehmanniae Radix) and *xuán shēn* (Scrophulariae Radix). To treat heat entering blood level in warm disease, manifested as high fever, loss of consciousness, macula and hematemesis, it is often combined with *lián qiáo* (Forsythiae Fructus) and *shēng dì huáng* (Rehmanniae Radix).

3. 热毒血痢　本品能清热解毒，凉血止痢。用治热毒痢疾，下痢脓血，可单用浓煎服，或与黄连、白头翁等同用。

(3) Blood dysentery due to heat toxin　It has functions of clearing heat and removing toxin, cooling blood and arresting dysentery. To treat dysentery with pus and blood due to heat-toxin, it can be used alone by processing the fresh one into condensed decoction for oral taking, or combined with *huáng lián* (Coptidis Rhizoma) and *bái tóu wēng* (Pulsatillae Radix).

本品经蒸制成金银花露，有清解暑热作用，可用于暑热烦渴及小儿热疖、痱子等。

It can be processed into distillate to clear heat, relieve summer-heat, and can be applied to treat vexation and thirst due to summer-heat, infantile simplex and heat rash.

【用法用量 / Usage and dosage】

煎服，6~15g。清热解毒、疏散风热以生品为佳；炒炭宜用于热毒血痢。

Decoction, 6-15g. The raw form is more suitable for clearing heat and removing toxin, as well as dissipating wind-heat; stir-baked with charcoal for blood dysentery caused by heat-toxin.

【使用注意 / Precaution】

脾胃虚寒者慎用。

It should be used with caution for those suffering deficiency cold of spleen and stomach.

【现代研究 / Modern research】

本品主要含绿原酸、异绿原、木犀草苷、忍冬苷，以及挥发油、环烯醚萜苷及三萜皂苷等。具有抑菌、抗病毒、解热、保肝、抗过敏、降血脂、降血糖、抗肿瘤等作用。

It mainly contains chlorogenic acid, isochlorogenic acid, luteoloside, lonicerin, volatile oil, iridoid glucosides and triterpenoidsaponins. It has functions of inhibiting bacteria, antivirus, relieving fever, protecting the liver, anti-allergy, reducing blood fat and blood sugar, as well as antitumor.

连翘　*Lián qiáo* (Forsythiae Fructus)

《神农本草经》

Shen Nong's Classic of the Materia Medica (Shén Nóng Běn Cǎo Jīng)

【来源 / Origin】

为木犀科植物连翘 *Forsythia suspensa*（Thunb.）Vahl 的干燥果实。主产于山西、河南、陕西等省。秋季果实初熟尚带绿色时采收晒干，习称"青翘"；果实熟透时采收，晒干，习称"老翘"；青翘蒸熟晒干，筛选籽实作"连翘心"。生用。本品气微香，味苦。《中国药典》规定，含连翘苷（$C_{27}H_{34}O_{11}$）不得少于 0.15%，连翘酯苷 A（$C_{29}H_{36}O_{15}$）不得少于 0.25%。

Lián qiáo is the dried fruit of *Forsythia suspensa* (Thunb.) Vahl, pertaining to Oleaceae. It is mainly produced in Shanxi, Henan and Shaanxi Province in China, collected in autumn when the primarily ripened fruit is still green and dried in the sun, which is usually called *qīng qiáo*; or collected when the fruit is fully ripened and dried in the sun, which is called *lǎo qiáo*; *qīng qiáo* is fully steamed and dried in the sunlight, its seeds are picked out as *lián qiáo xīn*. It is used in the raw. *Lián qiáo* has slight fragrance and tastes bitter. According to *Chinese Pharmacopoeia*, the content of phillyrin ($C_{27}H_{34}O_{11}$) should be no less than 0.15%, while that of forsythiaside A ($C_{29}H_{36}O_{15}$) should be no less than 0.25%.

【性味归经 / Medicinal properties】

苦，微寒。归肺、心、小肠经。

Bitter and slightly cold; act on the lung, heart and small intestine meridians.

【主要功效 / Medicinal efficacies】

清热解毒，消肿散结，疏散风热。

Clear heat and resolve toxins, subside swelling and dissipate masses, dissipate wind-heat.

【临床应用 / Clinical application】

1. 痈肿疮毒，瘰疬痰核　本品苦泄辛散，性寒清热，入心经，长于清心火，解热毒，并有消痈散结之效，故有"疮家圣药"之称。用治疮痈初起，红肿热痛，常与蒲公英、金银花等同用。用治疮痈溃烂、脓出不畅，常与穿山甲、皂角刺、天花粉等同用。用治瘰疬痰核，常配伍夏枯草、浙贝母、昆布等。用治乳痈肿痛，常与蒲公英、漏芦等同用。用治热毒咽喉肿痛，常配伍金银花、马勃等。

(1) Carbuncle, swelling, sore and toxin, scrofula and phlegm nodule It is bitter for draining, acrid for dispersing and cold in nature for clearing heat. It acts on heart meridian and is good at clearing heart fire, as well as resolving heat-toxin. It also function to eliminate carbuncles and dissipate masses, which is known as "the most effective medicinal to treat sores". To treat early stage of sores and carbuncles with red, swelling, heat and pain, it is often combined with *pú gōng yīng* (Taraxaci Herba) and *jīn yín huā* (Lonicerae Japonicae Flos). To treat carbuncle fester with unsmooth discharge of pus, it is often used with *chuān shān jiǎ* (Manitis Squama), *zào jiǎo cì* (Gleditsiae Spina) and *tiān huā fěn* (Trichosanthis Radix). For scrofula and phlegm nodule, it is often combined with *xià kū cǎo* (Prunellae Spica), *zhè bèi mǔ* (Fritillariae Thunbergii Bulbus) and *kūn bù* (Laminariae Thallus; Eckloniae Thallus). To treat mammary abscess with swelling and pain, it is often used with *pú gōng yīng* (Taraxaci Herba) and *lòu lú* (Rhapontici Radix). To treat sore throat due to heat-toxin, it is often combined with *jīn yín huā* (Lonicerae Japonicae Flos) and *mǎ bó* (Lasiosphaera seu Calvatia).

2. 风热表证，温病发热　本品苦寒，外能疏散风热，内能清热解毒，功似金银花，亦常用治风热表证及温热病的各个阶段。若治外感风热或温病初起，发热、咽痛、口渴等，常配伍金银花、薄荷、牛蒡子等。若治温病热入营分，常配伍地黄、玄参等。若治温病热入血分，多与金银花、地黄等同用。本品轻宣疏散之力不及金银花，但苦寒清降之性较强，尤长于清泻心火，用治温病热陷心包，高热、烦躁、神昏等，常与黄连、莲子心等同用。

(2) Wind-heat exterior syndrome, warm disease with fever It is bitter and cold with efficacies of dispelling wind-heat externally, clearing heat and resolving toxin internally. Its functions are similar to that of *jīn yín huā* (Lonicerae Japonicae Flos), and can also be used to treat wind-heat exterior syndrome, as well as all stages of warm disease. To treat external contraction of wind-heat or early stage of warm disease with symptoms of fever, sore throat and thirst, it is often combined with *jīn yín*

huā (Lonicerae Japonicae Flos), *bò he* (Menthae Herba) and *niú bàng zǐ* (Arctii Fructus). To treat heat entering nutritive level in warm disease, it is often combined with *dì huáng* (Rehmanniae Radix) and *xuán shēn* (Scrophulariae Radix). To treat heat entering blood level in warm disease, it is often combined with *jīn yín huā* (Lonicerae Japonicae Flos) and *dì huáng* (Rehmanniae Radix). The effect of *lián qiáo* in dispelling and dispersing is inferior to *jīn yín huā* (Lonicerae Japonicae Flos), but it has stronger effect of clearing and descending. It is especially good at clearing heart fire. To treat high fever, vexation, loss of consciousness caused by heat entering the pericardium, it is often combined with *huáng lián* (Coptidis Rhizoma) and *lián zǐ xīn* (Nelumbinis Plumula).

3. 热淋涩痛　本品有清心利尿之功。用治热淋，小便短赤涩痛，多与车前子、淡竹叶等同用。

(3) Heat strangury with difficult and painful urination　It has action of clearing heart fire and promoting urination. To treat heat strangury with scanty and brown urine, astringent pain, it is often combined with *chē qián zǐ* (Plantaginis Semen) and *dàn zhú yè* (Lophatheri Herba).

【用法用量 / Usage and dosage】

煎服，6~15g。青翘清热解毒之力较强，老翘长于疏散风热，连翘心长于清心泻火。

Decoction, 6-15g. *Qīng qiáo* is more suitable for clearing heat and removing toxin; *lǎo qiáo* is for dissipating wind-heat; *lián qiáo xīn* is for clearing and reducing heart fire.

【使用注意 / Precaution】

脾胃虚寒者不宜用。

It is not proper for those suffering deficiency cold of spleen and stomach.

【现代研究 / Modern research】

本品主要含连翘苷、连翘酯苷元、连翘酯苷 A、连翘酚、齐墩果酸、芦丁、熊果酸、咖啡酸、维生素 P 以及挥发油等。具有广谱抗菌、抗病毒、解热、抗炎、保肝、镇吐、强心、降压、抗肿瘤等作用。

It mainly contains phillyrin, phillygenin, forsythiaside A, forsythol, oleanic acid, rutinum, uosolic acid, caffeic acid, vitamin P and volatile oil. It has a broad-spectrum antibacterial effect. It also has the functions of antivirus, relieving fever, antagonizing inflammation, protecting the liver, antiemetic, strengthening cadiac action, reducing blood pressure and antitumor.

大青叶　*Dà qīng yè* (Isatidis Folium)
《名医别录》
Miscellaneous Records of Famous Physicians (Míng Yī Bié Lù)

【来源 / Origin】

为十字花科植物菘蓝 *Isatis indigotica* Fort. 的干燥叶。主产于河北、陕西、江苏等省。夏、秋二季分 2~3 次采收，鲜用或晒干，生用。本品气微，味微酸、苦、涩。《中国药典》规定，含靛玉红（$C_{16}H_{10}N_2O_2$）不得少于 0.020%。

Dà qīng yè is the leaf of *Isatis indigotica* Fort., pertaining to Cruciferae. It is mainly produced in Hebei, Shaanxi and Jiangsu Province in China. It is collected twice or three times in summer and fall, and used in fresh or dried in the sunlight. It is used in the raw. It has a slight flavor, tastes slightly sour, bitter and astringent. According to *Chinese Pharmacopoeia*, the content of indigo red ($C_{16}H_{10}N_2O_2$) should be no less than 0.020%.

【性味归经 / Medicinal properties】

苦，寒。归心、胃经。

Bitter and cold; act on the heart and stomach meridians.

【主要功效 / Medicinal efficacies 】

清热解毒，凉血消斑。

Clear heat and resolve toxins, cool blood and resolve macula.

【临床应用 / Clinical application 】

1. 温病发热，风热表证 本品苦寒，既入气分能清热泻火，又入血分能凉血消斑，具有表里两清、气血双解之效，常用于温病各个阶段以及风热表证。用治温病初起，邪在卫分或外感风热，发热头痛，口渴咽痛等，可与葛根、柴胡、牛蒡子等同用。用治温病热入营血，或气血两燔，高热神昏，发斑发疹，常配伍玄参、地黄、栀子等。

(1) **Warm disease with fever, wind-heat exterior syndrome** It is bitter and cold with efficacies of entering qi level to clear heat and reduce fire, as well as acting on blood level to cool blood and resolve macula. It has functions of clearing heat in the exterior and interior, relieving disorders in qi and blood level, which is often used to treat all stages of warm disease and wind-heat exterior syndrome. To treat early stage of warm disease, pathogenic factors entering defense aspect, or external contraction of wind-heat, manifested as fever, headache, thirst and sore throat, it is often combined with *gé gēn* (Puerariae Lobatae Radix), *chái hú* (Bupleuri Radix) and *niú bàng zǐ* (Arctii Fructus). To treat heat entering ying-blood aspect in warm disease, or flaring heat in qi level and blood level, manifested as high fever, loss of consciousness, rashes and macula, it is often combined with *dì huáng* (Rehmanniae Radix), *xuán shēn* (Scrophulariae Radix) and *zhī zǐ* (Gardeniae Fructus).

2. 痄腮，丹毒，口疮，咽痛 本品苦寒，既能清心胃实火，又善解瘟疫时毒，有解毒利咽、凉血消肿之效。用治疮痈、丹毒，常与蒲公英、紫花地丁、野菊花等同用。用治瘟毒上攻，痄腮、喉痹，可与金银花、黄芩等同用。用治心胃火盛，咽喉肿痛，口舌生疮，常与生地黄、大黄、升麻等同用。

(2) **Mumps, erysipelas, aphtha, sore throat** It is bitter and cold with effect of clearing excess fire of heart and stomach, relieving epidemic infectious disease. It has efficacies of resolving toxin and relieving sore throat, cooling the blood and removing swelling. To treat carbuncles and erysipelas, it is often used with *pú gōng yīng* (Taraxaci Herba), *zǐ huā dì dīng* (Violae Herba) and *yě jú huā* (Chrysanthemi Indici Flos). To treat mumps, throat *bì* due to the up-attacking of pestilential toxin, it is often used with *jīn yín huā* (Lonicerae Japonicae Flos) and *huáng qín* (Scutellariae Radix). To treat swollen and painful throat due to exuberant fire of heart and stomach, it is often combined with *shēng dì huáng* (Rehmanniae Radix), *dà huáng* (Rhei Radix et Rhizoma) and *shēng má* (Cimicifugae Rhizoma).

【用法用量 / Usage and dosage 】

煎服，9~15g。外用适量。

Decoction, 9-15g. A proper amount is used for external application.

【使用注意 / Precaution 】

脾胃虚寒者忌用。

It should be contraindicated for those suffering deficiency cold of spleen and stomach.

【现代研究 / Modern research 】

本品主要含靛玉红、靛蓝、菘蓝苷、5-羟基吲哚酮、靛红烷 B 和铁、钛、锰、锌等无机元素及挥发性成分等。具有广谱抑菌、抗病毒、抗肿瘤、解热、抗炎、抗内毒素、增强免疫、保肝、利胆等作用。

It mainly contains indigo red, indigo blue, isatan, 5-hydroxy indolinone, isatan B, inorganic elements, such as iron, titanium, manganese and zinc, as well as volatile oil. It has a broad-spectrum antibacterial effect. It also has the functions of antivirus, antitumor, relieving fever, antagonizing inflammation, antiendotoxin, enhancing immunity, protecting the liver and promoting gallbladder action.

板蓝根 *Bǎn lán gēn* (Isatidis Radix)
《新修本草》
Newly Revised Materia Medica (*Xīn Xīu Běn Cǎo*)

【来源 / Origin】

为十字花科植物菘蓝 *Isatis indigotica* Fort. 的干燥根。主产于江苏、河北。秋季采挖。切片，生用。本品气微，味微甜后苦涩。《中国药典》规定，含（R,S）- 告依春（C_5H_7NOS）不得少于 0.020%。

Bǎn lán gēn is the dried root of *Isatis indigotica* Fort., pertaining to Cruciferae. It is mainly produced in Jiangsu and Hebei Province in China, collected in autumn, and then cut into slices, and used raw. It has a slight flavor and tastes slightly sweet, bitter and astringent. According to *Chinese Pharmacopoeia*, the content of (R,S)-goitrin (C_5H_7NOS) should be no less than 0.020%.

【性味归经 / Medicinal properties】

苦，寒。归心、胃经。

Bitter and cold; act on the heart and stomach meridians.

【主要功效 / Medicinal efficacies】

清热解毒，凉血，利咽。

Clear heat and resolve toxins, cool blood, relieve sore throat.

【临床应用 / Clinical application】

1. 温病发热，风热表证　本品苦寒，功用与大青叶相近，亦为表里双解、气血两清之品，适用于温病各个阶段以及风热表证。用治温病初起，或外感风热，发热，咽痛，可单用或配伍大青叶、连翘、拳参等。用治温病气分实热，常与石膏、知母等同用。用治温病热入营血，或气血两燔，高热、发斑等，常与生地黄、玄参、紫草等同用。

(1) Warm disease with fever, wind-heat exterior syndrome　It is bitter and cold with effect of clearing heat in the exterior and interior, relieving disorders in qi and blood level. Which is similar to *dà qīng yè* (Isatidis Folium). It is often used to treat all stages of warm disease and wind-heat exterior syndrome. To treat early stage of warm disease, or external contraction of wind-heat, manifested as fever and sore throat, it can be used alone, or together with *dà qīng yè* (Isatidis Folium), *lián qiáo* (Forsythiae Fructus) and *quán shēn* (Bistortae Rhizoma). To treat excess heat in the qi level of warm disease, it is often used with *shí gāo* (Gypsum Fibrosum) and *zhī mǔ* (Anemarrhenae Rhizoma). To treat heat entering ying-blood aspect in warm disease, or flaring heat in qi level and blood level, manifested as high fever, rashes and macula, it is often combined with *shēng dì huáng* (Rehmanniae Radix), *xuán shēn* (Scrophulariae Radix) and *zǐ cǎo* (Arnebiae Radix).

2. 咽喉肿痛，大头瘟，痄腮，丹毒　本品善清肺胃之热而利咽喉，有清热解毒、凉血消肿之功，尤以利咽见长。用治肺胃热盛或风热郁肺所致的咽喉肿痛，常与玄参、薄荷、连翘等同用。用治大头瘟，头面红肿，咽喉不利，以及丹毒、痄腮等，常配伍连翘、黄芩、牛蒡子等。

(2) Swollen and painful throat, mumps, erysipelas　It is suitable to clear heat of the lung and stomach to relieve sore throat. It has efficacies of clearing heat and resolving toxin, as well as cooling the blood and removing swelling. Which is especially good at relieving sore throat. To treat swollen and painful throat caused by exuberant heat of the lung and stomach or wind-heat accumulating in the lung, it is often used with *xuán shēn* (Scrophulariae Radix), *bò he* (Menthae Herba) and *lián qiáo* (Forsythiae Fructus). To treat pestilence, red and swollen of head and face, obstructive sensation in the throat, mumps, and erysipelas, it is combined with *lián qiáo*, *huáng qín*, *niú bàng zǐ*.

【用法用量 / Usage and dosage】

煎服，9~15g。

Decoction, 9-15g.

【使用注意 / Precaution】

脾胃虚寒者慎用。

It should be used with caution for those suffering deficiency cold of spleen and stomach.

【现代研究 / Modern research】

本品主要含告依春、表告依春，以及靛玉红、靛蓝、羟基靛玉红、板蓝根乙素、板蓝根丙素、板蓝根丁素、β– 谷甾醇、植物性蛋白、树脂状物、糖类、多种氨基酸等。具有抑菌、抗病毒、抗肿瘤、解热、抗炎、增强免疫等作用。

It mainly contains goitrin, epigoitrin/(R,S)-goitrin, isatin, indigo, hydroxyindirubin, isatan B, isatan C, isatan D, β-sitosterol, vegetable proteins, resinous substance, carbohydrates and multiple amino acids. It has functions of inhibiting bacteria, antivirus, antitumor, relieving fever, antiinflammation and strengthening immunity.

青黛 *Qīng dài* (Indigo Naturalis)
《药性论》
Treatise on Medicinal Properties (Yào Xing Lùn)

【来源 / Origin】

为爵床科植物马蓝 *Baphicacanthus cusia*（Nees）Bremek.、蓼科植物蓼蓝 *Polygonumtinctorium* Ait. 或十字花科植物菘蓝 *Isatis indigotica* Fort. 的叶或茎叶经加工制得的干燥粉末、团块或颗粒。主产于福建、广东、江苏等地。秋季采收以上植物的落叶，加水浸泡至叶腐烂，捞去落叶，加适量石灰乳，充分搅拌至浸液由乌绿色转为深红色，捞取泡沫，晒干而成。研细用。本品微有草腥气，味淡。《中国药典》规定，含靛蓝（$C_{16}H_{16}N_2O_2$）不得少于 2.0%，含靛玉红（$C_{16}H_{10}N_2O_2$）不得少于 0.13%。

Qīng dài is the powder, conglomeration or granule processed from leaves or stems of *Baphicacanthus cusia* (Nees) Bremek., *Polygonumtinctorium* Ait. or *Isatis indigotica* Fort., pertaining to Acanthaceae. It is mainly produced in Fujian, Guangdong and Jiangsu Province in China. Leaves of above plants are selected in fall, and soaked in water until they are rotten. After the rotten leaves are removed, a proper amount of lime milk is added to the infusion, and is stirred until the infusion turns into deep red from dark green. The foam on the surface is collected, dried in the sun and ground into powder. It has a smell of grass, and tastes bland. According to *Chinese Pharmacopoeia*, the content of indigo ($C_{16}H_{16}N_2O_2$) should be no less than 2.0%, and the content of indigo red ($C_{16}H_{10}N_2O_2$) should be no less than 0.13%.

【性味归经 / Medicinal properties】

咸，寒。归肝经。

Salty and cold; act on the liver meridian.

【主要功效 / Medicinal efficacies 】
清热解毒，凉血消斑，泻火定惊。
Clear heat and resolve toxins, cool blood and resolve macula, drain fire and arrest convulsion.

【临床应用 / Clinical application 】

1. 温毒发斑，血热出血　本品苦寒清泄，咸入血分，其清热解毒、凉血消斑之功与大青叶、板蓝根相似，但解热之力较逊。用治温病温毒发斑，常与生地黄、石膏、栀子等同用。用治血热妄行之吐血、衄血、咯血等出血症，常与生地黄、白茅根等同用。

(1) **Warm-toxin macula, hemorrhages due to blood heat**　It is bitter and cold for clearing and draining, salty to act on blood aspect. Its efficacies of clearing heat and resolving toxins, cooling blood and resolving macula is similar to that of *dà qīng yè* (Isatidis Folium) and *bǎn lán gēn* (Isatidis Radix), but its effect of relieving fever is milder. To treat warm-toxin macula in warm disease, it is often combined with *dì huáng* (Rehmanniae Radix), *shí gāo* (Gypsum Fibrosum) and *zhī zǐ* (Gardeniae Fructus). To treat haematemesis, epistaxis and hemoptysis due to blood heat accelerating blood circulation, it is often combined with *dì huáng* (Rehmanniae Radix) and *bái máo gēn* (Imperatae Rhizoma).

2. 喉痹，痄腮，疮痈，丹毒　本品有清热解毒、凉血消肿之效。用治咽喉肿痛，口舌生疮，常配伍板蓝根、甘草等，或配伍黄连、冰片等吹敷患处。用治痄腮肿痛，可与黄芩、玄参等同用，又可单味水调外敷。用治疮痈、丹毒，多与蒲公英、紫花地丁等同用。

(2) **Sore throat, mumps, sores and ulcers, erysipelas**　It has functions of clearing heat and resolving toxins, cooling blood and removing swelling. To treat swollen and painful throat, stomatitis, it is often combined with *bǎn lán gēn* (Isatidis Radix) and *gān cǎo* (Glycyrrhizae Radix et Rhizoma); or combined with *huáng lián* (Coptidis Rhizoma) and *bīng piàn* (Borneolum Syntheticum) blown to the afflicted area. To treat mumps with swelling and pain, it can be used with *huáng qín* (Scutellariae Radix) and *xuán shēn* (Scrophulariae Radix); or used alone by mixing with water for external application. To treat sores and ulcers, erysipelas, it is usually combined with *pú gōng yīng* (Taraxaci Herba) and *zǐ huā dì dīng* (Violae Herba).

3. 肝火犯肺，咳嗽咯血　本品咸寒，长于清肝火，兼泻肺热，且能凉血止血。用治肝火犯肺，咳嗽胸痛，痰中带血，常与海蛤壳同用。用治肺热咳嗽，痰黄质稠，可与浙贝母、瓜蒌等同用。

(3) **Liver fire invading the lung, cough with hemoptysis**　It is salty and cold and good at clearing liver fire. It can also drain lung heat, stanch bleeding by cooling blood. To treat cough with chest pain and blood-tinged sputum due to liver fire invading the lung, it is often used with *hǎi gé qiào* (Meretricis Concha seu Cyclinae). To treat cough, yellowish and thick sputum due to lung heat, it is combined with *zhè bèi mǔ* (Fritillariae Thunbergii Bulbus) and *guā lóu* (Trichosanthis Fructus).

4. 肝热惊痫　本品有清肝泻火、定惊止痉之功，用治肝热生风，惊痫抽搐，多与钩藤、牛黄等同用。

(4) **Epilepsy and convulsion due to liver heat**　It functions to clear liver fire, arrest convulsion and relieve epilepsy. To treat frightened epilepsy, convulsion and spasm due to liver heat producing wind, it is often combined with *gōu téng* (Uncariae Cum Uncis Ramulus) and *niú huáng* (Calculus Bovis).

【用法用量 / Usage and dosage 】
1~3g, 宜入丸、散用。外用适量。
1-3g, it is used in pills or powder. A proper amount is used for external application.

【使用注意 / Precaution】

胃寒者慎用。

It should be used with caution for those suffering cold of stomach.

【现代研究 / Modern research】

本品主要含靛蓝、靛玉红、靛棕、靛黄、鞣酸、β–谷甾醇、蛋白质及大量无机盐等。具有抑菌、抗炎、抗肿瘤、保肝等作用。

It mainly contains indigo, indigo red, indigo palm, indigo yellow, tannic acid, β-sitosterol, protein and a large number of inorganic salts. It has the functions of inhibiting bacteria, antiinflammation, antitumor and protecting the liver.

蒲公英　*Pú gōng yīng* (Taraxaci Herba)
《新修本草》
Newly Revised Materia Medica (*Xīn Xiū Běn Cǎo*)

【来源 / Origin】

为菊科植物蒲公英 *Taraxacum mongolicum* Hand. -Mazz.、碱地蒲公英 *Taraxacum borealisinense* Kitag. 或同属数种植物的干燥全草。全国大部分地区均产。春至秋季花初开时采挖。鲜用或生用。本品气微，味微苦。《中国药典》规定，含咖啡酸（$C_9H_8O_4$）不得少于 0.020%。

Pú gong yīng is the entire plant of *Taraxacum mongolicum* Hand.-Mazz., *Taraxacum borealisinense* Kitag., pertaining to Composutae or other plants of the same genus, produced in large parts of China. It is collected from spring to autumn when it begins to blossom, and dried in the sun. It is used raw or fresh. It has a slight flavor and tastes slightly bitter. According to *Chinese Pharmacopoeia*, the content of caffeic acid ($C_9H_8O_4$) should be no less than 0.020%.

【性味归经 / Medicinal properties】

苦、甘，寒。归肝、胃经。

Salty and sweet, cold; act on the liver and stomach meridian.

【主要功效 / Medicinal efficacies】

清热解毒，消肿散结，利湿通淋。

Clear heat and resolve toxins, subside swelling and dissipate masses, remove damp and relieve strangury.

【临床应用 / Clinical application】

1. **热毒疮痈**　本品苦寒，善能清热解毒，消痈散结，凡是热毒疮痈，不论内痈外痈，均为常用之品。用治热毒疮痈肿热，常配伍金银花、紫花地丁、野菊花等。用治肠痈，常与大黄、牡丹皮同用。用治肺痈，常配伍鱼腥草、芦根等。因本品长于入肝、胃经，兼能通乳，故为治乳痈要药，可单用浓煎内服；或以鲜品捣汁内服，药渣外敷；或配伍瓜蒌、金银花、牛蒡子等。

(1) **Sores and carbuncles due to heat-toxin**　It is bitter and cold with effect of clearing heat and resolving toxins, removing ulcers and dissipating masses. It is a commonly used medicinal to treat sores and carbuncles due to heat-toxin, whether it is abscess of internal organs or carbuncles over the body surface. To treat sores and carbuncles with swelling and heat due to heat-toxin, it is often combined with *jīn yín huā* (Lonicerae Japonicae Flos), *zǐ huā dì dīng* (Violae Herba) and *yě jú huā* (Chrysanthemi Indici Flos). To treat intestinal abscess, it is often used with *dà huáng* (Rhei Radix et Rhizoma) and *mǔ dān pí* (Moutan Cortex). To treat lung abscess, it is often used with *yú xīng cǎo* (Houttuyniae Herba) and *lú gēn* (Phragmitis Rhizoma). Since it acts on the liver and stomach

meridians, it can also promote lactation, which serves as an essential medicinal to treat acute mastitis. To treat acute mastitis, the single concentrated decoction can be used for oral taking; or pound the fresh one into juice for oral administration, and the dregs are externally pasted on the afflected area; or combined with *guā lóu* (Trichosanthis Fructus), *jīn yín huā* (Lonicerae Japonicae Flos) and *niú bàng zǐ* (Arctii Fructus).

2. **湿热黄疸，热淋涩痛** 本品有清利湿热、利尿通淋之功。用治湿热黄疸，常与茵陈、栀子等同用。用治热淋涩痛，常与车前子、金钱草等同用。

(2) Jaundice due to damp-heat, heat strangury with astringent pain It has efficacies of clearing damp-heat, promoting urination and relieving strangury. To treat jaundice due to damp-heat, it is often combined with *yīn chén* (Artemisiae Scopariae Herba) and *zhī zǐ* (Gardeniae Fructus). To treat heat strangury with astringent pain, it is combined with *chē qián zǐ* (Plantaginis Semen) and *jīn qián cǎo* (Lysimachiae Herba).

此外，本品还有清肝明目作用，用治肝火上炎所致的目赤肿痛，可单用，或与菊花、夏枯草等同用。

In addition, it can also clearing liver fire and improve vision. To treat red and swollen eyes with pain due to upward flaming of liver fire, it can be used alone, or combined with *jú huā* (Chrysanthemi Flos) and *xià kū cǎo* (Prunellae Spica)

【用法用量 / Usage and dosage】

煎服，10~15g。外用鲜品适量，捣敷或煎汤熏洗患处。

Decoction, 10-15g. A proper amount of fresh one is used for external application, ground into pieces and pasted on the affected area or decocted for fumigation.

【使用注意 / Precaution】

用量过大可致缓泻。

Overdosage can cause mild diarrhea.

【现代研究 / Modern research】

本品主要含咖啡酸、绿原酸、蒲公英素、蒲公英甾醇、蒲公英苦素、木犀草素、槲皮素、挥发油等。具有抑菌、抗肿瘤、抗溃疡、提高免疫力、保肝、利胆、健胃、利尿作用。

It mainly contains caffeic acid, chlorogenic acid, taraxacin, taraxasterol, luteolin, quercetin and volatile oil. It has the functions of inhibiting bacteria, antitumor, antiulcer, enhancing immunity, protecting the liver, promoting gallbladder function, invigorating the stomach and promoting urination.

鱼腥草 *Yú xīng cǎo* (Houttuyniae Herba)

《名医别录》

Miscellaneous Records of Famous Physicians (Míng Yī Bié Lù)

【来源 / Origin】

为三白草科植物蕺菜 *Houttuynia cordata* Thunb. 的新鲜全草或干燥地上部分。主产于浙江、江苏、安徽等地。鲜品全年均可采割；干品夏季茎叶茂盛花穗多时采割，生用。本品具鱼腥气，味涩。

Yú xīng cǎo is the fresh whole plant or the aerial part of *Houttuynia cordata* Thunb., pertaining to Saururaceae. It is mainly produced in Zhejiang, Jiangsu and Anhui Province in China. Fresh *yú xīng cǎo* can be collected all year around and the dry one is often collected in summer when it is prosperous with more spikes. It is used raw. It has a fishy smell and tastes astringent.

【性味归经 / Medicinal properties】

辛，微寒。归肺经。

Salty and slightly cold; act on the lung meridian.

【主要功效 / Medicinal efficacies】

清热解毒，消痈排脓，利尿通淋。

Clear heat and resolve toxins, eliminate carbuncle and expel pus, promote urination and relieve strangury.

【临床应用 / Clinical application】

1. 肺痈吐脓，肺热咳嗽 本品性寒，专入肺经，长于清肺中热毒以消痈排脓，为治疗肺痈之要药。用治肺痈咳吐脓血，常与桔梗、芦根、薏苡仁等同用。若治肺热咳嗽，痰黄黏稠，常配伍黄芩、浙贝母等。

(1) **Lung abscess with expectoration of pus, cough due to lung heat** It is cold in nature and acts exclusively on the lung meridian. It is good at clearing heat-toxin in the lung to eliminate carbuncle and expel pus, which is regarded as an essential medicinal to treat lung abscess. To treat lung abscess with cough and expectoration of pus, it is often combined with *jié gěng* (Platycodonis Radix), *lú gēn* (Phragmitis Rhizoma) and *yì yǐ rén* (Coicis Semen). To treat cough due to lung heat, with symptoms of yellowish and thick sputum, it is often combined with *huáng qín* (Scutellariae Radix) and *zhè bèi mǔ* (Fritillariae Thunbergii Bulbus).

2. 热毒疮痈 本品有清热解毒之功。用治热毒疮痈，红肿热痛，可单用鲜品捣敷，或与连翘、野菊花、蒲公英等同用。

(2) **Sores and carbuncles due to heat-toxin** It has effect of clearing heat and resolving toxins. To treat sores and carbuncles due to heat-toxin with symptoms of red, swelling, heat and pain, the fresh one is pounded for external application, or combined with *lián qiáo* (Forsythiae Fructus), *yě jú huā* (Chrysanthemi Indici Flos) and *pú gōng yīng* (Taraxaci Herba).

3. 热淋热痢 本品有清热除湿、利尿通淋之效，兼能清热止痢。用治热淋涩痛，常与车前子、滑石等同用。用治湿热泻痢，可与黄连、白头翁等同用。

(3) **Heat strangury and dysentery of heat type** It has efficacies of clearing heat and removing damp, promoting urination and relieving strangury, as well as clearing heat to arrest dysentery. To treat heat strangury with astringent pain, it is often combined with *chē qián zǐ* (Plantaginis Semen) and *huá shí* (Talcum). To treat diarrhea and dysentery due to damp-heat, it is often combined with *huáng lián* (Coptidis Rhizoma) and *bái tóu wēng* (Pulsatillae Radix).

【用法用量 / Usage and dosage】

煎服，15~25g，不宜久煎；鲜品用量加倍，水煎或捣汁服。外用适量，捣敷或煎汤熏洗患处。

Decoction, 15-25g. It should not be decocted overtime. The dosage is doubled when the fresh one is decocted or pounded for juice. A proper amount is used for external application, or for fumigating and washing the affected area.

【现代研究 / Modern research】

本品主要含挥发油，如月桂烯、月桂醛、癸酰乙醛等，尚含阿福豆苷、金丝桃苷、槲皮素、槲皮苷、亚油酸、氯化钾等。具有抑菌、抗病毒、解热、抗炎、镇咳、镇痛、提高免疫力、利尿等作用。

It mainly contains volatile oil, such as myrcene, lauraldehyde, houttuynin. It also contains afzelin, hyperoside, quercetin, quercitrin, linoleic acid and potassium chloride. It has the functions of inhibiting bacteria, antivirus, relieving fever, antiinflammation, relieving cough, alleviating pain, enhancing immunity and promoting urination.

牛黄　*Niú huáng* (Bovis Calculus)
《神农本草经》
Shen Nong's Classic of the Materia Medica (Shén Nóng Běn Cǎo Jīng)

【来源 / Origin】

为牛科动物牛 *Bos taurus domesticus* Gmelin 的干燥胆结石。主产于华北、东北、西北。宰牛时，如发现有牛黄，即滤去胆汁，将牛黄取出，除去外部薄膜，阴干。《中国药典》规定，含胆酸（$C_{24}H_{40}O_5$）不得少于 4.0%，胆红素（$C_{33}H_{36}N_4O_6$）不得少于 25.0%。

Niú huáng is the dried gallstones of *Bos taurus domesticus* Gmelin, pertaining to Bovidae. It is mainly produced in north, northeast and northwest of China. If *niú huáng* is found in the butchered ox, filter out bile to take it, get rid of its external membrane, and then dry it in the shade. According to *Chinese Pharmacopoeia*, the content of cholanic acid ($C_{24}H_{40}O_5$) should be no less than 4.0%, and the content of bilirubin ($C_{33}H_{36}N_4O_6$) should be no less than 25.0%.

【性味归经 / Medicinal properties】

甘，凉。归心、肝经。

Sweet and cool; act on the heart and liver meridians.

【主要功效 / Medicinal efficacies】

清热解毒，清心豁痰，开窍醒神，凉肝息风。

Clear heat and resolve toxins, clear heart fire and eliminate sputum, induce resuscitation, cooling liver and extinguishing wind.

【临床应用 / Clinical application】

1. 热毒疮痈，咽喉肿痛　本品性凉，有良好的清热解毒作用。用治热毒内盛，咽喉肿痛、牙龈肿痛、口舌生疮，常配伍黄芩、黄连、大黄等。用治痈肿、疔疮、乳岩、瘰疬等，常配伍麝香、乳香、没药等。

(1) Sores and carbuncles due to heat-toxin, sore throat　It is cool in nature with favorable effect of clearing heat and resolving toxin. To treat sore throat, swollen and painful gum, aphtha of the mouth and tongue due to internal exuberance of heat-toxin, it is often combined with *huáng qín* (Scutellariae Radix), *huáng lián* (Coptidis Rhizoma) and *dà huáng* (Rhei Radix et Rhizoma). To treat carbuncle with swelling, furuncle and sores, breast cancer and scrofula, it is often combined with *shè xiāng* (Moschus), *rǔ xiāng* (Olibanum) and *mò yào* (Myrrha).

2. 热闭神昏　本品性凉，入心经，功能清心豁痰，开窍醒神，为凉开之品。用治温热病热入心包以及中风、惊风、癫痫等痰热阻闭心窍所致的高热烦躁，神昏谵语，常与麝香、冰片等同用。

(2) Loss of consciousness due to heat block　It is cool in nature and acts on the heart meridian. Which has efficacies of clearing heart fire and eliminating sputum as well as inducing resuscitation. To treat heat entering the pericardium, stroke, convulsion and epilepsy due to phlegm-heat blocking the heart, manifested as high fever, vexation, loss of consciousness, delirium speech, it is often combined with *shè xiāng* (Moschus) and *bīng piàn* (Borneolum Syntheticum).

3. 热极生风，癫痫发狂　本品性凉，入心、肝经，有清心凉肝、息风止痉之功。用治温热病壮热神昏，惊厥抽搐及小儿急惊风，常与钩藤、全蝎、朱砂等同用。若治癫痫发作，不知人事，常与琥珀、珍珠、钩藤等同用。

(3) Epilepsy and mania due to extreme heat generating wind It is cool in nature and acts on the heart and liver meridians. Which has efficacies of clearing heart fire and cooling the liver fire, as well as extinguishing wind to arrest convulsion. To treat warm disease with high fever, loss of consciousness, convulsion and spasm, and infantile convulsion, it is often combined with *gōu téng* (Uncariae Cum Uncis Ramulus), *quán xiē* (Scorpio) and *zhū shā* (Cinnabaris). To treat epileptic seizures, unconsciousness, it is often used with *hǔ pò* (Succinum), *zhēn zhū* (Margarita) and *gōu téng* (Uncariae Cum Uncis Ramulus).

【用法用量 / Usage and dosage】

入丸、散剂，0.15~0.35g。外用适量，研末敷患处。

It is used in pills and powder, 0.15-0.35g. A proper amount is used for external application, ground into powder for the affected area.

【使用注意 / Precaution】

非实热证不宜使用。孕妇慎用。

It should not be used in non-excess heat syndrome. It should be used with caution for pregnant women.

【现代研究 / Modern research】

本品主要含胆红素、胆酸、去氧胆酸、牛黄胆酸以及脂肪酸、卵磷脂、维生素 D 等。具有镇静、抗惊厥、解热、抗炎、镇痛、抗病原微生物、降压、利胆、保肝、降血脂等作用。

It mainly contains cholanic acid, bilirubin, deoxycholic acid, cholaic acid, fatty acid, lecithin and vitamin D. It has the functions of tranquilizing, anticonvulsion, relieving fever, relieving pain, antipathogenic microorganism, lowering blood pressure, promoting gallbladder function, protecting the liver and lowering blood fat.

白头翁 *Bái tóu wēng* (Pulsatillae Radix)
《神农本草经》
Shen Nong's Classic of the Materia Medica (Shén Nóng Běn Cǎo Jīng)

【来源 / Origin】

为毛茛科植物白头翁 *Pulsatilla chinensis*（Bge.）Regel 的干燥根。全国大部分地区均产。春、秋二季采挖。切薄片，生用。本品气微，味微苦涩。《中国药典》规定，含白头翁皂苷 B$_4$（C$_{59}$H$_{96}$O$_{26}$）不得少于 4.6%。

Bái tóu wēng is the root of *Pulsatilla chinensis* (Bge.) Regel, pertaining to Ranunculaceae. It is produced in most parts of China, collected in spring and autumn, cut into slices and used raw. It has a slight flavor and tastes slightly bitter and astringent. According to *Chinese Pharmacopoeia*, the content of anemoside B$_4$ (C$_{59}$H$_{96}$O$_{26}$) should be no less than 4.6%.

【性味归经 / Medicinal properties】

苦，寒。归胃、大肠经。

Bitter and cold; act on the stomach and large intestine meridians.

【主要功效 / Medicinal efficacies】

清热解毒，凉血止痢。

Clear heat and resolve toxins, cool the blood and stop dysentery.

【临床应用 / Clinical application】

1. **热毒血痢**　本品苦寒降泄，专入大肠经，功善清热解毒，凉血止痢，为治痢良药。无论热毒血痢还是湿热痢疾，症见下痢脓血、里急后重者均有较好的疗效，常与黄连、黄柏、秦皮等同用。若治赤痢下血，日久不愈，腹中冷痛，则与干姜、赤石脂等同用。

(1) Bloody dysentery due to heat-toxin　It is bitter and cold for descending and reducing, which exclusively acts on the large intestine. It functions to clear heat and resolve toxins, cool the blood and stop dysentery. It is an effective medicinal to treat dysentery. Whether it is bloody dysentery due to heat-toxin or dysentery caused by damp-heat, manifested as dysentery with pus and blood, tenesmus, it can be treated in combination with *huáng lián* (Coptidis Rhizoma), *huáng bó* (Phellodendri Chinensis Cortex) and *qín pí* (Fraxini Cortex) to reach favorable curative effect. To treat lingering bloody dysentery with cold pain in the abdomen, it is often combined with *gān jiāng* (Zingiberis Rhizoma) and *chì shí zhī* (Halloysitum Rubrum).

2. **阴痒带下**　本品性味苦寒，又具清热燥湿之效，亦可用治下焦湿热，阴痒带下，常与苦参、白鲜皮、秦皮等配伍，煎汤外洗。

(2) Pruritus vulvae, leukorrhea　It is bitter and cold with effect of clearing heat and drying damp. To treat pruritus vulvae, leukorrhea due to damp-heat in the lower energizer, it is often decocted with *kǔ shēn* (Sophorae Flavescentis Radix), *bái xiān pí* (Dictamni Cortex) and *qín pí* (Fraxini Cortex) for external washing.

【用法用量 / Usage and dosage】

煎服，9~15g。

Decoction, 9-15g.

【使用注意 / Precaution】

虚寒泻痢者忌服。

It should be contraindicated for those suffering diarrhea and dysentery due to deficient cold.

【现代研究 / Modern research】

本品主要含三萜皂苷、白头翁皂苷 B_4、白头翁素、原白头翁素、白桦脂酸、胡萝卜苷等。具有抗阿米巴原虫、抗阴道滴虫、抑菌、抗病毒、抗癌、镇静、镇痛等作用。

It mainly contains triterpenoidsaponins, anemoside B_4, anemonin, protoanemonin, betulinic acid and daucosterol. It has functions of resisting amebic protozoa, resisting trichomonadvaginitis, inhibiting bacteria, anticancer, tranquilizing, and relieving pain.

土茯苓　*Tǔ fú líng* (Smilacis Glabrae Rhizoma)
《本草纲目》
The Grand Compendium of Materia Medica (Běn Cǎo Gāng Mù)

【来源 / Origin】

为百合科植物光叶菝葜 *Smilax glabra* Roxb. 的干燥根茎。主产于广东、湖南、湖北等地。夏、秋二季采收。切片，生用。本品气微，味微甘、涩。《中国药典》规定，含落新妇苷（$C_{21}H_{22}O_{11}$）不得少于 0.45%。

Tǔ fú líng is the rhizome of *Smilax glabra* Roxb., pertaining to Liliaceae. It is mainly produced in Guangdong, Hunan and Hubei Province in China, collected in summer and autumn, cut into slices and used raw. It has a slight flavor and tastes slightly sweet and astringent. According to *Chinese Pharmacopoeia*, the content of astilbin ($C_{21}H_{22}O_{11}$) should be no less than 0.45%.

【性味归经 / Medicinal properties】

甘、淡，平。归肝、胃经。

Sweet, bland and neutral; act on the liver and stomach meridians.

【主要功效 / Medicinal efficacies】

解毒，除湿，通利关节。

Resolve toxins, remove damp, smooth joint movement.

【临床应用 / Clinical application】

1. **梅毒及汞中毒** 本品甘淡渗利，善能解毒利湿，又能通利关节，兼解汞毒，对梅毒或因治疗梅毒服汞剂中毒而致肢体拘挛、筋骨疼痛者，效果尤佳，故为治梅毒要药。可单味大剂量水煎服，或配伍金银花、薏苡仁、木瓜等。

(1) Syphilis and hydrargyrism It is sweet and bland with effect of resolving toxin and draining damp, smoothing joint movement, as well as removing hydrargyrism. It can treat syphilis or spasm of the limbs, pain in bones and muscles due to toxication caused by taking syphilitic amalgam. It is the most powerful medicinal for syphilis. It is decocted alone with large dosage for oral administration, or combined with *jīn yín huā* (Lonicerae Japonicae Flos), *yì yǐ rén* (Coicis Semen) and *mù guā* (Chaenomelis Fructus).

2. **热淋，带下，湿疹，疥癣** 本品性平偏凉，清热利湿，尤长于利湿，故可用治多种湿热病证。若治湿热淋证，可与车前子、木通等同用。若治湿热带下、阴痒，常与黄柏、苦参等同用。若治湿疹、疥癣瘙痒，可与苦参、白鲜皮等同用。

(2) Heat strangury, leukorrhea, eczema, scabies It is cool and neutral in nature with efficacies of clearing heat and draining damp. It is especially good at draining damp, and can be use to treat various diseases caused by damp-heat. To treat strangury caused by damp-heat, it can be used with *chē qián zǐ* (Plantaginis Semen) and *mù tōng* (Akebiae Caulis). To treat vaginal discharge caused by damp heat with symptoms of pruritus vulvae, it is often combined with *huáng bó* (Phellodendri Chinensis Cortex) and *kǔ shēn* (Sophorae Flavescentis Radix). To treat eczema, and itching scabies, it is combined with *kǔ shēn* (Sophorae Flavescentis Radix) and *bái xiān pí* (Dictamni Cortex).

此外，本品解毒除湿，也可用于疮痈红肿溃烂、瘰疬溃疡。

In addition, it can resolve toxin and remove damp, which can be used to treat sores and carbuncles with redness and swelling, as well as scrofula and ulcer.

【用法用量 / Usage and dosage】

煎服，15~60g。外用适量。

Decoction, 15-60g. A proper amount is used for external application.

【现代研究 / Modern research】

本品主要含落新妇苷、异黄杞苷、胡萝卜苷、生物碱、树脂、淀粉、多糖、挥发油、甾醇等。具有利尿、镇痛、抑菌、抗肿瘤、抗棉酚毒性作用。

It mainly contains astilbin, isoengelitin, daucosterol, alkaloid, resin, amylum, polysaccharide, volatile oil and sterol. It has the functions of promoting urination, relieving pain, inhibiting bacteria, antitumor and anti-gossypol toxicity.

山豆根 *Shān dòu gēn* (Sophorae Tonkinensis Radix et Rhizoma)

《开宝本草》

Materia Medica of the Kaibao Era (Kāi Bǎo Běn Cǎo)

【来源 / Origin】

为豆科植物越南槐 *Sophora tonkinensis* Gapnep. 的干燥根及根茎，又称广豆根。主产于广西。秋季采挖。切片，生用。本品有豆腥气，味极苦。《中国药典》规定，含苦参碱（$C_{15}H_{24}N_2O$）和

微课

医药大学堂
WWW.YIYAODXT.COM

氧化苦参碱（$C_{15}H_{24}N_2O_2$）不得少于 0.7%。

Shān dòu gēn is the root and rhizome of *Sophora tonkinensis* Gapnep., pertaining to Leguminosae, which is also called *guǎng dòu gēn*. It is mainly produced in Guangxi Zhuang Autonomous Region, collected in autumn and cut into slices, and used raw. It has a bean flavor and tastes extremely bitter. According to *Chinese Pharmacopoeia*, the content of matrine ($C_{15}H_{24}N_2O$) and oxymatrine ($C_{15}H_{24}N_2O_2$) should be no less than 0.7%.

【性味归经 / Medicinal properties】

苦，寒；有毒。归肺、胃经。

Bitter and cold; act on the lung and stomach meridians.

【主要功效 / Medicinal efficacies】

清热解毒，消肿利咽。

Clear heat and resolve toxins, remove swelling and relieve sore throat.

【临床应用 / Clinical application】

1. 咽喉肿痛 本品苦寒之性尤甚，长于清肺胃热毒以利咽消肿，为治疗热毒蕴结，咽喉红肿疼痛之要药，轻者可单用本品，水煎服或含漱；重者须配伍射干、玄参、板蓝根等。

(1) Swollen and sore throat It is extremely bitter with fairly cold nature, which is effective in treating swollen and sore throat due to heat-toxin accumulating in the lung and stomach. It is an essential medicinal to treat sore throat with swelling and pain. For the mild one, it can be used alone, decocted for oral taking or mouth washing, and for the severe one, it is combined with *shè gān* (Belamcandae Rhizoma), *xuán shēn* (Scrophulariae Radix) and *bǎn lán gēn* (Isatidis Radix).

2. 牙龈肿痛，口舌生疮 本品归胃经，有清胃热之功。用治胃火上攻，牙龈肿痛、口舌生疮，可单用煎汤漱口，或与石膏、黄连、升麻等同用。

(2) Swollen and painful gum, sore in the mouth and tongue *Shān dòu gēn* acts on the stomach meridian with effect of clearing stomach heat. To treat swollen and painful gum, sore in the mouth and tongue, it can be used alone, decocted for mouth washing, or combined with *shí gāo* (Gypsum Fibrosum), *huáng lián* (Coptidis Rhizoma) and *shēng má* (Cimicifugae Rhizoma).

【用法用量 / Usage and dosage】

煎服，3~6g。外用适量。

Decoction, 3-6g. A proper amount for external application.

【使用注意 / Precaution】

用量不宜过大，脾胃虚寒者慎用。

As it is toxic, overdosage can lead to vomiting, diarrhea, oppression in the chest and palpitation. It should be used with caution for those suffering deficient cold of spleen and stomach.

【现代研究 / Modern research】

本品主要含苦参碱、氧化苦参碱、臭豆碱、槐根碱、山豆根碱等，尚含柔枝槐酮、柔枝槐素、柔枝槐酮色烯等。具有抑菌、抗炎、抗肿瘤、保肝、强心、抗心律失常等作用。

It mainly contains matrine, oxymatrine, anagyrine, sophoridine and sophocarpidine. It also contains sophoranone, sophoradin and sophoranochromene. It has the functions of inhibiting bacteria, antiinflammation, antitumor, protecting the liver, increasing myocardial contractility and resisting arrhythmia.

射干　*Shè gān* (Belamcandae Rhizoma)
《神农本草经》
Shen Nong's Classic of the Materia Medica (Shén Nóng Běn Cǎo Jīng)

【来源 / Origin】

为鸢尾科植物射干 *Belamcanda chinensis*（L.）DC. 的干燥根茎。主产于湖北、江苏、河南等地。春初或秋末采挖，切片，生用。本品气微，味苦、微辛。《中国药典》规定，含次野鸢尾黄素（C$_{20}$H$_{18}$O$_8$）不得少于 0.1%。

Shè gān is the rhizome of *Belamcanda chinensis* (L.) DC., pertaining to Rutaceae, mainly produced in Hubei, Jiangsu and Henan Province in China. It is collected in the early spring or in late autumn, cut into slices, and used raw. It has a slight flavor and tastes bitter and slightly acrid. According to *Chinese Pharmacopoeia*, the content of irisflorentin (C$_{20}$H$_{18}$O$_8$) should be no less than 0.1%.

【性味归经 / Medicinal properties】

苦，寒。归肺经。

Bitter and cold; act on the lung meridian.

【主要功效 / Medicinal efficacies】

清热解毒，消痰，利咽。

Clear heat and resolve toxins, dissolve phlegm and relieve sore throat.

【临床应用 / Clinical application】

1. 咽喉肿痛　本品苦寒清泄，专入肺经，善能清热解毒、利咽消肿。因其兼能祛痰，故对痰热壅盛之咽喉肿痛较为适宜，可单用，或与桔梗、黄芩、甘草等同用。若治外感风热，咽痛音哑，可配伍蝉蜕、连翘、牛蒡子等。

(1) **Swollen and painful throat**　*Shè gān* is bitter and cold for clearing and draining heat. It specially acts on the lung meridian with efficacies of clearing heat and resolving toxins, as well as relieving swollen and sore throat. As it also has function of eliminating phlegm, it is suitable to treat swollen and sore throat caused by binding constraint of heat-toxin and phlegm. For the above-mentioned condition, it can be used alone, or combined with *jié gěng* (Platycodonis Radix), *huáng qín* (Scutellariae Radix) and *gān cǎo* (Glycyrrhizae Radix et Rhizoma). To treat sore throat hoarse voice caused by external contraction of wind-heat, it is often combined with *chán tuì* (Cicadae Periostracum), *lián qiáo* (Forsythiae Fructus) and *niú bàng zǐ* (Arctii Fructus).

2. 痰盛咳喘　本品苦寒降泄，能清肺泻火、降气消痰以止咳平喘。用治肺热咳喘，痰黄质稠，常配伍桑白皮、桔梗、马兜铃等。若治寒痰咳喘，痰多清稀，可配伍麻黄、细辛、半夏等。

(2) **Cough and panting due to phlegm congestion**　It is bitter and cold for descending and draining. It can clear lung fire, descend qi and eliminate phlegm to relieve cough and asthma. To treat cough, panting, yellowish and thick sputum caused by lung heat, it is combined with *sāng bái pí* (Mori Cortex), *jié gěng* (Platycodonis Radix) and *mǎ dōu líng* (Aristolochiae Fructus). To treat cough and panting due to accumulation of cold phlegm, manifested as profuse and thin sputum, it is combined with *má huáng* (Ephedrae Herba), *xì xīn* (Asari Radix et Rhizoma) and *bàn xià* (Pinelliae Rhizoma).

【用法用量 / Usage and dosage】

煎服，3~10g。

Decoction, 3-10g.

【使用注意 / Precaution】

脾虚便溏者不宜使用。孕妇慎用。

It should not be used with those suffering loose stool due to spleen deficiency. It should be used with caution for pregnant women.

【现代研究 / Modern research】

本品主要含次野鸢尾黄素、鸢尾黄素、鸢尾苷以及二苯乙烯类化合物、二环三萜及其衍生物等。具有抑菌、抗病毒、抗真菌、解热、抗炎、镇痛、镇咳、祛痰、利尿等作用。

It mainly contains irisflorentin, tectorigenin, tectoridin, stilbenes, dicyclic triperpenoids and their derivatives. It has the functions of inhibiting bacteria, antivirus, relieving fever, antiinflammation, relieving pain, relieving cough, eliminating sputum and promoting urination.

大血藤 *Dà xuè téng* (Sargentodoxae Caulis)
《本草图经》
Illustrated Classic of Materia Medica (Běn Cǎo Tú Jīng)

【来源 / Origin】

为木通科植物大血藤 *Sargentodoxa cuneata*（oliv.）Rehd.et wils. 的干燥藤茎。主产于江西、湖北、湖南等地。秋、冬二季采收。切厚片，生用。本品气微，味微涩。

Dà xuè téng is the dried ratan of *Sargentodoxa cuneata* (oliv.) Rehd.et wils., pertaining to Lardizabalaceae. It is mainly produced in Jiangxi, Hubei and Hunan Province in China, collected in autumn and winter, cut into thick slices and used raw. It has a slight flavor and tastes slightly astringent.

【性味归经 / Medicinal properties】

苦，平。归大肠、肝经。

Bitter and neutral; act on the large intestine and liver meridians.

【主要功效 / Medicinal efficacies】

清热解毒，活血，祛风止痛。

Clear heat and resolve toxins, activate blood, dispel wind and relieve pain.

【临床应用 / Clinical application】

1. 肠痈腹痛，热毒疮痈　本品清热解毒，活血消痈，无论内痈、外痈均可选用。因其主归大肠经，善清肠中热毒，行肠中瘀滞，故为肠痈腹痛之要药，常与败酱草、桃仁、大黄等同用。若治皮肤热毒疮痈，常配伍金银花、连翘等。

(1) **Abdominal pain due to intestinal abscess, sores and carbuncles due to heat-toxin** It has functions of clearing heat and resolving toxins, activating blood and removing carbuncles, which can be used to treat abscess of internal organs as well as carbuncle over the body surface. For it mainly acts on large intestine, it is especially effective in clearing heat-toxin in the intestines and removing intestinal stagnations, which serves as an essential medicinal to treat abdominal pain due to intestinal abscess, and is often combined with *bài jiàng cǎo* (Patriniae Herba), *táo rén* (Persicae Semen) and *dà huáng* (Rhei Radix et Rhizoma). To treat sores and carbuncles on the skin due to heat-toxin, it is often used with *jīn yín huā* (Lonicerae Japonicae Flos) and *lián qiào* (Forsythiae Fructus).

2. 跌打损伤，痛经，风湿痹痛　本品有活血祛瘀、消肿止痛之功。用治跌打损伤，瘀血肿痛，常配伍骨碎补、续断、赤芍等。用治血滞经闭、痛经，常与当归、红花、益母草等同用。用治风湿痹痛，腰膝疼痛，筋骨无力，屈伸不利等，常与独活、威灵仙、杜仲等同用。

(2) **Traumatic injuries, painful menstruation, wind-damp *bì* with pain** It has efficacies of

activating blood and removing stasis, as well as resolving swelling to relieve pain. To treat traumatic injuries, swelling and pain due to static blood, it is often combined with *gǔ suì bǔ* (Drynariae Rhizoma), *xù duàn* (Dipsaci Radix) and *chì sháo* (Paeoniae Rubra Radix). To treat amenorrhea and painful menstruation due to blood stagnation, it is often combined with *dāng guī* (Angelicae Sinensis Radix), *hóng huā* (Carthami Flos) and *yì mǔ cǎo* (Leonuri Herba). To treat wind-damp *bì* with pain, manifested as pain in the limb and legs, and unsmooth movement of joints, it is combined with *dú huó* (Angelicae Pubescentis Radix), *wēi líng xiān* (Clematidis Radix et Rhizoma) and *dù zhòng* (Eucommiae Cortex).

【用法用量 / Usage and dosage】

煎服，9~15g。外用适量。

Decoction, 9-15g. A proper amount is used for external application.

【使用注意 / Precaution】

孕妇慎用。

It should be used with caution for pregnant women.

【现代研究 / Modern research】

本品主要含大黄素、大黄素甲醚、大黄酚、胡萝卜苷、β-谷甾醇、硬脂酸、右旋丁香酚二葡萄糖苷、香草酸、鞣质等。具有抑菌、抗血小板聚集、增加冠脉血流量、扩张冠状动脉、抗血栓等作用。

It mainly contains emodin, physcion, chrysophanol, daucosterol, β-sitosterol, stearic acid, diverse phenols, phenolic glycosides, vanillic acid and tannins. It has the functions of inhibiting bacteria, antiplatelet aggregation, increasing the coronary flow, expanding coronary arteries and antithrombotic.

白花蛇舌草 *Bái huā shé shé cǎo* (Hedyotis Diffusae Herba)
《广西中药志》
Guangxi Chinese Materia Medica (Guǎng Xī Zhōng Yào Zhì)

【来源 / Origin】

为茜草科植物白花蛇舌草 *Oldenlandia diffusa*（willd.）Roxb. 的干燥全草。主产于云南、广东、广西等地。夏、秋二季采收。切段，生用。本品气微，味苦、淡。

Bái huā shé shé cǎo is the whole plant of *Oldenlandia diffusa* (willd.) Roxb., pertaining to Rubiaceae, and produced in Yunnan and Guangdong Province, and Guangxi Zhuang Autonomous Region. It is collected in summer and autumn, cut into segments and used raw. It has a slight flavor and tastes bitter and bland.

【性味归经 / Medicinal properties】

微苦、甘，寒。归胃、大肠、小肠经。

Slightly bitter, sweet and cold; act on the stomach, large intestine and small intestine meridians.

【主要功效 / Medicinal efficacies】

清热解毒，利湿通淋。

Clear heat and resolve toxins, eliminate damp and relieve strangury.

【临床应用 / Clinical application】

1. **痈肿疮毒，咽喉肿痛，毒蛇咬伤** 本品苦寒，既能清热解毒，消散痈肿，又能解蛇毒。用治皮肤痈肿疮毒，可单用捣烂外敷，也常配伍金银花、连翘、蒲公英等。用治肠痈腹痛，多与大血藤、败酱草等同用。用治咽喉肿痛，常与玄参、板蓝根、牛蒡子等同用。用治毒蛇咬伤，可单用鲜品捣烂绞汁内服或水煎服，渣敷伤口，或与半边莲、杠板归等同用。因其解毒消肿之力较强，也常用于各种癌肿的治疗。

(1) Abscess, swelling, sore and toxin, sore throat, bites by poisonous snakes It is bitter and cold with effects of clearing heat and resolving toxins, dissolving abscess and swelling, as well as resolving snake poison. To treat abscess, swelling, sore and toxin on the skin, it can be pounded alone to paste externally or combined with *jīn yín huā* (Lonicerae Japonicae Flos), *lián qiáo* (Forsythiae Fructus) and *pú gōng yīng* (Taraxaci Herba). To treat abdominal pain due to intestinal abscess, it is often combined with *dà xuè téng* (Sargentodoxae Caulis) and *bài jiàng cǎo* (Patriniae Herba). To treat swollen and sore throat, it is often combined with *xuán shēn* (Scrophulariae Radix), *bǎn lán gēn* (Isatidis Radix) and *niú bàng zǐ* (Arctii Fructus). To treat bites by poisonous snakes, the fresh one can be pounded into juice or decocted for oral taking, the dregs are pasted on the wound, or used with *bàn biān lián* (Lobeliae Chinensis Herba) and *gàng bǎn guī* (Polygonum perfoliatum). For its stronger effect in detoxicating and resolving swelling, it is also clinically used to treat various cancers.

2. **热淋涩痛**　本品有清热除湿、利尿通淋之效。用治膀胱湿热，小便淋沥涩痛，可单用或配伍泽泻、车前子等。

(2) Heat strangury with astringent pain It has actions of clearing heat and draining damp, promoting urination and relieving strangury. To treat dribbling, difficult and painful urination due to damp-heat in the bladder, it can be used alone or combined with *zé xiè* (Alismatis Rhizoma) and *chē qián zǐ* (Plantaginis Semen).

【用法用量 / Usage and dosage】

煎服，15~60g。外用适量。

Decoction, 15-60g. A proper amount for external application.

【使用注意 / Precaution】

阴疽及脾胃虚寒者忌用。

It is forbidden for those with dorsal furuncle and deficient cold of spleen and stomach.

【现代研究 / Modern research】

本品主要含车叶草苷酸、熊果酸、齐墩果酸、豆甾醇、β-谷甾醇、三十一烷、白花蛇舌草素、对位香豆苷等。具有抗炎、抑菌、抗肿瘤、镇痛、镇静、抑制生精、保肝、利胆等作用。

It mainly contains aperulosidic acid, ursolic acid, oleanic acid, stigmasterol, β-sitosterol, hentriacontane, hedyotis diffusin and coumarin para. It has the functions of antiinflammation, inhibiting bacteria, antitumor, relieving pain, tranquilizing, inhibiting spermatogenesis, protecting liver and promoting gallbladder function.

第四节　清热凉血药

Section 4　Heat-clearing and blood-cooling medicinals

本类药物味多苦或咸，性寒，主归肝、心经，以清解营分、血分热邪为主要功效，主治温病营分、血分证。温病热入营分主要表现为身热夜甚、心烦不寐、斑疹隐隐，舌绛等；热入血分主要表现为身热夜甚、躁扰不宁，甚或神昏谵语、斑疹显露、吐血衄血、尿血便血、舌深绛等。本类药物亦可用于内科杂病中各种血热出血证。

Medicinals of this category are mostly bitter, salty, cold in nature, and mainly act on the liver and heart meridians. Their main efficacies are to clear away pathogenic heat at nutrient and blood aspect. They are indicated to treat excess hear syndromes at nutrient and blood aspect in warm disease. For example, warm disease with heat entering nutrient aspect usually manifested as fever worsening at night, dysphoria, insomnia, macula and deep red tongue; warm disease with heat entering blood aspect usually manifested as fever worsening at night, restlessness, or even loss of consciousness, delirium speech, macula, hematemesis, epistaxis, hematuria, hematochezia and deep red tongue. Medicinals in this section can also be used to treat various hemorrhages caused by diseases of internal medicine.

生地黄　*Shēng dì huáng* (Rehmanniae Radix)
《神农本草经》
Shen Nong's Classic of the Materia Medica (*Shén Nóng Běn Cǎo Jīng*)

【 来源 / Origin 】

为玄参科植物地黄 *Rehmannia glutinosa* Libosch. 的干燥块根。主产于河南、河北、内蒙古等地，河南为道地产区。秋季采收。切片，鲜用或晒干生用。本品无臭，味微甜。《中国药典》规定，毛蕊花糖苷（$C_{29}H_{36}O_{15}$）含量不得少于 0.020%。梓醇（$C_{15}H_{22}O_{10}$）含量不得少于 0.20%，地黄苷 D（$C_{27}H_{42}O_{20}$）含量不得少于 0.10%。

Shēng dì huáng is the root tuber of *Rehmannia glutinosa* Libosch., pertaining to Scrophulariaceae, mainly produced in Henan and Hebei Province, and Inner Mongolia Autonomous Region in China. Henan is the genuine producing area of *dì huáng*. It is collected in autumn, cut into slices and used in fresh or dried in the sun and used raw. It has no fetid flavor and tastes slightly sweet. According to *Chinese Pharmacopoeia*, the content of acteoside ($C_{29}H_{36}O_{15}$) should be no less than 0.020%, the content of catalpol ($C_{15}H_{22}O_{10}$) should not be less than 0.20% and that of rehmanniae glycoside D ($C_{27}H_{42}O_{20}$) should not be less than 0.10%.

【 性味归经 / Medicinal properties 】

甘，寒。归心、肝、肾经。

Sweet and cold; act on the heart, liver and kidney meridians.

【 主要功效 / Medicinal efficacies 】

清热凉血，养阴生津。

Clear heat and cool the blood, nourish yin and generate fluid.

【 临床应用 / Clinical application 】

1. 温热病营血分证　本品甘寒，入心肝血分，为清热凉血的要药。用治温热病热入营分，身热夜甚，心烦不寐、斑疹隐隐，舌绛脉数者，常与玄参、连翘等同用。用治热入血分，身热发斑，神昏谵语，吐血衄血，尿血便血，舌深绛等，常与水牛角、赤芍、牡丹皮等同用。

(1) **Nutrient and blood syndromes in warm disease**　It is sweet and cold, and acts on the blood aspect of heart and liver, which is an essential medicinal for clearing heat and cooling blood. To treat fever worsening at night, dysphoria, insomnia, macula and deep red tongue due to heat entering nutrient aspect in warm disease, it is often combined with *xuán shēn* (Scrophulariae Radix) and *lián qiáo* (Forsythiae Fructus). To treat warm disease with heat entering blood level usually manifested as fever worsening at night, restlessness, or even loss of consciousness, delirium speech, macula, hematemesis,

epistaxis, hematuria, hematochezia and deep red tongue, it is often combined with *shuǐ niú jiǎo* (Bubali Cornu), *chì sháo* (Paeoniae Rubra Radix) and *mǔ dān pí* (Moutan Cortex).

2. **血热出血** 本品清热凉血且能止血。用治血热妄行之吐血、衄血，常与生侧柏叶、生荷叶、生艾叶同用。用治肠热便血，痔疮肿痛，常与黄连、槐角、地榆炭等同用。用治血热崩漏，可与茜草、苎麻根等同用。

(2) Bleeding due to blood heat It can clear heat and cool the blood, as well as stanch bleeding. To treat hematemesis and epistaxis due to blood heat, it is often combined with *cè bǎi yè* (Platycladi Cacumen), fresh *hé yè* (Nelumbinis Folium) and fresh *ài yè* (Artemisiae Argyi Folium). To treat bloody stool, hemorrhoid with swelling and pain due to heat accumulating in the intestines, it is often combined with *huáng lián* (Coptidis Rhizoma), *huái jiǎo* (Sophorae Fructus) and *dì yú tàn* (charred Sanguisorbae Radix). To treat uterine bleeding due to blood heat, it is often used with *qiàn cǎo* (Rubiae Radix et Rhizoma) and *zhù má gēn* (Boehmeriae Radix).

3. **津伤口渴，内热消渴，肠燥便秘** 本品甘寒质润，有养阴清热、生津止渴之功，可用于各脏腑的津伤阴亏病证。用治热病津伤，烦渴多饮，常与沙参、麦冬、玉竹等同用。用治热病伤津，肠燥便秘，常与玄参、麦冬等同用。用治内热消渴，多与葛根、天花粉、黄芪等同用。

(3) Thirst due to fluid consumption, *xiāo kě* due to internal heat, constipation caused by intestinal dryness It is sweet and cold with moistening nature. It functions to nourish yin and clear heat, generate fluid and relieve thirst, which can be used to treat fluid consumption and yin deficiency of various internal organs. To treat warm disease with fluid consumption, manifested as vexation, thirst and excessive drinking, it is often combined with *shā shēn* (Adenophorae seu Glehniae Radix), *mài dōng* (Ophiopogonis Radix) and *yù zhú* (Polygonati Odorati Rhizoma). To treat constipation due to intestinal dryness caused by fluid consumption, it is often combined with *xuán shēn* (Scrophulariae Radix) and *mài dōng* (Ophiopogonis Radix). To treat *xiāo kě* due to internal heat, it is often used with *gé gēn* (Puerariae Lobatae Radix), *tiān huā fěn* (Trichosanthis Radix) and *huáng qí* (Astragali Radix).

4. **阴虚发热** 本品甘寒，入肾经，能滋肾阴，退虚热。用治阴虚内热，骨蒸潮热，常与知母、地骨皮等同用。用治温热病后期，余热未清，阴津已伤，夜热早凉，常与青蒿、知母、鳖甲等同用。

(4) Fever due to yin deficiency It is sweet and cold, and acts on the kidney meridian, which functions to nourish kidney yin and relieve asthenia heat. To treat internal heat, steaming bone and tidal fever due to yin deficiency, it is often combined with *zhī mǔ* (Anemarrhenae Rhizoma) and *dì gǔ pí* (Lycii Cortex). In case of warm disease in late stage with afterheat and damaged yin fluid, manifested as night fever abating at dawn, it is often combined with *qīng hāo* (Artemisiae Annuae Herba), *zhī mǔ* (Anemarrhenae Rhizoma) and *biē jiǎ* (Trionycis Carapax).

【用法用量 / Usage and dosage】

煎服，10~15g。

Decoction, 10-15g.

【使用注意 / Precaution】

脾虚湿滞，腹满便溏者不宜使用。

It should be used with caution for those with abdominal fullness and loose stool due to spleen deficiency and damp accumulation.

【现代研究 / Modern research】

本品主要含梓醇、乙酰梓醇、益母草苷、毛蕊花糖苷、桃叶珊瑚苷、地黄苷、密力特苷、去羟栀子苷，以及多种糖类、甾醇、氨基酸等。具有抗炎、镇静、降压、增强免疫、降血糖、保肝、强心、利尿、抗癌、抗辐射、抑制真菌等作用。

It mainly contains catalpol, acetylcatalpol, leonuride, acteoside, aucubin, rehmannioside, melittoside, geniposide, sugar saccharide, sterol and amino acid. It has the functions of antiinflammation, tranquilizing, lowering blood pressure, enhancing immunity, reducing blood sugar, liver protection and anticancer. It also has cardiotonic and diuretic effects. In addition, it can enhance the phagocytic function of reticuloendothelial cells and resist radiation.

玄参　*Xuán shēn* (Scrophulariae Radix)
《神农本草经》
Shen Nong's Classic of the Materia Medica (*Shén Nóng Běn Cǎo Jīng*)

【来源 / Origin】

为玄参科植物玄参 *Scrophularia ningpoensis* Hemsl. 的干燥根。主产于长江流域、陕西、福建等地。冬季采挖，切片，生用。本品气特异，似焦糖，味苦、微甘。《中国药典》规定，含哈巴苷（$C_{15}H_{24}O_{10}$）和哈巴俄苷（$C_{24}H_{30}O_{11}$）的总量不得少于 0.45%。

Xuán shēn is the root of *Scrophularia ningpoensis* Hemsl., pertaining to Scrophulariaceae, mainly produced in Yangtze valley, Shaanxi and Fujian Province in China. It is collected in winter, cut into slices and used raw. It has a special flavor like caramel, and tastes bitter, slightly sweet. According to *Chinese Pharmacopoeia*, the total content of harpagide ($C_{15}H_{24}O_{10}$) and harpagoside ($C_{24}H_{30}O_{11}$) should be no less than 0.45%.

【性味归经 / Medicinal properties】

甘、苦、咸，微寒。归肺、胃、肾经。

Sweet, bitter, salty and slightly cold; act on the lung, stomach and kidney meridians.

【主要功效 / Medicinal efficacies】

清热凉血，滋阴降火，解毒散结。

Clear heat and cool the blood, nourish yin and reduce fire, resolve toxin and dissipate masses.

【临床应用 / Clinical application】

1. 温热病营血分证　本品性味甘苦咸寒而质润，入血分，清热凉血之功与生地黄相似而力稍逊，并有泻火解毒、养阴润燥之效。用治温热病热入营分，身热夜甚，心烦口渴，舌绛脉数，常与生地黄、连翘、黄连等同用。用治温热病热入心包，高热烦躁，神昏谵语，常配伍莲子心、连翘心等。用治温热病气血两燔，身发斑疹，常配伍石膏、知母等。

(1) **Nutrient and blood syndromes in warm disease**　It is sweet, bitter, salty and cold with moistening nature which enters blood aspect. Its effect of clearing heat and cooling the blood is inferior to *dì huáng* (Rehmanniae Radix). It can also drain fire and resolve toxin, nourish yin and moisten dryness. To treat heat entering nutrient aspect, manifested as fever aggravated at night, dysphoria, thirst, deep red tongue and rapid pulse, it is often combined with *dì huáng* (Rehmanniae Radix), *lián qiáo* (Forsythiae Fructus) and *huáng lián* (Coptidis Rhizoma). To treat heat invading pericardium, manifested as high fever, dysphoria, loss of consciousness and delirium speech, it is often combined with *lián zǐ xīn* (Nelumbinis Plumula) and *lián qiáo xīn* (Forsythiae Fructus Plumula). When treating blazing of both qi and blood in warm disease, manifested as macula and rashes, it is combined with *shí gāo* (Gypsum Fibrosum) and *zhī mǔ* (Anemarrhenae Rhizoma).

2. 咽喉肿痛，瘰疬痰核，痈肿疮毒　本品清热解毒，滋阴降火，利咽消肿，凡是咽喉肿痛，无论热毒壅盛，还是虚火上炎所致者，皆可应用。前者常配伍板蓝根、栀子、桔梗等；后者常与麦冬、桔梗、甘草等同用。本品苦寒泻火解毒，咸寒软坚散结，用治痰火郁结之瘰疬痰核，常与牡蛎、贝母等同用。用治热毒蕴结之痈疮肿毒，常与金银花、连翘、蒲公英等同用。若治热毒脱疽，常配伍金银花、当归、甘草等。

(2) Sore throat, scrofula and subcutaneous nodule, abscess, swelling, sores and toxin It has efficacies of clearing heat and resolving toxin, nourishing yin and reducing fire, as well as relieving sore throat and dissipating swelling. It can be used to treat sore throat with swelling caused by accumulation of heat-toxin or upward flaming of deficient fire. For sore throat due to accumulation of heat-toxin, it is usually combined with *bǎn lán gēn* (Isatidis Radix), *zhī zǐ* (Gardeniae Fructus) and *jié gěng* (Platycodonis Radix). For sore throat due to upward flaming of deficient fire, it is often combined with *mài dōng* (Ophiopogonis Radix), *jié gěng* (Platycodonis Radix) and *gān cǎo* (Glycyrrhizae Radix et Rhizoma). It is bitter and cold for reducing fire and resolving toxin, salty and cold for softening hardness and dissipating masses. To treat scrofula and subcutaneous nodule caused by congestion of phlegm-fire, it is often combined with *mǔ lì* (Ostreae Concha) and *bèi mǔ* (Fritillaria Bulbus). To treat abscess, swelling, sores and toxin due to accumulation of heat-toxin, it is often combined with *jīn yín huā* (Lonicerae Japonicae Flos), *lián qiáo* (Forsythiae Fructus) and *pú gōng yīng* (Taraxaci Herba). To treat finger-toe gangrene caused by heat-toxin, it is used with *jīn yín huā* (Lonicerae Japonicae Flos), *dāng guī* (Angelicae Sinensis Radix) and *gān cǎo* (Glycyrrhizae Radix et Rhizoma).

3. **劳嗽咯血，阴虚发热，消渴便秘** 本品甘寒质润，滋阴降火，生津润燥。用治阴虚劳嗽咯血，常与百合、川贝母等同用。用治阴虚发热，骨蒸劳热，常与知母、地骨皮等同用。用治内热消渴，多与麦冬、五味子等同用。用治津伤肠燥便秘，多与生地黄、麦冬配伍。

(3) Overstrain cough and hematemesis, fever due to yin deficiency, *xiāo kě* and constipation It is sweet and cold with moistening nature for nourishing yin and reducing fire, as well as generating fluid and moistening dryness. To treat overstrain cough and hematemesis caused by yin deficiency, it is usually combined with *bǎi hé* (Lilii Bulbus) and *chuān bèi mǔ* (Fritillariae Cirrhosae Bulbus). To treat fever, steaming bone and consumptive fever due to yin deficiency, it is usually combined with *zhī mǔ* (Anemarrhenae Rhizoma) and *dì gǔ pí* (Lycii Cortex). For treating *xiāo kě* due to internal heat, it is used with *mài dōng* (Ophiopogonis Radix) and *wǔ wèi zǐ* (Schisandrae Chinensis Fructus). To treat constipation due to intestinal dryness caused by damage of fluid, it is often used with *dì huáng* (Rehmanniae Radix) and *mài dōng* (Ophiopogonis Radix).

【用法用量 / Usage and dosage】

煎服，9~15g。

Decoction, 9-15g.

【使用注意 / Precaution】

脾虚便溏者不宜服用。不宜与藜芦同用。

It should be used with caution for those with loose stool due to spleen deficiency. It is mutual antagonistic with *lí lú* (Veratri Nigri Radix et Rhizoma).

【现代研究 / Modern research】

本品主要含哈巴苷、哈巴俄苷、玄参苷、桃叶珊瑚苷、梓醇、安格洛苷，尚含挥发油、植物甾醇、生物碱、脂肪酸等。具有抑菌、解热、抗炎、镇静、镇痛、降压、降血糖、扩张冠脉、保肝、利胆、免疫调节等作用。

It mainly contains harpagide, harpagoside, rhinanthin, aucubin, catalpol, angoroside. It also contains volatile oil, phytosterin, alkaloid and fatty acid. It has the functions of inhibiting bacteria, relieving fever, antiinflammation, tranquilizing, relieving pain, lowering blood pressure and blood sugar, enlarging coronary arteries, liver protection promoting gallbladder function and regulating immunity.

牡丹皮　*Mǔ dān pí* (Moutan Cortex)
《神农本草经》
Shen Nong's Classic of the Materia Medica (Shén Nóng Běn Cǎo Jīng)

【来源 / Origin】

为毛茛科植物牡丹 *Paeonia suffruticosa* Andr. 的干燥根皮。主产于安徽、河南、山东等地。秋季采挖。切片，生用或酒炙用。本品气芳香，味微苦而涩。《中国药典》规定，含丹皮酚（$C_9H_{10}O_3$）不得少于 1.2%。

Mǔ dān pí is the root bark of *Paeonia suffruticosa* Andr., pertaining to Ranunculaceae, mainly produced in Anhui, Henan and Shandong Province in China. It is collected in autumn, cut into slices, and used raw or stir-baked with wine. It is fragrant, and tastes slightly bitter and astringent. According to *Chinese Pharmacopoeia*, the content of paeonol ($C_9H_{10}O_3$) should be no less than 1.2%.

【性味归经 / Medicinal properties】

苦、辛，微寒。归心、肝、肾经。

Bitter, acrid and slightly cold; act on the heart, liver and kidney meridians.

【主要功效 / Medicinal efficacies】

清热凉血，活血化瘀，清虚热。

Clear heat and cool the blood, activate blood and remove stasis, clear deficiency heat.

【临床应用 / Clinical application】

1. **温热病营血分证**　本品苦寒清热，入血分，善清营分、血分实热。用治温热病热入营血，迫血妄行所致的斑疹紫暗、吐血衄血等，常与水牛角、生地黄、赤芍等同用。

(1) Nutrient and blood syndromes in warm disease　It is bitter and cold with effect of clearing heat, which enters blood aspect and is good at clearing excess heat in nutrient aspect and blood aspect. For heat entering nutrient-blood in warm disease, manifested as dark purple macula, hematemesis and epistaxis due to accelerated blood circulation, it is often combined with *shuǐ niú jiǎo* (Bubali Cornu), *dì huáng* (Rehmanniae Radix) and *chì sháo* (Paeoniae Rubra Radix).

2. **血瘀证**　本品辛行苦泄，能活血化瘀，散瘀消痈，适用于血瘀所致的多种病证。因其性寒，既能散瘀，又能凉血，故对血热瘀滞之证较为适宜。用治血滞经闭、痛经、癥瘕，常配伍桂枝、桃仁、川芎等。用治瘀血阻滞，月经不调兼肝郁化火者，常与栀子、白芍、柴胡等同用。用治跌打伤痛，常与红花、乳香、没药等同用。用治疮痈肿痛，可与金银花、蒲公英等同用。

(2) Blood stasis　It is acrid for moving and bitter for draining, which can activate blood and remove stasis, as well as dissolve stagnation and eliminate abscess. It can be used to treat various diseases caused by blood stasis. In addition, it is cold in nature with effect of dissipating stasis and cooling the blood, so it is suitable to treat stagnation caused by blood heat. To treat amenorrhea, painful menstruation and abdominal mass due to blood stagnation, it is often combined with *guì zhī* (Cinnamomi Ramulus), *táo rén* (Persicae Semen) and *chuān xiōng* (Chuanxiong Rhizoma). To treat irregular menstruation due to static blood, accompanied by liver constraint transforming into fire, it is often used together with *zhī zǐ* (Gardeniae Fructus), *bái sháo* (Paeoniae Alba Radix) and *chái hú* (Bupleuri Radix). To treat traumatic injury, it is combined with *hóng huā* (Carthami Flos), *rǔ xiāng* (Olibanum) and *mò yào* (Myrrha). To treat sores, carbuncle, swelling and pain, it can be combined with *jīn yín huā* (Lonicerae Japonicae Flos) and *pú gōng yīng* (Taraxaci Herba).

3. **阴虚发热** 本品苦辛而寒,清中有透,善于清透阴分伏热。用治温热病后期,余热未尽,阴液已伤,夜热早凉等,常与青蒿、鳖甲等同用。若治阴虚发热,骨蒸潮热,盗汗等,常与知母、熟地黄、黄柏等配伍。

(3) Fever due to yin deficiency It is bitter, acrid and cold, which is good at clearing away latent heat in yin level. To treat warm disease in late stage, manifested as lingered heat, damaged yin fluid, night fever abating at dawn, it is usually combined with *qīng hāo* (Artemisiae Annuae Herba) and *biē jiǎ* (Trionycis Carapax). To treat fever, steaming bone, tidal fever and night sweating due to yin deficiency, it is often used with *zhī mǔ* (Anemarrhenae Rhizoma), *shú dì huáng* (Rehmanniae Radix Praeparata) and *huáng bó* (Phellodendri Chinensis Cortex).

【用法用量 / Usage and dosage】

煎服,6~12g。清热凉血宜生用,活血祛瘀宜酒炙用。

Decoction, 6-12g. To clear heat and cool the blood, it is used in the raw. To invigorate blood and dissolve stasis, it is stir-baked with wine.

【使用注意 / Precaution】

孕妇慎用。

It should be used with caution for pregnant women.

【现代研究 / Modern research】

本品主要含丹皮酚、丹皮酚苷、牡丹酚原苷、牡丹酚新苷、芍药苷、氧化芍药苷、苯甲酰芍药苷、苯甲酰氧化芍药苷、没食子酸及挥发油等。具有抑菌、解热、抗炎、镇痛、镇静、降压、抗心脑缺血、抗动脉粥样硬化、抗过敏、保肝、调节免疫等作用。

It mainly contains paeonol, paeonoside, paeonolide, apiopaeonoside, paeoniflorin, oxypaeoniflora, benzoylpaeoniflorin, benzoyloxypaeoniflorin, gallic acid and volatile oil. It has the functions of inhibiting bacteria, relieving fever, antiinflammation, tranquilizing, relieving pain, lowering blood pressure. It also has effect of anticardio-cerebral ischemia, anti-atherosclerosis, anti-allergy, protecting liver and regulating immunity.

赤芍 *Chì sháo* (Paeoniae Rubra Radix)
《神农本草经》
Shen Nong's Classic of the Materia Medica (Shén Nóng Běn Cǎo Jīng)

【来源 / Origin】

为毛茛科植物芍药 *Paeonia lactiflora*. Pall. 的根。主产于内蒙古、河北、东北等地。春、秋二季采挖。切片,生用。本品气微香,味微苦、酸、涩。《中国药典》规定,芍药苷($C_{23}H_{28}O_{11}$)含量不得少于 1.8%。

Chì sháo is the root of *Paeonia lactiflora*. Pall., pertaining to Ranunculaceae. It is mainly produced in Inner Mongolia Autonomous Region, Hebei Province and northeast China, collected in spring and autumn, cut into slices and used raw. It is fragrant and tastes slightly bitter, sour and astringent. According to *Chinese Pharmacopoeia*, the content of paeoniflorin ($C_{23}H_{28}O_{11}$) should be no less than 1.8%.

【性味归经 / Medicinal properties】

苦,微寒。归肝经。

Bitter and slightly cold; act on liver meridian.

【主要功效 / Medicinal efficacies】

清热凉血,散瘀止痛。

Clear heat and cool the blood, resolve stasis and relieve pain.

【临床应用 / Clinical application】

1. 温热病营血分证　本品苦寒，入血分，清热凉血之功与牡丹皮相似而药力稍逊，活血化瘀，用治温热病热入营血，迫血妄行所致的斑疹紫暗、吐血衄血等，二者常相须为用。

(1) Nutrient and blood syndromes in warm disease　It is bitter and cold, and enters blood aspect. Its effect of clearing heat and cooling blood is inferior to that of *mǔ dān pí* (Moutan Cortex). To treat macula with dark purple color, hematemesis and epistaxis due to heat entering nutrient-blood to accelerate blood circulation, it is often combined with *mǔ dān pí* (Moutan Cortex) for mutual reinforcement.

2. 血瘀证　本品有较好的活血化瘀作用，尤长于祛瘀止痛，常用于瘀血阻滞诸痛证，因其药性微寒，故尤宜于血热瘀滞之证。用治血滞经闭痛经，癥瘕腹痛，常与当归、川芎、延胡索等同用。用治跌打损伤，瘀肿疼痛，常与乳香、没药等同用。用治热毒疮痈肿痛，常与金银花、天花粉、白芷等同用。

(2) Blood stasis　It is effective in activating blood and resolve stasis, especially good at removing stasis to relieve pain, which is often used to treat various pains caused by blood stagnation. For its slightly cold nature, it is especially suitable to treat blood stasis due to blood heat. To treat amenorrhea, painful menstruation and abdominal mass with abdominal pain due to blood stagnation, it is often combined with *dāng guī* (Angelicae Sinensis Radix), *chuān xiōng* (Chuanxiong Rhizoma) and *yán hú suǒ* (Corydalis Rhizoma). To treat traumatic injury with swelling and pain, it is combined with *rǔ xiāng* (Olibanum) and *mò yào* (Myrrha). To treat sores, carbuncle, swelling and pain, it can be combined with *jīn yín huā* (Lonicerae Japonicae Flos), *tiān huā fěn* (Trichosanthis Radix) and *bái zhǐ* (Angelicae Dahuricae Radix).

3. 目赤肿痛　本品苦寒入肝经，能清泻肝热。用治肝热目赤肿痛，羞明多眵，或目生翳障，可与菊花、夏枯草等同用。

(3) Red eyes with swelling and pain　It is bitter and cold, and acts on the liver meridian, which functions to clear and drain liver heat. To treat red eyes with swelling and pain, phengophobia and profuse gum in the eyes, or ocular due to liver heat, it is often combined with *jú huā* (Chrysanthemi Flos) and *xià kū cǎo* (Prunellae Spica).

【用法用量 / Usage and dosage】

煎服，6~12g。

Decoction, 6-12g.

【使用注意 / Precaution】

孕妇慎用。不宜与藜芦同用。

It should be used with caution for pregnant women. It is mutually antagonistic with *lí lú* (Veratri Nigri Radix et Rhizoma).

【现代研究 / Modern research】

本品主要含芍药苷、芍药内酯苷、氧化芍药苷、芍药吉酮、苯甲酰芍药苷、芍药新苷、没食子酸、丹皮酚、挥发油、糖类、β-谷甾醇等。具有抑菌、解热、抗炎、解痉、镇痛、镇静、扩张冠状动脉、增加冠状动脉血流量、抗血栓、抗惊厥等作用。

It mainly contains paeoniflorin, albiflorin, oxypaeoniflora, paeoniflorigenone, benzoylpaeoniflorin, lactiflorin, gallic acid, paeonol, volatile oil, carbohydrates and β-sitosterol. It has the functions of inhibiting bacteria, relieving fever, antiinflammation, relieving convulsion, tranquilizing, relieving pain, enlarging coronary arteries, increasing coronary blood flow, antithrombotic and anticonvulsion.

PPT

第五节 清虚热药

Section 5　Deficiency-heat-clearing medicinals

本类药物性味多甘寒，主入肝、肾经，以清虚热为主要功效，主治肝肾阴虚，虚火内扰所致的骨蒸潮热、午后发热、手足心热、虚烦不寐、遗精盗汗、舌红少苔、脉细数等症。亦可用于热病后期，余热未清，阴液已伤所致的夜热早凉、热退无汗、舌红绛、脉细数等症。

Deficiency-heat-clearing medicinals are mostly sweet and cold in property, and act on the liver and kidney meridians. Their main efficacy is to clear deficiency heat. They are often used to treat deficiency-heat harassing the interior due to yin-deficiency of the liver and kidney, manifested as steaming bone, tidal fever, afternoon fever, feverish sensation in the palms and soles, deficient vexation, insomnia, nocturnal emission and night sweating, red tongue with less coating, thin and rapid pulse. They also treat pathogenic heat incompletely eliminated, and consumption of body fluid due to damaged yin in the late stage of warm disease, manifested as night fever abating at dawn, fever relieved without sweating, crimson tongue, thin and rapid pulse.

> ### 青蒿　*Qīng hāo* (Artemisiae Annuae Herba)
> 《神农本草经》
> *Shen Nong's Classic of the Materia Medica (Shén Nóng Běn Cǎo Jīng)*

【来源 / Origin】

为菊科植物黄花蒿 *Artemisia annua* L. 的地上部分。全国大部分地区有产。秋季花盛开时采割，阴干，切段，生用。本品气香特异，味微苦。

Qīng hāo is the aerial part of *Artemisia annua* L., pertaining to Compositae, produced in most areas of China. It is collected in autumn when in full bloom, dried in the shade, cut into segments, used raw. *Qīng hāo* has a special fragrance and tastes slightly bitter.

【性味归经 / Medicinal properties】

苦、辛，寒。归肝、胆经。

Bitter, acrid and cold; act on liver and gallbladder meridians.

【主要功效 / Medicinal efficacies】

清虚热，除骨蒸，解暑，截疟，退黄。

Clear deficiency heat, treat steaming bone fever, relieve summer-heat, prevent attack of malaria, relieve jaundice.

【临床应用 / Clinical application】

1. **阴虚发热**　本品苦寒清热，辛香透散，长于清虚热、退骨蒸，为治疗阴虚发热之常用药。用治温热病后期，邪热未尽，阴液已伤，夜热早凉，热退无汗，或低热不退，常与鳖甲、生地黄、牡丹皮等同用。用治肝肾阴虚，骨蒸潮热，五心烦热，盗汗等，常与鳖甲、知母、地骨皮等同用。

(1) **Fever due to yin deficiency**　It is bitter and cold for clearing heat, acrid and fragrant for dispersing, which is effective in clearing deficiency heat, treating steaming bone fever. It is a commonly

used medicinal to treat fever due to yin deficiency. To treat warm disease in the late stage, manifested as unrelieved pathogenic heat, damaged yin fluid, night fever abating at dawn, fever relieved without sweating, or lingered low fever, it is often combined with *biē jiǎ* (Trionycis Carapax), *dì huáng* (Rehmanniae Radix) and *mǔ dān pí* (Moutan Cortex). To treat steaming bone and tidal fever, feverish sensation in the palms and soles, night sweating due to yin deficiency of liver and kidney, it is often combined with *biē jiǎ* (Trionycis Carapax), *zhī mǔ* (Anemarrhenae Rhizoma) and *dì gǔ pí* (Lycii Cortex).

2. 外感暑热　本品辛香发散，可外解暑热。用治外感暑热，发热烦渴，头痛头昏，常配伍连翘、西瓜翠衣、滑石等。

(2) External contraction of summer-heat　It is acrid and fragrant for dispersing, which can be used to relieve summer-heat. To treat fever, dysphoria, thirst, headache and dizziness due to external contraction of summer-heat, it is often combined with *lián qiáo* (Forsythiae Fructus), *xī guā cuì yī* (ExocarpiumCitrulli) and *huá shí* (Talcum).

3. 疟疾寒热　本品入肝、胆经，截疟之功较强，并善解热而缓解疟疾发作时的寒战壮热，为治疟疾寒热之要药，可单用大量鲜青蒿绞汁服用，或与草果、柴胡等同用。

(3) Malaria with alternating chills and fever　It acts on the liver and gallbladder meridians with strong effect of preventing attack of malaria. It is good at relieving fever to alleviate the chills and high fever during attack of malaria. It is an essential medicinal to treat malaria with alternating chills and fever. For this condition, a large dosage of fresh *qīng hāo* is pounded into juice with water for oral taking; or combined with *cǎo guǒ* (Tsaoko Fructus) and *chái hú* (Bupleuri Radix).

4. 湿热黄疸　本品有清泄湿热、利胆退黄之功。用于湿热黄疸，可与茵陈、栀子等同用。

(4) Jaundice due to damp-heat　It has efficacies of clearing and draining damp-heat, as well as promoting gallbladder function to relieve jaundice. To treat jaundice due to damp-heat, it is often combined with *yīn chén* (Artemisiae Scopariae Herba) and *zhī zǐ* (Gardeniae Fructus).

【用法用量 / Usage and dosage】

煎服，6~12g，后下。鲜品加倍。

Decoction, 6-12g, it is added later. The fresh one should be used in double dosage.

【使用注意 / Precaution】

脾胃虚弱，肠滑易泻者忌服。

It should be contraindicated in those suffering weak spleen and stomach, and diarrhea due to slippery intestines.

【现代研究 / Modern research】

本品主要含青蒿素、青蒿酸、青蒿内酯、青蒿醇、挥发油、黄酮类、香豆素类成分等。具有抑菌、抗病毒、抗疟、解热、镇痛、利胆、降压、抗肿瘤、抗血吸虫等作用。

It mainly contains artemisinin, artemisinic acid, artemisilactone, artemisinol, volatile oil, flavonoid and coumarines. It has the functions of inhibiting bacteria, antivirus, anti-malaria, relieving fever, relieving pain, promoting gallbladder function, reducing blood pressure, antitumor and antischistosome-agent.

地骨皮　*Dì gǔ pí* (Lycii Cortex)
《神农本草经》
Shen Nong's Classic of the Materia Medica (Shén Nóng Běn Cǎo Jīng)

【来源 / Origin】

为茄科植物枸杞 *Lycium chinense* Mill. 或宁夏枸杞 *L. barbarum* L. 的干燥根皮。南北各地均产。

春初或秋后采挖，晒干，切段，生用。本品气微，味微甘而后苦。

Dì gǔ pí is the dried root bark of *Lycium chinense* Mill. or *L. barbarum* L., pertaining to Solanaceae. It is produced in southern and northern parts of China, collected in the early spring or in late autumn, dried in the sun, cut into segments, and used raw. It has a slight flavor and tastes slightly sweet and bitter later on.

【性味归经 / Medicinal properties 】

甘，寒。归肺、肝、肾经。

Sweet and cold; act on the lung, liver and kidney meridians.

【主要功效 / Medicinal efficacies 】

凉血除蒸，清肺降火。

Cool the blood and relieve steaming bone fever, clear lung fire.

【临床应用 / Clinical application 】

1. 阴虚发热　本品甘寒清润，善清肝肾虚热，除有汗之骨蒸，为凉血退热除蒸之佳品。用治阴虚发热，潮热，心烦盗汗，常与银柴胡、鳖甲、知母等同用。

(1) **Fever due to yin deficiency**　It is sweet and cold for clearing and moistening, which is good at clearing deficiency heat of liver and kidney to treat steaming bone with sweat. It is an effective medicinal to cool blood and relieve steaming bone fever. To treat tidal fever, vexation and night sweating due to yin deficiency, it is often combined with *yín chái hú* (Stellariae Radix), *biē jiǎ* (Trionycis Carapax) and *zhī mǔ* (Anemarrhenae Rhizoma).

2. 肺热咳嗽　本品性寒，入肺经，能清泄肺热。用治肺火郁结，气逆不降，咳嗽气喘，常与桑白皮、甘草等同用。

(2) **Cough due to lung heat**　It is cold and acts on the lung meridian and functions to clear lung heat. To treat cough and dyspnea due to lung fire accumulation, it is often combined with *sāng bái pí* (Mori Cortex) and *gān cǎo* (Glycyrrhizae Radix et Rhizoma).

3. 血热出血证　本品甘寒，入血分，能清热凉血以止血。用治血热妄行之吐血、衄血、崩漏、尿血等，可与大蓟、白茅根、侧柏叶等同用。

(3) **Blood-heat bleeding**　It is sweet and cold, and enters blood level. It functions to clear heat and cool blood to stanch bleeding. To treat hematemesis, epistaxis, uterine bleeding and hematuria due to blood heat accelerating blood circulation, it is often combined with *dà jì* (Cirsii Japonici Herba), *bái máo gēn* (Imperatae Rhizoma) and *cè bǎi yè* (Platycladi Cacumen).

此外，本品还能泄热而生津止渴，可用治内热消渴，常与生地黄、天花粉、麦冬等同用。

In addition, *dì gǔ pí* can reduce heat and generate fluid to quench thirst. It can be used to treat *xiāo kě* due to internal heat, it is usually used with *dì huáng* (Rehmanniae Radix), *tiān huā fēn* (Trichosanthis Radix) and *mài dōng* (Ophiopogonis Radix).

【用法用量 / Usage and dosage 】

煎服，9~15g。

Decoction, 9-15g.

【使用注意 / Precaution 】

脾虚便溏者不宜用。

It should be used with caution for those suffering loose stool due to spleen deficiency.

【现代研究 / Modern research 】

本品主要含甜菜碱、莨菪亭、苦可胺 A、枸杞子酰胺、阿托品、天仙子胺以及有机酸、甾醇、酚类等。具有解热、抑菌、抗病毒、降压、降血糖、降血脂、兴奋子宫等作用。

It mainly contains betaine, scopoletin, kukoamine A, lyceum amide, atropine, hyoscyamine, organic acid, sterol and phenols. It has the functions of relieving fever, inhibiting bacteria, antivirus, reducing blood pressure, lowering blood sugar and blood fat, as well as stimulating uterus.

其他清热药功用介绍见表 7-1。

The efficacies of other heat-clearing medicinals are shown in table 7-1.

表 7-1　其他清热药功用介绍

分类	药物	药性	功效	应用	用法用量
清热泻火药	芦根	甘，寒。归肺、胃经	清热泻火，生津止渴，除烦，止呕，利尿	热病烦渴，肺热咳嗽，肺痈吐脓，胃热呕哕，热淋涩痛	煎服，15~30g，鲜品用量加倍；或捣汁用
	淡竹叶	甘，淡，寒。归心、小肠、胃经	清热泻火，除烦止渴，利尿通淋	热病烦渴，口舌生疮，热淋涩痛	煎服，6~10g
	竹叶	甘、辛、淡，寒。归心、胃、小肠经	清热除烦，生津利尿	热病烦渴，口舌生疮，小便短赤涩痛	煎服，6~15g；鲜品15~30g
	谷精草	辛、甘，平。归肝、肺经	疏散风热，明目退翳	风热目赤，肿痛羞明，眼生翳膜，风热头痛	煎服，5~10g
	密蒙花	甘，微寒。归肝经	清热泻火，养肝明目，退翳	目赤肿痛，羞明多泪，目生翳膜，肝虚目暗，视物昏花	煎服，3~9g
	青葙子	苦，微寒。归肝经	清肝泻火，明目退翳	肝热目赤，目生翳膜，视物昏花，肝火眩晕	煎服，9~15g
清热燥湿药	白鲜皮	苦，寒。归脾、胃、膀胱经	清热燥湿，祛风解毒	湿热疮毒，黄水淋漓，湿疹，风疹，疥癣疮癞，风湿热痹，黄疸尿赤	煎服，5~10g。外用适量，煎汤洗或研粉敷
	秦皮	苦，涩，寒。归肝、胆、大肠经	清热燥湿，收涩止痢，止带，明目	湿热泻痢，赤白带下，目赤肿痛，目生翳膜	煎服，6~12g。外用适量，煎洗患处
清热解毒药	野菊花	苦、辛，微寒。归肝、心经	清热解毒，泻火平肝	疔疮痈肿，咽喉肿痛，目赤肿痛，头痛眩晕	煎服，9~15g。外用适量，煎汤外洗或制膏外涂
	紫花地丁	苦、辛，寒。归心、肝经	清热解毒，凉血消肿	疔疮肿毒，丹毒，乳痈肠痈，毒蛇咬伤	煎服，15~30g。外用鲜品适量
	半边莲	辛，平。归心、小肠、肺经	清热解毒，利尿消肿	痈肿疔疮，蛇虫咬伤，水肿黄疸，湿疹湿疮	煎服，9~15g；鲜品，30~60g。外用适量
	穿心莲	苦，寒。归心、肺、大肠、膀胱经	清热解毒，凉血消肿，燥湿	风热感冒，温病初起，咽喉肿痛，口舌生疮，顿咳劳嗽，肺痈吐脓，痈肿疮疡，蛇虫咬伤，痢疾淋证，湿疹瘙痒	煎服，6~9g。多作丸、片剂服用。外用适量

续表

分类	药物	药性	功效	应用	用法用量
清热解毒药	马齿苋	酸，寒。归肝、大肠经	清热解毒，凉血止血，止痢	热毒血痢，痈肿疔疮，湿疹丹毒，蛇虫咬伤，便血崩漏	煎服，9~15g。外用适量
	败酱草	辛、苦，微寒。归胃、大肠、肝经	清热解毒，消痈排脓，祛瘀止痛	肠痈，肺痈，皮肤疮痈，产后瘀阻腹痛	煎服，6~15g。外用适量
	金荞麦	微辛、涩，凉。归肺经	清热解毒，排脓祛瘀	肺痈吐脓，肺热喘咳，瘰疬疮疖，乳蛾肿痛	煎服，15~45g，用水或黄酒隔水密闭炖服
	鸦胆子	苦，寒；有小毒。归大肠、肝经	清热解毒，止痢，截疟；外用腐蚀赘疣	血痢久痢，疟疾，赘疣鸡眼	内服，0.5~2g，龙眼肉包裹吞服。外用适量
	垂盆草	甘、淡，凉。归肝、胆、小肠经	利湿退黄，清热解毒	湿热黄疸，小便不利，疮疡咽痛，毒蛇咬伤，烧烫伤	煎服，15~30g
	马勃	辛，平。归肺经	清肺，解毒利咽，止血	咽痛音哑，咳嗽，鼻衄，出血	煎服，2~6g。外用适量
	木蝴蝶	苦、甘，凉。归肺、肝、胃经	清肺利咽，舒肝和胃	肺热咳嗽，喉痹音哑，肝胃气痛	煎服，1~3g
	半枝莲	辛、苦，寒。归肺、肝、肾经	清热解毒，化瘀利尿	疔疮肿毒，咽喉肿痛，跌仆伤痛，水肿黄疸，蛇虫咬伤	煎服，15~30g
清热凉血药	水牛角	苦，寒。归心、肝经	清热凉血，解毒，定惊	温病高热，神昏谵语，发斑发疹，吐血衄血，惊风，癫狂	煎服，15~30g，宜先煎3小时以上
清虚热药	白薇	苦、咸，寒。归胃、肝、肾经	清热凉血，利尿通淋，解毒疗疮	阴虚发热，产后虚热，热淋，血淋，疮痈肿毒，咽喉肿痛，阴虚外感	煎服，5~10g
	胡黄连	苦，寒。归肝、胃、大肠经	退虚热，除疳热，清湿热	骨蒸潮热，小儿疳热，湿热泻痢，黄疸尿赤，痔疮肿痛	煎服，3~10g
	银柴胡	甘，微寒。归肝、胃经	清虚热，除疳热	阴虚发热，骨蒸劳热，小儿疳热	煎服，3~10g

（杨 敏 余 娜）

第八章 泻 下 药
Chapter 8　Purgative medicinals

 学习目标 | Learning goals

1. **掌握** 泻下药在功效、主治、性能、配伍及使用注意方面的共性；大黄、芒硝的性能、功效、应用以及特殊的用法用量和特殊的使用注意。

2. **熟悉** 泻下药的分类；番泻叶、火麻仁、甘遂、巴豆霜、京大戟、芫花的功效、主治以及特殊的用法用量和特殊的使用注意。

3. **了解** 泻下、攻下、润下、峻下、逐水等功效术语的含义；芦荟、郁李仁、松子仁、牵牛子、千金子的功效以及特殊的用法用量和特殊的使用注意。

1. Master the commonness of purgative medicinals in efficacy, indications, property, compatibility and cautions; as well as the property, efficacy, application, special usage and dosage and special precautions of *dà huáng* and *máng xiāo*.

2. Familiar with the classifications of purgative medicinals; the efficacy, indications, special usage and dosage and special precautions of *fān xiè yè*, *huǒ má rén*, *gān suí*, *bā dòu shuāng*, *jīng dà jǐ*, and *yuán huā*.

3. Understand the definitions of purgation, moistening purgation, water expelling and drastic purgation; the efficacy, special usage and dosage and special precautions of *lú huì*, *yù lǐ rén*, *sōng zǐ rén*, *qiān niú zǐ*, and *qiān jīn zǐ*.

凡以泻下通便为主要功效，常用以治疗里实积滞证的药物，称为泻下药。

Medicinals with the main efficacy of promoting defecation by purgation and usually indicated for interior excess syndromes with accumulation and stagnation are known as purgative medicinals.

泻下药为沉降之品，主入大肠经，能引起腹泻，或滑利大肠，以促进排便，主要具有泻下通便作用，以排除胃肠积滞、燥屎及有害物质；或清热泻火，使实热火邪通过泻下而清解，起到"上病治下""釜底抽薪"的作用；或逐水退肿，使水湿停饮从大小便排除，达到祛除停饮、消退水肿的目的。主治大便秘结，胃肠积滞，实热内结及水肿停饮等里实证。部分药物兼有解毒、活血祛瘀等作用，还可用于疮痈肿毒及瘀血证。

Purgative medicinals usually have the efficacy to sink and descend, and act on large intestine meridian. They can cause diarrhea or lubricate large intestine to promote defecation. Their main efficacy is to promote defecation by purgation to remove retained food in the stomach and intestines, dry stool and other harmful substances. Some medicinals are indicated to clear away excess heat and reduce fire to reach the effect of "treating the lower for the upper diseases" and "raking the firewood from beneath the cauldron". Some others function to expel water and relieve edema to evacuate the water fluid, dampness and retained fluid through micturition and defecation so as to treat edema caused by retained fluid. These medicinals are indicated to treat various interior excess syndromes such as constipation, accumulation and stagnation of stomach and intestines, interior retention of excess heat and edema due to retained fluid. Some of the medicinals also have the functions of resolving toxin, activating blood and removing stasis, which can be used to treat sore, carbuncle, swelling as well as static blood syndrome.

根据泻下药的作用特点和作用强弱，可分为攻下药、润下药及峻下逐水药三类。

According to the different medicinal properties and efficacies, purgative medicinals can be classified into three categories: defecation-promoting purgative medicinals, defecation-promoting moistening-purgative medicinals and water-expelling drastic-purgative medicinals.

应用泻下药时，必须辨清证候，审查虚实，分别选用攻下药、润下药或峻下逐水药。同时，应根据饮食、痰湿、瘀血、寄生虫等不同积滞，分别与消食、化痰、祛湿、活血、驱虫等药同用。还应根据里实证的兼证及患者体质进行适当配伍。里实兼表邪者，应配伍解表药以表里同治，或先解表后攻里；里实而正虚者，应配伍补虚药，攻补兼施。若属热积便秘，应配伍清热药；寒积便秘，应配伍温里药。里实积滞，易阻滞气机，气机不畅，则加剧积滞，故泻下药常与行气药同用。

When using purgative medicinals, doctors are required to differentiate syndromes and identify excess or deficiency firstly to select defecation-promoting purgative medicinals, defecation-promoting moistening-purgative medicinals or water-expelling drastic-purgative medicinals accordingly. In addition, they should be combined appropriately with medicinals that have the efficacies of promoting digestion, dissolving phlegm, dispelling dampness, invigorating blood and expelling worm according to different accumulation and stagnation such as diet, phlegm and dampness, static blood as well as parasites. Proper combination should be considered based on the accompanied syndromes and physique. In case of interior excess accompanied by exterior pathogens, they should be used in combination with exterior-releasing medicinals to release both the interior and exterior, or first exterior-releasing medicinals and then interior-purging medicinals; for interior excess with healthy qi deficiency, deficiency-tonifying medicinals should be used to deal with both attack and supplementation. For constipation caused by heat accumulation, heat-clearing medicinals should be combined; while for constipation due to cold stagnation, they should be combined with interior-warming medicinals. Interior excessive accumulation tends to block qi movement which may aggravate stagnation, therefore, purgative medicinals are often applied in combination with qi-moving medicinals.

攻下药与峻下药容易损伤正气和脾胃，故小儿、老人及体虚患者慎用，妇女胎前产后及月经期忌用。使用作用较强的泻下药时，一般得泻即止，切勿过剂，以免损伤正气。对于峻猛而有毒的泻下药，应严格注意其炮制、配伍禁忌、用法用量的特殊要求，确保用药安全。

Defecation-promoting purgative medicinals and water-expelling drastic-purgative medicinals are easy to damage healthy qi and spleen and stomach qi, so they should be contraindicated before labor or after childbirth or during menstruation, and should be used with caution for children, the old or weak patients. Treatment of medicinals in this category should be discontinued as soon as the intended effect is obtained. Overdosage use would damage healthy qi. For those toxic purgative medicinals, the processing procedure, incompatibility, administration and dosage must be strictly controlled to ensure medication safety.

第一节　攻下药
Section 1　Defecation-promoting purgative medicinals

PPT

本类药物大多苦寒沉降，主入胃、大肠经，既有较强的攻下通便作用，又有较强的清热泻火或清热解毒功效，主治实热积滞，大便秘结，燥屎坚结；还可用治温热病高热神昏，谵语发狂；或火热上炎之头痛、目赤肿痛、咽喉肿痛、牙龈肿痛；血热妄行之吐血、衄血以及热毒疮痈等。上述病证无论有无便秘，均可使用本类药物，以清除实热或导热下行，起到"釜底抽薪"的作用。

Defecation-promoting purgative medicinals are usually bitter in flavor and cold in property. They function to sink and descend and act on stomach and large intestine meridians. Their major efficacy is to promote defecation by purgation, to clear heat and reduce fire or remove toxin. They are indicated to treat accumulation and stagnation of excess heat manifested as constipation, dry and hard stool, or warm-heat disease manifested as high fever, loss of consciousness, delirium speech and mania; or headache, red eyes, swelling and pain of throat and gum pain caused by fire-heat flaming upward, or nose bleeding and expectoration of blood due to blood heat, or sores and carbuncles due to fire toxin. Medicinals of this category can be used in the above symptoms whether constipation is presented or not to clear excess heat and induce heat to move downward so that function of "raking the firewood from beneath the cauldron" can be obtained.

大黄　*Dà huáng* (Rhei Radix et Rhizoma)
《神农本草经》
Shen Nong's Classic of the Materia Medica (Shén Nóng Běn Cǎo Jīng)

【来源 / Origin】

为蓼科植物掌叶大黄 *Rheum palmatum* L.、唐古特大黄 *Rheum tanguticum* Maxim.ex Balf. 或药用大黄 *Rheum officinale* Baill. 的干燥根和根茎。掌叶大黄和唐古特大黄药材称"北大黄"，主产于青海、甘肃等地；药用大黄药材称"南大黄"，主产于四川。秋末茎叶枯萎或次春发芽前采挖，切瓣或段，干燥。生用或酒炙、酒炖或蒸、炒炭用。本品气清香，味苦而微涩，嚼之粘牙，有沙粒感。《中国药典》规定，含总蒽醌以芦荟大黄素（$C_{15}H_{10}O_5$）、大黄酸（$C_{15}H_8O_6$）、大黄素（$C_{15}H_{10}O_5$）、大黄酚（$C_{15}H_{10}O_4$）和大黄素甲醚（$C_{16}H_{12}O_5$）的总量计，不得少于 1.5%。

Dà huáng is the root and rhizome of *Rheum palmatum* L., *Rheum tangutium* Maxim. ex Balf. or *Rheum officinale* Baill., pertaining to Polygonaceae. Medicinals from *Rheum palmatum* L., and *Rheum tanguticum* Maxim.ex Balf. are also called *běi* (north) *dà huáng*, which is mainly produced in Qinghai and Gansu Province in China. Midicinals from *Rheum officinale* Baill. are called *nán* (south) *dà huáng* and mainly produced in Sichuan Province in China. It is collected in late autumn after stem and leaves have withered or in the spring before the plants sprout, cut into slices and segments, dried in the sunshine, and used raw or stir-fried with wine, stewed with wine, or steamed, or stir-fried to scorch, has a delicate fragrance, and bitter and slightly astringent in taste. When chewed, it is sticky and induces a feeling of grittiness. According to *Chinese Pharmacopoeia*, the total content of anthraquinones such as aloe-emodin

$(C_{15}H_{10}O_5)$, rheinic acid $(C_{15}H_8O_6)$, emodin $(C_{15}H_{10}O_5)$, chrysophanol $(C_{15}H_{10}O_4)$ and physcion $(C_{16}H_{12}O_5)$ should be no less than 1.5%.

【性味归经 / Medicinal properties 】

苦，寒。归脾、胃、大肠、肝、心包经。

Bitter and cold; act on spleen, stomach, large intestine, liver and pericardium meridians.

【主要功效 / Medicinal efficacies 】

泻下攻积，清热泻火，凉血解毒，逐瘀通经，利湿退黄。

Attack accumulation by purgation; clear heat and drain fire; cool blood and resolve toxins; expel stasis and promote menstruation flow; drain dampness and relieve jaundice.

【临床应用 / Clinical application 】

1. **实热积滞便秘**　本品苦泄沉降，有较强的泻下通便、荡涤肠胃积滞作用，为治疗积滞便秘之要药。凡胃肠积滞，大便秘结，无论寒热虚实，均可配伍使用。因其性寒，故尤宜于热结便秘，常与芒硝、厚朴、枳实同用。若治里实热结而兼气血亏虚者，可与人参、当归等同用。若治热结津伤便秘，多与麦冬、生地黄、玄参等同用。若治脾阳不足，冷积便秘，须与附子、干姜等配伍。用治湿热痢疾，常与黄连、木香等同用，以清除肠道湿热积滞。

(1) **Constipation due to stagnation of excess heat**　*Dà huáng* is bitter with action to descend and sink. It has a strong effect in promoting defecation by purgation and cleaning up stagnation of stomach and intestines. Thus it is considered to be the major medicinal to treat constipation caused by accumulation and stagnation. It can be used in combination to deal with constipation caused by accumulation and stagnation without consideration of cold, heat, deficiency or excess. Because of its cold nature, it is especially effective for constipation due to stagnation of heat and usually combined with *máng xiāo* (Natrii Sulfas), *hòu pò* (Magnoliae Officinalis Cortex) and *zhǐ shí* (Aurantii Immaturus Fructus). To treat constipation due to heat accumulation accompanied by qi-blood deficiency, it is usually combined with *rén shēn* (Ginseng Radix et Rhizoma) and *dāng guī* (Angelicae Sinensis Radix). To treat constipation due to heat accumulation and fluid consumption, it is often combined with *mài dōng* (Ophiopogonis Radix), *shēng dì huáng* (Rehmanniae Radix) and *xuán shēn* (Scrophulariae Radix). To treat constipation due to cold accumulation accompanied by spleen yang insufficiency, it is often combined with *fù zǐ* (Aconiti Lateralis Radix Praeparata) and *gān jiāng* (Zingiberis Rhizoma). To treat damp-heat dysentery, it is often combined with *huáng lián* (Coptidis Rhizoma) and *mù xiāng* (Aucklandiae Radix) to eliminate damp-heat accumulation in the intestines.

2. **目赤咽肿，牙龈肿痛，血热吐衄**　本品苦降，能使上炎之火下泄，又具清热泻火、凉血止血之功。用治火热炎上之目赤肿痛、咽喉肿痛、牙龈肿痛等，常与黄芩、栀子等同用。用治血热妄行之吐血、衄血、咯血，常与黄连、黄芩同用。

(2) **Red eyes and swollen throat, pain gum, hematemesis due to blood heat**　*Dà huáng* is bitter for descending. It can discharge flaring of fire, clear heat and reduce fire, as well as cool blood and stop bleeding. To treat red eyes, swollen throat, swelling and pain of gingiva caused by fire-heat flaming upward, it is combined with *huáng qín* (Scutellariae Radix) and *zhī zǐ* (Gardeniae Fructus). To treat hematemesis, epistaxis, and hemoptysis due to blood heat, it can be combined with *huáng lián* (Coptidis Rhizoma) and *huáng qín*.

3. **痈肿疔疮，肠痈腹痛，烧烫伤**　本品有清热解毒、凉血消肿之功，并借其泻下通便作用，又能使热毒下泄。用治热毒痈肿疔疮，常与金银花、蒲公英、连翘等同用。用治肠痈腹痛，可与牡丹皮、桃仁、芒硝等同用。用治烧烫伤，可单用大黄粉，或配地榆粉，用麻油调敷。

(3) Pyocutaneous diseases, intestinal abscess with abdominal pain, burn and scald　*Dà huáng* functions to clear heat and remove toxin, cool blood and diminish swelling. It can also discharge heat toxin through promoting defecation with purgation. To treat carbuncle, sore, swelling and erysipelas due to heat toxin, it is often combined with *jīn yín huā* (Lonicerae Japonicae Flos), *lián qiáo* (Forsythiae Fructus) and *pú gōng yīng* (Taraxaci Herba). To treat intestinal abscess with abdominal pain, it is combined with *mǔ dān pí* (Moutan Cortex), *táo rén* (Persicae Semen) and *máng xiāo* (Natrii Sulfas). To treat burn and scald, it can be singly used in *dà huáng* powder, or combined with *dì yú* (Sanguisorbae Radix) powder, and mixed with sesame oil for external application.

4. 瘀血证　本品有较好的活血祛瘀作用，为治疗瘀血证的常用药。用治妇女瘀血经闭，可与红花、当归等同用；用治妇女产后瘀阻腹痛、恶露不尽，常与桃仁、土鳖虫等同用；用治跌打损伤，瘀血肿痛，可与当归、红花、穿山甲等同用。

(4) Blood stasis　*Dà huáng* can activate blood and remove stasis, so it is a commonly used medicinal to treat blood stasis syndrome. For female menstrual block due to blood stagnation, it is often used with *hóng huā* (Carthami Flos) and *dāng guī* (Angelicae Sinensis Radix); for postpartum abdominal pain due to blood stasis, and consistent flow of lochia, it is combined with *táo rén* (Persicae Semen) and *tǔ biē chóng* (Eupolyphaga seu Steleophaga). For injury from fall accompanied by swelling and pain with blood stasis, it can be used together with *dāng guī* (Angelicae Sinensis Radix), *hóng huā* (Carthami Flos) and *chuān shān jiǎ* (Manitis Squama).

5. 黄疸，淋证　本品泻下通便，兼利小便，导湿热从二便分消，可用治湿热蕴结诸证。若治湿热黄疸，常配伍茵陈、栀子；若治湿热淋证，多与木通、车前子、栀子等同用。

(5) Jaundice and stranguria　*Dà huáng* functions to promote defecation by purgation and induce diuresis so as to drain damp heat downward, so it can be used to treat various damp-heat accumulation syndromes. To treat damp-heat jaundice, it is often combined with *yīn chén* (Artemisiae Scopariae Herba) and *zhī zǐ* (Gardeniae Fructus). To treat damp-heat stranguria, it is combined with *mù tōng* (Akebiae Caulis), *chē qián zǐ* (Plantaginis Semen) and *zhī zǐ* (Gardeniae Fructus).

【用法用量 / Usage and dosage】

煎服，3~15g；用于泻下不宜久煎。外用适量，研末敷于患处。生大黄泻下力较强，欲攻下者宜生用，入汤剂宜后下；酒大黄善清上焦血分热毒，用于目赤咽肿、牙龈肿痛；熟大黄泻下力缓，可泻火解毒，用于热毒疮疡；大黄炭凉血化瘀止血，用于血热有瘀之出血证。

Decoction, 3-15g. It should not be decocted for a long time when used for purgation. An appropriate amount is ground into powder for applying on the afflicted area. The crude one with stronger purgative action should be used in purgation, and later added to the decoction. When prepared with wine, it is able to clear heat-toxin of blood phase in the upper energizer to treat red eyes, swollen throat, pain and swelling gingiva. The processed *dà huáng* has weaker purgative action, which discharges fire and resolves toxins can be used to treat skin ulcers caused by heat toxin. The carbonized form is usually used for bleeding syndrome to cool blood, remove stasis and stanch bleeding.

【使用注意 / Precaution】

孕妇及月经期、哺乳期妇女慎用。

It should be used with caution for pregnant women, or women during menstruation and lactation.

【现代研究 / Modern research】

本品主要含芦荟大黄素、大黄酸、大黄酚、大黄素甲醚、大黄素、大黄素甲醚 –8– 葡萄糖苷，芦荟大黄素 –8– 葡萄糖苷、番泻苷 A~D，尚含挥发油及鞣质等。具有加强肠蠕动、促进排便、抗急性胰腺炎、抗病原微生物、抗肾衰竭、保肝、利胆、抗溃疡、抗纤维化、降脂、抗动脉粥样硬化、抗炎、抗肿瘤等作用。

It mainly contains aloe-emodin, rhein acid, chrysophanol, physcion, emodin, chrysophanol ether-8-glucoside, aloe-emodin aloe-8-glucoside, sennoside A, B, C, D. *Dà huáng* also contains essential oil and tannin. It has the functions of increasing enterocinesia, promoting defecation, promoting pancreatic secretion, restraining trypsogen activity, anti-pathogenic microorganism, ameliorating renal function, hepatoprotection, cholaneresis, anti-ulcer, anti-fibrosis, decreasing blood fat, anti-arteriosclerosis, anti-inflammatory, inhibiting tumor.

芒硝 *Máng xiāo* (Natrii Sulfas)
《名医别录》
Miscellaneous Records of Famous Physicians (Míng Yī Bié Lù)

【来源 / Origin】

为硫酸盐类矿物芒硝族芒硝经加工精制而成的结晶体，主含含水硫酸钠（$Na_2SO_4 \cdot 10H_2O$）。主产于河北、河南、山东等地。全年均可采集提炼。本品气微，味咸。《中国药典》规定，含硫酸钠不得少于 99.0%。

Máng xiāo is the refined crystalline sodium sulphate, pertaining to the mirabilite family. It mainly contains aqueous sodium sulfate ($Na_2SO_4 \cdot 10H_2O$), mainly produced in Hebei, Henan and Shandong Province in China, and collected all around the year. It has a slight odor and is salty in flavor. According to *Chinese Pharmacopoeia*, the content of sodium sulphate should be no less than 99.0%.

【性味归经 / Medicinal properties】

咸、苦，寒。归胃、大肠经。

Salty, bitter and cold; act on stomach and large intestine channels.

【主要功效 / Medicinal efficacies】

泻下通便，润燥软坚，清火消肿。

Promote defecation by purgation; moisten dryness and soften hard masses; clear fire and relieve swelling.

【临床应用 / Clinical application】

1. **实热积滞，大便燥结** 本品苦寒泻热通便，味咸润燥软坚，长于软化坚硬燥结之大便。对实热积滞，腹满胀痛，大便燥结者尤为适宜，常与大黄相须为用。

(1) **Constipation due to stagnation of excess heat** *Máng xiāo* is bitter and cold in nature, which functions to promote defecation by purging heat. It is salty and good at moistening dryness and softening hard masses. It is suitable for softening hard and dry feces, especially for the constipation due to stagnation of excess heat accompanied by abdominal fullness, distension and pain; it is often combined with *dà huáng*.

2. **咽痛口疮，目赤肿痛，痈疮肿痛** 本品外用有清热消肿作用，可治疗多种热毒证。用治咽喉肿痛、口舌生疮，可与硼砂、冰片、朱砂等配伍。用治目赤肿痛，可用本品化水点眼，或煎汤熏洗。用治乳痈初起，可用本品化水或用纱布包裹外敷。用治肠痈初起，可与大黄、大蒜同用，捣烂外敷。用治痔疮肿痛，可单用本品煎汤外洗。

(2) **Sore throat and aphthae, red eyes with swelling and pain, ulcerative carbuncle** External use of this medicinal can clear heat and subside swelling, as well as various heat toxin syndrome. To treat sore throat and aphthae, it is usually combined with *péng shā* (Borax), *bīng piàn* (Borneolum

Syntheticum) and *zhū shā* (Cinnabaris). To treat red eyes with swelling and pain, it can be dissolved with water as eye-drops, or decocted for fumigation and washing. To treat mammary abscess in the initial stage, it can be dissolved in water or wrapped with gauze for external application. For intestinal abscess in the initial stage, it can be combined with *dà huáng* and garlic, which are ground into pieces for external use. For hemorrhoids with swelling and pain, it can be decocted singly with water for external wash.

【用法用量 / Usage and dosage】

冲入药汁内或开水溶化后服，6~12g。外用适量。

It is taken infused with decoction or dissolved with boiling water for oral use with the dosage of 6-12g. An appropriate amount is used externally.

【使用注意 / Precaution】

孕妇及哺乳期妇女慎用。不宜与硫黄、三棱同用。

It should be used with caution for pregnant women and women during menstruation. It is improper to be combined with *liú huáng* (Sulphur) and *sān léng* (Sparganii Rhizoma).

【现代研究 / Modern research】

本品主要含含水硫酸钠，尚含少量氯化钠、硫酸镁、硫酸钙等。具有阻止肠内水分吸收、促进肠蠕动而致泻、抗炎、溶石、利尿等作用。

Máng xiāo mainly contains aqueous sodium sulfate. It also contains small amount of magnesium sulfate, calcium sulfate and sodium chloride. It has the functions of preventing water absorption in the bowels, promoting bowel movement to induce purgation, antiinflammation, cholaneresis, and promoting urination.

番泻叶　*Fān xiè yè* (Sennae Folium)

《饮片新参》

New Reference of Prepared Medicines (*Yǐn Piàn Xīn Cān*)

【来源 / Origin】

为豆科植物狭叶番泻 *Cassia angustifolia* Vahl 或尖叶番泻 *Cassia acutifolia* Delile 的干燥小叶。前者主产于印度、埃及和苏丹；后者主产于埃及，我国广东、广西及云南亦有栽培。9 月采收，晒干，生用。本品气微弱而特异，味微苦，稍有黏性。《中国药典》规定，含番泻苷 A（$C_{42}H_{38}O_{20}$）和番泻苷 B（$C_{42}H_{38}O_{20}$）的总量，不得少于 1.1%。

Fān xiè yè is from the dry leaf of *Cassia angustifolia* Vahl and *Cassia acutifolia* Delile, family Leguminosae. The former is mainly produced in India, Egypt and Sudan, while the latter is mainly produced in Egypt, and it is also cultivated in Guangdong Province, Guangxi Zhuang Autonomous Region and Yunnan Province in China. It is usually collected in September, dried in the sunshine, and use raw. It has a slight odor with specificity, and is slightly bitter in flavor and a bit sticky. According to *Chinese Pharmacopoeia*, the total content of sennosides A($C_{42}H_{38}O_{20}$) and sennosides B ($C_{42}H_{38}O_{20}$) should be no less than 1.1%.

【性味归经 / Medicinal properties】

甘、苦，寒。归大肠经。

Sweet, bitter and cold; act on large intestine meridian.

【主要功效 / Medicinal efficacies】

泻热行滞，通便，利水。

Reduce heat and remove stagnation, promote defecation, clear dampness.

【临床应用 / Clinical application】

1. **热结便秘** 本品苦寒通降，有较强的泻下导滞、清导实热功效。小剂量缓泻通便，大剂量攻下。适用于热结便秘，也可用于习惯性便秘和老人便秘，大多单味泡服。若治热结便秘，腹满胀痛者，可与枳实、厚朴等同用。

(1) **Constipation due to heat stagnation** *Fān xiè yè* is bitter in flavor and cold in property for descending. It also has strong effect in purging and removing stagnation. Small dosage can be used for mild purgation, and large dosage for drastic purgation. It is suitable for constipation caused by heat stagnation, habitual constipation and constipation of the aging, and usually soaked singly in boiling water for oral use. To treat constipation due to heat stagnation accompanied by abdominal fullness, distension and pain, it is combined with *zhǐ shí* (Aurantii Immaturus Fructus) and *hòu pò* (Magnoliae Officinalis Cortex).

2. **水肿胀满** 本品能泻下行水消胀。用治水肿胀满，可单味泡服，或与牵牛子、大腹皮等同用。

(2) **Edema, abdominal fullness and distension** *Fān xiè yè* has actions of purging, clearing dampness and relieving distension. To treat edema and abdominal fullness and distension, it is soaked singly in boiling water for oral use, or combined with *qiān niú zǐ* (Pharbitidis Semen) and *dà fù pí* (Arecae Pericarpium).

【用法用量 / Usage and dosage】

2~6g，后下，或开水泡服。

2~6g, it is added later or soaked in boiling water for oral use.

【使用注意 / Precaution】

哺乳期、月经期妇女及孕妇慎用。

It should be used with caution for women during pregnancy, lactation and menstruation.

【现代研究 / Modern research】

本品主要含番泻苷 A~D 等。具有泻下、抗菌、止血等作用。

It mainly contains sennosides A-D, and has the functions of purging, antisepsis and stopping bleeding.

第二节　润下药

Section 2　Defecation-promoting moistening-purgative medicinals

PPT

本类药物多为植物的种子或种仁，富含油脂，味甘质润，药性平和，能润滑大肠，使大便软化易于排出。主要用治年老、体弱、久病、产后所致之津枯、阴虚、血虚肠燥便秘。

Defecation-promoting moistening-purgative medicinals are usually plant seeds and kernels, which are rich in oil, sweet in flavor and moistening in nature. They are neutral in medicinal nature and mainly function to lubricate intestine to moisten dried feces. Medicinals in this section are suitable for the treatment of constipation due to fluid consumption, yin deficiency and blood deficiency in the old, the weak, the patients with chronic diseases, or postpartum women.

火麻仁　*Huǒ má rén* (Cannabis Fructus)
《神农本草经》
Shen Nong's Classic of the Materia Medica (Shén Nóng Běn Cǎo Jīng)

【来源 / Origin】

为桑科植物大麻 *Cannabis sativa* L. 的干燥成熟果实。主产于山东、河北、黑龙江等地。秋季采收，晒干，生用或炒用。本品气微，味淡。

Huǒ má rén is the ripe fruits of *Cannabis sativa* L., pertaining to Moraceae. It is mainly produced in Shandong, Hebei and Heilongjiang Province in China, collected in autumn, dried in the sun, and used raw or stir-fried. It has a slight odor and is bland in flavor.

【性味归经 / Medicinal properties】

甘，平。归脾、胃、大肠经。

Sweet and neutral; act on spleen, stomach and large intestine meridians.

【主要功效 / Medicinal efficacies】

润肠通便。

Moisten the intestines to promote defecation.

【临床应用 / Clinical application】

肠燥便秘　本品甘平，多脂质润，能润肠通便，且略兼滋养之力。用治津血不足之肠燥便秘，可单用，或与大黄、厚朴等同用。

Constipation due to dryness of intestine　*Huǒ má rén* is sweet in flavor and neutral in nature, rich in oil and moistening in nature. It has efficacies of moistening the intestine to promote defecation as well as nourishing effect. To treat constipation due to intestinal dryness and insufficiency of the body fluids and blood, it can be used singly or combined with *dà huáng* and *hòu pò* (Magnoliae Officinalis Cortex).

【用法用量 / Usage and dosage】

煎服，10~15g。

Decoction, 10~15g.

【现代研究 / Modern research】

本品主要含葫芦巴碱、甜菜碱、胆碱、木犀草素、牡荆素、荭草苷以及酚类、蛋白质、多种脂肪酸等。具有缓泻、降脂、抗动脉粥样硬化、抗氧化、延缓衰老、降血压等作用。

It mainly contains trigonelline, betaine, choline, luteolin, vitexin and orientin. It also contains phenols, protein and various fatty acids. It has the functions of purging mildly, reducing blood fat, anti-arteriosclerosis, antagonizing oxidation, delaying senility and reducing blood pressure.

郁李仁　*Yù lǐ rén* (Pruni Semen)
《神农本草经》
Shen Nong's Classic of the Materia Medica (Shén Nóng Běn Cǎo Jīng)

【来源 / Origin】

为蔷薇科植物欧李 *Prunus humilis* Bge.、郁李 *Prunus japonica* Thunb. 或长柄扁桃 *Prunus pedunculata* Maxim. 的干燥成熟种子。前两种习称"小李仁"，后一种习称"大李仁"。主产于内蒙古、河北、辽宁等地。夏、秋二季采收，干燥，生用。本品气微，味微苦。《中国药典》规定，苦杏仁苷（$C_{20}H_{27}NO_{11}$）的含量，不得少于 2.0%。

The source is from dried ripe seeds of *Prunus humilis* Bge., *Prunus japonica* Thunb. or *Prunus*

pedunculata Maxim.. The former two are commonly called *xiǎo lǐ rén* and the latter one named *dà lǐ rén*. It is mainly produced in Inner Mongolia Autonomous Region, Hebei and Liaoning Province. The ripe fruits are collected in the summer and autumn, dried in the sun, and used raw. It has a slight ordor and is a bit bitter in flavor. According to *Chinese Pharmacopoeia*, the content of amygdalin ($C_{20}H_{27}NO_{11}$) should be no less than 2.0%.

【性味归经 / Medicinal properties】

辛、苦、甘，平。归脾、大肠、小肠经。

Acrid, bitter, sweet and neutral; act on spleen, large intestine and small intestine meridians.

【主要功效 / Medicinal efficacies】

润肠通便、下气利水。

Moisten the intestine to relieve constipation, move qi downward and promote diuresis.

【临床应用 / Clinical application】

1. 肠燥便秘　本品甘平质润，辛行苦降，功似火麻仁润肠通便，兼行大肠气滞。用治气滞腹胀，肠燥便秘，常与柏子仁、杏仁、桃仁等同用。用治血虚津枯，肠燥便秘，可与当归、火麻仁等同用。

(1) Constipation due to dryness of intestine　*Yù lǐ rén* is sweet and neutral, moistening in nature. It is acrid for regulating qi and bitter for descending. Apart from moistening intestine to promote defecation as *huǒ má rén*, it can also regulate qi stagnation in large intestine. To treat constipation due to intestinal dryness, qi stagnation and abdominal distension, it is often combined with *bǎi zǐ rén* (Platycladi Semen), *xìng rén* (Armeniacae Amarum Semen) and *táo rén* (Persicae Semen). To treat constipation caused by intestinal dryness and insufficiency of the body fluids and blood, it is combined with *dāng guī* (Angelicae Sinensis Radix) and *huǒ má rén*.

2. 水肿，小便不利，脚气浮肿　本品能利水消肿。用治水肿胀满，小便不利，多与桑白皮、赤小豆等同用。用治脚气肿痛，可与木瓜、蚕沙等配伍。

(2) Edema, beriberi and dysuria　*Yù lǐ rén* can promote diuresis and relieve edema. To treat edema and abdominal dullness and distension, as well as dysuria, it is combined with *sāng bái pí* (Mori Cortex) and *chì xiǎo dòu* (Phaseoli Semen). To treat beriberi with swelling and pain, it is used together with *mù guā* (Chaenomelis Fructus) and *cán shā* (Bombycis Faeces).

【用法用量 / Usage and dosage】

煎服，6~10g。

Decocted, 6-10g.

【使用注意 / Precaution】

孕妇慎用。

It should be used with caution on pregnant women.

【现代研究 / Modern research】

本品主要含阿弗则林、苦杏仁苷、山柰苷、郁李仁苷、香草酸、熊果酸、原儿茶酸以及脂肪油、皂苷、纤维素等。具有促进肠蠕动、抗炎、镇痛等作用。

It mainly contains afzelin, amygdalin, kaempferitrin, bunge cherry seed glycosides, vanillic acid, uosolic acid, protocate-chuic acid, fatty oil, saponin and cellulose. It has the functions of promoting bowels movement, antiinflammation and alleviating pain.

PPT

第三节 峻下逐水药
Section 3 Water-expelling drastic-purgative medicinals

本类药物大多苦寒有毒，泻下作用峻猛，服后能引起剧烈腹泻，使体内留滞的水湿从大便排出体外，消除肿胀。部分药物兼能利尿。主治全身水肿、胸腹积水及痰饮积聚、喘满壅实等形证俱实，或用一般利水消肿药难以奏效者。

Water-expelling drastic-purgative medicinals are usually bitter and cold in nature, toxic, and with drastic efficacy. They can cause severe diarrhea after oral taking. It discharges the retained water fluid and dampness inside body through defecation to relieve edema. Some can also promote urination. Medicinals in this section are suitable for general edema, water accumulated in the chest and abdomen, phlegm-rheum accumulation, and excessive panting and fullness with no decline of healthy qi, or symptoms that general diuretic detumescence medicinals fail to reach effects.

本类药攻伐力强，副作用大，易伤正气，临床应用当"中病即止"，不可久服，使用时常配伍补益药以固护正气。体虚者慎用，孕妇忌用。还要注意本类药物的炮制、剂量、用法及禁忌等，以确保用药安全、有效。

Medicinals in this section have drastic purgative effects and strong side effects, which are likely to damage healthy qi. So in clinical application, the medication should be discontinued as soon as getting effect. They should not be taken for a long time. When in use, they should be combined with tonifying medicinals to consolidating healthy qi. They should be used with caution in weak patients, and be contraindicated in pregnant women. The processing procedure, dosage, usage and contraindication of medicinals of this category should be paid attention in order to ensure medication safety and efficacy.

甘遂 *Gān suí* (Kansui Radix)
《神农本草经》
Shen Nong's Classic of the Materia Medica (Shén Nóng Běn Cǎo Jīng)

【来源 / Origin】

为大戟科植物甘遂 *Euphorbia kansui* T.N.Liou ex T.P.Wang 的干燥块根。春季开花前或秋末茎叶枯萎后采挖，晒干，生用或醋炙用。本品气微，味微甘而辣。《中国药典》规定，含大戟二烯醇（$C_{30}H_{50}O$）不得少于 0.12%。

Gān suí is the root tuber of *Euphorbia kansui* T.N.Liou ex T.P.Wang, pertaining to Euphorbiaceae. It is collected either before bloom in spring or when the stem and leaves have withered in late autumn, and dried in the sun, and used raw or stir-fried with vinegar. *Gān suí* has a slight odor, and is slightly sweet and acrid in taste. According to *Chinese Pharmacopoeia*, the content of euphadienol ($C_{30}H_{50}O$) should not be less than 0.12%.

【性味归经 / Medicinal properties】

苦，寒；有毒。归肺、肾、大肠经。

Bitter, cold and poisonous; act on lung, kidney and large intestine meridians.

【主要功效 / Medicinal efficacies】

泻水逐饮，消肿散结。

Expel fluid retention by drastic purgation; relieve swelling and dissipate masses.

【临床应用 / Clinical application】

1. 水肿胀满，胸腹积水，痰饮积聚 本品苦寒性降，泻水逐饮之力峻猛，服后可连续泻下，使体内留滞的水湿迅速排出。用治水肿、鼓胀、胸胁停饮而正气未衰者，可单用研末服，或与大戟、芫花为末，枣汤送服。

(1) Edema, accumulated water in the chest and abdomen, and accumulation of phlegm rheum *Gān suí* is bitter and cold with action of descending. It has drastic efficacy of expelling water and fluid retention, which can cause consistent purgation after oral taking so as to discharge the water fluid and dampness inside the body rapidly. To treat edema with fullness and distension, accumulated water in the chest and abdomen and accumulation of phlegm rheum without decline of healthy qi, it is used alone and ground into powder for oral use, or it is combined with *dà jǐ* (Euphorbiae Pekinensis Radix), and *yuán huā* (Genkwa Flos) and ground into powder for taking with Chinese date decoction.

2. 风痰癫痫 本品尚有攻逐痰涎作用，治风痰癫痫，可用甘遂为末，入猪心煨后，与朱砂末为丸服。

(2) Epilepsy with wind-phlegm *Gān suí* also has an efficacy of expelling phlegm and spittle. To treat epilepsy with wind-phlegm, it can be used singly and pounded into powder, added to a pork heart and roasted, then it is prepared with *zhū shā* (Cinnabaris) to make pills for oral use.

3. 痈肿疮毒 本品外用能消肿散结，治疮痈肿毒，可用甘遂末水调外敷。

(3) Sores and carbuncles with swelling and toxin *Gān suí* can relieve swelling and dissipate masses. To treat sores and carbuncles with swelling and toxin, it can be ground into powder and mixed with water for external application.

【用法用量 / Usage and dosage】

炮制后多入丸、散用，0.5~1.5g。外用适量，生用。

It is usually made into pills or powder for use after processing, 0.5~1.5g. An appropriate amount of the raw form is used externally.

【使用注意 / Precaution】

孕妇禁用。不宜与甘草同用。

It should be contraindicated in pregnant women. It is not proper to be combined with *gān cǎo*.

【现代研究 / Modern research】

本品主要含大戟二烯醇、甘遂醇、α- 大戟醇和 γ- 大戟醇、巨大戟萜醇、甘遂萜酯 A 和 B 以及棕榈酸、枸橼酸、草酸等。具有泻下、利尿、抗急性胰腺炎、镇痛、中止妊娠、免疫抑制、抗白血病等作用。

Gān suí mainly contains euphadienol, tirucallol, α-euphorbol and γ-euphorbol, ingenol, kansuinine A and kansuinine B, and also contains palmitinic acid, citric acid and oxalic acid. It has the functions of purging, promoting urination, inhibiting acute pancreatitis, relieving pain, antagonizing fertility, immunosuppression and anti-leukemia.

京大戟　*Jīng dà jǐ* (Euphorbiae Pekinensis Radix)
《神农本草经》
Shen Nong's Classic of the Materia Medica (Shén Nóng Běn Cǎo Jīng)

【来源 / Origin】

为大戟科植物大戟 *Euphorbia pekinensis* Rupr. 的干燥根。主产于江苏、四川、江西等地。秋、冬二季采挖，晒干，生用或醋煮用。本品气微，味微苦涩。《中国药典》规定，含大戟二烯醇（C$_{30}$H$_{50}$O）不得少于 0.60%。

Jīng dà jǐ is the root of *Euphorbia pekinensis* Rupr., pertaining to Euphorbiaceae. It is mainly produced in Jiangsu, Sichuan and Jiangxi Province in China, collected in autumn and winter, dried in the sun, and used raw or stir-fried with vinegar. It has a slight odor, slightly bitter and astringent in taste. According to *Chinese Pharmacopoeia*, the content of euphadienol (C$_{30}$H$_{50}$O) should not be less than 0.60%.

【性味归经 / Medicinal properties】

苦，寒；有毒。归肺、脾、肾经。

Bitter, cold and toxic, act on the lung, spleen and kidney meridians.

【主要功效 / Medicinal efficacies】

泻水逐饮，消肿散结。

Expel fluid retention by drastic purgation, relieve swelling and dissipate masses.

【临床应用 / Clinical application】

1. 水肿胀满，胸腹积水，痰饮积聚　本品泻水逐饮功似甘遂而力稍逊，用治水肿、鼓胀、胸胁停饮而正气未衰者，常与甘遂、芫花同用。用治痰饮积聚，气逆咳喘，可配伍甘遂、白芥子等。

(1) Edema, accumulated water in the chest and abdomen, and accumulation of phlegm rheum　The function of *jīng dà jǐ* in expelling fluid retention by drastic purgation is similar but inferior to that of *gān suí*. To treat edema, tympanites and accumulated water in the chest and abdomen without decline of healthy qi, it can be decocted with *gān suí* and *yuán huā* (Genkwa Flos). To treat accumulation of phlegm rheum with panting and cough due to qi counterflow, it is combined with *gān suí* and *bái jiè zǐ* (Sinapis Semen).

2. 痈肿疮毒，瘰疬痰核　本品消肿散结，内服外用均可。用治热毒痈肿疮毒，可鲜品捣烂外敷。用治痰火凝结之瘰疬痰核，可与鸡蛋同煮，食鸡蛋。

(2) Sores and carbuncles with swelling and toxin, scrofula and phlegm node　*Jīng dà jǐ* has efficacies of removing swelling and dissipating masses, which can be used externally and orally. To treat swollen carbuncle and sore toxin due to heat toxin, the fresh can be pounded to pieces for external application. To treat scrofula and phlegm node (subcutaneous nodule) due to phlegm-fire, it can be decocted with eggs and the eggs should also be eaten.

【用法用量 / Usage and dosage】

煎服，1.5~3g。入丸、散服，每次 1g。内服醋制用。外用适量，生用。

Decoction, 1.5-3g; pills or powder, 1g each time. It is stir-fried with vinegar for oral taking. An appropriate amount of the raw form is used externally.

【使用注意 / Precaution】

孕妇禁用。不宜与甘草同用。

It should be contraindicated in pregnant women. It is not proper to be combined with *gān cǎo*.

【现代研究 / Modern research】

本品主要含京大戟素、大戟醇、大戟酸、大戟苷以及生物碱、有机酸、鞣质、多糖等成分。具有泻下、镇痛、镇静、抗肿瘤、抗白血病等作用。

Jīng dà jǐ mainly contains euphorbia pekiensis, euphorbol, euphorbic acid, and euphorbon, and also contains alkaloids, organic acids, tannin and polysaccharides. It has the functions of purging, relieving pain, tranquilizing, antagonizing tumor and inhibiting leukemia.

芫花　*Yuán huā* (Genkwa Flos)

《神农本草经》

Shen Nong's Classic of the Materia Medica (Shén Nóng Běn Cǎo Jīng)

【来源 / Origin】

为瑞香科植物芫花 *Daphne genkwa* Sieb.et Zucc. 的干燥花蕾。主产于安徽、江苏、浙江等地。春季采收，干燥。生用或醋制用。本品气微，味甘、微辛。《中国药典》规定，含芫花素（$C_{16}H_{12}O_5$）不得少于 0.20%。

Yuán huā is the dried flower bud of *Daphne genkwa* Sieb.et Zucc., pertaining to Thymelaeaceae. It is mainly produced in Anhui, Jiangsu, Zhejiang Province in China, collected in spring, dried in the sun, and used raw or after stir-fried with vinegar. It has a slight odor and is slightly acrid. According to *Chinese Pharmacopoeia*, the content of genkwanin ($C_{16}H_{12}O_5$) should be no less than 0.20%.

【性味归经 / Medicinal properties】

苦、辛，温；有毒。归肺、脾、肾经。

Bitter, acrid, warm and toxic; act on the lung, spleen and kidney meridians.

【主要功效 / Medicinal efficacies】

泻水逐饮；外用杀虫疗疮。

Expel fluid retention by drastic purgation; kill worms and cure sores for external use.

【临床应用 / Clinical application】

1. 水肿胀满，胸腹积水，痰饮积聚　本品泻水逐饮功似甘遂、大戟而药力稍逊，三者常相须为用。因其兼能祛痰止咳，长于泻胸胁水饮，故多用治胸胁停饮所致的喘咳痰多、胸胁引痛，可单用或与大枣煎服。

(1) Edema, accumulated water in the chest and abdomen, and accumulation of phlegm rheum　The function of *yuán huā* in expelling fluid retention by drastic purgation is similar but inferior to that of *gān suí* and *dà jǐ*. They are often combined to reinforce the effects. *Yuán huā* has the efficacies of eliminating phlegm to relieve cough and expelling accumulated water in the chest and abdomen. To treat cough and panting due to fluid retention in the chest and abdomen, as well as thoracic and hypochondriac pain caused by fluid retention, it can be used singly or decocted with *dà zǎo*.

2. 疥癣，秃疮，痈肿　本品外用能杀虫疗疮，用治头疮、白秃、顽癣等皮肤病及痈肿，可研末单用，或配雄黄研末，猪脂调敷。

(2) Scabies, tinea (ringworm), favus, swollen carbuncle and chilblain　*Yuán huā* can kill worms and core sores for external use. To treat skin diseases such as scabies, tinea (ringworm) and favus, and swollen carbuncle and chilblain, it is ground into powder and used alone, or combined with *xióng huáng* (Realgar), both are ground into powder and mixed with pork fat for external application.

【用法用量 / Usage and dosage 】

煎服，1.5~3g。研末吞服，每次 0.6~0.9g，每日 1 次。内服醋炙用。外用适量，生用。

Decoction, 1.5-3g. Stir-fried with vinegar and ground into powder for swallowing, 0.6-0.9g each time, once a day. An appropriate amount is used raw for external application.

【使用注意 / Precaution 】

孕妇禁用。不宜与甘草同用。

It should be contraindicated in pregnant women; it is not proper to be combined with *gān cǎo*.

【现代研究 / Modern research 】

本品主要含芫花素、3′− 羟基芫花素、芹菜素、木犀草素、芫根苷、芫花萜、芫花酯乙、芫花酯丙、芫花酯丁、芫花酯戊、芫花瑞香宁以及脂肪酸、挥发油等。具有泻下、利尿、祛痰、镇咳、镇静、抗菌、抗肿瘤等作用。

It mainly contains genkwanin, 3′-hydroxygenkwanin, apigenin, luteolin, yuenkanin, yuanhuacine, yuanhuadine, yuanhuafine, yuanhuatine, yuanhuapine, and genkwadaphnin. It also contains fatty acid and volatile oil. It has the functions of purging, promoting urination, eliminating phlegm, relieving cough, tranquilizing, antagonizing bacterium and tumor.

巴豆霜　*Bā dòu shuāng* (Crotonis Semen Pulveratum)
《神农本草经》
Shen Nong's Classic of the Materia Medica (Shén Nóng Běn Cǎo Jīng)

【来源 / Origin 】

为大戟科植物巴豆 *Croton tiglium* L. 干燥净仁的炮制加工品。主产于四川、广西、云南等地。秋季采收。制霜用。本品气微，味辛辣。《中国药典》规定，含巴豆苷（$C_{10}H_{13}N_5O_5$）不得少于 0.80%。

Bā dòu shuāng is the processed product of dried ripe fruit of *Croton tiglium* L., pertaining to Euphorbiaceae. It is mainly produced in Sichuan Province, Guangxi Zhuang Autonomous Region and Yunnan Province in China, collected in autumn when the fruits are ripe. The kernel is selected and prepared into frost-like powder. It has a slight odor and is acrid in taste. According to *Chinese Pharmacopoeia*, the content of crotonoside ($C_{10}H_{13}N_5O_5$) should not be less than 0.80%.

【药性】

辛，热；有大毒。归胃、大肠经。

Acrid, hot and extremely toxic; act on stomach and large intestine meridians.

【功效】

峻下冷积，逐水退肿，祛痰利咽；外用蚀疮。

Dredge the cold accumulation by drastic purgation, expel water and relieve edema, dispel phlegm and relieve sore throat; erode sores for external use.

【应用】

1. **寒积便秘**　本品辛热，能峻下冷积，开通肠道闭塞。用治腹满胀痛，大便不通，气急口噤，属寒邪食积阻滞肠道，气血未衰者，可单用本品装胶囊服，或与大黄、干姜同用。若治小儿冷积，停乳停食，秘结腹胀，痰壅惊悸者，可峻药轻投，与六神曲、天南星、朱砂共为末服。

(1) Constipation due to cold accumulation　*Bā dòu shuāng* is acrid and hot with drastic efficacy of dredging cold accumulation to smooth intestinal tract. To treat excess cold or cold accumulation accompanied by abdominal fullness and distending pain, and inhibited defecation without decline of qi and blood, it can be used alone and put in capsules for oral use, or combined with *dà huáng* and *gān jiāng* (Zingiberis Rhizoma). To treat infantile cold accumulation, stagnation and accumulation of milk and food, constipation with abdominal distension, even palpitation due to fright, small amount of *bā dòu* is combined with *liù shén qū* (Medicata Fermentata Massa), *tiān nán xīng* (Arisaematis Rhizoma) and *zhū shā* (Cinnabaris) making into powder for oral use.

2. 腹水鼓胀，二便不通　本品峻泻，有较强的逐水退肿作用。用治腹水鼓胀，二便不通之水湿实证，常与杏仁为丸服。

(2) Abdominal dropsy and tympanites, blockage of defecation and micturition　*Bā dòu shuāng* has drastic purging effect, especially in expelling water and relieving edema. To treat abdominal dropsy and tympanites, blockage of defecation and micturition due to excess syndrome of water fluid and dampness, it is combined with *xìng rén* (Armeniacae Amarum Semen) and made into pills for oral use.

3. 喉风，喉痹　本品能祛痰利咽，使呼吸畅通。用治喉痹痰阻，呼吸困难，甚则窒息欲死者，可单用适量吹入喉部，引吐痰涎，开通气道；或与朱砂、雄黄等同用。

(3) Throat *bi*(pharyngitis) with phlegm obstruction　*Bā dòu shuāng* can eliminate phlegm and relieve sore throat to make breathing easier. To treat throat *bi* with phlegm obstruction, dyspnea, even suffocation verging on death, it can be administered orally or by nasal feeding in order to induce spitting of phlegm-drool and open airway. Or it is combined with *zhū shā* (Cinnabaris) and *xióng huáng* (Realgar).

4. 痈肿，疥癣，恶疮　本品外用有蚀腐肉、疗疮毒作用。用治疮痈脓成未溃，或溃后腐肉不脱，或疥癣恶疮、疣痣等，可研末涂患处，或捣烂以纱布包擦患处。

(4) Carbuncle-abscess, scabies and tinea, ulcer　*Bā dòu shuāng* functions to erode carrion and cure sores for external use. To treat carbuncle-abscess with pus formed but without ulceration, or with ulceration and slough without falling off, or scabies and tinea, and warts, it can be pounded into pieces for afflicted area, or wrapped in gauze to wipe the afflicted area.

【用法用量 / Usage and dosage】
入丸、散，0.1~0.3g。外用适量。
It is made into pills or powder for oral use, 0.1-0.3g. An appropriate amount is used externally.

【使用注意 / Precaution】
孕妇禁用。不宜与牵牛子同用。
It should be contraindicated for pregnant women; it is not proper to be combined with *qiān niú zǐ* (Pharbitidis Semen).

【现代研究 / Modern research】
本品主要含脂肪油、巴豆苷，尚含巴豆毒素、巴豆异鸟嘌呤、β- 谷甾醇及酶等。具有泻下、促进平滑肌运动、抗肿瘤、抗菌、抗炎等作用。

Bā dòu shuāng mainly contains fatty oil, hydroxyadenosine, crotonallin toxin, croton tiglium, β-sitosterol and enzymes. It has the functions of purging, promoting smooth muscles movement, antagonizing tumor, antagonizing bacterium and inhibiting inflammation.

其他泻下药功用介绍见表 8-1。
The efficacies of other purgative medicinals are shown in table 8-1.

表 8-1　其他泻下药功用介绍

分类	药物	药性	功效	应用	用法用量
攻下药	芦荟	苦，寒。归肝、胃、大肠经	泻下通便，清肝泻火，杀虫疗疳	热结便秘，惊痫抽搐，小儿疳积；外治癣疮	宜入丸、散，2~5g。外用适量，研末敷患处
润下药	松子仁	甘，微温。归肝、肺、大肠经	润肠通便，润肺止咳	肠燥便秘，肺燥干咳	煎服，5~10g
峻下逐水药	牵牛子	苦、寒；有毒。归肺、肾、大肠经	泻水通便，消痰涤饮，杀虫攻积	水肿胀满，二便不通，痰饮积聚，气逆喘咳，虫积腹痛	煎服，3~6g。入丸、散服，每次 1.5~3g
	千金子	辛、温；有毒。归肝、肾、大肠经	泻下逐水，破血消癥；外用疗癣蚀疣	二便不通，水肿，痰饮，积滞胀满，血瘀经闭；外治顽癣，赘疣	1~2g，去壳用，多入丸、散服。外用适量，捣烂敷患处

题库

（林海燕）

第九章　祛风湿药
Chapter 9　Wind-damp expelling medicinals

 学习目标 | Learning goals

1. 掌握 祛风湿药在性能、功效、主治、配伍及使用注意方面的共性；独活、木瓜、秦艽、防己、五加皮、桑寄生的性能、功效、应用以及特殊的用法用量和特殊的使用注意。

2. 熟悉 祛风湿药的分类；威灵仙、川乌、蕲蛇、雷公藤、豨莶草、桑枝的功效、主治以及特殊的用法用量和特殊的使用注意。

3. 了解 祛风湿药、祛风寒湿药、祛风湿热药、祛风湿强筋骨药等相关功效术语的含义；草乌、香加皮、海风藤、乌梢蛇、蚕沙、伸筋草、青风藤、穿山龙、丝瓜络、路路通、络石藤、臭梧桐、千年健的功效以及特殊的用法用量和特殊的使用注意。

1. Master the commonness of wind-damp expelling medicinals in efficacy, indications, property, compatibility and cautions; as well as the property, efficacy, application, special usage and dosage and special precautions of *dú huó*, *mù guā*, *qín jiāo*, *fáng jǐ*, *wǔ jiā pí*, and *sāng jì shēng*.

2. Familiar with their classifications; as well as the efficacy, indications, special usage and dosage and special precautions of *wēi líng xiān*, *chuān wū*, *qí shé*, *léi gōng téng*, *xī xiān cǎo*, and *sāng zhī*.

3. Understand the definitions of wind-damp expelling medicinals, wind-cold-damp expelling medicinals, wind-damp-heat expelling medicinals, wind-damp expelling and sinew-bone strengthening medicinals and related efficacy terms; as well as the efficacy, special usage and dosage and special precautions of *cǎo wū*, *xiāng jiā pí*, *hǎi fēng téng*, *wū shāo shé*, *cán shā*, *shēn jīn cǎo*, *qīng fēng téng*, *chuān shān lóng*, *sī guā luò*, *lù lù tōng*, *luò shí téng*, *chòu wú tóng*, and *qiān nián jiàn*.

凡以祛除风湿邪气为主要功效，常用以治疗痹证的药物，称为祛风湿药。

Medicinals with efficacies of expelling wind and removing dampness in order to treat *bi* syndrome due to wind-damp, are known as wind-damp expelling medicinals.

祛风湿药多具有辛、苦味，性或温或凉，入肝、肾、脾经。辛能发散，苦以燥湿，善能祛除留滞于肌肉、筋骨、关节的风寒湿邪或风湿热邪，缓解或消除痹证的各种症状。主要用治痹证，表现为肢体筋骨、关节、肌肉等处疼痛、酸楚、重着、麻木或屈伸不利、僵硬、肿大、变形及活动障碍等。部分药物还适用于腰膝酸软、下肢痿弱等。

Wind-damp expelling medicinals are usually acrid and bitter in flavor, and cold or warm or cool in nature, act on liver, kidney and spleen meridians. They are acrid for dispersing, and bitter for drying, and good at expelling pathogenic wind-cold-damp or pathogenic wind-damp-heat from muscles, sinews and bones, and joints, and relieving or eliminating different symptoms of *bì* syndrome. They are mainly used to treat *bì* syndrome (impediment or arthralgia) manifested as pain, soreness, heaviness, numbness, or inhibited bending and stretching, stiffness, swelling, deformity and difficulty in moving, in the limbs, sinews and bones, joints and muscles. Some of them are also used to treat soreness and weakness of the waist and knees, and flaccidity of the lower limbs.

根据祛风湿药的药性及功效主治差异，可分为祛风寒湿药、祛风湿热药及祛风湿强筋骨药三类。

According to the different medicinal properties and efficacies, they are classified into three categories: wind-cold-damp expelling medicinals, wind-damp-heat expelling medicinals and wind-damp expelling and sinew-bone strengthening medicinals.

应用祛风湿药时，必须针对痹证的性质、部位、新久的不同，选用适宜的药物并行适当配伍。如风邪偏盛的行痹，应选择祛风为主的祛风湿药，配伍活血养营之品；湿邪偏盛的着痹，应选用温燥的祛风湿药，配伍燥湿健脾之品；寒邪偏盛的痛痹，应选用温性较强的祛风湿药，配伍温经止痛之品；风湿热痹者，应选用性质寒凉的祛风湿药，配伍清热解毒之品。若感邪初期，病邪在表者，当配伍祛风胜湿的解表药。若痹证日久，累及肝肾，筋骨不健，或气血亏虚，筋骨失养者，应配伍补益肝肾或益气养血之品。

Proper combination depends on the particular syndrome, the affected location and the course of disease process. For abnormal exuberance of pathogenic wind, wind-damp expelling medicinals should be used in combination with blood-invigorating and nutrient-nourishing medicinals. For abnormal exuberance of pathogenic dampness, they should be used in combination with spleen-fortifying and dampness-percolating medicinals. For abnormal exuberance of pathogenic cold, they should be used in combination with meridian-warming and cold-dissipating medicinals. For abnormal exuberance of pathogenic heat, they should be used in combination with heat-clearing medicinals. In the early stage of the disease, if the pathogens exist in the exterior, they should be combined with exterior-releasing medicinals that can remove wind-damp. To treat prolonged *bì* syndrome involving liver and kidney manifested as weakness of sinews and bones or qi-blood insufficiency, and sinews and bones without being nourished, they should be combined with liver-kidney supplementing medicinals or qi-blood boosting medicinals.

痹证属慢性疾病，为了服用方便，祛风湿药一般制成酒剂或丸剂。本类药多辛温性燥，易伤阴耗血，阴血亏虚者应慎用。

Bì syndrome (compediment) usually belongs to chronic disease so wind-damp expelling medicinals can be made into wine preparation or pills for the convenience of taking orally. For they are usually acrid, warm and dry in nature, which tend to damage yin and consume blood, wind-damp expelling medicinals should be used with caution for patients with yin-blood depletion.

第一节　祛风寒湿药
Section 1　Wind-cold-damp expelling medicinals

本类药物味多辛苦而性温，辛能散风，苦能燥湿，温通祛寒，以祛风除湿、散寒止痛为主要功效，适用于风寒湿痹。其中疼痛部位游走不定者为行痹；疼痛剧烈，痛有定处，遇寒加重者为痛痹；关节酸痛、重着者为着痹。

Wind-cold-damp expelling medicinals are usually acrid, bitter in flavor and warm in nature. They are acrid for wind-dispersing, bitter for dampness-drying, and warm for cold-dispelling. Their major efficacies are to expel wind, remove dampness, dissipate cold and relieve pain. They are indicated to wind-cold-damp *bì* syndrome: migratory arthralgia is marked by migratory pains in the limbs and joints; agonizing arthralgia is marked by fixed pains in the limbs and joints, which will aggravate when encountering cold; fixed arthralgia is marked by swelling with heavy sensation in the joints with fixed or localized pain.

独活　*Dú huó* (Angelicae Pubescentis Radix)

《神农本草经》

Shen Nong's Classic of the Materia Medica (Shén Nóng Běn Cǎo Jīng)

【来源 / Origin】

为伞形科植物重齿毛当归 *Angelica pubescens* Maxim. f. *biserrata* Shan et Yuan 的干燥根。主产于四川、湖北。春初苗刚发芽或秋末茎叶枯萎时采挖，切片，生用。本品有特异香气，味苦、辛、微麻舌。《中国药典》规定，含蛇床子素（$C_{15}H_{16}O_3$）不得少于0.50%，含二氢欧山芹醇当归酸酯（$C_{19}H_{20}O_5$）不得少于0.080%。

Dú huó is the dry root of *Angelica pubescens* Maxim. f. *biserrata* Shan et Yuan, pertaining to Umbelliferae. It is mainly produced in Sichuan and Hubei Province in China, collected in early spring and late autumn, cut into pieces and used raw. It has peculiar fragrance, and is bitter and acrid in taste and can slightly benumb the tongue. According to *Chinese Pharmacopoeia*, the content of osthole ($C_{15}H_{16}O_3$) should be no less than 0.50%, and the content of dihydrocresol angelic acid ester ($C_{19}H_{20}O_5$) should be no less than 0.080%.

【性味归经 / Medicinal properties】

辛、苦，微温。归肾、膀胱经。

Acrid, bitter, slightly warm; act on kidney and bladder meridians.

【主要功效 / Medicinal efficacies】

祛风除湿，通痹止痛，解表。

Dispel wind and eliminate dampness; unblock *bì* and relieve pain; release the exterior.

【临床应用 / Clinical application】

1. 痹证　本品辛散苦燥，性温散寒，善能祛风、散寒、胜湿、止痛，凡风寒湿痹，无论新久，均可应用。因其主入肾经，性善下行，故善治下半身痛证，症见腰膝、腿足关节疼痛属寒湿者，常与附子、羌活、威灵仙等同用。若痹证日久，肝肾亏损，气血不足，腰膝酸软，筋骨无力者，常配伍桑寄生、杜仲、人参等。

(1) Bì syndrome　*Dú huó* is acrid for dispersing and bitter for drying, warm for dissipating cold. It can dispel wind, dissipate cold, remove dampness, and relieve pain. It is used to treat wind-cold-damp *bì* syndrome, both the new onset and chronic pattern. Mainly acting on kidney meridian, and focusing on the lower part of the body, it can be especially used for painful *bì* syndrome in lower half of the body with cold-damp pattern, manifested as pain in the waist, knees and joints of legs and feet, often combined with *fù zǐ*, *qiāng huó*, and *wēi líng xiān*. To treat liver-kidney depletion and qi-blood insufficiency manifested as soreness and weakness of the waist and knees, flaccidity of sinew and bone due to prolonged *bì*

syndrome, it is often used with *sāng jì shēng*, *dù zhòng* and *rén shēn*.

2. 风寒夹湿表证　本品入足太阳膀胱经，可散在表之风寒湿邪，功似羌活而药力稍逊。用治外感风寒夹湿之表证，症见恶寒发热、无汗、头痛身重者，常与羌活、防风等同用。

(2) Exterior pattern with wind-cold complicated by dampness　*Dú huó* acts in the bladder meridian. It can dispel exterior pathogenic wind-cold-damp. Its efficacies are similar to *qiāng huó* but weaker than it. To treat externally-contracted wind-cold complicated by dampness manifested as aversion to cold, fever, absence of sweating, headache and heaviness of body, it is often combined with *qiāng huó* and *fáng fēng*.

此外，本品尚能祛风止痛、止痒，还可用治少阴头痛、皮肤瘙痒等。

In addition, it can dispel wind, relieve pain and itching, and also relieving Shaoyin headache and cutaneous pruritus.

【用法用量 / Usage and dosage】

煎服，3~10g。

Decoction, 3~10g.

【现代研究 / Modern research】

本品主要含蛇床子素、东莨菪素、异欧前胡素、东莨菪内酯、二氢欧山芹醇当归酸酯、二氢山芹醇、当归醇及甾醇类等。具有抗炎、镇痛、镇静、抗心律失常、降压等作用。

Dú huó mainly contains osthole, scopoletin, isoimperatorin, scopolactone, dihydrocresol angelic acid ester, dihydrocresol, angelinol and sterols. It has the functions of inhibiting inflammation, relieving pain, tranquilizing the mind, antagonizing arrhythmia and reducing blood pressure.

威灵仙　*Wēi líng xiān* (Clematidis Radix et Rhizoma)
《新修本草》
Newly Revised Materia Medica (*Xīn Xīu Běn Cǎo*)

【来源 / Origin】

为毛茛科植物威灵仙 *Clematis chinensis* Osbeck、棉团铁线莲 *Clematis hexapetala* Pall. 或东北铁线莲 *Clematis manshurica* Rupr. 的干燥根和根茎。产于辽宁、吉林、黑龙江等地。秋季采挖，切段，生用。威灵仙气微，味淡；棉团铁线莲味咸；东北铁线莲味辛辣。《中国药典》规定，含齐墩果酸（$C_{30}H_{48}O_3$）不得少于 0.30%。

Wēi líng xiān is the dry root and rhizome of *Clematis chinensis* Osbeck, *Clematis hexapetala* Pall., or *Clematis manshurica* Rupr., pertaining to Ranunculaceae. It is mainly produced in Liaoning, Jilin and Heilongjiang Province, collected in autumn, cut into segments and used raw. *Wēi líng xiān* has slight odor and is bland in taste, *Clematis hexapetala* Pall. is salty, and *Clematis manshurica* Rupr. is acrid and spicy. According to *Chinese Pharmacopoeia*, the content of oleanolic acid ($C_{30}H_{48}O_3$) should be no less than 0.30%.

【性味归经 / Medicinal properties】

辛、咸，温。归膀胱经。

Acrid, salty and warm; act on the bladder meridian.

【主要功效 / Medicinal efficacies】

祛风湿，通经络，止痛，消骨鲠。

Dispel wind and dampness, unblock the meridians and collaterals, relieve pain, and remove the fishbone stuck in the throat.

【临床应用 / Clinical application 】

1. 痹证 本品辛温行散，其性善走，既能祛风湿，又能通经络，止痹痛。凡风湿痹痛，肢体麻木，筋脉拘挛，屈伸不利，无论上下均可应用，为治风湿痹痛之要药，尤宜于风邪偏胜的行痹，可单用为末，或配伍羌活、独活、川芎等。

(1) *Bì* syndrome *Wēi líng xiān* is acrid and warm with the functions of dispersing and moving. It can dispel wind-dampness, unblock the meridians and collaterals, and relieve *bì* pain. To treat *bì* syndrome due to wind-damp manifested as numbness of limbs, spasms of the sinews, inflexibility of tendons, no matter in the upper or lower body, especially spasm and pain with wind predominance, it can be ground into powder and used alone, or combined with *qiāng huó*, *dú huó* and *chuān xiōng*.

2. 骨鲠咽喉 本品味咸，有软化骨鲠作用，用治诸骨鲠喉，可单用或与砂糖、醋煎后，慢慢咽下。

(2) The fishbone stuck in the throat *Wēi líng xiān* is salty and can soften hardness to remove the fishbone stuck in the throat. It can be decocted alone or in combination with sugar and vinegar for slow swallow.

【用法用量 / Usage and dosage 】

煎服，6~10g。消骨鲠 30~50g。

Decoction, 6-10g. If used to remove the fishbone stuck in the throat, 30-50g.

【使用注意 / Precaution 】

气血虚弱者慎用。

It should be used with caution for patients with weakness of qi and blood.

【现代研究 / Modern research 】

本品主要含齐墩果酸、威灵仙皂苷 A 和 B、常春藤皂苷、橙皮苷、柚皮素及挥发油等。具有镇痛、抗炎、利胆、保肝、松弛平滑肌、促进尿酸排泄等作用。

Wēi líng xiān mainly contains oleanolic acid, wilfordside A and B, ivy saponin, hesperidin, naringin, and volatile oil. It has the functions of relieving pain, inhibiting inflammation, promoting gallbladder function, protecting liver, relaxing smooth muscle, and promoting discharge of uric acid.

川乌 *Chuān wū* (Aconiti Radix)
《神农本草经》
Shen Nong's Classic of the Materia Medica (Shén Nóng Běn Cǎo Jīng)

【来源 / Origin 】

为毛茛科植物乌头 *Aconitum carmichaelii* Debx. 的干燥母根。主产于四川、云南、陕西。6月下旬至 8月上旬采挖，切片，生用或制后用。本品气微，味辛辣、麻舌。《中国药典》规定，含乌头碱（$C_{34}H_{47}NO_{11}$）、次乌头碱（$C_{33}H_{45}NO_{10}$）和新乌头碱（$C_{33}H_{45}NO_{11}$）的总量应为 0.050%~0.17%。

Chuān wū is the dry root of *Aconitum carmichaelii* Debx., pertaining to Ranunculaceae. It is mainly produced in Sichuan, Yunnan and Shaanxi Province in China, collected from the last ten-day period of June to the first ten-day period of August, cut in to pieces, and used in the raw form or processed. It has slight odor and is acrid in flavor, and can benumb the tongue. According to *Chinese Pharmacopoeia*, the content of aconitine ($C_{34}H_{47}NO_{11}$), hypaconine ($C_{33}H_{45}NO_{10}$) and mesaconitine ($C_{33}H_{45}NO_{11}$) should be 0.050%-0.17%.

【性味归经 / Medicinal properties 】

辛、苦，热；有大毒。归心、肝、肾、脾经。

微课

Acrid, bitter, hot and extremely poisonous; act on heart, liver, kidney and spleen meridians.

【主要功效 / Medicinal efficacies】

祛风除湿，温经止痛。

Dispel wind and eliminate dampness; warm the meridians and relieve pain.

【临床应用 / Clinical application】

1. 痹证 本品辛苦燥热，善能祛风除湿，散寒止痛，为治风寒湿痹证之佳品。因其性热，温经散寒止痛之力尤为显著，故尤宜于寒邪偏盛之痛痹，常与制马钱子、全蝎、蜈蚣等同用。若治寒湿瘀血留滞经络，肢体筋脉挛痛，关节屈伸不利，日久不愈者，常配伍地龙、天南星、乳香等。

(1) *Bì* syndrome *Chuān wū* is acrid and bitter in flavor. It can dispel wind and eliminate dampness, dissipate cold and relieve pain. Because it is hot in nature, it has strong effect of warm the meridians, dissipate cold and relieve pain, and is especially suitable for the treatment of painful *bì* syndrome due to wind-damp with abnormal exuberance of pathogenic cold, often combined with *zhì mǎ qián zǐ*, *quán xiē* and *wú gōng*. To treat stagnation of cold-damp and static blood in the meridians and collaterals manifested as spasms and pain of the limb sinews, inflexibility of the joints, lasting for a long period, it is combined with *dì lóng*, *tiān nán xīng* and *ru xiāng*.

2. 心腹冷痛，寒疝作痛 本品辛散温通，功善温煦脏腑，散寒止痛。适用于寒凝诸痛。用治阴寒内盛，心痛彻背、背痛彻心，常配伍附子、干姜、蜀椒等。用治寒疝，脐腹疼痛，手足厥冷，多与蜂蜜同煎。

(2) Cold pain in the heart and abdomen, and pain due to cold hernia *Chuān wū* is acrid for dispersing and warm for dredging. It can warm *zang-fu* organs, dissipate cold and relieve pain, and is used for different pains due to congealing cold. To treat internal exuberance of yin cold manifested as chest pain involving the back, back pain involving the heart, it is often combined with *fù zǐ*, *gān jiāng* and *shǔ jiāo*. To treat abdominal pain and reversal cold of the hands and feet due to cold hermia, it is often decocted with honey.

此外，本品止痛之力较佳，可用治跌打损伤，骨折瘀肿疼痛。古方也常以本品外用作麻醉止痛药。

In addition, it can relieve pain effectively and be used for injury from knocks and falls, and bone fracture with stasis and swollen pain. In ancient times, it was usually used as anesthetics to relieve pain.

【用法用量 / Usage and dosage】

1.5~3g，先煎、久煎，内服炮制后用。生品外用，适量。

Decoction, 1.5-3g. It should be decocted first and for a long time, and processed for oral taking. Also an appropriate amount is used externally.

【使用注意 / Precaution】

内服应炮制用，生品内服宜慎；孕妇禁用。不宜与半夏、瓜蒌、瓜蒌子、瓜蒌皮、天花粉、川贝母、浙贝母、平贝母、伊贝母、湖北贝母、白蔹、白及同用。

Chuān wū should be processed before oral use, the raw form should be used with caution for oral use. It should be contraindicated in pregnant women. It is not proper to be combined with *bàn xià*, *guā lóu*, *guā lóu zǐ*, *guā lóu pí*, *tiān huā fěn*, *chuān bèi mǔ*, *zhè bèi mǔ*, *píng bèi mǔ*, *yī bèi mǔ*, *hú běi bèi mǔ*, *bái liǎn* and *bái jí*.

【现代研究 / Modern research】

本品主要含乌头碱、次乌头碱、新乌头碱等多种生物碱，以及乌头多糖 A~D 等。制川乌主要含苯甲酰乌头原碱、苯甲酰次乌头原碱、苯甲酰新乌头原碱等。具有镇痛、抗炎、强心等作用。

Chuān wū mainly contains various alkaloids such as aconitine, hypaconine and mesaconitine, aconitane A, aconitane B, aconitane C, and aconitane D. *Zhì chuān wū* mainly contains benzoylaconitine, benzoylhypoaconitine and benzoylneoaconitine. It has the functions of relieving pain and inhibiting inflammation, and it also has cardiotonic effect.

蕲蛇　*Qí shé* (Agkistrodon)
《雷公炮炙论》
Master Lei's Discourse on Medicinal Processing (Léi Gōng Páo Zhì Lùn)

【来源 / Origin】

为蝰科动物五步蛇 *Agkistrodon acutus*（Güenther）的干燥体。产于浙江、湖北、江西等地。夏、秋二季捕捉，切段，生用或酒炙用，或制成蕲蛇肉用。本品气腥，味微咸。

Qí shé is the dried body of *Agkistrodon acutus* (Güenther), pertaining to Grotalidae. It is mainly produced in Zhejiang, Hubei and Jiangxi Province in China, caught in summer and autumn, cut into segments, and used raw or stir-fried with wine. It is also processed into meat. It has a fishy smell and is salty in taste.

【性味归经 / Medicinal properties】

甘、咸，温；有毒。归肝经。

Sweet, salty, warm and toxic; act on the liver meridian.

【主要功效 / Medicinal efficacies】

祛风，通络，止痉。

Dispel wind; unblock the collaterals; arrest convulsion.

【临床应用 / Clinical application】

1. 痹证，中风半身不遂　本品性善走窜，内入脏腑，外达肌肤，透骨搜风，祛风湿之力颇强，兼善通经活络，风寒湿痹诸证均宜使用，尤宜用于风湿顽痹，日久难愈，关节拘挛，肢体麻木不仁者，常配伍当归、防风、天麻等。若治中风口眼歪斜，半身不遂，手足麻木，常与黄芪、地龙、当归等同用。

(1) *Bì* syndrome and wind-strike with half-body paralysis　*Qí shé* has the property of moving and scurrying to interior of *zang-fu* organs and to exterior of the body, and is effective at promoting actions to bone, removing wind-damp, and unblocking meridians and activating collaterals, suitable for various symptoms of wind-cold-damp *bì* syndromes. It is especially effective at treating obstinate *bì* syndrome due to wind-damp manifested as contracture of the joints and numbness of the limbs, often combined with *dāng guī*, *fáng fēng* and *tiān má*. To treat stoke with wry eye and mouth, hemiplegia (half-body paralysis) and numbness of the hands and feet, it is often combined with *huáng qí*, *dì lóng* and *dāng guī*.

2. 小儿惊风，破伤风　本品入肝经，既能祛外风，又能息内风，善能定惊止痉，为治痉挛抽搐常用药。用治小儿惊风，高热惊厥，四肢抽搐，常与全蝎、牛黄等同用。用治破伤风，项背强直，角弓反张，抽搐痉挛者，常与蜈蚣、乌梢蛇等同用。

(2) Infantile convulsion and tetanus　*Qí shé* acts on liver meridian with the functions of dispelling external wind and extinguishing internal wind. It is good at stopping convulsions and is a commonly used medicinal for spasms and convulsions. To treat infantile convulsion, febrile convulsion and convulsion of the limbs, it is often combined with *quán xiē* and *niú huáng*. To treat tetanus with rigidity of the nape and back, opisthotonos, spasms and convulsions, it is often used with *wú gōng* and *wū shāo shé.*

3．麻风，疥癣 本品外走肌肤，有较好的祛风止痒作用，可用于多种皮肤病之皮肤瘙痒。用治麻风，常配伍大黄、蝉蜕等。用治疥癣，常与薄荷、天麻、荆芥等同用。用治风癣疮，皮肤瘙痒而有湿热者，可与苦参、白鲜皮、防风等同用。

(3) Leprosy, scabies and tinea *Qí shé* acts on the exterior skin and has a good effect of dispelling wind and relieving itching, so it can be used for various cutaneous pruritus. To treat leprosy, it is often combined with *dà huáng* and *chán tuì*. To treat scabies and tinea, it is often used with *bò he*, *tiān má* and *jīng jiè*. To treat wind tinea and sores, cutaneous pruritus with dampness-heat, it is used with *ku shēn*, *bái xiān pí* and *fáng fēng*.

【用法用量 / Usage and dosage】

煎服，3~9g；研末吞服，1 次 1~1.5g，1 日 2~3 次；或酒浸、熬膏，或入丸、散服。

Decoction, 3-9g; it is ground into powder for swallowing, 1-1.5g each time, 2-3 times a day; or it is steeped in wine, decocted into paste, or made into pills or powder for use.

【使用注意 / Precaution】

阴虚内热者慎用。

It should be used with caution for patients with yin deficiency and internal heat.

【现代研究 / Modern research】

本品主要含蛋白质及脂肪类成分，蕲蛇酶等蛇毒成分为蛋白质类成分。具有抗血栓、降血压、抗肿瘤以及镇静、镇痛等作用。

It mainly contains proteins and fats, and snake venoms such as acutase is mainly protein. It has the functions of antagonizing thrombus, decreasing blood pressure, inhibiting tumor, tranquilizing and relieving pain.

木瓜 *Mù guā* (Chaenomelis Fructus)
《名医别录》
Miscellaneous Records of Famous Physicians (Míng Yī Bié Lù)

【来源 / Origin】

为蔷薇科植物贴梗海棠 *Chaenomeles speciosa*（Sweet）Nakai 的干燥近成熟果实。主产于安徽、湖南、湖北等地。夏、秋二季采收，切片，生用。本品气微清香，味酸。《中国药典》规定，含齐墩果酸（$C_{30}H_{48}O_3$）和熊果酸（$C_{30}H_{48}O_3$）的总量不得少于 0.50%。

Mù guā is the nearly mature fruit of *Chaenomeles speciosa* (Sweet) Nakai, pertaining to Rosaceae. It is mainly produced in Anhui, Hunan and Hubei Province in China, collected in summer and autumn, cut into pieces and used in the raw form. It has fragrance and is sour in flavor. According to *Chinese Pharmacopoeia*, the content of oleanolic acid ($C_{30}H_{48}O_3$) and ursolic acid ($C_{30}H_{48}O_3$) should be no less than 0.50%.

【性味归经 / Medicinal properties】

酸，温。归肝、脾经。

Sour and warm; act on the liver and spleen meridians.

【主要功效 / Medicinal efficacies】

舒筋活络，和胃化湿。

Relax the sinews and quicken the collaterals; harmonize the stomach and remove dampness.

【临床应用 / Clinical application】

1．痹证，筋脉拘挛 本品酸温入肝经，长于舒筋活络，化湿除痹，乃痹证常用之品，为治湿痹，筋脉拘挛、关节屈伸不利之要药，常与羌活、独活、秦艽等同用。若治筋急项强，不可转侧，常与乳香、没药配伍。

(1) Bì syndrome and spasms of the sinews *Mù guā* is sour and warm, acting on the liver meridian. It is good at relaxing the sinews and activating the collaterals, resolving dampness and eliminating *bì*. It is an essential medicinal to treat damp *bì* syndrome with spasms of the sinews and inhibited bending and stretching of the joints, often combined with *qiāng huó*, *dú huó* and *qín jiāo*. To treat spasms of the sinews and stiff neck, it is often used with *rǔ xiāng* and *mò yào*.

2．吐泻转筋　本品酸温气香，入肝、脾经，既能化湿和脾胃，又能舒筋缓挛急。用于湿浊中阻，吐泻不止，足腓转筋，挛急疼痛，无论寒热均可配伍使用，若属寒湿者，常与吴茱萸、小茴香等同用；若属湿热者，常与蚕沙、黄芩等同用。

(2) Vomiting and diarrhea with spasm *Mù guā* is sour, warm and fragrant, acting on the liver and spleen meridians. It can resolve dampness, harmonize the stomach, relax the sinews and relieve spasm. It is used to treat damp-turbidity obstructing the middle energizer manifested as continuous vomiting and diarrhea, spasm and pain of fibula cruris in combination due to either cold or heat. For predominance of cold-dampness, it is combined with *wú zhū yú* and *xiǎo huí xiāng*. For predominance of dampness-heat, it is combined with *cán shā* and *huáng qín*.

3．脚气水肿　本品化湿舒筋，为治脚气水肿常用药。用治脚气水肿，疼痛不可忍，常配伍槟榔、吴茱萸、紫苏叶等。

(3) Foot qi (tinea pedis) with edema *Mù guā* resolves dampness and relaxes the sinews. To treat tinea pedis with edema and intolerable pain, it is combined with *bīng láng*, *wú zhū yú* and *zǐ sū yè*.

此外，本品有消食之功，可用治消化不良；能生津止渴，尚可用治津伤口渴。

In addition, it has the effects of promoting digestion and promoting fluid production to quench thirst, so it can be used to help digestion and quench thirst.

【用法用量 / Usage and dosage】

煎服，6~9g。

Decoction, 6-9g.

【使用注意 / Precaution】

胃酸过多者不宜用。

It should be contraindicated in patients with profuse stomach acid.

【现代研究 / Modern research】

本品主要含齐墩果酸、熊果酸、苹果酸、枸橼酸、琥珀酸、酒石酸等。具有镇痛、抗炎、保肝、松弛胃肠道平滑肌、抑菌等作用。

Mù guā mainly contains oleanolic acid, ursolic acid, malic acid, citric acid, succinic acid and tartaric acid. It has the effects of relieving pain, inhibiting inflammation, protecting the liver, relaxing smooth muscle of the gastrointestinal tract, and inhibiting bacterium.

第二节　祛风湿热药

Section 2　Wind-damp-heat expelling medicinals

本类药物多味辛苦而性寒，辛能行散，苦寒泄热，以祛风除湿、清热通络为主要功效。适用于风湿热痹，关节红肿热痛等，经配伍也可用治风寒湿痹。

Wind-damp-heat expelling medicinals are usually acrid and bitter in flavor, and cold in nature. They are acrid for dispersing and bitter for discharging heat. Their major efficacies are to expel wind, remove dampness, clear heat and unblock the collaterals. They are indicated to wind-damp-heat *bì* syndrome with red swelling and hot pain of the joints, and also can be used for wind-cold-damp *bì* syndrome through combination.

秦艽 *Qín jiāo* (Gentianae Macrophyllae Radix)
《神农本草经》
Shen Nong's Classic of the Materia Medica (Shén Nóng Běn Cǎo Jīng)

【来源 / Origin】

为龙胆科植物秦艽 *Gentiana macrophylla* Pall.、麻花秦艽 *Gentiana straminea* Maxim.、粗茎秦艽 *Gentiana crassicaulis* Duthie ex Burk. 或小秦艽 *Gentiana dahurica* Fisch. 的干燥根。主产于甘肃、青海、内蒙古等地。春、秋二季采挖，切厚片，生用。本品气特异，味苦、微涩。《中国药典》规定，含龙胆苦苷（$C_{16}H_{20}O_9$）和马钱苷酸（$C_{16}H_{24}O_{10}$）的总量不得少于 2.5%。

Qín jiāo is the dry root of of *Gentiana macrophylla* Pall., *Gentiana straminea* Maxim., *Gentiana crassicaulis* Duthie ex Burk, or *Gentiana.dahurica* Fisch., pertaining to Gentianaceae. It is mainly produced in Gansu and Qinghai Province and Inner Mongolia Autonomous Region of China, collected in spring and autumn, cut into thick pieces and used raw. It has peculiar fragrance, and it is bitter and slightly astringent in flavor. According to *Chinese Pharmacopoeia*, the content of gentiopicroside ($C_{16}H_{20}O_9$) and loganic acid ($C_{16}H_{24}O_{10}$) should be no less than 2.5%.

【性味归经 / Medicinal properties】

辛、苦，平。归胃、肝、胆经。

Acrid, bitter and bland; act on the stomach, liver and gallbladder meridians.

【主要功效 / Medicinal efficacies】

祛风湿，清湿热，止痹痛，退虚热。

Dispel wind and dampness; clear damp-heat; relieve *bì* pain; abate deficiency heat.

【临床应用 / Clinical application】

1. 痹证 本品辛能散风，苦能燥湿，既能祛风湿，止痹痛，又能舒筋活络，其药性平和，质润不燥，素有"风药中之润剂"之称。凡是痹证，关节疼痛，筋脉拘挛，无问新久寒热，均可应用。因其性平偏凉，兼能清热，故尤宜于热痹，关节红肿热痛者，常与防己、桑枝、络石藤等同用。若与羌活、川芎、天麻等同用，可用治风寒湿痹。

(1) *Bì* syndrome *Qín jiāo* is acrid for wind-dispersing, bitter for dampness-drying. Its major efficacies are to expel wind, remove dampness, relieve *bì* pain and relax the sinews and quicken the collaterals. It is neutral and moistening but not dry in nature, and also known as lubricant formula in wind-expelling medicinals. It is indicated to *bì* syndrome with pain in the joints and spasms of the sinews, both the new onset and chronic pattern. It is neutral and tends to be cool in nature, and has the effect of clearing heat. It is especially suitable for the treatment of wind-damp-heat *bì* syndrome with red swelling, hot pain of the joints, and usually combined with *fáng jǐ*, *sāng zhī* and *luò shí téng*. To treat wind-cold-damp *bì* syndrome, it is combined with *qiāng huó*, *chuān xiōng* and *tiān má*.

2. 中风半身不遂 本品有祛风通络之功。用治中风半身不遂，口眼㖞斜等，常与防风、当归、葛根等同用。

(2) Wind-strike with hemiplegia (half-body paralysis) *Qín jiāo* has the effects of dispelling wind and unblocking the collaterals. To treat wind-strike with half-body paralysis and wry eye and mouth, it is often combined with *fáng fēng*, *dāng guī* and *gé gēn*.

3．湿热黄疸 本品苦平偏凉，入肝经，能清肝胆湿热而退黄。用治湿热黄疸，常与茵陈、栀子、大黄等同用。

(3) Damp-heat Jaundice *Qín jiāo* is bitter, neutral and cool, acting on the liver meridian. It can clear the damp-heat of the liver and gallbladder to eliminate jaundice. To treat damp-heat jaundice, it is often used with *yīn chén*, *zhī zǐ* and *dà huáng*.

4．骨蒸潮热，疳积发热 本品尚能退虚热，除骨蒸，清疳热，为治虚热证常用药。用治阴虚内热，骨蒸潮热，常与鳖甲、青蒿、知母等同用。若治小儿疳积发热，可与银柴胡、胡黄连等同用。

(4) Steaming bone fever, tidal fever and malnutrition fever *Qín jiāo* is an essential medicinal to treat deficiency-heat pattern with the functions of relieving steaming bone fever and clear malnutrition fever. To treat steaming bone fever or afternoon tidal fever due to yin deficiency with internal heat, it is often combined with *biē jiǎ*, *qīng hāo* and *zhī mǔ*. To treat infantile malnutrition fever, it is often combined with *yín chái hú* and *hú huáng lián*.

【用法用量 / Usage and dosage】
煎服，3~10g。
Decoction, 3-10g.

【现代研究 / Modern research】
本品主要含龙胆苦苷、马钱苷酸、秦艽苷、当归苷、獐牙菜苦苷、秦艽碱甲、秦艽碱乙、有机酸类、糖类及挥发油等。具有抗炎、镇痛、镇静、解热、降压、保肝、免疫调节等作用。

Qín jiāo mainly contains gentiopicroside, loganic acid, gentiopicroside, angelic glycoside, swertiamarin, gentiana alkaloid A, gentiana alkaloid B, organic acids, sugars and volatile oil. It has the functions of inhibiting inflammation, relieving pain, tranquilizing, clearing heat, decreasing blood pressure, protecting the liver and regulating immunity.

防己 *Fáng jǐ* (Stephaniae Tetrandrae Radix)
《神农本草经》
Shen Nong's Classic of the Materia Medica (Shén Nóng Běn Cǎo Jīng)

【来源 / Origin】
为防己科植物粉防己 *Stephania tetrandra* S. Moore 的干燥根。产于浙江、江西、安徽等地。秋季采挖，切厚片，生用。本品气微，味苦。《中国药典》规定，含粉防己碱（$C_{38}H_{42}N_2O_6$）和防己诺林碱（$C_{37}H_{40}N_2O_6$）的总量不得少于1.6%，饮片不得少于1.4%。

Fáng jǐ is the dry root of *Stephania tetrandra* S.Moore, pertaining to Menispermaceae. It is mainly produced in Zhejiang, Jiangxi and Anhui Province in China, collected in autumn, cut into thick pieces and used in the raw form. It has slight odor and is bitter in flavor. According to *Chinese Pharmacopoeia*, the content of tetrandrine ($C_{38}H_{42}N_2O_6$) and fangchinoline ($C_{37}H_{40}N_2O_6$) should be no less than 1.6%, and no less than 1.4% in decoction pieces.

【性味归经 / Medicinal properties】
苦，寒。归膀胱、肺经。
Bitter and cold; act on the bladder and lung meridians.

【主要功效 / Medicinal efficacies 】

祛风湿，止痛，利水，消肿。

Dispel wind-damp, relieve pain, promote urination and alleviate edema.

【临床应用 / Clinical application 】

1. 痹证　本品苦寒之性较甚，既能祛风湿，止痹痛，又能清热，故宜于风湿热痹，关节疼痛，局部灼热红肿，屈伸不利者，常与薏苡仁、滑石、蚕沙等同用。若治风寒湿痹，关节疼痛，可与制川乌、肉桂、白术等同用。

(1) *Bì* syndrome　*Fáng jǐ* is extremely bitter and cold with the functions of dispelling wind-damp, relieving pain and clearing heat. To treat wind-damp-heat *bì* syndrome with pain, local burning and red swelling, and inhibited bending and stretching of the joints, it is often combined with *yì yǐ rén*, *huá shí* and *cán shā*. To treat wind-cold-damp *bì* syndrome with pain of the joints, it is combined with *zhì chuān wū*, *ròu guì* and *bái zhú*.

2. 水肿脚气，小便不利　本品苦寒降泄，入膀胱经，善走下焦，长于泄下焦膀胱湿热而利水消肿，较宜于下部水湿停留的水肿、小便不利。若治湿热腹胀水肿，小便不利，常配伍椒目、葶苈子、大黄等。若治风湿，脉浮、身重、汗出、恶风之风水证，常与黄芪、白术、甘草等同用。若治脚气足胫肿痛、重着、麻木，可与吴茱萸、木瓜、槟榔等同用。

(2) Edema, foot qi (tinea pedis), and difficulty in micturition　*Fáng jǐ* descends and discharges with bitter cold. It acts on the bladder meridian and the lower energizer. It can discharge the damp-heat in the bladder to promote urination and relieve edema, and is used for edema and difficulty in micturition due to retention of water and dampness in the lower part of the body. For damp-heat abdominal dropsy and difficulty in micturition, it is often combined with *jiāo mù*, *tíng lì zǐ* and *dà huáng*. To treat wind edema manifested as wind-dampness, floating pulse, heavy body, sweating, and aversion to wind, it is often combined with *huáng qí*, *bái zhú* and *gān cǎo*. To treat foot qi and algesic edema of feet and legs with heaviness sensation and numbness, it is combined with *wú zhū yú*, *mù guā* and *bīng láng*.

【用法用量 / Usage and dosage 】

煎服，5~10g。

Decoction, 5-10g.

【使用注意 / Precaution 】

胃纳不佳及阴虚体弱者均当慎用。

It should be used with caution for patients with poor appetite, yin deficiency and weak body.

【现代研究 / Modern research 】

本品主要含粉防己碱、防己诺林碱、轮环藤酚碱、氧防己碱、防己斯任碱，尚含黄酮苷、有机酸、挥发油等。具有抗炎、解热、镇痛、抗心肌缺血、抗心律失常、抗过敏、降压、抑制免疫等作用。

Fáng jǐ mainly contains tetrandrine, fangchinoline, cyclanoline, oxytetrandrine, tetrandrine, flavonoid glycoside, organic acid, and volatile oil. It has the functions of inhibiting inflammation, clearing heat, relieving pain, antagonizing myocardial ischemia and arrhythmia, anti-allergy, decreasing blood pressure and regulating immunity.

雷公藤　*Léi gōng téng* (Tripterygii Wilfordii Radix)
《本草纲目拾遗》
Supplement to The Grand Compendium of Materia Medica (Běn Cǎo Gāng Mù Shí Yí)

【来源 / Origin】

为卫矛科植物雷公藤 *Tripterygium wilfordii* Hook. f. 的干燥根或根的木质部。产于浙江、安徽、福建等地。秋季采挖，切厚片，生用。本品气微特异，味苦、微辛。

Léi gōng téng is the dry root or the hadromestome of roots of *Tripterygium wlfordii* Hook. f., pertaining to Celastraceae. It is mainly produced in Zhejiang, Anhui and Fujian Province in China, collected in autumn, cut into thick pieces and used raw. It has a slight and peculiar odor, and is bitter and slightly acrid in taste.

【性味归经 / Medicinal properties】

苦、辛，寒；有大毒。归肝、肾经。

Bitter, acrid, cold and extremely toxic; act on the liver and kidney meridians.

【主要功效 / Medicinal efficacies】

祛风除湿，活血通络，消肿止痛，杀虫解毒。

Dispel wind and eliminate dampness; invigorate blood and unblock the collaterals; relieve edema and pain; kill worms and resolve toxins.

【临床应用 / Clinical application】

1. 痹证　本品性猛功著，有较强的祛风除湿、活血通络作用，为治风湿顽痹之要药。其苦寒清热，又善消肿止痛，故尤宜于关节红肿热痛、肿胀难消、僵硬、功能受限，甚至关节变形的顽痹，可单用，或与独活、威灵仙、防风等同用。

(1) *Bì* syndrome　*Léi gōng téng* is drastic with the functions of dispelling wind and eliminating dampness, invigorating blood and unblocking the collaterals, and is an essential medicinal to treat obstinate *bì* syndrome due to damp-heat. It can clear heat with bitter cold, and is good at relieving edema and pain, especially suitable to treat obstinate *bì* syndrome with red swelling and hot pain of the joints, stubborn swelling, stiffness, dysfunction, and even deformity of the joints, and is used alone, or combined with *dú huó*, *wēi líng xiān* and *fáng fēng*.

2. 麻风，顽癣，湿疹，疥疮　本品苦燥除湿，以毒攻毒，既能祛风止痒，又能杀虫解毒，可用治多种皮肤病。用治麻风，可单用煎服，或配伍黄柏、金银花、当归等。用治顽癣，可单用，或与荆芥、防风、刺蒺藜等同用。用治湿疹、疥疮等，可与苦参、白鲜皮等同用。

(2) Leprosy, stubborn dermatitis, eczema and scabies　*Léi gōng téng* is expelling dampness with bitter dryness, fighting poison with poison. It has the functions of dispelling wind and relieving itching, and killing worms and resolving toxins. It can be used for various skin diseases. To treat leprosy, it can be used alone or combined with *huáng bó*, *jīn yín huā* and *dāng guī*. To treat stubborn dermatitis, it can be used alone or combined with *jīng jiè*, *fáng fēng* and *cì jí lí*. To treat eczema and scabies, it is combined with *kǔ shēn* and *bái xiān pí*.

【用法用量 / Usage and dosage】

煎服，1~3g，先煎。外用适量。

Decoction, 1-3g. It should be decocted first. An appropriate amount is used externally.

【使用注意 / Precaution】

心、肝、肾功能不全和白细胞减少者均慎用。孕妇禁用。

It should be contraindicated for pregnant women, and be used with caution for patients with heart, liver or kidney insufficiency, or leucopenia.

【现代研究 / Modern research】

本品主要含雷公藤碱、雷公藤次碱、雷公藤戊碱、雷公藤新碱、雷公藤碱乙、雷公藤碱丁、雷公藤碱戊、雷公藤甲素、雷公藤乙素、雷公藤酮以及挥发油、蒽醌和多糖等。具有免疫抑制、抗炎、镇痛、改善血液流变学、抗肿瘤和抗生育等作用。

Léi gōng téng mainly contains wilforine, pureonebio, evonimine, triptolide B, tripterygium aldaoid, triptolide, tripdiolide, triptolone. It also contains volatile oil, anthraquinone and polysaccharide. It has the functions of inhibiting immunity, inhibiting inflammation, relieving pain, improving blood rheology, inhibiting tumor and fertility.

第三节　祛风湿强筋骨药

Section 3　Wind-damp expelling and sinew-bone strengthening medicinals

PPT

本类药物味多辛苦而性温，入肝、肾经，除祛风湿外，兼有一定的补肝肾、强筋骨作用，主要用于痹证日久，肝肾亏虚，腰膝酸软，足弱无力等，亦可用于肾虚腰痛，骨痿，软弱无力等。

Wind-damp expelling and sinew-bone strengthening medicinals are usually acrid and bitter in flavor and warm in nature, acting in the liver and kidney meridians. Their major efficacies are to expel wind and dampness, supplement the liver and kidney, and strengthen the sinews and bones. They are indicated to long-term *bì* syndrome with liver-kidney deficiency manifested as soreness and weakness of the waist and knees, and flaccidity of the feet, and also can be used for the treatment of lumbago and bone flaccidity due to deficiency of the kidney with weakness and lack of strength.

五加皮　*Wǔ jiā pí* (Acanthopanacis Cortex)

《神农本草经》

Shen Nong's Classic of the Materia Medica (Shén Nóng Běn Cǎo Jīng)

【来源 / Origin】

为五加科植物细柱五加 *Acanthopanax gracilistylus* W. W. Smith 的干燥根皮。主产于湖北、湖南、浙江等地。夏、秋二季采挖，切厚片，生用。本品气微香，味微辣而苦。

Wǔ jiā pí is the dry root bark of *Acanthopanax gracilistylus* W.W.Smith, pertaining to Araliaceae. It is mainly produced in Hubei, Hunan and Zhejiang Province. It is collected in summer and autumn, cut into thick pieces and used raw. It has slight fragrance and is slightly acrid and bitter in taste.

【性味归经 / Medicinal properties】

辛、苦，温。归肝、肾经。

Acrid, bitter and warm; act on the liver and kidney meridians.

【主要功效 / Medicinal efficacies】

祛风除湿，补益肝肾，强筋壮骨，利水消肿。

Dispel wind and eliminate dampness; supplement and boost the liver and kidney; strengthen the sinews and bones; promote urination and relieve edema.

【临床应用 / Clinical application】

1. 痹证　本品辛能散风，苦则燥湿，性温除寒，入肝、肾经，既能祛风除湿散寒，又兼能补肝肾、强筋骨，适用于风寒湿痹证，腰膝疼痛，筋脉拘挛，关节屈伸不利等。尤宜于痹证日久，肝肾不足，腰膝酸软，筋骨无力者，可单用浸酒服，或与桑寄生、牛膝、独活等同用。

(1) **Bì syndrome**　*Wǔ jiā pí* is acrid for dispersing wind and bitter for drying dampness and warm for eliminating cold, acting in the liver and kidney meridians. It has the effects of dispelling wind, eliminating dampness, dissipating cold, and supplementing the liver and kidney, strengthening the sinews and bones. It can treat wind-cold-damp *bì* syndrome with pain of the waist and knees, spasms of the sinews and inhibited bending and stretching of the joints. It is especially suitable for long-term *bì* syndrome with liver-kidney deficiency manifested as soreness and weakness of the waist and knees, and flaccidity of sinews and bones, and can be soaked in wine alone, or combined with *sāng jì shēng*, *niú xī* and *dú huó*.

2. 筋骨痿软，小儿行迟　本品能补肝肾、强筋骨。用治肝肾不足，筋骨痿软，常与杜仲、牛膝等同用。用治小儿行迟，可与龟甲、熟地黄、牛膝等同用。

(2) **Flaccidity of sinew and bone, and infantile walk retardation**　*Wǔ jiā pí* can supplement the liver and kidney, and strengthen the sinews and bones. To treat insufficiency of liver and kidney with flaccidity of sinew and bone, it is often combined with *dù zhòng* and *niú xī*. To treat infantile walk retardation, it is combined with *guī jiǎ*, *shú dì huáng* and *niú xī*.

3. 水肿，脚气　本品能利尿消肿。用治水湿内停之水肿、小便不利，常与茯苓皮、大腹皮、生姜皮等同用。用治寒湿壅滞之脚气肿痛，可与木瓜、吴茱萸、蚕沙等同用。

(3) **Edema and foot qi**　*Wǔ jiā pí* can promote urination and relieve edema. To treat edema and difficulty in micturition due to retention of water and dampness, it is often used with *fú líng pí*, *dà fù pí* and *shēng jiāng pí*. To treat weak foot qi due to cold-dampness accumulation and stagnation, it is combined with *mù guā*, *wú zhū yú* and *cán shā*.

【用法用量 / Usage and dosage】

煎服，5~10g；或酒浸、入丸散服。

Decoction, 5-10g; or it is steeped in wine or made into pills or powder for use.

【现代研究 / Modern research】

本品主要含紫丁香苷、刺五加苷 B_1、无梗五加苷 A~D、无梗五加苷 K_2、无梗五加苷 K_3，尚含萜类、多糖、脂肪酸、挥发油等。具有抗炎、镇痛、镇静、调节免疫、抗疲劳等作用。

Wǔ jiā pí mainly contains syringin, acanthopanax glycoside B_1, and acanthoside A-D, acanthoside K_2, acanthoside K_3. It also contains terpenoids, polysaccharides, fatty acids and volatile oils. It has the functions of inhibiting inflammation, relieving pain, tranquilizing, regulating immunity and antagonizing fatigue.

桑寄生　*Sāng jì shēng* (Taxilli Herba)
《神农本草经》
Shen Nong's Classic of the Materia Medica (Shén Nóng Běn Cǎo Jīng)

【来源 / Origin】

为桑寄生科植物桑寄生 *Taxillus chinensis*（DC.）Danser 的干燥带叶茎枝。主产于广西、广东。冬季至次春采割，切段，生用。本品气微，味涩。

Sāng jì shēng is the dry stem and branch with leaves of *Taxillus chinensis* (DC.) Danser, pertaining to Loranthaceae. It is mainly produced in Guangxi Zhuang Autonomous Region and Guangdong Province, collected from winter to the next spring, cut into segments and used raw. It has slight odor and is astringent in taste.

【性味归经 / Medicinal properties 】

苦、甘，平。归肝、肾经。

Bitter, bland and neutral; act on the liver and kidney meridians.

【主要功效 / Medicinal efficacies 】

祛风湿，补肝肾，强筋骨，安胎元。

Dispel wind and dampness; supplement the liver and kidney; strengthen the sinews and bones; calm the fetus.

【临床应用 / Clinical application 】

1．痹证　本品味甘性平，苦而不燥，功用与五加皮相似，但祛风湿之力稍逊，长于补肝肾以强健筋骨，尤宜于痹证日久，损伤肝肾，腰膝酸软，筋骨无力者，常配伍杜仲、牛膝、独活等。

(1) *Bì* syndrome　*Sāng jì shēng* is bland in flavor and neutral in nature, bitter but not dry. Its efficacies are similar to *Wǔ jiā pí*, but has weaker effect of repelling wind-damp. It can supplement the liver and kidney to strengthen the sinews and bones. It is especially suitable for the treatment of long-term *bì* syndrome with liver-kidney deficiency manifested as soreness and weakness of the waist and knees, and flaccidity of sinew and bone, often combined with *dù zhòng*, *niú xī* and *dú huó*.

2．崩漏经多，妊娠漏血，胎动不安　本品补益肝肾，兼能养血，可收固冲任、安胎之效。用治肝肾亏虚，冲任不固，崩漏，月经过多，妊娠下血，胎动不安等，常与续断、菟丝子、阿胶等。

(2) Flooding and spotting, profuse menstruation, vaginal bleeding during pregnancy, and restless fetus　*Sāng jì shēng* can supplement and boost the liver and kidney and nourish blood with the functions of securing thoroughfare and conception and preventing miscarriage. To treat depletion of the liver and kidney with flooding and spotting, profuse menstruation, vaginal bleeding during pregnancy and restless fetus, it is often combined with *xù duàn*, *tù sī zǐ* and *ē jiāo*.

【用法用量 / Usage and dosage 】

煎服，9~15g。

Decoction, 9-15g.

【现代研究 / Modern research 】

本品主要含广寄生苷、槲皮素、槲皮苷、金丝桃苷、苯甲酰、苯二烯、芳姜黄烯等。具有抗炎、镇痛、调节免疫、抗疲劳、降血糖、降血压、扩张冠状动脉、抗肿瘤等作用。

Sāng jì shēng mainly contains mistletoe glycoside, quercetin, quercitrin, hyperoside, benzoyl, phenyldiene and curcumene. It has the functions of inhibiting inflammation, relieving pain, regulating immunity, antagonizing fatigue, decreasing blood sugar and pressure, expand the coronary artery and antagonizing tumor.

其他祛风湿药功用介绍见表 9-1。

The efficacies of other wind-damp expelling medicinals are shown in table 9-1.

表 9-1　其他祛风湿药功用介绍

分类	药物	药性	功效	应用	用法用量
祛风寒湿药	草乌	辛，苦，热；有大毒。归心、肝、肾、脾经	祛风除湿，温经止痛	风湿痹痛，心腹冷痛，寒疝疼痛，跌打损伤	煎服，1.5~3g，先煎、久煎
	海风藤	辛、苦，微温。归肝经	祛风湿，通经络，止痹痛	风寒湿痹，肢节疼痛，筋脉拘挛，屈伸不利，跌打损伤	煎服，6~12g
	乌梢蛇	甘，平。归肝经	祛风，通络，止痉	风湿顽痹，麻木拘挛，中风口眼喎斜，半身不遂，破伤风，麻风，疥癣	煎服，6~12g。研末，每次 2~3g
	蚕沙	甘、辛，温。归肝、脾、胃经	祛风除湿，和胃化湿	风湿痹痛，吐泻转筋，风疹、湿疹瘙痒	煎服，5~15g，包煎
	伸筋草	微苦、辛，温。归肝、脾、肾经	祛风除湿，舒筋活络	风寒湿痹，关节疼痛，屈伸不利，跌打损伤	煎服，3~12g
	青风藤	苦、辛，平。归肝、脾经	祛风湿，通经络，利小便	风湿痹痛，关节肿胀，麻木不仁，水肿，脚气，皮肤瘙痒	煎服，6~12g。外用适量
	穿山龙	甘、苦，温。归肝、肾、肺经	祛风除湿，活血通络，止咳平喘	风湿痹痛，关节肿胀，疼痛麻木，跌打损伤，闪腰岔气，咳嗽气喘	煎服，9~15g。也可以制成酒剂用
	丝瓜络	甘，平。归肺、胃、肝经	祛风，通络，活血，下乳	风湿痹痛，筋脉拘挛，胸胁胀痛，乳汁不通，乳痈肿痛	煎服，5~12g。外用适量
	路路通	苦，平。归肝、肾经	祛风活络，利水，通经	风湿痹痛，麻木拘挛，中风半身不遂；水肿胀满，经行不畅，经闭，乳少，乳汁不通	煎服，5~10g。外用适量
祛风湿热药	豨莶草	辛、苦，寒。归肝、肾经	祛风湿，利关节，解毒	风湿痹痛，中风半身不遂；风疹，湿疹，痈肿疮毒	煎服，9~12g。外用适量
	桑枝	微苦，平。归肝经	祛风湿，利关节	风湿痹证，肩臂、关节酸痛麻木	煎服，9~15g
	臭梧桐	辛、苦、甘，凉。归肝经	祛风湿，通经络，平肝	风湿痹痛，中风半身不遂；风疹，湿疮；肝阳上亢，头痛眩晕	煎服，5~15g。研末，每次 3g
	络石藤	苦，微寒。归心、肝、肾经	祛风通络，凉血消肿	风湿热痹，筋脉拘挛，腰膝酸痛；喉痹，痈肿，跌打损伤	煎服，6~12g
祛风湿强筋骨药	香加皮	辛、苦，温；有毒。归肝、肾、心经	祛风湿，强筋骨，利水消肿	风寒湿痹，腰膝酸软；下肢浮肿，心悸气短	煎服，3~6g
	千年健	苦、辛，温。归肝、肾经	祛风湿，强筋骨	风寒湿痹，腰膝冷痛，拘挛麻木，筋骨痿软	煎服，5~10g；或酒浸服

（刘立萍）

第十章 化 湿 药
Chapter 10　Damp-resolving medicinals

PPT

 学习目标 ┊ Learning goals

1. **掌握** 化湿药在性能、功效、主治、配伍及使用注意方面的共性；广藿香、苍术、厚朴、砂仁的性能、功效、应用以及特殊的用法用量和特殊的使用注意。

2. **熟悉** 佩兰、豆蔻的功效、主治以及特殊的用法用量和特殊的使用注意。

3. **了解** 化湿药及相关功效术语的含义；草豆蔻、草果的功效以及特殊的用法用量和特殊的使用注意。

1. Master the commonness of damp-resolving medicinals in efficacy, indications, property, compatibility and cautions; as well as the property, efficacy, application, special usage and dosage and special precautions of *guǎng huò xiāng*, *cāng zhú*, *hòu pò*, and *shā rén*.

2. Familiar with the efficacy, indications, special usage, dosage and special precautions of *pèi lán* and *dòu kòu*.

3. Understand the definitions of damp-resolving medicinals and related efficacy terms; and the efficacy, special usage and dosage and special precautions of *cǎo dòu kòu* and *cǎo guǒ*.

凡以化湿运脾为主要功效，常用以治疗湿阻中焦证的药物，称为化湿药，又称芳香化湿药。

Medicinals with efficacies of resolving dampness and improving the spleen's transportation are known as damp-resolving medicinals or aromatic damp-resolving medicinals. Those medicinals are usually used to treat syndromes of dampness obstructing the middle energizer.

化湿药多辛香温燥，主入脾、胃经，辛香化浊，苦温燥湿，能使湿浊消散；脾喜燥恶湿，土爱暖而喜芳香，辛香又能行散，调理中焦气机，促进脾的运化，故可收化湿运脾之效。主治湿浊内阻，脾为湿困，运化失常的湿阻中焦证，症见脘腹痞满、呕吐泛酸、大便溏薄、食少体倦、口甘多涎、舌苔白腻等。部分药物也可用于湿温和暑湿。

Damp-resolving medicinals are mostly acrid, aromatic, warm and dry, and act on the spleen and stomach meridians. They are acrid and aromatic with actions of resolving turbidity, and bitter and warm with efficacy of drying the dampness, so damp-resolving medicinals can diffuse and resolve damp-turbidity. The spleen prefers dryness and is aversion to dampness. It prefers warm and fragrant flavor. Acrid and fragrant taste have functions of moving and dispersing and regulating qi flow in the middle energizer to promote transportation and transformation of spleen. Thus, the effect of resolving dampness and improving the spleen's transportation can be achieved. Damp-resolving medicinals are mainly indicated to treat failure of spleen in transportation and transformation due to dampness encumbering the spleen because of damp-turbidity obstructing the middle energizer, manifested as epigastric and abdominal stuffiness and fullness, vomiting, regurgitation, loose stool, poor appetite, fatigue, sweet taste in the mouth with profuse saliva, and white and greasy coating. Besides, they also proper for damp-warm and summer-damp.

使用化湿药时，应针对湿浊内阻的不同情况进行适当的配伍。湿为阴邪，易阻遏气机，行气有助于化湿，故化湿药常与行气药同用，以增强疗效。湿证有寒湿和湿热之分，若寒湿困脾，应配伍温中祛寒药；若湿热中阻，应配伍清热燥湿药。若脾虚湿盛，应配伍补气健脾药。"治湿不利小便，非其治也"，湿邪较盛者，使用化湿药常配伍利水渗湿药，使邪有去路。

When using damp-resolving medicinals, doctors should make proper compatibility according to different symptoms and signs of damp harassment. Damp belongs to yin pathogenic factors and tends to obstruct qi flow. Moving qi can help to resolve dampness. Therefore, when damp harassment is accompanied by qi stagnation, damp-resolving medicinals are usually used with qi-moving medicinals to strengthen curative effect. Damp syndrome is differentiated into cold-damp and damp-heat. To treat cold-damp encumbering spleen, damp-resolving medicinals are usually used with medicinals that can warm the middle energizer and disperse cold; to treat damp-heat obstructs the middle energizer, damp-resolving medicinals are usually used with those that can clear heat and dry dampness. When damp harassment is accompanied by spleen deficiency and damp exuberance, it is usually used with medicinals that can replenish qi and invigorate spleen. "Promoting urination is the most effective way in the treatment of dampness", when the dampness is exuberant, damp-resolving medicinals are usually used with medicinals that can promote urination and remove dampness.

化湿药气味芳香，多含挥发油，入汤剂宜后下，以免有效成分挥发而降低药效。本类药物多为辛香温燥之品，易于耗气伤阴，阴虚津亏及气虚者慎用。

Damp-resolving medicinals are mostly fragrant and contain volatile oil, so they should be added later to avoid loss of effective components and reducing the efficacies. They are mostly acrid, fragrant, warm and dry, and are likely to consume qi and damage yin, so they should be used with caution for those with yin deficiency, shortage of body fluid and qi deficiency.

广藿香 *Guǎng huò xiāng* (Pogostemonis Herba)
《名医别录》
Miscellaneous Records of Famous Physicians (Míng Yī Bié Lù)

【来源 / Origin】

为唇形科植物广藿香 *Pogostemon cablin*（Blanco）Benth. 的干燥地上部分。主产于广东。枝叶茂盛时采收，切段，生用。本品气香特异，味微苦。《中国药典》规定，含百秋李醇（$C_{15}H_{26}O$）不得少于 0.10%。

Guǎng huò xiāng is the aerial part of *Pogostemon cablin* (Blanco) Benth., pertaining to Labiatae, mainly produced in Guangdong Province. It is collected in summer and autumn when its branches and leaves are exuberant, cut into segments, and used raw. It has peculiar fragrance, and is slightly bitter in taste. According to *Chinese Pharmacopoeia*, the content of patchouli alcohol ($C_{15}H_{26}O$) should be no less than 0.10%.

【性味归经 / Medicinal properties】

辛，微温。归脾、胃、肺经。

Acrid and slightly warm; act on the spleen, stomach and lung meridians.

【主要功效 / Medicinal efficacies】

芳香化浊，和中止呕，发表解暑。

Resolve dampness due to its aromatic nature, harmonize the center and arrest vomiting, release the exterior and clear summer-heat.

【临床应用 / Clinical application】

1. 湿阻中焦证　本品芳香之气浓烈，善能化湿醒脾，开胃和中，为芳香化湿之要药。常用于湿阻中焦，脾失健运之脘腹痞闷、食欲不振、呕恶泄泻、神疲体倦、舌苔厚腻者，其性偏温，尤宜于寒湿中阻者，常配伍苍术、厚朴、陈皮等。

(1) Damp obstruction in the middle energizer　With strong fragrant nature, *huò xiāng* is good at resolving damp and activating spleen, promoting appetite and harmonizing the center. It is an essential medicinal to resolve dampness due to aromatic nature. It is usually used to treat epigastric and abdominal stuffiness and fullness, poor appetite, vomiting and diarrhea, spiritual and physical lassitude, thick and greasy tongue coating due to failure of spleen to transport because of damp obstructing the middle energizer. *Huò xiāng* is warm in nature, so it is especially suitable to treat cold-damp obstructing the middle energizer and often combined with *cāng zhú* (Atractylodis Rhizoma), *hòu pò* (Magnoliae Officinalis Cortex), and *chén pí* (Citri Reticulatae Pericarpium).

2. 呕吐　本品既能化湿，又能和胃止呕。凡呕吐之证，不论寒热虚实皆可选用，尤宜用于湿浊中阻之呕吐。若属寒湿中阻者，常配伍半夏、生姜等。若属湿热中阻者，常与黄连、竹茹等同用。若属脾胃虚弱者，常配伍党参、白术等。若治妊娠呕吐，常与砂仁、紫苏梗等同用。

(2) Vomiting　*Guǎng huò xiāng* can not only resolve damp, but also harmonize stomach to arrest vomiting. It is can be selected to treat vomiting syndromes without consideration of cold, heat, deficiency or excess. It is especially effective at arresting vomiting caused by turbid-damp obstructing the middle energizer. To treat vomiting due to cold-damp obstructing the middle energizer, it is often combined with *bàn xià* (Pinelliae Rhizoma) and *shēng jiāng* (Zingiberis Recens Rhizoma). To treat vomiting due to damp-heat obstructing the middle energizer, it is often combined with *huáng lián* (Coptidis Rhizoma) and *zhú rú* (Bambusae Caulis in Taenia). To treat vomiting caused by deficiency of spleen and stomach, it is often combined with *dǎng shēn* (Codonopsis Radix) and *bái zhú* (Atractylodis Macrocephalae Rhizoma). To treat vomiting due to pregnancy, it is often combined with *shā rén* (Amomi Fructus) and *zǐ sū gěng* (Perillae Caulis).

3. 暑湿表证，湿温初起　本品辛温芳香，外能发散风寒，内能化湿和中。用治暑月外感风寒、内伤湿浊之恶寒发热、头痛、脘腹痞满、呕恶吐泻，常配伍紫苏、厚朴、半夏等。用治湿温初起，湿重于热者，常与厚朴、半夏、茯苓等同用；若湿热并重者，常与黄芩、茵陈、滑石等同用。

(3) Exterior syndrome of summer-damp, damp-warm in the early stage　*Guǎng huò xiāng* is acrid and warm with aroma. It can disperse wind-cold and resolve damp as well as harmonize the center. To treat fever, aversion to cold, headache, epigastric fullness and stuffiness, vomiting, nausea and diarrhea due to attack of wind-cold and internal impairment by turbid-damp, it is often combined with *zǐ sū* (Perillae), *hòu pò* (Magnoliae Officinalis Cortex) and *bàn xià* (Pinelliae Rhizoma). To treat damp-warm in the early stage, when damp is severer than heat, it is often combined with *hòu pò* (Magnoliae Officinalis Cortex), *bàn xià* (Pinelliae Rhizoma) and *fú líng* (Poria). If damp and heat are of equal severity, it is usually used together with *huáng qín* (Scutellariae Radix), *yīn chén* (Artemisiae Scopariae Herba) and *huá shí* (Talcum).

【用法用量 / Usage and dosage】

煎服，3~10g。

Decoction, 3-10g.

【现代研究 / Modern research】

本品主要含广藿香醇、广藿香酮、百秋李醇、丁香油酚、桂皮醛、藿香黄酮醇、芹菜素、鼠李素等。具有促进胃液分泌、增强消化、调节胃肠功能、保护胃黏膜、止泻、抗病原微生物、抗炎、镇痛、镇咳、祛痰、平喘等作用。

Guǎng huò xiāng mainly contains patchouli alcohol, pogostone, eugenol, cinnamaldehyde, pachypodol, apigenin and rhamnetin. It has the functions of promoting the secretion of gastric juice, enhancing digestion, regulating gastrointestinal functions, protecting gastric mucosa, stopping diarrhea, resisting pathogenic microorganism, antagonizing inflammation, relieving pain, eliminating phlegm and alleviating asthma.

佩兰 *Pèi lán* (Eupatorii Herba)
《神农本草经》
Shen Nong's Classic of the Materia Medica (Shén Nóng Běn Cǎo Jīng)

【来源 / Origin】

为菊科植物佩兰 *Eupatorium fortunei* Turcz. 的干燥地上部分。主产于江苏、浙江、河北。夏、秋二季分两次采割。切段，生用。本品气芳香，味微苦。《中国药典》规定，含挥发油不得少于0.30%（ml/g），饮片不得少于0.25%（ml/g）。

Pèi lán is the aerial part of *Eupatorium fortunei* Turcz., pertaining to Compositae. It is mainly produced in Jiangsu, Zhejiang and Hebei Province in China. It is collected in the summer and autumn, cut into segments and used raw. It is fragrant and slightly bitter in taste. According to *Chinese Pharmacopoeia*, the content of volatile oil should be no less than 0.30% (ml/g), and that in decoction pieces should be no less than 0.25% (ml/g).

【性味归经 / Medicinal properties】

辛，平。归脾、胃、肺经。

Acrid and neutral; act on the spleen, stomach and lung meridians.

【主要功效 / Medicinal efficacies】

芳香化湿，醒脾开胃，发表解暑。

Resolve dampness due to its aromatic nature, activate the spleen and promote appetite, release the exterior and clear summer-heat.

【临床应用 / Clinical application】

1. 湿阻中焦证　本品气味芳香，化湿和中之功与广藿香相似，治疗湿阻中焦证，常与广藿香相须为用，并配伍苍术、厚朴等。本品药性平和，不偏温燥，善能化湿浊，去陈腐，故长于治疗脾经湿热，口中甜腻多涎、口臭的脾瘅证，可单用煎服，或配伍黄芩、甘草、白芍等。

(1) Damp obstruction in the middle energizer　*Pèi lán* is aromatic. Its action of resolving damp and harmonizing the middle is similar to *guǎng huò xiāng* (Pogostemonis Herba), and both are usually used together for mutual reinforcement to treat damp obstruction in the middle energizer in combination with *cāng zhú* (Atractylodis Rhizoma) and *hòu pò* (Magnoliae Officinalis Cortex). It is neutral in nature and good at resolving turbid-damp, removing odor smell. So it is especially effective to treat spleen-heat syndrome (*pǐ dān zhèng*) caused by damp-heat in the spleen meridian, manifested as sweetness and greasiness in the mouth, profuse saliva and foul breath. To treat this morbid condition, it can be used alone or combined with *huáng qín* (Scutellariae Radix), *gān cǎo* (Glycyrrhizae Radix et Rhizoma) and *bái sháo* (Paeoniae Alba Radix).

2. 暑湿表证，湿温初起　本品气香辛散，既化湿，又解表，功似广藿香而解表之力稍逊，也用治暑湿表证或湿温初起，前者常与广藿香、陈皮、厚朴等同用；后者常与广藿香、滑石、薏苡仁等同用。

(2) Exterior syndrome of summer-damp, early stage of damp-warm　*Pèi lán* is aromatic and acrid in taste with dispersing effect. Its functions of resolving damp and relieving the exterior is similar to *guǎng huò xiāng* (Pogostemonis Herba), but it is inferior to *guǎng huò xiāng* (Pogostemonis Herba) in relieving the exterior. To treat exterior syndrome of summer-damp, it is combined with *guǎng huò xiāng* (Pogostemonis Herba), *chén pí* (Citri Reticulatae Pericarpium) and *hòu pò* (Magnoliae Officinalis Cortex); to treat early stage of damp-warm, it is often combined with *guǎng huò xiāng* (Pogostemonis Herba), *huá shí* (Talcum) and *yì yǐ rén* (Coicis Semen).

【用法用量 / Usage and dosage】

煎服，3~10g。

Decoction, 3-10g.

【现代研究 / Modern research】

本品主要含对聚伞花素、乙酸橙醇酯、百里香酚甲醚、宁德洛菲碱、蒲公英甾醇、蒲公英甾醇乙酸酯、延胡索酸、琥珀酸等。具有刺激胃肠运动、促进胃肠排空、抗炎、抑菌、祛痰等作用。

Pèi lán mainly contains p-cymen, neryl acetate, methyl thymyl ether, lindelofine, taraxasterol, taraxasteryl acetate, fumaric acid, succinic acid. It has the functions of stimulating gastrointestinal motility and promoting gastrointestinal emptying, antagonizing inflammation, inhibiting bacteria and eliminating phlegm.

苍术　*Cāng zhú* (Atractylodis Rhizoma)
《神农本草经》
Shen Nong's Classic of the Materia Medica (Shén Nóng Běn Cǎo Jīng)

【来源 / Origin】

为菊科植物茅苍术 *Atractylodes lancea*（Thunb.）DC. 或北苍术 *Atractylodes chinensis*（DC.）Koidz. 的干燥根茎。前者主产于江苏茅山一带，质量最好，故称茅苍术；后者主产于内蒙古、山西、陕西等地。春、秋二季采挖，切厚片，生用或麸炒用。茅苍术气香特异，味微甘、辛、苦；北苍术香气较淡，味辛、苦。《中国药典》规定，含苍术素（$C_{13}H_{10}O$）不得少于 0.30%，麸炒苍术不得少于 0.20%。

Cāng zhú is the rhizome of *Atractylodes lancea* (Thunb.) DC. or *Atractylodes chinensis* (DC.) Koidz., pertaining to Compositae. The former is mainly produced in Maoshan, Jiangsu Province with the best quality, which is called *Máo cāng zhú*. The latter is mainly produced in Inner Mongolia Autonomous Region, Shanxi and Shaanxi Province in China. It is collected in spring and autumn, cut into thick pieces, and used raw or stir-fried with wheat bran. *Máo cāng zhú* smells especially fragrant and tastes slightly sweet, acrid and bitter; while *běi cāng zhú* has a peculiar fragrance and is acrid and bitter in taste. According to *Chinese Pharmacopoeia*, the content of atractylodin ($C_{13}H_{10}O$) should be no less than 0.30%, while that in stir-fried with wheat bran should be no less than 0.20%.

【性味归经 / Medicinal properties】

辛、苦，温。归脾、胃、肝经。

Acrid, bitter and warm; act on the spleen, stomach and liver meridians.

【主要功效 / Medicinal efficacies】

燥湿健脾，祛风散寒，明目。

Dry dampness and fortify the spleen, dispel wind and dissipate cold, improve vision.

【临床应用 / Clinical application】

1. 湿阻中焦证　本品苦温燥湿，辛香运脾，为燥湿健脾之要药，善治湿阻中焦，脾失健运所致的脘腹胀满、不思饮食、恶心呕吐、大便溏泄、舌苔白腻等症，常配伍厚朴、陈皮、甘草等。若治脾虚失运，水湿停聚之痰饮、水肿，常与茯苓、猪苓、泽泻等同用。

(1) Damp obstruction in the middle energizer　*Cāng zhú* is bitter and warm with effect of drying dampness, and it is acrid and aromatic with effect of strengthening the spleen. So, it is regarded as an essential medicinal to dry dampness and fortify spleen. It is especially effective to treat failure of spleen to transport soundly due to damp obstruction in the middle energizer, manifested as epigastric distension and fullness, poor appetite, nausea, vomiting, loose stool, whitish and greasy tongue coating. For this pathological condition, it is often combined with *hòu pò* (Magnoliae Officinalis Cortex), *chén pí* (Citri Reticulatae Pericarpium) and *gān cǎo* (Glycyrrhizae Radix et Rhizoma). To treat retention of water fluid and dampness caused by spleen deficiency, manifested as phlegm, retained fluid and edema, it is often combined with *fú líng* (Poria), *zhū líng* (Polyporus) and *zé xiè* (Alismatis Rhizoma).

2. 痹证　本品辛散苦燥，温通祛寒，能祛风散寒除湿，尤长于祛湿，对于湿邪偏盛的着痹尤为适宜，常与独活、羌活、薏苡仁等同用。若治湿热下注之脚气肿痛或痿软无力，常与黄柏同用。

(2) *Bì* syndrome　Since it is acrid for dispersing, bitter for drying and warm for dissipating cold, it is effective in dispelling wind, dissipating cold and eliminating dampness. It is especially suitable to eliminate dampness. For treating stationary *bì* caused by exuberant damp, it is often combined with *dú huó* (Angelicae Pubescentis Radix), *qiāng huó* (Notopterygii Rhizoma et Radix) and *yì yǐ rén* (Coicis Semen). To treat beriberi with swelling and pain due to downward flow of damp-heat, or flaccidity, it is often combined with *huáng bó* (Phellodendri Chinensis Cortex).

3. 风寒夹湿表证　本品辛散苦燥，既善胜湿，又能开腠理，发汗解表，外散风寒，适用于外感风寒夹湿表证，症见恶寒发热、头痛身痛、无汗鼻塞者，常配伍羌活、白芷、防风等。

(3) Exterior syndrome of coexistence of wind-cold and damp　It is acrid for dispersing and bitter for drying. It has efficacies of overcoming dampness, opening striae and interstices, promoting sweating and relieving the exterior, and dispersing wind-cold. It is suitable to treat exterior syndrome of coexistence of wind-cold and damp, manifested as fever, aversion to cold, headache and body pain, anhidrosis and stuffy nose. In this condition, it is often combined with *qiāng huó* (Notopterygii Rhizoma et Radix), *bái zhǐ* (Angelicae Dahuricae Radix) and *fáng fēng* (Saposhnikoviae Radix).

此外，本品尚能明目，用于夜盲、眼目昏涩，可单用，或与羊肝、猪肝等煎煮同食。

In addition, *cāng zhú* can also improve vision. To treat night blindness, blurred vision and dry eyes, it can be used alone or together with livers of goats and pigs.

【用法用量 / Usage and dosage】

煎服，3~9g。

Decoction, 3-9g.

【现代研究 / Modern research】

本品主要含β- 橄榄烯、苍术素、苍术酮、茅苍术醇、丁香烯、广藿香烯、白术内酯、苍术烯内酯丙等。具有调节胃肠道功能、抗溃疡、镇静、镇痛、抗炎、降压、降血糖、保肝、促进胆汁分泌、抑菌、抗病毒等作用。

Cāng zhú mainly contains β-maaliene, atractylodin, atractyline, hinesol, caryophyllene, patchoulene, atractylenolide, atractylenotide Ⅲ. It has the functions of regulating gastrointestinal motility, antagonizing ulcer, tranquilizing, relieving pain, antagonizing inflammation, reducing blood pressure and blood glucose, protecting the liver, promoting secretion of bile, inhibiting bacteria and antagonizing virus.

厚朴 *Hòu pò* (Magnoliae Officinalis Cortex)
《神农本草经》
Shen Nong's Classic of the Materia Medica (Shén Nóng Běn Cǎo Jīng)

【来源 / Origin】

为木兰科植物厚朴 *Magnolia officinalis* Rehd. et Wils. 或凹叶厚朴 *Magnolia officinalis* Rehd. et Wils. var. *biloba* Rehd. et Wils. 的干燥干皮、根皮及枝皮。主产于四川、湖北、浙江。4~6 月剥取，切丝，生用或姜汁炙用。本品气香，味辛辣、微苦。《中国药典》规定，含厚朴酚（$C_{18}H_{18}O_2$）与和厚朴酚（$C_{18}H_{18}O_2$）的总量不得少于 2.0%，姜厚朴不得少于 1.6%。

Hòu pò is the dried bark, root bark and branch bark of *Magnolia officinalis* Rehd. et Wils. or *Magnolia officinalis* Rehd. et Wils. var. *biloba* Rehd. et Wils., pertaining to Magnoliaceae. It is mainly produced in Sichuan, Hubei and Zhejiang Province, collected from April to June, cut into thread-like strips, and used raw or prepared with ginger. *Hòu pò* is fragrant, acrid and slightly bitter in taste. According to *Chinese Pharmacopoeia*, the content of magnolol ($C_{18}H_{18}O_2$) and honokiol ($C_{18}H_{18}O_2$) should be no less than 2.0%, and no less than 1.6% in *jiāng hòu pò*.

【性味归经 / Medicinal properties】

苦、辛，温。归脾、胃、肺、大肠经。

Bitter, acrid and warm; act on the spleen, stomach, lung and large intestine meridians.

【主要功效 / Medicinal efficacies】

燥湿，行气，消积，消痰平喘。

Dry dampness, move qi, remove stagnation, eliminate phlegm and relieve asthma.

【临床应用 / Clinical application】

1. 湿阻中焦证 本品苦温燥湿，辛香行散，既能燥湿运脾，又能行气除胀，为消除胀满之要药。用治湿阻中焦，脾胃气滞之脘腹胀满、不思饮食、呕吐泄泻等，常配伍苍术、陈皮等。

(1) Obstruction of damp in the middle energizer It is bitter and warm for drying dampness, and acrid with fragrance for driving qi downward. It functions to dry dampness to activate the spleen and move qi to remove distension, which is regarded as an essential medicinal to eliminate distension and fullness. To treat distension and fullness in the stomach cavity and abdomen, poor appetite, vomiting and diarrhea due to qi stagnation of spleen and stomach caused by obstruction of damp in the middle energizer, it is often combined with *cāng zhú* (Atractylodis Rhizoma) and *chén pí* (Citri Reticulatae Pericarpium).

2. 食积气滞，腹胀便秘 本品有行气宽中、消积导滞之功。用治饮食积滞，脘腹胀满，嗳腐吞酸，多与枳实、麦芽等同用。用治实热积滞，大便秘结，脘腹胀痛，常与大黄、芒硝、枳实等同用。若治脾虚气滞，食少体倦，脘腹胀满，常与人参、白术等同用。

(2) Food accumulation and qi stagnation, abdominal distension and constipation *Hòu pò* has efficacies of moving qi and loosening the center, promoting digestion and guiding out food stagnation.

To treat distension and fullness in the stomach cavity and abdomen, eructation with fetid odor and acid regurgitation caused by food retention, it is often combined with *zhǐ shí* (Aurantii Immaturus Fructus) and *mài yá* (Hordei Germinatus Fructus). To treat constipation, distension and pain in the stomach cavity and abdomen due to accumulation of excess heat, it is often combined with *dà huáng* (Rhei Radix et Rhizoma), *máng xiāo* (Natrii Sulfas) and *zhǐ shí* (Aurantii Immaturus Fructus). To treat poor appetite, fatigue, distension and fullness in the stomach cavity and abdomen due to spleen deficiency and qi stagnation, it is often combined with *rén shēn* (Ginseng Radix et Rhizoma) and *bái zhú* (Atractylodis Macrocephalae Rhizoma).

3. 痰饮喘咳 本品苦燥而降，能燥湿消痰，降气平喘。用治痰饮阻肺，肺气不降之咳喘胸闷，常与苏子、半夏等同用。若治寒饮化热，胸闷气喘，喉间痰声漉漉，烦躁不安者，常与石膏、麻黄、杏仁等同用。若治宿有喘病，又外感风寒而诱发者，多与桂枝、杏仁配伍。

(3) Cough and asthma due to phlegm rheum *Hòu pò* is bitter with effect of drying and descending. It has efficacies of drying damp and eliminating phlegm, descending qi and relieving asthma. To treat cough, asthma and tight chest caused by failure of lung qi to move downward due to obstruction of phlegm rheum in the lung, it is often combined with *sū zǐ* (Perillae Fructus) and *bàn xià* (Pinelliae Rhizoma). To treat tight chest and panting, gurgling sound of phlegm in the throat and dysphoria due to transformation of cold fluid into heat, it is often combined with *shí gāo* (Gypsum Fibrosum), *má huáng* (Ephedrae Herba) and *xìng rén* (Armeniacae Amarum Semen). To treat panting due to external contraction of wind-cold, it is combined with *guì zhī* (Cinnamomi Ramulus) and *xìng rén* (Armeniacae Amarum Semen).

此外，取本品燥湿消痰、下气宽中之功，可用治情志郁结，痰气互阻，咽中如有物阻，咽之不下，吐之不出的梅核气，常配伍半夏、茯苓、生姜等。

In addition, with its efficacies of drying damp and eliminating phlegm, moving qi downward to loosen the center, *hòu pò* is also used to treat plum pit qi, which is manifested as a subjective sensation of blockage or constriction of the throat, and usually caused by mental depression and intermingling of phlegm and qi. Under this condition, it is often combined with *bàn xià* (Pinelliae Rhizoma), *fú líng* (Poria) and *shēng jiāng* (Zingiberis Recens Rhizoma).

【用法用量 / Usage and dosage】

煎服，3~10g。

Decoction, 3-10g.

【使用注意 / Precaution】

气虚津亏者及孕妇慎用。

It should be used with caution for pregnant women and those suffering qi deficiency and body fluid consumption.

【现代研究 / Modern research】

本品主要含厚朴酚、和厚朴酚、桉醇、β-桉叶醇、木脂素、去甲木脂素、双木脂素等。具有调节胃肠功能、抗炎、抑菌、镇静、镇痛、止泻、保肝、抗溃疡、降压等作用。

Hòu pò mainly contains magnolol, honokiol, eudesmol , β-eudesmol, lignans, norlignane and haedoxane. It has the functions of regulating gastrointestinal actions, antagonizing inflammation, inhibiting bacteria, tranquilizing, relieving pain, stopping diarrhea, protecting liver, antiulcer and reducing blood pressure.

砂仁 *Shā rén* (Amomi Fructus)
《药性论》
Treatise on Medicinal Properties (Yào Xing Lùn)

【来源 / Origin】

为姜科植物阳春砂 *Amomum villosum* Lour.、绿壳砂 *Amomum villosum* Lour. var. *xanthioides* T. L. Wu et Senjen 或海南砂 *Amomum longiligulare* T. L.Wu 的干燥成熟果实。主产于广东、广西、云南等地。夏、秋二季果实成熟时采收，生用，用时捣碎。阳春砂、绿壳砂气芳香而浓烈，味辛凉、微苦；海南砂气味稍淡。《中国药典》规定，阳春砂、绿壳砂种子团含挥发油不得少于 3.0%（ml/g），海南砂种子团含挥发油不得少于 1.0%（ml/g）；含乙酸龙脑酯（$C_{12}H_{20}O_2$）不得少于 0.90%。

Shā rén is the ripe fruit of *Amomum villosum* Lour., *Amomum villosum* Lour. var. *xanthioides* T. L. Wu et Senjen, or *Amomum longiligulare* T. L.Wu, pertaining to Zingiberaceae. It is mainly produced in Guangdong Province, Guangxi Zhuang Autonomous Region and Yunnan Province, collected in summer and autumn when the fruits are ripe. Raw *shā rén* is ground into pieces for medication. *Yáng chūn shā* and *lǜ ké shā* have strong fragrance, and are cool, acrid, slightly bitter in taste; while *hǎi nán shā* has a milder taste. According to *Chinese Pharmacopoeia*, the content of volatile oil in *yáng chūn shā* and *lǜ ké shā* seeds group should be no less than 3.0%(ml/g), while that in *hǎi nán shā* seeds group should be no less than 1.0% (ml/g); the content of bomyl acetate ($C_{12}H_{20}O_2$) should be no less than 0.90%.

【性味归经 / Medicinal properties】

辛，温。归脾、胃、肾经。

Acrid and warm; act on the spleen, stomach and kidney meridians.

【主要功效 / Medicinal efficacies】

化湿开胃，温脾止泻，理气安胎。

Resolve dampness and increase appetite, warm the spleen to arrest diarrhea, rectify qi to calm the fetus.

【临床应用 / Clinical application】

1. 湿阻中焦证，脾胃气滞证 本品辛温气香，入脾、胃经，化湿开胃、行气温中之功俱佳。凡湿阻中焦及脾胃气滞证皆可使用，尤宜用于寒湿气滞者。若治湿阻中焦，脘腹痞闷，食欲不振，呕吐泄泻，常与厚朴、豆蔻等同用。若治寒湿中阻，脘腹胀满冷痛，食少腹泻，常配伍干姜、厚朴、草豆蔻等。若治脾虚气滞，脘腹痞闷，食少纳呆，大便溏泄，可与白术、枳实、木香等同用。

(1) **Damp obstruction in the middle energizer, qi stagnation of spleen and stomach** *Shā rén* is acrid and warm with fragrance and acts on the spleen and stomach meridians. It is effective in resolving damp and stimulating appetite, moving qi and warming the spleen and stomach. It can be used to treat disorders caused by damp obstructing the middle energizer and qi stagnation of spleen and stomach, especially to treat diseases due to cold-damp and qi stagnation. To treat stuffiness and fullness in the stomach cavity and abdomen, poor appetite, vomiting and diarrhea due to obstruction of damp in the middle energizer, it is combined with *hòu pò* and *dòu kòu* (Amomi Rotundus Fructus). To treat distension, fullness and cold pain in the stomach cavity and abdomen, poor appetite and diarrhea caused by obstruction of cold-damp in the middle energizer, it is combined with *gān jiāng* (Zingiberis Rhizoma), *hòu pò* and *cǎo dòu kòu* (Alpiniae Katsumadai Semen). To treat stuffiness and fullness in the stomach cavity and abdomen, poor appetite and loose stool, it is combined

with *bái zhú* (Atractylodis Macrocephalae Rhizoma), *zhǐ shí* (Aurantii Immaturus Fructus) and *mù xiāng* (Aucklandiae Radix).

2. 脾胃虚寒，呕吐泄泻　本品性温，有温中健脾、止呕止泻之功，尤善于温脾止泻。用治脾胃虚寒，呕吐泄泻，可单用研末服，或与干姜、附子等同用。

(2) Vomiting and diarrhea due to deficiency-cold of spleen and stomach　It is warm in nature for warming the middle energizer and invigorating spleen, as well as arresting vomiting and diarrhea. It is especially good at warming the spleen to arrest diarrhea. To treat vomiting and diarrhea due to deficiency-cold of spleen and stomach, it can be used alone and ground into powder, or combined with *gān jiāng* (Zingiberis Rhizoma) and *fù zǐ* (Aconiti Lateralis Radix Praeparata).

3. 胎动不安　本品能行气和中，止呕安胎。用治妊娠气滞，呕逆不能食或胎动不安，常与紫苏、白术等同用。若治气血不足，胎动不安，多与人参、白术、当归配伍。若治肾虚胎元不固，胎动不安，常与杜仲、续断、桑寄生等同用。

(3) Restless fetus　*Shā rén* has efficacies of moving qi and harmonizing the center, arresting vomiting and calming fetus. To treat vomiting with no desire to eat or restless fetus due to qi stagnation during pregnancy, it is used together with *zǐ sū* (Perillae Fructus) and *bái zhú* (Atractylodis Macrocephalae Rhizoma). To treat restless fetus caused by insufficiency of qi and blood, it is often combined with *rén shēn* (Ginseng Radix et Rhizoma), *bái zhú* (Atractylodis Macrocephalae Rhizoma) and *dāng guī* (Angelicae Sinensis Radix). To treat restless fetus caused by liability to be abortion due to kidney deficiency, it is combined with *dù zhòng* (Eucommiae Cortex), *xù duàn* (Dipsaci Radix) and *sāng jì shēng* (Taxilli Herba).

【用法用量 / Usage and dosage】

煎服，3~6g，后下。

Decoction, 3-6g. It should be added later.

【使用注意 / Precaution】

阴虚血燥者慎用。

It should be used with caution for those suffering yin deficiency and blood dryness.

【现代研究 / Modern research】

本品主要含乙酸龙脑酯、樟脑、樟烯等挥发油，尚含黄酮等。具有调节胃肠功能、抗炎、镇痛、止泻、抗溃疡、利胆等作用。

Shā rén mainly contains volatile oil, such as bornyl acetate, camphor and camphene. It also contains flavone. It has the functions of regulating gastrointestinal actions, antagonizing inflammation, relieving pain, stopping diarrhea, antiulcer and promoting the function of gallbladder.

豆蔻　*Dòu kòu* (Amomi Fructus Rotundus)
《名医别录》
Miscellaneous Records of Famous Physicians (Míng Yī Bié Lù)

【来源 / Origin】

为姜科草本植物白豆蔻 *Amomum kravanh* Pierre ex Gagnep. 或爪哇白豆蔻 *Amomum compactum* Soland ex Maton 的干燥成熟果实，又称白豆蔻。按产地不同分为"原豆蔻"和"印尼白蔻"。前者主产于泰国、柬埔寨、越南等地，后者主产于印度尼西亚。我国云南、广东、广西等地有栽培。秋季果实由绿色转成黄绿色时采收，生用，用时捣碎。原豆蔻气芳香，味辛凉；印尼豆蔻气味较弱。《中国药典》规定，原豆蔻仁含挥发油不得少于 5.0%（ml/g），印尼豆蔻仁不得少于

4.0%（ml/g）；本品的仁中含桉油精（C$_{10}$H$_{18}$O）不得少于 3.0%。

Dòu kòu is the ripe fruit of *Amomum kravanh* Pierre ex Gagnep. or *Amomum compactum* Soland ex Maton, pertaining to Zingiberaceae, and is also called *bái dòu kòu*. It is classified into *yuán dòu kòu* and *yìn ní dòu kòu* according to different origins. The former is mainly produced in Thailand, Cambodia and Vietnam, and the latter in Indonesia. *Dòu kòu* is also cultivated in Yunnan, Guangdong Province and Guangxi Zhuang Autonomous Region in China. It is collected in autumn when the fruits turn from green to yellow-green. It is used raw and ground into pieces. *Yuán dòu kòu* is fragrant, acrid and cool; while *yìn ní dòu kòu* has milder aroma. According to *Chinese Pharmacopoeia*, the content of volatile oil in *yuán dòu kòu* fructus should be no less than 5.0%(ml/g), while that in *yìn ní dòu kòu* fructus should be no less than 4.0%(ml/g); the content of cineole (C$_{10}$H$_{18}$O) in *dòu kòu* fructus should be no less than 3.0%.

【性味归经 / Medicinal properties 】

辛，温。归肺、脾、胃经。

Acrid and warm; act on the lung, spleen and stomach meridians.

【主要功效 / Medicinal efficacies 】

化湿行气，温中止呕，开胃消食。

Resolve dampness and move qi, warm the spleen and stomach to arrest vomiting, increase appetite and promote digestion.

【临床应用 / Clinical application 】

1. 湿阻中焦证，脾胃气滞证　本品辛温气香，入脾胃经，善化中焦湿浊，行脾胃气滞。用治湿阻中焦，脾胃气滞，脘腹胀满，不思饮食等，常配伍苍术、厚朴、陈皮等。若治脾虚湿阻气滞所致的胸腹虚胀，食少纳呆，倦怠无力，常与人参、白术、黄芪等同用。

(1) Damp obstruction in the middle energizer, qi stagnation of spleen and stomach　*Dòu kòu* is acrid and warm with fragrance, and acts on spleen and stomach meridians. It is effective in resolving turbid-damp in the middle energizer and moving qi stagnation of spleen and stomach. To treat distension and fullness in the stomach cavity and abdomen as well as poor appetite due to damp obstruction in the middle energizer and qi stagnation of spleen and stomach, it is often combined with *cāng zhú* (Atractylodis Rhizoma), *hòu pò* (Magnoliae Officinalis Cortex) and *chén pí* (Citri Reticulatae Pericarpium). To treat flatulence of chest and abdomen, poor appetite, weakness and fatigue caused by spleen deficiency and qi stagnation due to obstruction of damp, it is often combined with *rén shēn* (Ginseng Radix et Rhizoma), *bái zhú* (Atractylodis Macrocephalae Rhizoma) and *huáng qí* (Astragali Radix).

2. 湿温初起　本品辛温，入肺、脾经，善除上、中二焦之湿浊。用治湿温初起，湿邪偏重之胸闷不饥、头痛身重，常配伍苦杏仁、薏苡仁等。若热重于湿，常与黄芩、滑石等同用。

(2) Damp-warm in the early stage　*Dòu kòu* is acrid and warm, and acts on spleen and stomach meridians. It is good at resolving turbid-damp in the upper and middle energizer. To treat chest distress without hunger sensation, headache, heavy sensation of the body caused by damp-warm in the early stage with exuberant dampness, it is often used with *kǔ xìng rén* (Armeniacae Amarum Semen) and *yì yǐ rén* (Coicis Semen). If heat is severer, it is used with *huáng qín* (Scutellariae Radix) and *huá shí* (Talcum).

3. 寒湿呕吐　本品能化湿醒脾，行气宽中，温胃止呕，适宜于胃寒湿阻气滞之呕吐，可单用为末服，或与砂仁、广藿香、半夏等同用。用治小儿胃寒，吐乳不食者，常与砂仁、甘草等同用。

(3) Vomiting due to cold-damp　*Dòu kòu* has efficacies of resolving damp and activating spleen, moving qi and loosening the center as well as warm the stomach to arrest vomiting. It is suitable to treat vomiting caused by stomach cold and qi stagnation due to obstruction of damp. It can be used alone and ground into pieces, or combined with *shā rén* (Amomi Fructus), *guǎng huò xiāng* (Pogostemonis Herba) and *bàn xià* (Pinelliae Rhizoma). *To* treat infantile stomach cold, manifested as milk vomiting, it is used with *shā rén* (Amomi Fructus) and *gān cǎo* (Glycyrrhizae Radix et Rhizoma).

【用法用量 / Usage and dosage 】

煎服，3~6g，后下。

Decoction, 3-6g. It should be added later.

【使用注意 / Precaution 】

阴虚血燥者慎用。

It should be used with caution for those suffering yin deficiency and blood dryness.

【现代研究 / Modern research 】

本品主要含桉油精、β- 蒎烯、α- 蒎烯、丁香烯、乙酸龙脑酯等挥发油。具有促进胃液分泌、增进胃肠蠕动、制止肠内异常发酵、祛除胃肠积气、止呕、解酒等作用。

Dòu kòu mainly contains volatile oil, such as cineole, β-pinene, α-pinene, caryophyllene and bomyl acetate. It has the functions of promoting secretion of gastric juice, promoting gastrointestinal motility, preventing abnormal fermentation in the intestines, eliminating gas in the stomach and intestines, relieving nausea and neutralizing the effect of alcoholic drinks.

其他化湿药功用介绍见表 10-1。

The efficacies of other damp-resolving medicinals are shown in table 10-1.

表 10-1　其他化湿药功用介绍

分类	药物	药性	功效	应用	用法用量
化湿药	草豆蔻	辛，温。归脾、胃经	燥湿行气，温中止呕	寒湿中阻证，脾胃气滞证，寒湿呕吐	煎服，3~6g
	草果	辛，温。归脾、胃经	燥湿温中，截疟除痰	寒湿中阻证，脾胃气滞证，疟疾	煎服，3~6g

（刘立萍）

题库

第十一章　利水渗湿药
Chapter 11　Damp-draining diuretic medicinals

 学习目标 | Learning goals

　　1. 掌握　利水渗湿药在性能、功效、主治、配伍及使用注意方面的共性；茯苓、泽泻、薏苡仁、车前子、木通、滑石、茵陈、金钱草的性能、功效、应用以及特殊的用法用量和特殊的使用注意。

　　2. 熟悉　利水渗湿药的分类；猪苓、萆薢、通草、石韦、海金沙、瞿麦、萹蓄的功效、主治以及特殊的用法用量和特殊的使用注意。

　　3. 了解　利水渗湿药、利水消肿药、利尿通淋药、利湿退黄药及相关功效术语的含义；冬瓜皮、玉米须、枳椇子、地肤子、冬葵子、灯心草、广金钱草、连钱草的功效以及特殊的用法用量和特殊的使用注意。

　　1. Master the commonness of damp-draining diuretic medicinals in efficacy, indications, property, compatibility and cautions; as well as the property, efficacy, application, special usage and dosage and special precautions of *fú líng, zé xiè, yì yǐ rén, chē qián zǐ, mù tōng, huá shí, yīn chén*, and *jīn qián cǎo*.

　　2. Familiar with the classification of the damp-draining diuretics, and the efficacy, indications, special usage, dosage and special precautions of *zhū líng, bì xiè, tōng cǎo, shí wéi, hǎi jīn shā, qú mài*, and *biǎn xù*.

　　3. Understand the definitions of damp-draining diuretics, edema-alleviating diuretics, stranguria-relieving diuretics and damp-excreting anti-icteric medicinals, and related efficacy terms; and the efficacy, special usage and dosage and special precautions of *dōng guā pí, yù mǐ xū, zhī jǔ zǐ, dì fū zǐ, dōng kuí zǐ, dēng xīn cǎo, guǎng jīn qián cǎo*, and *lián qián cǎo*.

　　凡以通利水道、渗泄水湿为主要功效，常用以治疗水湿内停证的药物，称为利水渗湿药。

　　Medicinals with the main functions of regulating water passages, as well as draining water and dampness and usually indicated for retention of water and dampness syndromes are called damp-draining diuretic medicinals.

　　利水渗湿药味多甘淡或苦，性平或偏寒凉，多入膀胱、小肠、肾、脾经。能渗利水湿，畅通小便，增加尿量，使体内的水湿邪气从小便排出。主治小便不利、水肿、泄泻、痰饮、淋证、黄疸、湿疮、带下、湿温等水湿所致的病证。

　　These medicinals are mostly sweet and bland, or bitter in flavor, as well as neutral or slightly cold in nature, mainly acting on bladder, small intestine, kidney and spleen meridians. They have the ability to drain the dampness, induce diuresis, and increase the amount of urine, so the removal of water and dampness, accumulated inside the body, is accomplished through the process of increased urination. They are indicated for dysuria, edema, diarrhea, phlegm-fluid retention, stranguria, jaundice, eczema, leukorrhea and damp-warm diseases.

根据利水渗湿药的功效主治差异，可分为利水消肿药、利尿通淋药及利湿退黄药三类。

According to the different medicinal properties and efficacies, these medicinals are mainly divided into three types: edema-alleviating diuretics, stranguria-relieving diuretics, and damp-excreting anti-icteric medicinal.

使用利水渗湿药时应根据水湿之邪所致的不同病证选用适宜的药物，并行适当的配伍。如水肿骤起兼有表证者，配伍宣肺发汗药；水肿日久，脾肾阳虚者，配伍温补脾肾药；脾虚泄泻、痰饮者，配伍健脾化湿药；湿热合邪者，配伍清热燥湿药；寒湿并重者，配伍温里散寒药；热伤血络尿血者，配伍凉血止血药。气行则水行，气滞则水停，由于水湿易阻滞气机，故利水渗湿药常与行气药配伍。

In clinical practice, medicinals that induce diuresis and drain dampness should be combined together with appropriate medicinals according to different syndromes. For example, to treat edema in the initial stages with exterior syndromes, these medicinals should be combined with those that can ventilate lung and promote sweating. In cases of prolonged edema, due to the deficiency of spleen-kidney yang, they should be used together with medicinals that warm and tonify the spleen and kidney. In cases of diarrhea due to spleen deficiency, phlegm-fluid retention, they are combined with medicinals that invigorate spleen to resolve dampness. For the dampness-heat with pathogens, they are combined with heat-clearing dampness-drying medicinals. For cold-dampness patterns, they are combined with medicinals that warm the interior and dispel cold. To treat heat stranguria and bloody urine due to blood collaterals injuried by heat, they should be used together with blood-cooling hemostatic medicinals. Qi flow promotes water transportation, while qi stagnation leads to water retention. Because water and dampness stops qi movement, damp-draining diuretic medicinals are usually combined with qi-moving medicinal.

本类药物易耗伤津液，阴虚津亏者慎用或忌用。部分药物有较强的通利作用，孕妇慎用或忌用。

These medicinals are able to consume body fluids, thus, they should be used with caution or avoided for syndromes of yin-deficiency and decreased body fluids. Certain medicinals have a strong function to induce diuresis, so they should be used with caution or avoided for pregnant women.

第一节 利水消肿药
Section 1　Edema-alleviating diuretic medicinals

本类药物味多甘淡，性平或微寒，服药能使小便通畅，尿量增多，具有利水消肿的功效，主治水湿内停之水肿、小便不利及泄泻、痰饮等，也可用于水湿内停所致的其他病证。

These medicinals are mostly sweet and bland in flavor and neutral or slightly cold in nature, with the functions of inducing diuresis, increasing the amount of urine, and promoting the flow of water to relieve edema. They are indicated for edema, dysuria, diarrhea, phlegm-fluid retention and other syndromes due to water and damp retention inside the body.

微课

茯苓 *Fú líng* (Poria)
《神农本草经》
Shen Nong's Classic of the Materia Medica (Shén Nóng Běn Cǎo Jīng)

【来源 / Origin】

为多孔菌科真菌茯苓 *Poria cocos*（Schw.）Wolf 的干燥菌核。野生或栽培，主产于云南、安徽、湖北等地。产于云南者称"云苓"，质较优。多于 7~9 月采挖，阴干，生用。本品气微，味淡，嚼之粘牙。

Fú líng is the dried sclerotium of *Poria cocos* (Schw.) Wolf, pertaining to Polyporaceae. Wild or cultivated, it is mainly produced in Yunnan, Anhui and Hubei Province. It is also called *yún líng* since it is produced in Yunnan Province with superior quality. It is mainly collected between July and September, dried in the shade and used raw. It has a slight odor and is bland in taste. When chewed, it is sticky.

【性味归经 / Medicinal properties】

甘、淡，平。归心、肺、脾、肾经。

Sweet, bland and neutral; act on the heart, lung, spleen and kidney meridians.

【主要功效 / Medicinal efficacies】

利水渗湿，健脾，宁心。

Promote diuresis to drain dampness; invigorate the spleen; and sedate the mind.

【临床应用 / Clinical application】

1. 水肿、小便不利　本品淡渗甘补，既可渗湿祛邪，又可健脾扶正，利水而不伤阴，且性质平和，不偏寒热，为利水消肿之要药，凡是水肿、小便不利，不论寒热虚实皆可用之。用治水湿内停所致的水肿、小便不利，常与泽泻、猪苓、白术等配伍。若治脾肾阳虚水肿，可与附子、生姜等同用。若治水热互结，阴虚小便不利、水肿，多与滑石、阿胶、泽泻等同用。

(1) Edema and dysury　*Fú líng* is draining with bland and tonifying with sweet, with the functions of draining dampness and eliminating the pathogenic, as well as invigorating the spleen and reinforcing the healthy qi. *Fú líng* can promote diuresis without damaging yin. It is neutral, neither cold nor heat, and is the principal medicinal to induce diuresis and alleviate edema. It can be used to treat any kind of edema or dysuria, whether it is due to cold or heat, deficiency or excess. To edema or dysuria due to water and damp retention, it is often combined with *zé xiè*, *zhū líng* and *bái zhú*. To treat edema due to the deficiency of the spleen-kidney yang, it is combined with *fù zǐ* and *shēng jiāng*. To treat dysuria or edema due to the accumulation of dampness and heat, it should be combined with *huá shí*, *ē jiāo* and *zé xiè*.

2. 脾虚食少，便溏泄泻　本品入脾经，能健脾补中，渗湿而止泻。适宜于脾虚湿盛之便溏泄泻，常与白术、山药、薏苡仁等同用。若治脾胃虚弱，脘腹胀满，倦怠乏力，食少便溏等，常与人参、白术、陈皮等同用。

(2) Poor appetite, loose stool and diarrhea due to spleen deficiency　*Fú líng* acts in spleen meridian, can invigorate the spleen and replenish the middle qi, drain dampness and stop diarrhea. To treat loose stool and diarrhea due to spleen deficiency with profuse dampness, it is combined with *bái zhú*, *shān yào* and *yì yǐ rén*. To treat spleen-stomach weakness, fullness in stomach and abdomen, languid, fatigue, poor appetite, and loose stool, it is combined with *rén shēn*, *bái zhú* and *chén pí*.

3. 痰饮　本品善能渗湿、健脾，使湿无所聚，痰无由生。用治湿痰咳嗽，痰多色白，常配伍半夏、陈皮、甘草。用治痰饮之目眩心悸，常与桂枝、白术、甘草同用。用治饮停于胃而呕吐者，多与半夏、生姜等配伍。

(3) Phlegm-fluid retention *Fú líng* is good at draining dampness and invigorate the spleen, preventing the accumulation of dampness and phlegm. To treat cough with dampness-phlegm, profuse phlegm with white color, it is combined with *bàn xià.*, *chén pí* and *gān cǎo*. To treat dizziness or palpitation due to phlegm-fluid retention, it is combined with *guì zhī*, *bái zhú* and *gān cǎo*. To treat vomiting due to fluid retention in the stomach, it is combined with *bàn xià* and *shēng jiāng*.

4．心悸失眠　本品入心经，能补益心脾而宁心安神。用治心脾两虚，气血不足之心悸怔忡、健忘失眠，常与人参、当归、酸枣仁等同用。若治心肾不交之神志不宁、惊悸健忘、失眠等，可配伍党参、远志、石菖蒲等。

(4) Palpitation and insomnia *Fú líng* acts on heart meridian, with the functions of tonifying heart and spleen, calming the heart and sedating the mind. For palpitation, insomnia and poor memory due to deficiency of heart and spleen, deficiency of qi and blood, it is often combined with *rén shēn*, *dāng guī* and *suān zǎo rén*. For mental restlessness, fright palpitations, amnesia, and insomnia due to non-interaction between heart and kidney, it is often combined with *dǎng shēn*, *yuǎn zhì* and *shí chāng pú*.

【用法用量 / Usage and dosage】

煎服，10~15g。

Decoction, 10-15g.

【现代研究 / Modern research】

本品主要含 β– 茯苓聚糖、茯苓酸、麦角甾醇等，尚含树胶、甲壳质、蛋白质、脂肪、卵磷脂、腺嘌呤及钙、镁、铁、钠、钾等。具有调节免疫、利尿、保肝、抗白血病、抗肿瘤、抗菌、降血糖、抗疲劳、改善大脑记忆力及抗衰老等作用。

It mainly contains β-pachyman, poria acid, ergosterol, as well as gum, chitin, protein, fat, lecithin, adenine, calcium, magnesium, iron, sodium, potassium, etc. It has the functions of regulating immunity, diuresis, protecting liver, anti-leukemia, anti-tumor, anti-bacteria, reducing blood sugar, anti-fatigue, improving brain memory and anti-aging.

薏苡仁　*Yì yǐ rén* (Coicis Semen)
《神农本草经》
Shen Nong's Classic of the Materia Medica (Shén Nóng Běn Cǎo Jīng)

【来源 / Origin】

为禾本科植物薏苡 *Coix lacryma-jobi* L.var.*ma-yuen*（Roman.）Stapf 的干燥成熟种仁。主产于福建、河北、辽宁等地。秋季采收，晒干，收集种仁，生用或炒用。本品气微，味微甜。《中国药典》规定，含甘油三油酸酯（$C_{57}H_{104}O_6$）不得少于 0.50%，麸炒薏苡仁不得少于 0.40%。

Yì yǐ rén is the dried seed of *Coix lacryma-jobi* L. var. *ma-yuen* (Roman.) Stapf, pertaining to Gramineae, mainly produced in Fujian, Hebei and Liaoning Province, collected when the fruit is ripe in autumn, dried in the sunshine, and used raw or the stir-fried. It has a slight odor and is slightly sweet in taste. According to *Chinese Pharmacopoeia*, the content of triglyceride ($C_{57}H_{104}O_6$) should be no less than 0.50%, and that in *yì yǐ rén* stir-fried with bran should be no less than 0.40%.

【性味归经 / Medicinal properties】

甘、淡，凉。归脾、胃、肺经。

Sweet, bland and cool; act on spleen, stomach and lung meridians.

【主要功效 / Medicinal efficacies】

利水渗湿，健脾止泻，除痹，排脓，解毒散结。

Promote urination and drain dampness, invigorate spleen to relieve diarrhea; eliminate impediment; expel pus; remove toxins and dissolve a mass.

【临床应用 / Clinical application】

1. 水肿，脚气，小便不利　本品淡渗甘补，既能利水，又能健脾，功似茯苓而力稍弱。用治脾虚湿盛之水肿，多与茯苓、白术、黄芪等同用。若治脚气浮肿，可与防己、木瓜、苍术等同用。

(1) **Edema, beriberi and dysuria**　*Yì yǐ rén* is draining with bland and tonifying with sweet, with the functions of promoting urination and tonifying spleen, similar but inferior to *fú líng*. For edema due to excessive dampness and spleen deficiency, it is often combined with *fú líng*, *bái zhú* and *huáng qí*. To treat beriberi and edema, it is combined together with *fáng jǐ*, *mù guā* and *cāng zhú*.

2. 脾虚泄泻　本品渗利水湿，健脾止泻。用治脾虚湿盛之便溏泄泻，常与人参、白术、茯苓等同用。

(2) **Diarrhea due to deficiency of spleen**　*Yì yǐ rén* can promote urination and drain dampness, invigorate spleen to relieve diarrhea. To treat loose stool and diarrhea due to spleen deficiency with profuse dampness, it is combined with *rén shēn*, *bái zhú* and *fú líng*.

3. 湿痹拘挛　本品既能渗湿除痹，又能利关节，舒筋脉，有缓和筋脉挛急的作用。用治湿痹而筋脉拘急疼痛者，可与独活、防风、苍术同用。若治风湿热痹，关节红肿热痛，肌肉酸楚，可与防己、忍冬藤、石膏等同用。若治风湿日久，筋脉挛急，水肿，可单用本品煮粥服，或与木瓜、苍术等同用。

(3) **Dampness impediment and spasm of sinews**　*Yì yǐ rén* can drain dampness and eliminate impediment, as well as dredge joints, relax tendons and activate collaterals to relieve spasms. For dampness impediment manifesting as spasm of the sinews, it is usually combined with *dú huó*, *fáng fēng* and *cāng zhú*. To treat wind-dampness-heat impediment manifesting as red and swollen joints with heat pain, and muscle soreness, it is combined with *fáng jǐ*, *rěn dōng téng* and *shí gāo*. To treat spasm of the sinews, and edema for a long time, it can be cooked alone as porridge or combined with *mù guā* and *cāng zhú*.

4. 肺痈，肠痈　本品性凉，能清肺肠之热，排脓消痈。用治肺痈咳吐脓痰者，常与苇茎、桃仁等配伍；用治肠痈腹痛，常与附子、败酱草、丹皮等同用。

(4) **Pulmonary and intestinal abscess**　*Yì yǐ rén* is cold in nature and can clear away heat of lung and intestines, expel pus and disperse abscess. For pulmonary abscess with cough and thick phlegm, it is usually combined with *wěi jīng* and *táo rén*. For intestinal abscess with abdominal pain, it is combined with *fù zǐ*, *bài jiàng cǎo* and *dān pí*.

此外，本品尚能解毒散结，用治赘疣、癌肿等。

In addition, it can also remove toxins and dissolve masses and is used to treat wart and cancer.

【用法用量 / Usage and dosage】

煎服，9~30g。清利湿热宜生用，健脾止泻宜炒用。

Decoction, 9~30g. The raw form is utilized for clearing heat and draining dampness, while the stir-fried form is utilized for invigorating spleen and relieving diarrhea.

【使用注意 / Precaution】

孕妇慎用。

It should be used with caution for pregnant women.

【现代研究 / Modern research】

本品主要含甘油三油酸酯、α-单油酸甘油酯、α-单亚麻酯、薏苡素、薏苡内酯、薏苡仁多糖等。具有抗肿瘤、调节免疫、降血糖、降血钙、抗炎、镇痛、解热、镇静、兴奋子宫等作用。

Yì yǐ rén mainly contains triglyceride, α-monooleate, α-monolinolenate, coixol, coixenolide, coixenopolysaccharide, etc. It has the functions of anti-tumor, regulating immunity, lowering blood sugar, reducing blood calcium, anti-inflammatory, analgesic, antipyretic, sedative, stimulating uterus, etc.

猪苓 *Zhū líng* (Polyporus)
《神农本草经》
Shen Nong's Classic of the Materia Medica (Shén Nóng Běn Cǎo Jīng)

【来源 / Origin】

为多孔菌科真菌猪苓 *Polyporus umbellatus*（Pers.）Fries 的干燥菌核，寄生于桦树、枫树、柞树的根上。主产于陕西、山西、河北等地。春秋采挖，干燥，切片，生用。本品气微，味淡。《中国药典》规定，含麦角甾醇（$C_{28}H_{44}O$）不得少于 0.070%。

Zhū líng is the dried sclerotium of *Polyporus umbellatus* (Pers.) Fries, pertaining to Polyporaceae, parasitic on the roots of birch, maple and tussah. It is mainly produced in Shaanxi, Shanxi and Hebei Province, mainly collected in spring and autumn, sliced into thick pieces, dried in the shade and used raw. It has slight odor and bland in flavor. According to *Chinese Pharmacopoeia*, the content of ergosterol ($C_{28}H_{44}O$) should be no less than 0.070%.

【性味归经 / Medicinal properties】

甘、淡，平。归肾、膀胱经。

Sweet, bland and neutral; act on kidney and bladder meridians.

【主要功效 / Medicinal efficacies】

利水渗湿。

Promote diuresis and drain dampness.

【临床应用 / Clinical application】

水肿，泄泻，淋浊，带下　本品甘淡渗泄，药性沉降，功专通水道，利小便，祛水湿，其作用强于茯苓，凡水湿停滞之证均可选用。若治水湿内停之小便不利、水肿，常与茯苓、泽泻、桂枝等配伍。若治水湿泄泻，可与茯苓、苍术、厚朴等同用。若治水热互结，阴虚小便不利、水肿，多与滑石、泽泻、阿胶等同用。若治湿热淋证，可与木通、滑石等同用。若治湿热带下，可与茯苓、车前子、泽泻等配伍。

Edema, diarrhea, turbid stranguria, and leucorrhea　*Zhū líng* is sweet and bland in flavor, draining and purgative, functioning to sink and descend. It can regulate water passages, promote diuresis as well as drain water and dampness and usually indicated for retention of water and dampness with the efficacy superior to *fú líng*. To treat dysuria and edema due to retention of water and dampness, it is combined with *fú líng*, *zé xiè* and *guì zhī*. To treat diarrhea due to water and dampness, it is combined with *fú líng*, *cāng zhú* and *hòu pò*. To treat dysuria or edema due to dampness-heat interaction and yin deficiency, it is combined with *huá shí*, *zé xiè* and *ē jiāo*. For stranguria due to dampness-heat, it is used together with *mù tōng* and *huá shí*. To treat leucorrhea due to dampness-heat, it is combined together with *fú líng*, *chē qián zǐ* and *zé xiè*.

【用法用量 / Usage and dosage】

煎服，6~12g。

Decoction, 6-12g.

【现代研究 / Modern research】

本品主要含麦角甾醇、猪苓多糖、猪苓聚糖、猪苓酸、猪苓酮、氨基酸等。具有利尿、抗肿瘤、保肝、调节免疫、抗肾结石形成、抗辐射、抗衰老等作用。

Zhū líng mainly contains ergosterol, polyporusus bellatus, polyporus polysaccharide, polyporus acid, polyporus ketone, amino acid, etc. It has the functions of promoting urination, anti-tumor, protecting liver, regulating immunity, resisting kidney stone formation, resisting radiation, anti-aging and so on.

泽泻 *Zé xiè* (Alismatis Rhizoma)
《神农本草经》
Shen Nong's Classic of the Materia Medica (Shén Nóng Běn Cǎo Jīng)

【来源 / Origin】

为泽泻科植物东方泽泻 *Alisma orientalis*（Sam.）Juzep. 或泽泻 *Alisma Plantago-aquatica* Linn. 的干燥块茎。主产于福建、四川、江西等地。冬季采挖，切厚片，晒干，麸炒或盐水炒用。本品气微，味微苦。《中国药典》规定，含 23-乙酰泽泻醇 B（$C_{32}H_{50}O_5$）和 23-乙酰泽泻醇 C（$C_{32}H_{48}O_6$）的总量不得少于 0.10%。

Zé xiè is the dried stem tuber of *Alisma orientalis* (Sam.)Juzep., or *Alisma Plantago-aquatica* Linn., pertaining to Alismataceae, mainly produced in Fujian, Sichuan and Jiangxi Province, collected in winter, sliced into thick pieces, dried in the sunshine, and used raw or stir-fried with bran or salt. It has slight odor and slightly bitter in flavor. According to *Chinese Pharmacopoeia*, the total content of 23-acetylalisol B ($C_{32}H_{50}O_5$) and 23-acetylalisol C ($C_{32}H_{48}O_6$) should be no less than 0.10%.

【性味归经 / Medicinal properties】

甘、淡，寒。归肾、膀胱经。

Sweet, bland and cold; act on the kidney and bladder meridians.

【主要功效 / Medicinal efficacies】

利水渗湿，泄热，化浊降脂。

Promote diuresis and drain dampness; expel heat; resolve turbidity and lower lipid.

【临床应用 / Clinical application】

1. 水肿，小便不利，泄泻，痰饮 本品甘淡渗利，入膀胱经，善于渗泄水湿，通利小便，其作用较茯苓为强，凡是水湿为患的病证均可选用。若治水湿内停之水肿、小便不利，常与茯苓、猪苓同用。若治痰饮内停，头目昏眩，常与白术同用。若治脾湿过盛，浮肿泄泻，可与厚朴、苍术、猪苓等同用。

(1) Edema, dysuria, diarrhea and phlegm-fluid retention *Zé xiè* is sweet and bland in flavor, acting on bladder meridian with the main functions of draining water and dampness, and promoting diuresis, and is especially useful for water and dampness accumulation syndromes with efficacies superior to *fú líng*. To treat edema and dysuria due to retention of water and dampness, it is combined with *fú líng* and *zhū líng*. To treat diarrhea and dizziness due to phlegm retention, it is combined with *bái zhú*. To treat edema and diarrhea due to profuse dampness in spleen, it is combined with *hòu pò*, *cāng zhú* and *zhū líng*.

2. 淋证，带下，遗精 本品药性寒凉，既能渗湿，又善清肾与膀胱之热，下焦湿热者尤为适宜。用治湿热淋证，常与木通、车前子等同用。用治湿热带下，常与车前子、木通、龙胆等同用。用治肾阴不足，相火亢盛之遗精、潮热、盗汗等，可与熟地黄、知母、黄柏等同用。

(2) Stranguria, leucorrhea and seminal emission *Zé xiè* is cold in nature. It can drain dampness, eliminate heat in kidney and bladder and is especially useful for lower-energizer dampness-heat syndrome. To treat stranguria due to dampness-heat, it is often combined with *mù tōng* and *chē qián zǐ*.

For leukorrhea due to dampness-heat, it is often combined with *chē qián zǐ*, *mù tōng* and *lóng dǎn*. For seminal emission, tidal fever and night sweat due to the deficiency of kidney yin or excess of ministerial fire, it is combined with *shú dì huáng*, *zhī mǔ* and *huáng bó*.

3. 高脂血症 本品利水渗湿，又化浊降脂。常用治高脂血症，可与决明子、荷叶、何首乌等同用。

(3) Hyperlipidemia *Zé xiè* can induce diuresis and drain dampness, as well as resolve turbidity and lower lipid. For hyperlipidemia, it is combined with *jué míng zǐ*, *hé yè* and *hé shǒu wū*.

【用法用量 / Usage and dosage 】

煎服，6~10g。

Decoction, 6-10g.

【现代研究 / Modern research 】

本品主要含四环三萜酮醇类成分：泽泻醇 A、泽泻醇 B、泽泻醇 C、泽泻醇 A 乙酸酯、泽泻醇 B 单乙酸酯、23- 乙酰泽泻醇等，尚含少量挥发油、生物碱、黄酮、蛋白质等。具有利尿、降血脂、抗脂肪肝、抗动脉硬化、降血压、保肝、抗炎、调节免疫等作用。

It mainly contains tetracyclic triterpenol ketones: alisol A, B, C, alisol A acetate, alisol B monoacetate, 23-acetylalisol, etc., and a small amount of volatile oil, alkaloids, flavonoids, proteins, etc. It has the functions of promoting urination, lowering blood lipid, resisting fatty liver, anti arteriosclerosis, lowering blood pressure, protecting liver, anti inflammation, regulating immunity, etc.

第二节 利尿通淋药

Section 2 Stranguria-relieving diuretic medicinals

PPT

本类药物多味苦或甘淡，性偏寒凉，主入膀胱、小肠经，善走下焦，长于清利下焦湿热，以利尿通淋为主要功效，主要用于湿热蕴结下焦所致的热淋、血淋、石淋、膏淋，症见小便频数短涩，滴沥刺痛，欲出未尽，小腹拘急，或痛引腰腹者。

These medicinals are mostly bitter, or sweet and bland in flavor, slightly cold in nature, acting on bladder and small intestine meridians, with the main functions of clearing heat and draining dampness in lower energizer to induce diuresis to treat stranguria. They are indicated for heat stranguria, blood stranguria, stony stranguria and chylous stranguria due to the accumulation of dampness and heat in lower energizer, manifested as frequent, short, difficult and painful dribbling urination, contraction in stomach, or pain in waist and stomach.

车前子　*Chē qián zǐ* (Plantaginis Semen)

《神农本草经》

Shen Nong's Classic of the Materia Medica (Shén Nóng Běn Cǎo Jīng)

【来源 / Origin 】

为车前科植物车前 *Plantago asiatica* L. 或平车前 *Plantago depressa* Willd. 的干燥成熟种子。前者分布于全国各地，后者分布于北方各省。夏、秋采收，晒干，生用或盐水炙用。本品气微，味淡。《中国药典》规定，含京尼平苷酸（$C_{16}H_{22}O_{10}$）不得少于 0.50%，毛蕊花糖苷（$C_{29}H_{36}O_{15}$）不得少于 0.40%。

Chē qián zǐ is the dried mature seed of *Plantago asiatica* L. or *Plantago depressa* Willd., pertaining to Plantaginaceae. The former is produced all over the country; the latter is mainly produced in northern provinces. It is collected in spring and autumn, dried in the sunshine, and used raw or stir-fried with salty water. It has slight odor and bland in flavor. According to *Chinese Pharmacopoeia*, the content of geniposide ($C_{16}H_{22}O_{10}$) should be no less than 0.50%, and the content of mullein glycoside ($C_{29}H_{36}O_{15}$) should be no less than 0.40%.

【性味归经 / Medicinal properties 】

甘，微寒。归肝、肾、肺、小肠经。

Sweet and slightly cold; act on liver, kidney, lung and small intestine meridians.

【主要功效 / Medicinal efficacies 】

清热利尿通淋，渗湿止泻，明目，祛痰。

Clear heat, promote diuresis to relive stranguria; drain dampness, stop diarrhea; improve vision; expel phlegm.

【临床应用 / Clinical application 】

1. 淋证，水肿　本品甘寒滑利，善通利水道，清膀胱热结，导湿热下行从小便而出，为治湿热下注之淋证、水肿的常用药。用治热淋，常配伍木通、滑石、瞿麦等。用治血淋，常与小蓟、白茅根、蒲黄等同用。用治石淋，常与金钱草、海金沙、滑石等同用。用治膏淋，可与萆薢、石韦、萹蓄等同用。用治水湿内停之水肿胀满、小便不利，常与茯苓、猪苓、泽泻等配伍。

(1) Stranguria and edema　*Chē qián zǐ* is sweet, cold and slippery in nature, with the function of regulating water passages, clearing heat accumulation in bladder, and clear dampness-heat through urination. It is a commonly used medicinal to treat stranguria and edema due to downpour of dampness-heat. For heat stranguria, it is often combined with *mù tōng*, *huá shí* and *qú mài*. For blood stranguria, it is often combined with *xiǎo jì*, *bái máo gēn* and *pú huáng*. For stony stranguria, it is often combined with *jīn qián cǎo*, *hǎi jīn shā* and *huá shí*. For chylous stranguria, it is often combined with *bì xiè*, *shí wéi* and *biǎn xù*. For edema and dysuria due to retention of water and dampness, it is often combined with *fú líng*, *zhū líng* and *zé xiè*.

2. 泄泻　本品能利水湿、分清浊而止泻，即利小便以实大便。尤宜于湿盛之水泻，可单用本品研末，米饮送服；或与白术、茯苓、泽泻等同用。

(2) Diarrhea　*Chē qián zǐ* can drain water and dampness, stop diarrhea based on clarity and turbidity, and treat diarrhea with diuretics. It is good at treating diarrhea due to exuberant dampness. It is used alone and ground into powder for taking orally with rice water or combined together with *bái zhú*, *fú líng* and *zé xiè*.

3. 目赤肿痛　本品性寒清热，主入肝经，善清肝热而能明目。用治肝热目赤肿痛，常与菊花、夏枯草、决明子等配伍。用治肝肾阴亏，两目昏花，须配伍菟丝子、熟地黄等。

(3) Conjunctivitis　*Chē qián zǐ* is cold in nature and can clear heat, acting on liver meridian with the function of clearing liver-fire to improve vision. In treating conjunctivitis due to liver heat, it is often combined with *jú huā*, *xià kū cǎo* and *jué míng zǐ*. For blurry and poor vision or nebula due to liver-kidney yin deficiency, it is combined with *tù sī zǐ* and *shú dì huáng*.

4. 痰热咳嗽　本品性寒入肺，能清肺化痰止咳。用治肺热咳嗽，痰黄黏稠，常与瓜蒌、浙贝母、黄芩等同用。

(4) Cough of phlegm-heat type　*Chē qián zǐ* is cold in nature and acts on lung meridian, clear lung to resolve phlegm, and stop cough. For cough, yellow and sticky phlegm due to lung-heat, it is combined with *guā lóu*, *zhè bèi mǔ* and *huáng qín*.

【用法用量 / Usage and dosage】

煎服，9~15g，包煎。

Decocted, 9-15g, wrap-decocting.

【使用注意 / Precaution】

孕妇及肾虚精滑者慎用。

It should be used with caution for pregnant women and those with spermatorrhea due to kidney deficiency.

【现代研究 / Modern research】

本品主要含桃叶珊瑚苷、京尼平苷酸、都桷子苷酸，尚含毛蕊花糖苷、消旋－车前子苷、车前子酸、琥珀酸、脂肪油、维生素A和B等。具有利尿、排石、祛痰、镇咳、抗炎、缓泻、降血糖等作用。

It mainly contains aucubin, geniposide, dauricoside, mullein glycoside, racemic plantain, succinic acid, fatty oil, vitamin A and B, etc. It has the functions of promoting urination, expelling stone, expelling phlegm, relieving cough, anti-inflammation, relieving diarrhea, and decreasing blood glucose.

滑石　*Huá shí* (Talcum)
《神农本草经》
Shen Nong's Classic of the Materia Medica (Shén Nóng Běn Cǎo Jīng)

【来源 / Origin】

为硅酸盐类矿物滑石族滑石，主含含水硅酸镁〔Mg₃（Si₄O₁₀）(OH)₂〕。主产于山东、江西、山西等地。全年可采，粉碎成细粉用，或水飞晾干用。本品气微，味淡。

Huá shí is the steatite of the silicate mineral, pertaining to Talcum. The main medicinal component is magnesium silicate hydrate〔$Mg_3 (Si_4O_{10})(OH)_2$〕. It is mainly produced in Shandong, Jiangxi and Shanxi Province, collected all the year round, ground into powder, or refined with water. It has slight odor and bland in taste.

【性味归经 / Medicinal properties】

甘、淡，寒。归膀胱、肺、胃经。

Sweet, bland and cold; act on bladder, lung and stomach meridians.

【主要功效 / Medicinal efficacies】

利尿通淋，清热解暑；外用祛湿敛疮。

Promote diuresis to relive stranguria; clear heat and resolve summer-heat; dispel dampness and promote healing sores.

【临床应用 / Clinical application】

1. **热淋，石淋**　本品性寒滑利，寒能清热，滑能利窍，善于开通下窍，清利膀胱湿热，有良好的利尿通淋之功，为治疗淋证的常用药，尤宜于热淋、石淋。若治热淋，小便淋沥涩痛，常与木通、车前子、瞿麦等同用。若治石淋，可与海金沙、金钱草、木通等同用。

(1) **Heat stranguria and stony stranguria**　*Huá shí* is cold and acts for clearing heat and benefit orifices. It is good at opening lower orifices, clearing heat and draining dampness in bladder with good efficacies of inducing diuresis to treat stranguria. It is a commonly used medicinal for stranguria, especially for heat stranguria and stony stranguria. To treat heat stranguria, painful dribbling urination, it

is combined with *mù tōng*, *chē qián zǐ* and *qú mài*. To treat stony stranguria, it is combined with *hǎi jīn shā*, *jīn qián cǎo* and *mù tōng*.

2. 暑湿，湿温，湿热水泻　本品甘淡性寒，既能利水，又能解暑热，为治暑湿、湿温的常用药。用治暑热烦渴，小便短赤，常与甘草同用。用治湿温初起或暑温夹湿，头痛恶寒，身重胸闷，常与杏仁、白蔻仁、薏苡仁等同用。若治湿热水泻，可与茯苓、车前子、薏苡仁等同用。

(2) Summer-heat dampness, damp-warmth and watery diarrhea due to dampness-heat *Huá shí* is sweet, bland and cold in nature with the functions of inducing diuresis and resolving summer-heat. It is a commonly used medicinal for summer-heat dampness and damp-warmth. In treating restlessness and thirst due to summer-heat-dampness, scanty and brown urine, it is often combined with *gān cǎo*. To treat damp-warmth at the beginning, or summer-heat with dampness, manifested as headache, aversion to cold, and oppression of the chest, it is combined with *xìng rén*, *bái kòu rén* and *yì yǐ rén*. For watery diarrhea due to dampness-heat, it is combined with *fú líng*, *chē qián zǐ* and *yì yǐ rén*.

3. 湿疹，湿疮，痱子　本品外用有清热、祛湿敛疮作用，为治湿疹、湿疮的常用药，可单用，或与黄柏、煅石膏、枯矾等配伍，外敷或撒布于患处。若治痱子，常与薄荷、甘草等配制成痱子粉外用。

(3) Eczema, damp sores, miliaria *Huá shí* has functions of clearing heat, expelling dampness and astringing sores for external use and is often used to treat eczema and damp sores alone or combined with *huáng bó*, *duàn shí gāo* and *kū fán* for external application on the affected area. To treat miliaria, it is combined with *bò he* and *gān cǎo* to make prickly-heat powder for external use.

【用法用量 / Usage and dosage】

煎服，10~20g，先煎。外用适量。

Decocted, 10-20g, to be decocted first. Appropriate amount for external use.

【现代研究 / Modern research】

本品主要含含水硅酸镁，尚含氧化铝、氧化镍等成分。具有利尿、吸附、收敛、抑菌等作用，内服能保护肠壁，有止泻作用；外用有保护创面、吸收分泌物、促进结痂的作用。

It mainly contains magnesium silicate hydrate, alumina, nickel oxide and other components. It has diuretic, adsorption, astringent and bacteriostatic effects. Oral administration can protect the intestinal wall and relieve diarrhea. External use can protect wound, absorb secretion and promote scab formation.

> ## 木通　*Mù tōng* (Akebiae Caulis)
> ### 《神农本草经》
> *Shen Nong's Classic of the Materia Medica* (*Shén Nóng Běn Cǎo Jīng*)

【来源 / Origin】

为木通科植物木通 *Akebia quinata*（Thunb.）Decne.、三叶木通 *Akebia trifoliata*（Thunb.）Koidz. 或白木通 *Akebia trifoliata*（Thunb.）Koidz.var.*australis*（Diels）Rehd. 的干燥藤茎。主产于江苏、湖南、湖北等地。秋季采收，阴干，切片，生用。本品气微，味微苦而涩。《中国药典》规定，含木通苯乙醇苷 B（$C_{23}H_{26}O_{11}$）不得少于 0.15%。

Mù tōng is the rattan and stalk of *Akebia quinata* (Thunb.) Decne., *Akebia trifoliata* (Thunb.) Koidz. or *Akebia trifbliata* (Thunb.) Koidz. var.*australis*(Diels)Rehd., pertaining to Akebiaceae, mainly produced in Jiangsu, Hunan and Hubei Province, collected in autumn, dried in the shade, sliced and used raw. It has slight odor and slightly bitter, astringent in flavor. According to *Chinese Pharmacopoeia*, the content of paeonoside B ($C_{23}H_{26}O_{11}$) should be no less than 0.15%.

【性味归经 / Medicinal properties】

苦，寒。归心、小肠、膀胱经。

Bitter and cold; act on heart, small intestine and bladder meridians.

【主要功效 / Medicinal efficacies】

利尿通淋，清心除烦，通经下乳。

Promote diuresis to relieve stranguria, clear heart-heat and relieve vexation, promote menstruation and lactation.

【临床应用 / Clinical application】

1. **淋证，水肿**　本品苦寒性降，善清膀胱湿热，具有较强的清热利尿之功。治疗膀胱湿热，小便短赤，淋沥涩痛，常与车前子等同用。本品尚能利尿消肿，用治水肿，小便不利，脚气肿胀，可与猪苓、桑白皮等同用。

(1) Stranguria and edema　*Mù tōng* descends with bitter cold and is good at clearing dampness-heat in bladder and induce diuresis. For dampness-heat in bladder, short voiding of dark urine, and painful dribbling urination, it is combined with *chē qián zǐ*. It can also induce diuresis to alleviate edema. To treat edema, difficulty in urination, and beriberi, it is combined with *zhū líng* and *sāng bái pí*.

2. **心烦尿赤，口舌生疮**　本品苦寒泄热，主入心、小肠经，能上清心经之火，下导小肠之热，以利尿通淋。常用治心火上炎，口舌生疮，或心火下移小肠之心烦、尿赤，常配伍生地黄、甘草、竹叶等。

(2) Vexation and dark urine, sore in mouth and tongue　*Mù tōng* is bitter in flavor and cold in nature, acting on heart and small intestine meridians with the function of inducing diuresis to treat stranguria by clearing heart-meridian fire in the upper energizer, and eliminating small intestine heat in the lower energizer. It is suitable for treating sores in mouth and tongue due to heart fire flaming upward, or vexation and dark urine due to heart fare moving downward to the small intestine usually combined with *shēng dì huáng*, *gān cǎo* and *zhú yè*.

3. **经闭乳少，湿热痹痛**　本品入血分，能通血脉、下乳汁。用治血瘀经闭，与红花、桃仁、丹参等同用。用治产后乳少或不通，可与王不留行、穿山甲等同用。本品尚能清湿热，通经脉，利关节，用治湿热痹痛，可与秦艽、防己、薏苡仁等同用。

(3) Amenorrhea and insufficient lactation, dampness-heat type impediment　*Mù tōng* enters the blood aspect, promotes blood circulation and lactation. In treating amenorrhea due to blood stasis, it is combined with *hóng huā*, *táo rén* and *dān shēn*. To treat post-partum galactostasis, it is often combined with *wáng bù liú xíng* (Vaccariae Semen) and *chuān shān jiǎ* (Manitis Squama). It also can clear dampness-heat, dredge the collaterals and joints, so it is able to treat dampness-heat type impediment in combination with *qín jiāo*, *fáng jǐ* and *yì yǐ rén*.

【用法用量 / Usage and dosage】

煎服，3~6g。

Decoction, 3-6g.

【使用注意 / Precaution】

孕妇慎用。不宜大量或长期服用。

It should be used with caution when treating pregnant women. It should not be taken in a large amount or for a long time.

【现代研究 / Modern research】

本品主要含常春藤皂苷元、齐墩果酸、木通皂苷、白桦脂醇、木通苯乙醇苷 B，尚含豆甾醇、β-谷甾醇、胡萝卜苷、钾盐等。具有利尿、抗炎、抗菌等作用。

It mainly contains ivy sapogenin, oleanolic acid, Mutong sapogenin, betulin, Mutong phenylethanolic glycoside B, and also includes stigmasterol, β-sitosterol, carotene, potassium salt, etc. It has diuretic, anti-inflammatory and antibacterial effects.

萆薢 *Bì xiè* (Dioscoreae Rhizoma)
《神农本草经》
Shen Nong's Classic of the Materia Medica (Shén Nóng Běn Cǎo Jīng)

【来源 / Origin】

为薯蓣科植物绵萆薢 *Dioscorea spongiosa* Thunb. 或福州薯蓣 *Dioscorea futschauensis* Uline ex R. Kunth 和粉背薯蓣 *Dioscorea hypoglauca* Palibin 的干燥根茎。前两种称"绵萆薢"，主产于浙江、福建；后者称"粉萆薢"，主产于安徽、浙江、江西等地。秋、冬季采挖，切片，晒干，生用。绵萆薢气微，味微苦；粉萆薢味辛、微苦。

Bì xiè is the dry rhizome of *Dioscorea spongiosa* Thunb. or *Dioscorea futschauensis* Uline ex R. Kunth and *Dioscorea hypoglauca* Palibin. The first two species are called *mián bì xiè* mainly produced in Zhejiang and Fujian Province; the latter is called *fěn bì xiè* mainly produced in Anhui, Zhejiang, and Jiangxi Province. It is collected in autumn and winter, sliced, dried in the sun, and used raw. *Mián bì xiè* has a slight odor and slightly bitter taste, while *fěn bì xiè* is acrid and slightly bitter.

【性味归经 / Medicinal properties】

苦，平。归肾、胃经。

Bitter and neutral; act on the kidney and stomach meridians.

【主要功效 / Medicinal efficacies】

利湿去浊，祛风除痹。

Drain dampness and remove turbidity; dispel wind and relieve impediment.

【临床应用 / Clinical application】

1. **膏淋，白浊，白带过多** 本品苦降下行，善能利湿而分清去浊，为治膏淋、白浊之要药，常与益智仁、石菖蒲、乌药等同用。若治妇女湿盛白带过多者，可与薏苡仁、白术、泽泻等同用。

(1) Chylous stranguria, whitish and turbid urine and leucorrhea *Bì xiè* is bitter and functions to descend, good at promoting urination and removing turbidity. It is the principal medicinal to treat chylous stranguria and whitish and turbid urine combined with *yì yǐ rén*, *shí chāng pú* and *wū yào*. For leucorrhea due to profuse dampness, it is combined with *yì yǐ rén*, *bái zhú* and *zé xiè*.

2. **风湿痹痛，关节不利，腰膝疼痛** 本品能祛风除湿，通络止痛，可用治风湿痹痛，关节不利，腰膝疼痛。因其性平，长于除湿，故寒热皆宜，但尤宜于湿盛着痹。若治寒湿痹痛，可与附子、牛膝等同用。若治湿热痹痛，常与防己、黄柏、忍冬藤等配伍。

(2) Wind-dampness arthralgia, joint stiffness, pain in the loins and knees *Bì xiè* can eliminate wind and remove dampness, activate meridians to stop pain, with the function of treating wind-dampness arthralgia, joint stiffness, and pain in the loins and knee. For it is neutral in nature, it is good at removing dampness and suitable for chills and fever, especially for arthralgia due to profuse dampness. For cold-dampness arthralgia, it is combined with *fù zǐ* and *niú xī*. For dampness-heat arthralgia, it is often combined with *fáng jǐ*, *huáng bó* and *rěn dōng téng*.

【用法用量 / Usage and dosage】

煎服，9~15g。

Decoction, 9-15g.

【使用注意 / Precaution】

肾阴亏虚，遗精滑泄者慎用。

It should be used with caution for those with deficiency of kidney yin, spermatorrhea and efflux diarrhea.

【现代研究 / Modern research】

本品主要含薯蓣皂苷等多种甾体皂苷，尚含鞣质、淀粉、蛋白质等。具有抗痛风、抗骨质疏松、抗心肌缺血、抗肿瘤、抗菌等作用。

It mainly contains diosgenin and other steroidal saponins, as well as tannin, starch, protein and so on. It has the functions of anti gout, anti osteoporosis, anti myocardial ischemia, anti-tumor and anti-bacterial.

石韦　*Shí wéi* (Pyrrosiae Folium)
《神农本草经》
Shen Nong's Classic of the Materia Medica (Shén Nóng Běn Cǎo Jīng)

【来源 / Origin】

为水龙骨科植物庐山石韦 *Pyrrosia sheareri*（Bak.）Ching、石韦 *Pyrrosia lingua*（Thunb.）Farwell 或有柄石韦 *Pyrrosia petiolosa*（Christ）Ching 的干燥叶。主产于浙江、湖北、河北等地。全年均可采收，晒干或阴干，切段，生用。本品气微，味微涩苦。《中国药典》规定，含绿原酸（$C_{16}H_{18}O_9$）不得少于 0.20%。

Shí wéi is the dried leaf of *Pyrrosia sheareri* (Bak.) Ching, or *Pyrrosia lingua* (Thunb.) Farwell, or *Pyrrosia patiolosa* (Christ) Ching, pertaining to Polypodiaceae, mainly produced in Zhejiang, Hubei and Hebei Province, collected all the year round, dried in the sunshine or in the shade, cut into segments, and used raw. It has slight odor and slightly astringent and bitter in flavor. According to *Chinese Pharmacopoeia*, the content of chlorogenic acid ($C_{16}H_{18}O_9$) should be no less than 0.20%.

【性味归经 / Medicinal properties】

甘、苦，微寒。归肺、膀胱经。

Sweet, bitter and slightly cold; act on the lung and bladder meridians.

【主要功效 / Medicinal efficacies】

利尿通淋，清肺止咳，凉血止血。

Promote urination to relieve stranguria; clear lung to stop cough; cool blood to stop bleeding.

【临床应用 / Clinical application】

1. 淋证　本品苦寒性降，善能清利膀胱湿热，具有清热利尿通淋之功，为治疗淋证的常用品。因其兼能凉血止血，故治血淋尤宜，常与白茅根、小蓟等同用。若治热淋，可与滑石、车前子等同用。若治石淋，常配伍鸡内金、海金沙、金钱草等。

(1) **Stranguria**　*Shí wéi* is bitter and cold, functioning to descend, and can clear heat and drain dampness in bladder to induce urination to treat stranguria. It is a commonly used medicinal for stranguria. Since it can cool blood to stop bleeding, it is suitable to treat blood stranguria in combination with *bái máo gēn* and *xiǎo jì*. For heat stranguria, it is used with *huá shí* and *chē qián zǐ*, for stony stranguria, it is combined with *jī nèi jīn, hǎi jīn shā, jīn qián cǎo*.

2. 肺热咳喘　本品入肺，能清肺热，止咳喘。用治肺热咳喘，可与鱼腥草、黄芩、芦根等同用。

(2) Dyspnea and cough due to lung heat *Shí wéi* acts on lung meridian and can clear lung heat, stop dyspnea and cough. For dyspnea and cough due to lung heat, it is combined with *yú xīng cǎo*, *huáng qín* and *lú gēn*.

3. 吐血、衄血、尿血、崩漏　本品性寒，入血分，能凉血止血。用治血热妄行之吐血、衄血、尿血、崩漏等多种出血，可单用，或随证配伍侧柏叶、栀子、小蓟等。

(3) Hematemesis, nose-bleeding, hematuria, metrorrhagia and metrostaxis *Shí wéi* is cold in nature, enters the blood aspect, and can cool blood to stop bleeding. In treating hematemesis, nose-bleeding, hematuria, metrorrhagia and metrostaxis due to blood-heat, it can be used alone or combined with *cè bǎi yè*, *zhī zǐ* and *xiǎo jì*.

【用法用量 / Usage and dosage】

煎服，6~12g。

Decoction, 6-12g.

【现代研究 / Modern research】

本品主要含绿原酸、山奈素、槲皮素、异槲皮素、三叶豆苷、甘草苷、芒果苷等。具有抑菌、保护肾脏、镇咳祛痰、降血糖、抗Ⅰ型单纯疱疹病毒（HSVⅠ）、抑制血小板聚集等作用。

It mainly contains chlorogenic acid, kaempferol, quercetin, isoquercetin, trifolioside, liquiritigenin, mangiferin, etc. It has the functions of inhibiting bacteria, protecting kidney, relieving cough, dispelling phlegm, reducing blood glucose, anti herpes simplex virus Ⅰ (HSVⅠ) and inhibiting platelet aggregation.

海金沙　*Hǎi jīn shā* (Lygodii Spora)
《嘉祐本草》
Materia Medica of Jiayou Era (Jiā Yòu Běn Cǎo)

【来源 / Origin】

为海金沙科植物海金沙 *Lygodium japonicum*（Thunb.）Sw. 的干燥成熟孢子。主产于广东、浙江等地。秋季采收，晒干，生用。本品气微，味淡。

Hǎi jīn shā is the dried mature spore of *Lygodium japonicum* (Thunb.) Sw., pertaining to Lygodiaceae. It is mainly produced in Guangdong and Zhejiang Province, collected in autumn, dried in the sunshine, and used raw. It has slight odor and bland flavor.

【性味归经 / Medicinal properties】

甘、咸，寒。归膀胱、小肠经。

Sweet, salty and cold; act on the bladder and small intestine meridians.

【主要功效 / Medicinal efficacies】

清热利湿，通淋止痛。

Clear heat and drain dampness, relieve stranguria and pain.

【临床应用 / Clinical application】

诸淋涩痛　本品甘寒性降，善通水道，清泄小肠、膀胱湿热，功专利尿通淋，尤善止尿道疼痛，为治诸淋尿道涩痛之要药。若治热淋，可与车前子、木通等同用。若治石淋，常与金钱草、鸡内金等配伍。若治血淋，多与小蓟、石韦等同用。若治膏淋，则与滑石、甘草等同用。

Stranguria syndromes accompanied with astringent pain *Hǎi jīn shā* is sweet and cold, functioning to descend, and can promote water passages, dissipate and discharge dampness-heat in small intestine and bladder. It is good at inducing diuresis to relieve stranguria, especially treating pain of the urethra, and it is the principal medicinal for treating different stranguria syndromes with astringent pain. For heat stranguria, it is often combined with *chē qián zǐ* and *mù tōng*. For stony stranguria, it is combined with *jīn qián cǎo* and *jī nèi jīn*. For bloody stranguria, it is used together with *xiǎo jì* and *shí wéi*. For creamy stranguria, it is combined together with *huá shí* and *gān cǎo*.

此外，本品又能利尿消肿，也可用治水肿、小便不利。

In addition, it induces diuresis to relieve edema, so it can treat edema and inhibited urination.

【用法用量 / Usage and dosage 】

煎服，6~15g，包煎。

Decoction, 6-15g, wrap-decocting.

【使用注意 / Precaution 】

肾阴亏虚者慎服。

It should be used with caution for those with deficiency of kidney yin.

【现代研究 / Modern research 】

本品主要含棕榈酸、油酸、亚油酸以及金沙素等。具有抑菌、利胆、增加输尿管蠕动频率等作用。

It mainly contains palmitic acid, oleic acid, linoleic acid and kinshasin. It has the functions of inhibiting bacteria, promoting gallbladder function and increasing the frequency of ureteral peristalsis.

瞿麦 *Qú mài* (Dianthi Herba)
《神农本草经》
Shen Nong's Classic of the Materia Medica (Shén Nóng Běn Cǎo Jīng)

【来源 / Origin 】

为石竹科植物瞿麦 *Dianthus superbus* L. 或石竹 *Dianthus chinensis* L. 的干燥地上部分。主产于河北、河南、辽宁等地。夏、秋采收，干燥，切段，生用。本品气微，味淡。

Qú mài is the dried portion above the ground of *Dianthus superbus* L. or *Dianthus chinensis* L., pertaining to Caryophyllaceae, mainly produced in Hebei, Henan and Liaoning Province, collected in summer and autumn, cut into segments, dried in the sunshine, and used raw. It has slight odor and is bland in flavor.

【性味归经 / Medicinal properties 】

苦，寒。归心、小肠经。

Bitter and cold; act on the heart and small intestine meridians.

【主要功效 / Medicinal efficacies 】

利尿通淋，活血通经。

Promote urination and relieve stranguria, activate the blood and promote menstruation.

【临床应用 / Clinical application 】

1. **淋证**　本品苦寒降泄，能清心与小肠之火，导热下行，有利尿通淋之功，为治淋证常用药。用治热淋，多与木通、车前子等同用。用治血淋，常与小蓟、白茅根等同用。用治石淋，常与金钱草、滑石等配伍。

(1) **Stranguria**　*Qú mài* is bitter and cold, functioning to descend and purge, can clear heat in heart and small intestine, and induce diuresis to treat stranguria. It is a commonly used medicinal for stranguria. For heat stranguria, it is combined with *mù tōng* and *chē qián zǐ*. For bloody stranguria, it is combined with *xiǎo jì* and *bái máo gēn*. For stony stranguria, it is combined with *jīn qián cǎo* and *huá shí*.

2. 经闭瘀阻　本品苦泄下行，有活血通经之功。用治血热瘀阻之经闭或月经不调，多与益母草、赤芍、丹参等同用。

(2) Blood-stasis due to amenorrhea　*Qú mài* is bitter, functioning to descend and purge, and can activate the blood and promote menstruation. To treat amenorrhea and dysmenorrheal due to blood-stasis, it is combined with *yì mǔ cǎo*, *chì sháo* and *dān shēn*.

【用法用量 / Usage and dosage 】

煎服，9~15g。

Decoction, 9-15g.

【使用注意 / Precaution 】

孕妇慎用。

It should be used with caution for pregnant women.

【现代研究 / Modern research 】

本品主要含丁香酚、苯乙醇、苯甲酸苄酯、水杨酸苄酯、石竹皂苷及糖类等。具有利尿、抗衣原体、抑菌、兴奋肠道平滑肌、兴奋子宫、抑制心脏、降压等作用。

It mainly contains eugenol, phenylethanol, benzyl benzoate, benzyl salicylate, carnation saponin and sugar, etc. It has the functions of promoting urination, anti chlamydia, inhibiting bacteria, exciting intestinal smooth muscle, exciting uterus, inhibiting heart, reducing blood pressure, etc.

第三节　利湿退黄药

Section 3　Damp-excreting anti-icteric medicinals

PPT

本类药物性味多苦寒，入脾、胃、肝、胆经，以清利湿热、利胆退黄为主要功效。主治湿热黄疸，症见目黄、身黄、小便黄等，寒湿偏盛之阴黄亦可配伍使用。部分药物还可用治湿疮、湿疹、湿温等。

Damp-excreting anti-icteric medicinals are usually bitter in flavor and cold in property, acting on spleen, stomach, liver and gallbladder meridians with the main functions of clearing heat, draining dampness, and normalizing gallbladder to cure jaundice. They are indicated for jaundice due to dampness-heat, such as yellowish sclera, yellow skin and yellow urine, for yin jaundice due to abnormal exuberance of cold-dampness through combination. Some medicinals also treat eczema and dampness-warmth.

> ### 茵陈　*Yīn chén* (Artemisiae Scopariae Herba)
> 《神农本草经》
> *Shen Nong's Classic of the Materia Medica (Shén Nóng Běn Cǎo Jīng)*

【来源 / Origin 】

为菊科植物茵陈蒿 *Artemisia capillaris* Thunb. 或滨蒿 *Artemisia scoparia* Waldst. et Kit. 的干燥地上部分。主产于陕西、山西、安徽等地。春季或秋季采割，春季采收的习称"绵茵陈"，秋季采割的称"花茵陈"。晒干，切碎，生用。绵茵陈气清香，味微苦；花茵陈气芳香，味微苦。《中国药典》规定，绵茵陈含绿原酸（$C_{16}H_{18}O_9$）不得少于 0.50%；花茵陈含滨蒿内酯（$C_{11}H_{10}O_4$）不得少于 0.20%。

Yīn chén is the dried part above the ground of *Artemisia capillaris* Thunb. or *Artemisia scoparia* Waldst. et Kit., pertaining to Chrysanthemum. It is mainly produced in Shaanxi, Shanxi and Anhui Province, collected in spring or autumn. It is called *mián yīn chén* collected in spring, and *huā yīn chén* collected in autumn. It is dried in the sunshine, cut up and used raw. *Mián yīn chén* has delicate fragrance, slightly bitter in taste; *huā yīn chén* is fragrant and slightly bitter. According to *Chinese Pharmacopoeia*, the content of chlorogenic acid ($C_{16}H_{18}O_9$) in *mián yīn chén* should be no less than 0.50%; the content of scoparone ($C_{11}H_{10}O_4$) in *huā yīn chén* should be no less than 0.20%.

【性味归经 / Medicinal properties】

苦、辛，微寒。归脾、胃、肝、胆经。

Bitter, pungent and slightly cold; act on the spleen, stomach, liver and gallbladder meridians.

【主要功效 / Medicinal efficacies】

清利湿热，利胆退黄。

Clear and drain dampness-heat; promote gallbladder function to relieve jaundice.

【临床应用 / Clinical application】

1. 黄疸尿少　本品苦能燥湿，性寒清热，善能清利脾、胃、肝、胆湿热，使之从小便排出，具有良好的清利湿热、利胆退黄作用，为治黄疸之要药，无论湿热阳黄、寒湿阴黄皆可用之。因其性寒，以清利湿热见长，故尤善治湿热黄疸之身目发黄、黄色鲜明者，常与栀子、大黄同用。若治寒湿黄疸之黄色晦暗、畏寒腹胀者，则常与附子、干姜等配伍。

(1) **Jaundice and oliguria**　*Yīn chén* is bitter to dry dampness and cold to clear heat with the functions of clearing heat and eliminating dampness in spleen, stomach, liver and gallbladder through urine. The major efficacy is to clear away heat, eliminate dampness, and drain the gallbladder to relieve jaundice. It is main medicinal for treating jaundice, suitable for yang jaundice due to dampness-heat or yin jaundice due to cold-dampness. For it is cold in nature, it is especially used in the treatment of damp-heat jaundice with bright yellow eyes and body in combination with *zhī zǐ* and *dà huáng*. To treat cold-damp jaundice with dark yellow color, aversion to cold and abdominal distention, it is combined with *fù zǐ* and *gān jiāng*.

2. 湿温暑湿　本品气清芳香，清热利湿，兼可芳化湿浊。用治外感湿温或暑湿，发热困倦、胸闷腹胀、小便不利者，常与黄芩、滑石、广藿香等同用。

(2) **Dampness-warmth and summerheat-dampness**　*Yīn chén* is fragrant, clearing heat, eliminating dampness and transforming damp turbidity with aromatics. For dampness-warmth and summerheat-dampness, fever and drowsiness, thoracic oppression and abdominal distention, and inhibited urination, it is combined with *huáng qín*, *huá shí* and *guǎng huò xiāng*.

3. 湿疮瘙痒　本品能清利湿热，解毒疗疮。用治湿热内蕴之湿疮瘙痒，可与黄柏、苦参、地肤子等同用。

(3) **Eczema and pruritus**　*Yīn chén* is able to clear and eliminate dampness-heat, resolve toxins and relieve sores. To treat eczema and pruritus due to internal accumulation of dampness-heat, it is combined with *huáng bó*, *kǔ shēn* and *dì fū zǐ*.

【用法用量 / Usage and dosage】

煎服，6~15g。外用适量，煎汤熏洗。

Decoction, 6-15g. The appropriate amount is decocted for fumigating and washing externally.

【使用注意 / Precaution】

蓄血发黄及血虚萎黄者慎用。

It should be used with caution for patients with jaundice due to blood amassment and sallow yellow due to blood deficiency.

【现代研究 / Modern research】

本品主要含滨蒿内酯、东莨菪素、茵陈黄酮、蓟黄素、绿原酸、水杨酸等，尚含挥发油、三萜、甾体等。具有利胆、保肝、解热、利尿、降血压、抑菌、抗病毒、抗炎、抗肿瘤等作用。

It mainly contains scoparone, scopolamine, artemisia flavonoids, thistle flavin, chlorogenic acid, salicylic acid, etc., and also volatile oil, triterpenoids, steroids, etc. It has the functions of promoting gallbladder function, protecting liver, clearing heat, promoting urination, reducing blood pressure, inhibiting bacteria and virus, inhibiting inflammatory and antagonizing tumor.

金钱草　*Jīn qián cǎo* (Lysimachiae Herba)
《本草纲目拾遗》
Supplement to the Grand Compendium of Materia Medica (Běn Cǎo Gāng Mù Shí Yí)

【来源 / Origin】

为报春花科植物过路黄 *Lysimachia christinae* Hance 的干燥全草，习称大金钱草。主产于四川。夏、秋采收，晒干，切段，生用。本品气微，味淡。《中国药典》规定，含槲皮素（$C_{15}H_{10}O_7$）和山奈素（$C_{15}H_{10}O_6$）总量不得少于 0.10%。

Jīn qián cǎo is the dried whole plant of *Lysimachia christinae* Hance, pertaining to Primulaceae, also known as *dà jīn qián cǎo*. It is mainly produced in Sichuan province, collected in summer and autumn, cut into segments, dried in the sunshine, and used raw. It has a slight odor and is bland in flavor. According to *Chinese Pharmacopoeia*, the total content of quercetin ($C_{15}H_{10}O_7$) and kaempferol ($C_{15}H_{10}O_6$) should be no less than 0.10%.

【性味归经 / Medicinal properties】

甘、咸，微寒。归肝、胆、肾、膀胱经。

Sweet, salty and slightly cold; act on liver, gallbladder, kidney and bladder meridians.

【功效】

利湿退黄，利尿通淋，解毒消肿。

Eliminate dampness and relieve jaundice, promote urination and relieve stranguria, resolve toxins and relieve swelling.

【临床应用 / Clinical application】

1. 湿热黄疸，胆胀胁痛　本品甘淡渗湿，微寒清热，入肝胆经，能清湿热，退黄疸，排结石。用治湿热黄疸，常与茵陈、栀子、虎杖等配伍。用治肝胆结石，胆胀胁痛，常与郁金、茵陈、大黄等同用。

(1) **Damp-heat jaundice, gallbladder distension and hypochondriac pain**　*Jīn qián cǎo* is sweet and bland to drain dampness, slightly cold to clear heat, and acts in liver and gallbladder meridians with the functions of clearing dampness-heat, relieve jaundice, and expelling calculi. To treat damp-heat jaundice, it is often combined with *yīn chén*, *zhī zǐ* and *hǔ zhàng*. For calculi in liver and gallbladder, gallbladder distension, and hypochondriac pain, it is often combined with *yù jīn*, *yīn chén* and *dà huáng*.

2. 石淋，热淋　本品通利下窍，有清热利尿、通淋排石之功，为治石淋、热淋之要药。用治石淋，可单用大剂量煎汤代茶饮，或配伍海金沙、鸡内金、滑石等。用治热淋，常与车前子、瞿麦等同用。

(2) **Heat stranguria and stony stranguria**　*Jīn qián cǎo* promotes lower orifices with the

functions of clearing heat, promoting urination, relieving stranguria and expelling calculi. It is the principal medicinal to treat heat stranguria and stony stranguria. For stony stranguria, it can be decocted alone in a large amount instead of tea, or combined with *hǎi jīn shā*, *jī nèi jīn* and *huá shí*. For heat stranguria, it is often combined with *chē qián zǐ* and *qú mài*.

3. 痈肿疔疮，蛇虫咬伤　本品有解毒消肿之效，内服外敷皆效。用治痈肿疔疮，蛇虫咬伤，常单用鲜品捣烂取汁服并以渣外敷，或配伍金银花、蒲公英、白花蛇舌草等。

(3) Swollen carbuncle, furuncle and sores, snake or insect bite　*Jīn qián cǎo* is with the functions of eliminating toxins and relieving swelling. It can be taken orally or used for external application. It is used to treat swollen carbuncle, furuncle and sores, snake or insect bite. Juice can be ground out the fresh form and taken orally, and the dregs can be used as external applications. It may be used in combination with *jīn yín huā*, *pú gōng yīng* and *bái huā shé shé cǎo*.

【用法用量 / Usage and dosage】

煎服，15~60g，鲜品加倍。外用适量。

Decoction, 15-60g, it is doubled for oral use. An appropriate amount is used for external use.

【现代研究 / Modern research】

本品主要含槲皮素、山奈素等，尚含苷类、鞣质、挥发油、氨基酸、胆碱、甾醇等。具有促进胆汁分泌、利尿、排石、镇痛、抑菌、抗炎等作用。

It mainly contains quercetin, kaempferol, glycosides, tannins, volatile oil, amino acids, choline, sterols, etc. It has the functions of promoting bile secretion and urination, removing stones, analgesia, inhibiting bacteria and inflammation.

其他利水渗湿药功用介绍见表 11-1。

The efficacies of other damp-draining diuretic medicinals are shown in table 11-1.

表 11-1　其他利水渗湿药功用介绍

分类	药物	药性	功效	应用	用法用量
利水消肿药	冬瓜皮	甘，凉。归脾、小肠经	利尿消肿，清热解暑	水肿，小便不利，暑热烦渴	煎服，9~30g
	玉米须	甘，平。归膀胱、肝、胆经	利尿消肿，利湿退黄	水肿，小便不利，淋证，黄疸	煎服，30~60g。鲜品加倍
	枳椇子	甘，酸，平。归脾经	利水消肿，解酒毒	水肿，醉酒	煎服，10~15g
利尿通淋药	通草	甘，淡，微寒。归肺、胃经	清热利尿，通气下乳	湿热淋证，水肿尿少，产后乳汁不下	煎服，3~5g
	萹蓄	苦，微寒。归膀胱经	利尿通淋，杀虫，止痒	热淋涩痛，小便短赤；虫积腹痛，皮肤湿疹，阴痒带下	煎服，9~15g。外用适量
	地肤子	辛、苦，寒。归肾、膀胱经	清热利湿，祛风止痒	小便涩痛，阴痒带下，风疹，湿疹，皮肤瘙痒	煎服，9~15g。外用适量，煎汤熏洗
	冬葵子	甘，寒。归大肠、小肠、膀胱经	清热利尿，下乳，润肠	淋证，水肿，乳汁不通，乳房胀痛，肠燥便秘	煎服，10~15g
	灯心草	甘，淡，微寒。归心、肺、小肠经	清心火，利小便	心烦失眠，尿少涩痛，口舌生疮	煎服，1~3g

题库

续表

分类	药物	药性	功效	应用	用法用量
利湿退黄药	广金钱草	甘、淡，凉。归肝、肾、膀胱经	利湿退黄，利尿通淋	黄疸尿赤，热淋，石淋，小便涩痛，水肿尿少	煎服，15~30g
	连钱草	辛、微苦，微寒。归肝、肾、膀胱经	利湿通淋，清热解毒，散瘀消肿	热淋，石淋，湿热黄疸，疮痈肿痛，跌打损伤	煎服，15~30g。外用适量，煎汤洗

（林海燕　金素安）

第十二章 温 里 药
Chapter 12   Interior-warming medicinals

 学习目标 | Learning goals

1. 掌握 温里药在性能、功效、主治、配伍及使用注意方面的共性；附子、肉桂、干姜、吴茱萸的性能、功效、应用以及特殊的用法用量和特殊的使用注意。

2. 熟悉 小茴香、丁香的功效、主治以及特殊的用法用量和特殊的使用注意。

3. 了解 温里药以及散寒止痛、回阳救逆等相关功效术语的含义；花椒、高良姜、荜茇的功效以及特殊的用法用量。

1. Master the commonness of interior-warming medicinals in efficacy, indications, property, compatibility and cautions; as well as the property, efficacy, application, special usage and dosage and special precautions of *fù zǐ*, *ròu guì*, *gān jiāng* and *wú zhū yú*.

2. Familiar with the efficacy, indications, special usage, dosage and special precautions of *xiǎo huí xiāng* and *dīng xiāng*.

3. Understand the definitions of related efficacy terms, such as interior-warming medicinals, dissipate cold and relieve pain as well as restore yang and rescue from counterflow; and the efficacy, special usage and dosage of *huā jiāo gāo liáng jiāng* and *bì bá*.

凡以温里祛寒为主要功效，常用于治疗里寒证的药物，称为温里药，又称祛寒药。

Medicinals with major efficacies of warming the interior and dissipating cold are known as interior-warming medicinals, or cold-dispelling medicinals, which are usually used to treat interior-cold syndrome.

温里药味辛而性温热，多归脾、胃经，部分药物兼归肾、肝、心、肺经。辛能行散，温热祛寒，善走脏腑而温散在里的寒邪，温煦脏腑阳气之不足，多具有温里祛寒、温经止痛的功效，部分药物兼能助阳、回阳，主治里寒证。由于里寒证有部位之分、虚实之别，故里寒证又表现出不同的证候特点。如脾胃寒证，症见脘腹冷痛、呕吐泄泻、食欲不振等；肺寒痰饮证，症见咳喘痰鸣、痰白清稀等；寒滞肝脉，症见少腹冷痛、寒疝腹痛、厥阴头痛等；肾阳虚证，症见腰膝冷痛、阳痿宫冷、遗精遗尿、夜尿频多等；心肾阳虚证，症见畏寒肢冷、心悸怔忡、小便不利、肢体浮肿等；亡阳证，症见四肢厥逆、脉微欲绝等。

Interior-warming medicinals are acrid and warm and hot in nature, and mainly act on the spleen and stomach meridians. Some act on the kidney, liver, heart and lung meridians. It is acrid to dissipate, and warm-heat to dispel cold. They tend to work on *zang-fu* organs to warm and dissipate internal pathogenic cold, and warm insufficient yang qi of *zang-fu* organs. Their major efficacy is to warm interior and dispel cold, warm meridian and relieve pain. Some of them can also assist and restore yang, mainly indicated to interior-cold syndrome. Since there are different parts, deficiency or excess, interior-cold syndrome shows different syndrome characteristics, such as cold syndrome of spleen and stomach manifested as cold pain of epigastric-abdomen, vomiting and diarrhea, and poor appetite; syndrome of lung cold with phlegm-fluid retention manifested as asthmatic cough and wheezing, white and thin sputum; syndrome of cold invasion in liver meridian manifested as abdominal cold pain, colic of cold type with abdominal pain or Jueyin headache; syndrome of kidney-yang deficiency manifested as pain and coldness of waist and knees, impotence and uterine cold, spermatorrhea, enuresis, and frequent urination at night; syndrome of heart-kidney yang deficiency manifested as aversion to cold, cold limbs, palpitation, difficulty in urination and limbs edema; and yang collapse syndrome manifested as reversal cold of limbs, indistinct and faint pulse.

使用温里药应根据里寒证的虚实及不同兼证行适当的配伍。寒为阴邪，易伤阳气，虚寒相兼，故温里药常配伍补阳药。治外寒内侵而表寒未解者，当与发散风寒药同用。治寒凝经脉，气滞血瘀者，宜与温通经脉或行气活血药同用。寒性主痛，治寒凝疼痛较甚者，当与止痛药配伍。治寒湿内阻者，配伍化湿药。治脾肾阳虚者，宜配伍温补脾肾药。治亡阳气脱者，须与大补元气药配伍。

Interior-warming medicinals should be appropriately combined with other medicinals according to deficiency or excess of interior cold syndrome and different accompanied symptoms and signs. Cold belongs to yin pathogen and tends to damage yang qi, deficiency and cold are accompanied, so interior-warming medicinals are often used in combination with yang-tonifying medicinals. For external pathogenic cold invading inside and exterior cold without releasing, they should be used in combination with wind-cold dispersing-dissipating medicinals; for qi stagnation and blood stasis due to cold congealing in the meridians, with medicinals for warming and unblocking meridians or moving qi and invigorating blood; for severe pain due to cold congealing, with pain-relieving medicinals; for internal obstruction of cold-dampness, with dampness-resolving medicinals; for spleen-kidney yang deficiency, with medicinals for warming and tonifying spleen and kidney; and for yang and qi collapse, with medicinals of powerful tonification of primordial qi.

温里药多辛热燥烈，易助火伤阴，实热证、阴虚火旺、津血亏虚者忌用；孕妇慎用。部分药物有毒，应注意炮制、剂量及用法，避免中毒。

Interior-warming medicinals are mostly acrid, hot, dry and drastic, and tend to assist fire and damage yin, so they are contraindicated in patients with excess heat, vigorous fire due to yin deficiency, and fluid-blood depletion; and they should be used with caution for pregnant women. Some medicinals are toxic, so attention should be paid to the processing procedure, dosage and usage to avoid poisoning.

附子　*Fù zǐ* (Aconiti Lateralis Radix Praeparata)
《神农本草经》
Shen Nong's Classic of the Materia Medica (Shén Nóng Běn Cǎo Jīng)

【来源 / Origin】

为毛茛科植物乌头 *Aconitum carmichaelii* Debx. 的子根的加工品。主产于四川。6月下旬至 8 月上旬采收，加工炮制为盐附子、黑顺片及白附片。其中，盐附子气微，味咸而麻，刺舌；黑顺片气微，味淡；白附片气微，味淡。《中国药典》规定，含苯甲酰新乌头原碱（$C_{31}H_{43}NO_{10}$）、苯甲酰乌头原碱（$C_{32}H_{45}NO_{10}$）和苯甲酰次乌头原碱（$C_{31}H_{43}NO_9$）的总量，不得少于 0.010%。

Fù zǐ is the daughter root of *Aconitum carmichaelii* Debx., pertaining to Ranunculaceae, mainly

217

produced in Sichuan Province in China. It is collected from late June to early August. The processed materials are named *yán fù zǐ* (salty-prepared), *hēi shùn piàn* (black-*fù zǐ* pieces) and *bái fù piàn* (white-*fù zǐ* pieces). *Yán fù zǐ* has a slight flavor and tastes salty and numbing with sensation of tongue-pricking; *hēi shùn piàn* has a slight flavor and tastes bland; *bái fù piàn* has a slight flavor and tastes bland. According to *Chinese Pharmacopeia*, the total content of benzoylmesaconine ($C_{31}H_{43}NO_{10}$), benzoylaconitine ($C_{32}H_{45}NO_{10}$) and benzoylhypacoitine ($C_{31}H_{43}NO_9$) should be no less than 0.010%.

【性味归经 / Medicinal properties】

辛、甘，大热；有毒。归心、肾、脾经。

Acrid, sweet, hot and poisonous; act on the heart, kidney and spleen meridians.

【作用功效】

回阳救逆，补火助阳，散寒止痛。

Restore yang to rescue from counterflow, supplement fire and assist yang, dissipate cold and relieve pain.

【临床应用 / Clinical application】

1. 亡阳证　本品辛甘大热，为纯阳之品，能助心阳以复脉，补命门之火以救散失之元阳，为"回阳救逆第一品药"。用治久病阳气亏虚，阴寒内盛，或大汗、大吐、大泻所致的亡阳证，症见四肢厥逆、脉微欲绝者，常与干姜、甘草同用。若治亡阳兼气虚欲脱者，常与人参同用。

(1) Yang collapse　*Fù zǐ* is acrid, sweet and extremely hot in nature, and is a medicinal of pure yang. It can assist heart yang to restore pulse, tonify fire of life gate to save primordial yang. It is the first choice to restore yang to rescue from counterflow. For the decline of yang due to enduring illness, internal exuberance of yin cold, or yang collapse due to profuse sweating, severe vomiting or severe diarrhea manifested as counterflow cold of four limbs, indistinct and faint pulse, it is often used with *gān jiāng* and *gān cǎo*. For yang collapse complicated by qi deficiency verging on desertion, it is often used with *rén shēn*.

2. 阳虚证　本品主归心、肾、脾经，能上助心阳，下补肾阳，中温脾阳，故肾、脾、心等多种阳虚证皆可选用。用治肾阳不足，命门火衰，阳痿滑精、宫寒不孕、腰膝冷痛、夜尿频多，常与肉桂、山茱萸、熟地黄等同用。用治脾胃虚寒较甚或脾肾阳虚，脘腹冷痛，呕吐泄泻，多与党参、白术、干姜等同用。用治脾肾阳虚，水湿内停，小便不利、肢体浮肿，常与茯苓、白术等同用。用治心阳衰弱，心悸气短、胸痹心痛，可与人参、三七、红花等同用。若治阳虚外感风寒，每与麻黄、细辛同用。

(2) Yang deficiency　*Fù zǐ* mainly acts on heart, kidney and spleen meridians, and can assist heart yang in the upper, tonify kidney yang in the lower and warm spleen yang in the middle, so it can be selected for various yang deficiency syndromes like kidney, spleen and heart. For kidney insufficiency and decline of the fire of life gate manifested as impotence and seminal emission, cold uterus and infertility, cold pain of waist and knees, and frequent nocturia, it is often combined with *ròu guì*, *shān zhū yú* and *shú dì huáng*. For severe spleen-stomach deficiency cold or spleen-kidney yang deficiency, manifested as cold pain in the stomach cavity and abdomen, vomiting and diarrhea, it is often used with *dāng shēn*, *bái zhú* and *gān jiāng*. For spleen-kidney yang deficiency and internal stagnation of water-dampness manifested as difficulty in urination and limb edema, it is used with *fú líng* and *bái zhú*. For heart yang insufficiency manifested as palpitations and short breath, chest impediment and cardiac pain, it is used with *rén shēn*, *sān qī* and *hóng huā*. For external-contraction wind-cold due to yang deficiency, it is used with *má huáng* and *xì xīn*.

3. 寒湿痹痛　本品辛散温通，善逐经络之风寒湿邪，有较强的散寒止痛作用。凡风寒湿痹，

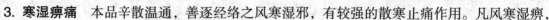

周身骨节疼痛均可使用，尤善治寒痹痛剧者，常与桂枝、白术、甘草同用。

(3) Cold-damp painful *bì* syndrome　*Fù zǐ* is acrid dispersing and warm dredging, good at expelling wind-cold pathogens in channels and collaterals with a strong effect of dispersing cold and relieving pain. It can be used for all wind-damp painful *bì* syndromes with general pain of the joints, especially cold *bì* with *bì* syndromes with severe pain, in combination with *guì zhī*, *bái zhú* and *gān cǎo*.

【用法用量 / Usage and dosage 】

煎服，3~15g，先煎、久煎。

Decoction, 3-15g, it should be decocted first and for a long time.

【使用注意 / Precaution 】

孕妇慎用。不宜与半夏、瓜蒌、瓜蒌仁、瓜蒌皮、天花粉、川贝母、浙贝母、平贝母、伊贝母、湖北贝母、白蔹、白及同用。

It should be used with caution for pregnant women. It is not proper to be combined with *bàn xià* (Pinelliae Rhizoma), *guā lóu* (Trichosanthis Fructus), *guā lóu rén* (Trichosanthis Semen), *guā lóu pí* (Trichosanthis Pericarpium), *tiān huā fěn* (Trichosanthis Radix), *chuān bèi mǔ* (Fritillariae Cirrhosae Bulbus), *zhè bèi mǔ* (Fritillariae Thunbergii Bulbus), *píng bèi mǔ* (Fritillariae Ussuriensis Bulbus), *yī bèi mǔ* (Fritillariae Pallidiflorae Bulbus), *hú běi bèi mǔ* (Fritillariae Hupehensis Bulbus), *bái liǎn* (Ampelopsis Radix) and *bái jí* (Bletillae Rhizoma).

【现代研究 / Modern research 】

本品主要含乌头碱、新乌头碱、次乌头碱、去甲乌头碱、新乌宁碱等双酯型生物碱，尚含苯甲酰乌头原碱、苯甲酰新乌头原碱、苯甲酰次乌头原碱等单酯型生物碱。双酯型生物碱是附子的主要活性和毒性成分。具有强心、抗炎、镇痛、扩血管、抗衰老等作用。

It mainly contains diester-type alkaloids, such as aconitine, aconitane, hypaconitine, hydroxybenzyl and neoline. It also contains monoester aconitum alkaloids, such as benzoylmesaconine, benzoylaconitine and benzoylhypacoitine. Diester-type alkaloids are the main active and poisonous ingredients of *fù zǐ*. It has the functions of strengthening the heart, anti-inflammation, relieving pain, enlarging blood vessels and antagonizing aging.

干姜　*Gān jiāng* (Zingiberis Rhizoma)
《神农本草经》
Shen Nong's Classic of the Materia Medica (*Shén Nóng Běn Cǎo Jīng*)

【来源 / Origin 】

为姜科植物姜 *Zingiber officinale* Rosc. 的干燥根茎。产于四川、广东、广西等地。冬季采收，切厚片或块，干燥，生用。本品气香特异，味辛辣。《中国药典》规定，含挥发油不得少于 0.8%（ml/g），6- 姜辣素（$C_{17}H_{26}O_4$）不得少于 0.60%；姜炭含 6- 姜辣素不得少于 0.050%。

Gān jiāng is the rhizome of *Zingiber officinale* Rosc., pertaining to Zingiberaceae, and is mainly produced in Sichuan, Guangdong Province and Guangxi Zhuang Autonomous Region in China. It is collected in winter, cut into thick slices or masses, dried in the sun and used raw. It has unique fragrance and tastes acrid. According to *Chinese Pharmacopeia*, the content of volatile oil should be no less than 0.8%(ml/g), and that of 6-gingerol ($C_{17}H_{26}O_4$) should be no less than 0.60%, and that in *jiāng tàn* (Zingiber offcinale Rose) should be no less than 0.050%.

【性味归经 / Medicinal properties 】

辛，热。归脾、胃、肾、心、肺经。

Acrid and hot; act on the spleen, kidney, heart and lung meridians.

【主要功效 / Medicinal efficacies】

温中散寒，回阳通脉，温肺化饮。

Warm the center and dissipate cold, restore yang to unblock the vessels, warm the lung and dissolve rheum.

【临床应用 / Clinical application】

1. 脘腹冷痛，呕吐泄泻　本品辛热燥烈，主归脾、胃经，长于温暖中焦、健运脾胃，为温中散寒之主药，凡是脾胃寒证，不论外寒内侵的实证，还是阳气不足的虚证皆宜选用。若治脾胃虚寒，脘腹冷痛，食欲不振，呕吐泄泻，常与党参、白术等同用。若治脾胃实寒，腹痛呕吐，可单用本品研末服，或与高良姜、吴茱萸等同用。

(1) Chills and pain of stomach cavity and abdomen, vomiting and diarrhea　It is acrid, hot, dry and acts on the spleen and stomach meridians. It is effective in warming middle energizer and strengthening spleen and stomach, which is a principal medicinal to warm the center and dispel cold. It can be used to treat spleen-stomach cold, both excess-cold syndrome due to internal invasion of exogenous cold and deficiency-cold syndrome due to yang qi deficiency. To treat deficiency-cold of spleen and stomach, manifested as cold pain of stomach cavity and abdomen, poor appetite, vomiting and diarrhea, it is often combined with *dǎng shēn* (Codonopsis Radix) and *bái zhú* (Atractylodis Macrocephalae Rhizoma). To treat abdominal pain and vomiting due to excess-cold of spleen and stomach, it can be ground into powder for oral taking, or combined with *gāo liáng jiāng* (Alpiniae Officinarum Rhizoma) and *wú zhū yú* (Evodiae Fructus).

2. 亡阳证　本品辛热，入心、肾经，有回阳通脉的功效。用治心肾阳虚，阴寒内盛之亡阳证，症见四肢厥逆、脉微欲绝者，常与附子相须为用。

(2) Yang collapse syndrome　It is acrid and hot, and acts on the heart and kidney meridians with effects of restoring yang and unblocking meridians. To treat yang collapse syndrome due to yang deficiency of heart and kidney, and internal exuberance of yin-cold, manifested as reversal counterflow cold of four limbs and faint pulse verging on expiry, it is often combined with *fù zǐ* (Aconiti Lateralis Radix Praeparata) for mutual reinforcement.

3. 寒饮喘咳　本品归肺经，有温肺化饮之功。用治寒饮伏肺，咳嗽喘息，形寒背冷，痰多清稀，常与细辛、五味子、麻黄等同用。

(3) Cough and panting due to cold fluid-retention　It acts on the lung meridian with effect of warming the lung and resolving fluid retention. To treat latent cold fluid retention in the lung, manifested as cough, panting, cold body and back, profuse and thin sputum, it is often combined with *xì xīn* (Asari Radix et Rhizoma), *wǔ wèi zǐ* (Schisandrae Chinensis Fructus) and *má huáng* (Ephedrae Herba).

【用法用量 / Usage and dosage】

煎服，3~10g。

Decoction, 3-10g.

【使用注意 / Precaution】

阴虚内热，血热妄行者忌用。孕妇慎用。

It should be contraindicated in patients with yin deficiency and internal heat and bleeding due to blood-heat. It should be used with caution for pregnant women.

【现代研究 / Modern research】

本品主要含挥发油 6- 姜辣素、α- 姜烯、牻牛儿醇、β- 甜没药烯等，其中，6- 姜辣素是其辛辣成分。具有调节胃肠运动、镇吐、抗消化性溃疡、利胆、抗炎、镇静、镇痛、升血压等作用。

It mainly contains volatile oil, such as 6-gingerol, α-zingiberene, geraniol and β-bisabolene. 6-gingerol is the acrid ingredient. It has the functions of regulating gastrointestinal motility, arresting vomiting, anti-gastric ulcer, promoting gallbladder functions, anti-inflammation, tranquilizing, relieving pain and elevating blood pressure.

肉桂　*Ròu guì* (Cinnamomi Cortex)
《神农本草经》
Shen Nong's Classic of the Materia Medica (Shén Nóng Běn Cǎo Jīng)

【来源 / Origin】

为樟科植物肉桂 *Cinnamomum cassia* Presl. 的干燥树皮。主产于广东、广西、海南等地。多于秋季剥取，阴干，生用。本品气香浓烈，味甜、辣。《中国药典》规定，含挥发油不得少于 1.2%（ml/g），桂皮醛（C_9H_8O）不得少于 1.5%。

Ròu guì is the bark of *Cinnamomum cassia* Presl., pertaining to Lauraceae, and is mainly produced in Guangdong, Hainan Province and Guangxi Zhuang Autonomous Region in China. It is mostly peeled off and collected in autumn, dried in the shade and used raw. It has strong peculiar fragrance and tastes sweet and acrid. According to *Chinese Pharmacopeia*, the content of volatile oil should be no less than 1.2%(ml/g), and cinnamaldehyde (C_9H_8O) should be no less than 1.5%.

【性味归经 / Medicinal properties】

辛、甘，大热。归肾、脾、心、肝经。

Acrid, sweet and hot; act on the kidney, spleen, heart and liver meridians.

【主要功效 / Medicinal efficacies】

补火助阳，散寒止痛，温经通脉，引火归元。

Supplement fire and assist yang, dissipate cold and relieve pain, warm and unblock the channels, return fire to its source.

【临床应用 / Clinical application】

1. 阳虚证　本品辛甘大热，补火助阳，能够温助肾、脾、心三脏之阳气，功似附子而作用温和。尤其长于补肾阳，益命门之火，为治命门火衰之要药。用治肾阳不足，命门火衰之阳痿宫冷、腰膝冷痛、夜尿频多、滑精遗尿等，常配附子、熟地黄、山茱萸等。若治元阳亏虚，虚阳上浮之面赤、眩晕、虚喘、汗出、脉微弱，多与山茱萸、五味子、人参等同用。用治脾肾阳虚，四肢逆冷，食少神疲，大便溏泄，常与附子、人参、白术等同用。用治心阳不足，心悸气短，胸闷不舒，常与人参、黄芪、薤白等同用。

(1) Yang deficiency syndrome It is acrid and hot with effects of supplementing fire and assisting yang. It can warm and assist the yang qi of kidney, spleen and heart. Its efficacies is similar to *fù zǐ* (Aconiti Lateralis Radix Praeparata), but it is milder. *Ròu guì* is effective in supplementing kidney yang and strengthening vital gate fire, which is an essential medicinal to treat decline of vital gate fire. To treat deficiency of kidney yang and decline of vital gate fire, manifested as impotence, cold uterus, chills and pain of waist and knees, frequent nocturnal urine, spermatorrhea and enuresis, it is often combined with *fù zǐ* (Aconiti Lateralis Radix Praeparata), *shú dì huáng* (Rehmanniae Radix Praeparata) and *shān zhū yú* (Corni Fructus). To treat insufficiency of the kidney-yang and rising of deficiency-yang, manifested as flushed complexion, dizziness, deficiency-type panting, sweating and weak or feeble pulse, it is often combined with *shān zhū yú* (Corni Fructus), *wǔ wèi zǐ* (Schisandrae Chinensis Fructus) and *rén shēn* (Ginseng Radix et Rhizoma). To treat yang deficiency of spleen and stomach, with symptoms of reversal cold of limbs, poor appetite, spiritual lassitude and loose stool, it is often used together with *fù zǐ* (Aconiti Lateralis Radix Praeparata), *rén shēn* (Ginseng Radix et Rhizoma) and *bái zhú* (Atractylodis Macrocephalae Rhizoma). To treat palpitation, short breath and chest distress due to deficiency of heart yang, it is often combined with *rén shēn* (Ginseng Radix et Rhizoma), *huáng qí* (Astragali Radix) and *xiè bái* (Allii Macrostemi Bulbus).

2. 寒凝疼痛证　本品辛散温通，既能温通经脉，又能散寒止痛，为治寒凝诸痛之要药。用治寒邪内侵或脾胃虚寒的脘腹冷痛，可单用研末，酒煎服；或与干姜、高良姜、荜茇等同用。用治胸阳不振，寒邪内侵的胸痹心痛，可与附子、川芎、丹参等同用。用治寒疝腹痛，多与吴茱萸、小茴香等同用。用治风寒湿痹痛，尤宜于寒痹腰痛，常与独活、杜仲、桑寄生等同用。若治阳虚寒凝的阴疽肿痛，常与鹿角胶、炮姜、麻黄等同用。

(2) **Pain syndromes due to congealing cold**　It is acrid and warm for warming and unblocking, which functions to warm and unblock meridians, dispel cold and relieve pain. It is an important medicinal to treat pain syndromes due to congealing cold. To treat chills and pains of stomach cavity and abdomen due to invasion of pathogenic cold or deficiency-cold of spleen and stomach, it can be ground into powder and decocted with wine for oral taking; or combined with *gān jiāng* (Zingiberis Rhizoma), *gāo liáng jiāng* (Alpiniae Officinarum Rhizoma) and *bì bá* (Piperis Longi Fructus). To treat chest *bì* and heart pain due to hypofunction of yang qi in the chest and internal invasion of pathogenic cold, it can be combined with *fù zǐ* (Aconiti Lateralis Radix Praeparata), *chuān xiōng* (Chuanxiong Rhizoma) and *dān shēn* (Salviae Miltiorrhizae Radix et Rhizoma). To treat cold *shàn* with abdominal pain, it is often combined with *wú zhū yú* (Evodiae Fructus) and *xiǎo huí xiāng* (Foeniculi Fructus). To treat wind-cold-damp *bì*, especially cold *bì* with lumbar pain, it is often combined with *dú huó* (Angelicae Pubescentis Radix), *dù zhòng* (Eucommiae Cortex) and *sāng jì shēng* (Taxilli Herba). To treat dorsal furuncle with swelling and pain due to yang deficiency and cold congealing, it is often combined with *lù jiǎo jiāo* (Cervi Cornus Colla), *páo jiāng* (Zingiberis Praeparatum Rhizoma) and *má huáng* (Ephedrae Herba).

3. 寒凝血瘀证　本品能温通血脉，促进血行，常用于寒邪凝滞的瘀血证。用治冲任虚寒，寒凝血滞之月经不畅、闭经、痛经，常与红花、当归、香附等同用。用治产后瘀阻腹痛，可与当归、川芎等同用。用治气滞血瘀的癥瘕积聚，可与莪术、赤芍、枳壳等同用。若治跌打损伤，瘀肿疼痛，可与当归、川芎等同用。

(3) **Cold congealing and blood stasis**　It has functions of warming and unblocking meridians to promote blood circulation, and is often used to treat static blood syndrome due to congealing of pathogenic cold. To treat deficiency-cold of thoroughfare and conception vessels, cold congealing and blood stasis, manifested as menstrual disorders, amenorrhea and painful menstruation, it is often combined with *hóng huā* (Carthami Flos), *dāng guī* (Angelicae Sinensis Radix) and *xiāng fù* (Cyperi Rhizoma). To treat postpartum abdominal pain due to blood stasis and qi stagnation, it is often combined with *dāng guī* (Angelicae Sinensis Radix) and *chuān xiōng* (Chuanxiong Rhizoma). To treat aggregation and accumulation due to qi stagnation and blood stasis, it is often combined with *é zhú* (Curcumae Rhizoma), *chì sháo* (Paeoniae Rubra Radix) and *zhǐ qiào* (Aurantii Fructus). To treat traumatic injury with swelling and pain, it is often combined with *dāng guī* (Angelicae Sinensis Radix) and *chuān xiōng* (Chuanxiong Rhizoma).

此外，久病体虚，气血不足者，在补益气血方中加入少量肉桂，有温运阳气，鼓舞气血生长之效。

In addition, small amount of *ròu guì* is added in formulas that supplement and boost qi and blood to treat deficiency of qi and blood after prolonged chronic disease, which can warm up and transport yang qi, as well as promote production of qi and blood.

【用法用量 / Usage and dosage】

煎服，1~5g。

Decoction, 1-5g.

【使用注意 / Precaution】

阴虚火旺者忌服。有出血倾向者及孕妇慎用。不宜与赤石脂同用。

It should be contraindicated in patients with exuberant fire due to yin deficiency. It should be used with caution for patients with tendency of bleeding and pregnant women. It is not proper to be combined with *chì shí zhī* (Halloysitum Rubrum).

【现代研究 / Modern research】

本品主要含挥发油（桂皮油或肉桂油），其中主要成分为桂皮醛、乙酸桂皮酯、乙酸丙酯、肉桂酸等，尚含香豆素、鞣质等。具有扩张血管、促进血液循环、增加冠脉及脑血流量、抗血小板凝集、镇静、镇痛、解热、增强消化功能、缓解胃肠痉挛性疼痛等作用。

It mainly contains volatile oil (which is known as cinnamon oil), including cinnamaldehyde, cinnamyl acetate, propyl acetate and cinnamic acid. It also contains coumarin and tannin. It has the functions of enlarging blood vessels, promoting blood circulation, increasing coronary and cerebral blood flow, anti-platelet aggregation, tranquilizing, relieving fever, strengthening digestive function, relieving gastrointestinal spastic pain.

吴茱萸 *Wú zhū yú* (Evodiae Fructus)

《神农本草经》

Shen Nong's Classic of the Materia Medica (Shén Nóng Běn Cǎo Jīng)

【来源 / Origin】

为芸香科植物吴茱萸 *Evodia rutaecarpa*（Juss.）Benth.、石虎 *Evodia rutaecarpa*（Juss.）Benth. var. *officinalis*（Dode）Huang 或疏毛吴茱萸 *Evodia rutaecarpa*（Juss.）Benth. var. *bodinieri*（Dode）Huang 的干燥近成熟果实。产于贵州、广西、湖南等地。8~11月果实尚未开裂时采收，晒干或低温烘干，生用或制用。本品气芳香浓郁，味辛辣而苦。《中国药典》规定，含吴茱萸碱（$C_{19}H_{17}N_3O$）和吴茱萸次碱（$C_{18}H_{13}N_3O$）的总量不得少于 0.15%，柠檬苦素（$C_{26}H_{30}O_8$）不得少于 0.20%。

Wú zhū yú is the nearly-mature fruit of *Evodia rutaecarpa* (Juss.) Benth., *Evodia rutaecarpa* (Juss.) Benth. var. *officinalis* (Dode) Huang or *Evodia rutaecarpa* (Juss.) Benth. var. *bodinieri* (Dode) Huang. It is mainly produced in Guizhou, Hunan Province and Guangxi Zhuang Autonomous Region in China. It is collected when the fruit are not ruptured from August to November, dried in the sun, or baked in low temperature. It is used in the raw or processed form. It has strong fragrance and tastes acrid and bitter. According to *Chinese Pharmacopeia*, the total content of evodiamine ($C_{19}H_{17}N_3O$) and rutaecarpine ($C_{18}H_{13}N_3O$) should be no less than 0.15%, and the content of limonin ($C_{26}H_{30}O_8$) should be no less than 0.20%.

【性味归经 / Medicinal properties】

辛、苦，热；有小毒。归肝、脾、胃、肾经。

Acrid, bitter, hot and slightly poisonous; act on the liver, spleen, stomach and kidney meridians.

【主要功效 / Medicinal efficacies】

散寒止痛，降逆止呕，助阳止泻。

Dissipate cold and relieve pain, direct counterflow downward and arrest vomiting, assist yang and arrest diarrhea.

【临床应用 / Clinical application】

1. 寒滞肝经诸痛　本品辛散苦泄，性热祛寒，主入肝经，既散肝经之寒邪，又解肝气之郁滞，并有良好的止痛功效，为治寒滞肝经诸痛之主药。用治寒侵肝经，疝气疼痛，常与小茴香、川楝子、木香等配伍。用治厥阴头痛，呕吐涎沫，常与人参、生姜、大枣同用。用治冲任虚寒，瘀血阻滞之痛经，常与桂枝、当归、川芎等同用。用治寒湿脚气肿痛，或上冲入腹，常与木瓜、苏叶、槟榔等配伍。

(1) **All pains due to cold congealing in the liver meridian**　It is acrid for dispersing and bitter for discharging, and hot for eliminating cold. It mainly acts on the liver meridian with efficacies of dispelling pathogenic cold of liver meridian, relieving liver qi stagnation, as well as alleviating pain. *Wú zhū yú* is considered to be a vital medicinal to treat all pains due to cold congealing in the liver meridian. To treat *shàn qì* with pain due to cold invading liver meridian, it is often combined with *xiǎo huí xiāng* (Foeniculi Fructus), *chuān liàn zǐ* (Toosendan Fructus) and *mù xiāng* (Aucklandiae Radix). To treat Jueyin headache, vomiting with spittle, it is often combined with *rén shēn* (Ginseng Radix et Rhizoma), *shēng jiāng* (Zingiberis Recens Rhizoma) and *dà zǎo* (Jujubae Fructus). To treat painful menstruation due to insecurity of thoroughfare and conception vessels and stagnation of static blood, it is often used with *guì zhī* (Cinnamomi Ramulus), *dāng guī* (Angelicae Sinensis Radix) and *chuān xiōng* (Chuanxiong Rhizoma). To treat beriberi with swelling and pain, or upward flowing into the abdomen, it is often used with *mù guā* (Chaenomelis Fructus), *sū yè* (Perillae Folium) and *bīng láng* (Arecae Semen).

2. 呕吐吞酸　本品既能散寒止痛，又可疏肝解郁，降逆止呕，兼能制酸止痛，为治呕吐吞酸之良药。用治肝胃虚寒，脘腹胁痛，呕吐吞酸，常与人参、生姜等同用。用治外寒内侵，胃失和降之呕吐，常与半夏、生姜等配伍。若治肝郁化火，肝胃不和之胁痛口苦、呕吐吞酸，常与黄连同用。

(2) **Vomiting and acid regurgitation**　It has functions of dispelling cold and relieving pain, dispersing stagnated liver qi for relieving qi stagnation, directing counterflow downward and arresting vomiting. It can also inhibit acidity to relieve pain, which serves a powerful medicinal to treat vomiting and acid regurgitation. To treat pain of stomach cavity, abdomen and hypochondrium, vomiting and acid regurgitation caused by deficiency-cold of liver and stomach, it is usually combined with *rén shēn* (Ginseng Radix et Rhizoma) and *shēng jiāng* (Zingiberis Recens Rhizoma). To treat vomiting caused by invasion of exogenous pathogenic cold and counterflow rise of stomach qi, it is often used with *bàn xià* (Pinelliae Rhizoma) and *shēng jiāng* (Zingiberis Recens Rhizoma). To treat stagnated liver qi transforming into fire and disharmony of liver and stomach, manifested as hypochondriac pain, bitter taste in the mouth, vomiting and acid regurgitation, it is often combined with *huáng lián* (Coptidis Rhizoma).

3. 虚寒泄泻　本品性热祛寒，味苦燥湿，能温暖脾肾，散寒燥湿，助阳止泻，为治脾肾阳虚，五更泄泻之常用药，常与补骨脂、肉豆蔻、五味子同用。

(3) **Diarrhea due to deficiency-cold**　It is hot in nature for eliminating cold and bitter in taste for drying damp. It has efficacies of warming spleen and kidney, dissipating cold and drying damp, as well as assisting yang to arrest diarrhea, which is a commonly used medicinal to treat diarrhea before dawn due

to yang deficiency of spleen and stomach. For the diarrhea before dawn, it is often combined with *bǔ gǔ zhī* (Psoraleae Fructus), *ròu dòu kòu* (Myristicae Semen) and *wǔ wèi zǐ* (Schisandrae Chinensis Fructus).

【用法用量 / Usage and dosage】

煎服，2~5g。外用适量。

Decoction, 2-5g. A proper amount for external application.

【使用注意 / Precaution】

不宜多用、久服。阴虚有热者忌用。孕妇慎用。

It is not suitable for overdosage and long-term application. It should be contraindicated for patients with yin deficiency accompanied by fever. It should be used with caution for pregnant women.

【现代研究 / Modern research】

本品主要含吴茱萸碱、吴茱萸次碱、吴茱萸新碱等生物碱，以及挥发油、吴茱萸酸、吴茱萸啶酮、吴茱萸精、吴茱萸苦素等。具有抑制胃肠痉挛、抗胃溃疡、止泻、抗心肌缺血、抗炎、镇痛、抗血栓等作用。

It mainly contains alkaloids, such as evodiamine, rutaecarpine and evocarpine. It also contains volatile oil, goshuynic acid, evodinone, evogin and rutae-vine. It has the functions of inhibiting gastrointestinal spasm, anti-gastric ulcer, arresting diarrhea, anti-myocardial ischemia, anti-inflammation, relieving pain and antagonizing thrombus.

其他温里药功用介绍见表 12-1。

The efficacies of other interior-warming medicinals are shown in table 12-1.

表 12-1 其他温里药功用介绍

类别	药物	药性	功效	应用	用法用量
温里药	小茴香	辛，温。归肝、肾、脾、胃经	散寒止痛，理气和胃	寒疝腹痛，少腹冷痛，痛经；脘腹胀痛，食少吐泻	煎服，3~6g。外用适量
	丁香	辛，温。归脾、胃、肺、肾经	温中降逆，散寒止痛，温肾助阳	胃寒呕吐、呃逆，胃寒脘腹冷痛，肾虚阳痿，宫冷	煎服，1~3g
	花椒	辛，温。归脾、胃、肾经	温中止痛，杀虫止痒	脘腹冷痛，呕吐泄泻，虫积腹痛，湿疹，阴痒	煎服，3~6g。外用适量，煎汤熏洗
	高良姜	辛，热。归脾、胃经	温中止呕，散寒止痛	脘腹冷痛，胃寒呕吐，嗳气吞酸	煎服，3~6g
	荜茇	辛，热。归胃、大肠经	温中散寒，下气止痛	脘腹冷痛，呕吐，泄泻，寒凝气滞，胸痹心痛，头痛，牙痛	煎服，1~3g。外用适量，研末塞龋齿孔中

题库

（管家齐）

第十三章　理　气　药
Chapter 13　Qi-rectifying medicinals

学习目标 ¦ Learning goals

　　1. 掌握　理气药在性能、功效、主治、配伍及使用注意方面的共性；陈皮、枳实、木香、香附、川楝子的性能、功效、应用以及特殊的用法用量和特殊的使用注意。

　　2. 熟悉　青皮、枳壳、沉香、薤白的功效、主治以及特殊的用法用量。

　　3. 了解　理气药以及行气、降气、破气等相关功效术语的含义；乌药、佛手、香橼、甘松、大腹皮、檀香、柿蒂的功效。

1. Master the commonness of qi-rectifying medicinals in efficacy, indications, property, compatibility and cautions; as well as the property, efficacy, application, special usage and dosage and special precautions of *chén pí*, *zhǐ shí*, *mù xiāng*, *xiāng fù* and *chuān liàn zǐ*.

2. Familiar with the efficacy, indications, special usage and dosage of *qīng pí*, *zhǐ qiào*, *chén xiāng*, *wū yào* and *xiè bái*.

3. Understand the definitions of moving qi, descending qi and breaking stagnant-qi; the efficacy of *fó shǒu*, *xiāng yuán*, *gān sōng*, *dà fù pí* and *shì dì*.

　　凡以疏理气机为主要功效，常用于治疗气滞或气逆证的药物，称为理气药，又称行气药。理气作用较强者，又称破气药。

　　Medicinals with the major efficacy of regulating qi movement are known as qi-rectifying medicinals, also called qi-moving medicinals. They are usually used to treat qi stagnation or syndrome of counterflow of qi. Among them, medicinals that have strong effect of rectifying qi are also known as stagnant-qi breaking medicinals.

　　理气药多辛香苦温，主入脾、胃、肝、肺经。辛能行散，芳香走窜，苦能降泄，性温通畅，故有疏理气机的作用。因其作用部位和作用特点的不同，分别具有理气调中、疏肝解郁、理气宽胸、行气消胀、行气止痛和破气散结等不同的表述，部分药物还兼能降气，有止呕、止呃、平喘之功，主治气机失调之气滞、气逆证。具体来说，本类药物可用于治疗脾胃气滞之脘腹胀满疼痛、嗳气吞酸、恶心呕吐、大便秘结或泻痢不爽等，肝气郁滞之胁肋胀痛、急躁易怒、情志不舒、疝气疼痛、乳房胀痛、月经不调等，肺气壅滞之胸闷胸痛、咳嗽气喘等。

　　Qi-rectifying medicinals are usually acrid, fragrant and bitter in flavor and warm in nature, acting on spleen, stomach, liver and lung meridians. Medicinals with acrid and aromatic properties have the efficacies of moving and dispersing, and those bitter in taste have the efficacies of descending and discharging, and those warm in nature have the efficacy of unblocking and moving. Thus, medicinals in this category function to regulate qi movement. Because of the differences in action sites and

医药大学堂
WWW.YIYAODXT.COM

226

characteristics, there are expressions of rectifying qi and regulating the center, soothing liver to relieve depression, regulating qi to loosen chest, moving qi to dissolve distension, moving qi to relieve pain and breaking qi to dissipate masses. Some medicinals can also move qi downward to treat vomit, hiccup and relieve asthma. They are indicated to treat qi stagnation syndrome and qi counterflow syndrome due to disorder of qi movement. Specifically, they can be applied to treat symptoms caused by qi stagnation in the spleen and stomach such as fullness, distension and pain of epigastrium and abdomen, belching and acid regurgitation, nausea and vomit, constipation as well as diarrhea; to treat manifestations due to stagnation of liver qi, such as hypochondriac pain and distension, irritability, depression, hernia pain, distending pain in breast, irregular menstruation; or to treat oppression and pain in the chest, cough and dyspnea due to obstruction and stagnation of lung qi.

使用理气药，应针对病证选择适宜的药物，并进行相应的配伍。脾胃气滞者，宜选用长于理气调中的药物，因饮食积滞者，当配伍消食药；因脾胃气虚者，当配伍补气健脾药；因湿热阻滞者，当配伍清热除湿药；因寒湿困脾者，当配伍苦温燥湿药。肝郁气滞者，宜选用长于疏肝理气的药物，因肝血不足者，应配伍养血柔肝药；因肝经受寒者，应配伍暖肝散寒药；因瘀血阻滞者，应配伍活血祛瘀药。肺气壅滞者，宜选用长于理气宽胸的药物；因外邪客肺者，应配伍宣肺解表药；因痰饮阻肺者，应配伍化痰药。

When using qi-rectifying medicinals, we should select proper medicinals and make corresponding compatibility according to different syndromes. For qi stagnation in the spleen and stomach, qi-rectifying and center-regulating medicinals should be firstly selected and combined with digestion-promote medicinals, qi-tonifying and spleen-invigorating medicinals, heat-clearing and damp-removing medicinals, and medicinals that dry dampness with bitter and warm nature respectively according to different etiological factors such as food retention, qi deficiency, obstruction of damp-heat, and cold-damp encumbering spleen. When qi-rectifying medicinals are used to treat liver constraint and qi stagnation, liver-soothing and qi-regulating medicinals should be selected and combined with blood-nourishing and liver-softening medicinals, liver-warming and cold-dissipating medicinals, and blood-activating and stasis-removing medicinals respectively according to different etiological factors such as liver-blood insufficiency, cold congealing in the liver channel and stagnation caused by static blood. For lung qi obstruction and stagnation, qi-rectifying and chest-loosening medicinals should be selected and combined with exterior-releasing and lung-dispersing medicinals, and phlegm-dissolving medicinals respectively according to different etiological factors, such as exogenous pathogens attacking the lung, and phlegm obstruction.

理气药多辛温香燥，易耗气伤阴，故气阴不足者慎用。破气药作用峻猛而更易耗气，故孕妇慎用。

Medicinals with acrid, warm, aromatic and dry nature have disadvantages of consuming qi and yin, they should be contraindicated for patients with insufficiency of qi and yin. Stagnant-qi breaking medicinals have fierce effects and tend to consume qi, so they should be used with caution for pregnant women.

陈皮 *Chén pí* (Citri Reticulatae Pericarpium)
《神农本草经》
Shen Nong's Classic of the Materia Medica (*Shén Nóng Běn Cǎo Jīng*)

【来源 / Origin】

为芸香科植物橘 *Citrus reticulata* Blanco 及其栽培变种的成熟干燥果皮。主产于广东，其中，产于广东新会者称新会皮、广陈皮。秋末冬初果实成熟时采收，晒干或低温干燥，切丝，生用。以陈久者为佳，故称陈皮。本品气香，味辛、苦。《中国药典》规定，含橙皮苷（$C_{28}H_{34}O_{15}$）不得少于 3.5%；饮片不得少于 2.5%。

Chén pí is the pericarp of mature fruit of *Citrus reticulata* Blanco and its cultivated varieties, pertaining to Rutaceae. It is mainly produced in Guangdong Province in China. Those produced in Xinhui, Guangdong Province are called *xīn huì pí* or *guǎng chén pí*. It is collected when the fruits are mature in autumn, and dried in the sun or in low temperature. It is cut into shreds and used raw. The old one is of better quality and that is the reason why it is called *chén pí*. It has fragrance and is acrid and bitter in flavor. According to *Chinese Pharmacopoeia*, the content of hesperidin ($C_{28}H_{34}O_{15}$) should be no less than 3.5%, and no less than 2.5% in decoction pieces.

【性味归经 / Medicinal properties】

辛、苦，温。归脾、肺经。

Bitter, acrid and warm; act on the spleen and lung meridians.

【主要功效 / Medicinal efficacies】

理气健脾，燥湿化痰。

Rectify qi and fortify the spleen, dry dampness and dissolve phlegm.

【临床应用 / Clinical application】

1. **脾胃气滞证** 本品辛温气香，主入中焦，作用温和，长于理气宽中，健运脾胃，适用于各种原因所致的脾胃气滞证。因其味苦，兼能降逆止呕、燥湿健脾，故对于脾胃气滞兼有呕恶者，以及寒湿阻滞中焦者最为适宜。用治脾胃气滞，脘腹胀满，痞闷疼痛，常与枳实、木香等同用。用治寒湿中阻之脾胃气滞，脘腹胀痛、恶心呕吐，常与苍术、厚朴等同用。用治脾虚气滞，腹痛喜按，不思饮食，食后腹胀、大便溏泄，常与党参、白术、茯苓等同用。用治肝郁乘脾，腹痛泄泻，常与白芍、白术、防风同用。用治食积气滞，脘腹胀痛，可与山楂、神曲、莱菔子等同用。

(1) **Qi stagnation in the spleen and stomach** *Chén pí* is aromatic and acrid, warm in nature. It mainly acts on the middle energizer and is good at regulating qi and loosening the center, as well as reinforcing the spleen and stomach. *Chén pí* is suitable to treat qi stagnation syndrome of stomach and spleen caused by various etiological factors. *Chén pí* is bitter in taste and can rectify adverse flow of qi and relieve nausea, as well as dry dampness and invigorate spleen. So it is especially good at treating qi stagnation in the spleen and stomach with vomit and nausea, as well as cold-damp stagnates in the middle energizer. To treat qi stagnation in the spleen and stomach with symptoms of distension pain and fullness in the stomach and abdomen, it is usually combined with *zhǐ shí* (Aurantii Immaturus Fructus) and *mù xiāng* (Aucklandiae Radix). To treat qi stagnation in the spleen and stomach due to cold-damp obstructing the middle energizer, with manifestations of distension and pain in stomach and abdomen, nausea and vomit, it is combined with *cāng zhú* (Atractylodis Rhizoma) and *hòu pò* (Magnoliae Officinalis Cortex). To treat spleen deficiency and qi stagnation manifested as abdominal pain and relief with pressure, poor appetite, postcibal abdominal distension and loose stool, it is often combined with *dǎng shēn* (Codonopsis

Radix), *bái zhú* (Atractylodis Macrocephalae Rhizoma) and *fú líng* (Poria). To treat abdominal pain and diarrhea due to liver qi over-restricting the spleen, it is often combined with *bái sháo* (Paeoniae Alba Radix), *bái zhú* (Atractylodis Macrocephalae Rhizoma) and *fáng fēng* (Saposhnikoviae Radix). To treat distension and pain in stomach and abdomen due to food retention and qi stagnation, it can be combined with *shān zhā* (Crataegi Fructus), *shén qū* (Medicata Fermentata Massa) and *lái fú zǐ* (Raphani Semen).

2. **湿痰、寒痰咳嗽**　本品辛行苦泄，温燥除湿，能行能降，既能燥湿化痰、温化寒痰，又能宣降肺气。用治湿痰咳嗽，痰多色白，胸闷呕恶，常与半夏、茯苓、甘草同用。用治寒痰咳嗽，痰多清稀，多与干姜、细辛、五味子等同用。

(2) Damp-phlegm, cough due to cold-phlegm　*Chén pí* is acrid and bitter in taste with actions of promoting qi movement and rectifying adverse flow of qi. It is warm in property to eliminate dampness. *Chén pí* can dry dampness and dissolve phlegm, warm and remove cold-phlegm, as well as disperse and descend lung qi. To treat cough due to phlegm-damp, manifested as excessive and white phlegm, oppression in the chest, nausea and vomit, it is usually combined with *bàn xià* (Pinelliae Rhizoma), *fú líng* (Poria) and *gān cǎo* (Glycyrrhizae Radix et Rhizoma). To treat cough due to cold-phlegm, manifested as profuse and thin phlegm, it is often combined with *gān jiāng* (Zingiberis Rhizoma), *xì xīn* (Asari Radix et Rhizoma) and *wǔ wèi zǐ* (Schisandrae Chinensis Fructus).

【用法用量 / Usage and dosage】

煎服，3~10g。

Decoction, 3-10g.

【现代研究 / Modern research】

本品主要含橙皮苷、新橙皮苷、川陈皮素、橙皮素以及辛弗林、挥发油等。具有抑制胃肠运动、扩张支气管、平喘、镇咳、祛痰、升血压、抗血小板聚集、强心、抗休克、抗过敏、抑菌、利胆、降低胆固醇、抗氧化等作用。

Chén pí mainly contains hesperidin, neohesperidin, nobiletin, hesperetin and synephrine, volatile oil. It has the functions of restraining bowel movement, expanding the trachea, relieving asthma, alleviating cough, dissipating phlegm, raising blood pressure, antiplatelet aggregation, cardiotonifying, antishock, ananaphylaxis, inhibiting bacteria, promoting gallbladder function, reducing cholesterol, and antioxidation.

青皮　*Qīng pí* (Citri Reticulatae Pericarpium Viride)

《本草图经》

Illustrated Classic of Materia Medica (Běn Cǎo Tú Jīng)

【来源 / Origin】

为芸香科植物橘 *Citrus reticulata* Blanco 及其栽培变种的幼果或未成熟果实的干燥果皮。产地同陈皮。5~6 月间收集自落的幼果，晒干，称为"个青皮"；7~8 月间采收未成熟的果实，在果皮上纵剖成四瓣至基部，除去瓤肉，晒干，习称"四花青皮"。切厚片或丝，生用或醋炙用。个青皮气清香，味酸、苦、辛；四花青皮气香，味苦、辛。《中国药典》规定，含橙皮苷（$C_{28}H_{34}O_{15}$）不得少于 5.0%。

Qīng pí is the dried pericarp of immature fruits of *Citrus reticulata* Blanco and its cultivated varieties, pertaining to Rutaceae. It is mainly produced in the same places as *Chén pí*. From May to June, the automatically-fallen young fruits are collected, dried in the sun and called *gè qīng pí*; from July to August, the immature fruits are collected, they are cut vertically into four parts with reservation of the base, and dried in the sun without pulp, which are called *sì huā qīng pí*. It is usually cut into thick slices or shreds, and used raw or stir-fried with vinegar. *Gè qīng pí* is delicate fragrant, and sour, bitter and acrid in taste. *Sì huā qīng pí* has fragrance and is bitter and acrid in taste. According to *Chinese Pharmacopoeia*, the content of hesperidin ($C_{28}H_{34}O_{15}$) should be no less than 5.0%.

【性味归经 / Medicinal properties】

苦、辛，温。归肝、胆、胃经。

Bitter, acrid and warm; act on the liver, gallbladder and stomach meridians.

【主要功效 / Medicinal efficacies】

疏肝破气，消积化滞。

Soothe the liver and break stagnant qi, disperse accumulation and resolve food stagnation.

【临床应用 / Clinical application】

1. 肝郁气滞证　本品辛散温通，苦泄下行，主入肝胆经，长于疏肝胆、破气滞，药性峻烈，适宜于肝郁气滞之重证。用治肝郁气滞，胁肋胀痛，常配伍柴胡、郁金、香附等。用治乳房胀痛或结块，可与柴胡、浙贝母、夏枯草等同用。用治乳痈肿痛，常与蒲公英、瓜蒌皮、金银花等同用。若治寒疝疼痛，多与乌药、小茴香、木香等同用。

(1) Liver constraint and qi stagnation *Qīng pí* is acrid in flavor with dispersing effect, warm in nature with unblocking effect, and bitter in flavor with discharging and descending effects. It acts on the liver and gallbladder meridians and can soothe liver and gallbladder, as well as break qi stagnation. It has drastic nature and is especially suitable to treat severe syndromes of liver constraint and qi stagnation. To treat distending pain in the chest and hypochondrium due to liver constraint and qi stagnation, it is often combined with *chái hú* (Bupleuri Radix), *yù jīn* (Curcumae Radix) and *xiāng fù* (Cyperi Rhizoma). To treat distending pain in the breast or breast lumps, it is often combined with *chái hú* (Bupleuri Radix), *zhè bèi mǔ* (Fritillariae Thunbergii Bulbus), and *xià kū cǎo* (Prunellae Spica). To treat mammary abscess with swelling and pain, it is often combined with *pú gōng yīng* (Taraxaci Herba), *guā lóu pí* (Trichosanthis Pericarpium) and *jīn yín huā* (Lonicerae Japonicae Flos). To treat pain from cold *shàn* (hernia), it is often combined with *wū yào* (Linderae Radix), *xiǎo huí xiāng* (Foeniculi Fructus) and *mù xiāng* (Aucklandiae Radix).

2. 食积气滞证　本品兼入胃经，能破气消积，和胃止痛。用治食积气滞，脘腹胀痛，常与山楂、神曲、麦芽等同用。若食积气滞较甚，脘腹胀痛较重而大便不通者，可与大黄、槟榔、枳实等同用。

(2) Syndrome of food accumulation and qi stagnation *Qīng pí* acts on stomach meridian. It has effects of breaking stagnant qi and resolving food stagnation, as well as harmonizing stomach and relieving pain. To treat distending pain in the stomach cavity and abdomen due to food accumulation and qi stagnation, it is often combined with *shān zhā* (Crataegi Fructus), *shén qū* (Medicata Fermentata Massa) and *mài yá* (Hordei Germinatus Fructus). To treat severe food accumulation and qi stagnation, manifested as serious distending pain in the stomach and abdomen as well as constipation, it is often combined with *dà huáng* (Rhei Radix et Rhizoma), *bīng láng* (Arecae Semen) and *zhǐ shí* (Aurantii Immaturus Fructus).

3. 气滞血瘀证　本品苦泄峻烈，辛散温通力强，有破气散结之功。用治气滞血瘀之癥瘕积聚、久疟痞块等，常与三棱、莪术、鳖甲等同用。

(3) Syndrome of qi stagnation and blood stasis *Qīng pí* is bitter and with drastic effect of discharging and descending. It is acrid in flavor with strong dispersing effect and warm in nature for unblocking qi. Thus, *qīng pí* functions to break stagnant qi and dissipate masses. It is commonly used for the treatment of concretions and conglomerations (*zhēng jiǎ*), accumulations and gatherings and chronic malaria with *pǐ* lumps due to qi stagnation and blood stasis, and is often combined with *sān léng* (Sparganii Rhizoma), *é zhú* (Curcumae Rhizoma) and *biē jiǎ* (Trionycis Carapax).

【用法用量 / Usage and dosage】

煎服，3~10g。

Decoction, 3-10g.

【使用注意 / Precaution】

气虚者慎用。

It should be used with caution for patients with qi deficiency.

【现代研究 / Modern research】

本品所含主要成分与陈皮相似，但含量不同，如辛弗林含量高于陈皮。尚含多种氨基酸，如天冬氨酸、谷氨酸、脯氨酸等。具有解痉、利胆、促进消化液分泌、促进胃肠运动、升高血压、强心、祛痰、平喘等作用。

The main components of *qīng pí* are similar to that of *chén pí*, but the content of oxedrine is higher than that of *chén pí*. It also contains amino acids, such as aspartic acid, glutamic acid and proline, etc. *Qīng pí* has the effects of relaxing spasm, promoting gallbladder function, promoting secretion of digestive juice and bowel movement, increasing blood pressure, eliminating phlegm, calming panting and cardiotonifying.

枳实　*Zhǐ shí* (Aurantii Fructus Immaturus)
《神农本草经》
Shen Nong's Classic of the Materia Medica (Shén Nóng Běn Cǎo Jīng)

【来源 / Origin】

为芸香科植物酸橙 *Citrus aurantium* L. 及其栽培变种或甜橙 *Citrus sinensis* Osbeck 的干燥幼果。主产于江西、四川、福建等地。5~6 月间采集自落的果实，晒干或低温干燥，切薄片，生用或麸炒用。本品气清香，味苦、微酸。《中国药典》规定，含辛弗林（$C_9H_{13}NO_2$）不得少于 0.30%。

Zhǐ shí is the dried young fruit of *Citrus aurantium* L. and its cultivated varieties or *Citrus sinensis* Osbeck, pertaining to Rutaceae. It is mainly produced in Sichuan, Jiangxi and Fujian Province in China. The automatically-fallen immature fruits are collected between May to June, dried in the sun or at low temperature. It is cut into slices and used raw or stir-fried with bran. It has delicate fragrance and is bitter and slightly sour in taste. According to *Chinese Pharmacopoeia*, the content of synephrine ($C_9H_{13}NO_2$) should be no less than 0.30%.

【性味归经 / Medicinal properties】

苦、辛、酸，微寒。归脾、胃经。

Bitter, acrid, sour and slightly cold; act on the spleen and stomach meridians.

【主要功效 / Medicinal efficacies】

破气消积，化痰散痞。

Break stagnant qi and disperse accumulation, dissolve phlegm and disperse *pǐ*.

【临床应用 / Clinical application】

1. **胃肠气滞证**　本品辛行苦降，性猛力强，善行中焦之气，以破气除痞、消积导滞，适用于

231

胃肠气滞，脘腹痞满者。用治饮食积滞，脘腹痞满胀痛，嗳腐吞酸，常与山楂、麦芽、神曲等同用。用治热结便秘，腹部胀满疼痛，常与大黄、芒硝、厚朴等同用。用治湿热积滞，脘痞腹满或泻痢后重，常与黄芩、黄连、大黄等同用。用治脾胃虚弱，脘腹痞满胀闷，常与白术配用。用治脾虚气滞，寒热互结，心下痞满，常与厚朴、黄连、半夏等同用。

(1) Qi stagnation in the stomach and intestines *Zhǐ shí* is acrid in flavor with moving effect and bitter in flavor with descending effect, has fierce flavor and nature. It is good at moving qi of middle energizer to break stagnant qi and disperse stuffiness as well as eliminate accumulation. It is especially suitable to treat stuffiness and fullness in the stomach and abdomen due to qi stagnation in the stomach and intestines. To treat food accumulation with distending pain in the stomach cavity and abdomen, fetid eructation and acid regurgitation, it is often combined with *shān zhā* (Crataegi Fructus), *mài yá* (Hordei Germinatus Fructus), and *shén qū* (Medicata Fermentata Massa). To treat constipation due to heat accumulation with stuffiness and fullness, and distending pain, it is often combined with *dà huáng* (Rhei Radix et Rhizoma), *máng xiāo* (Natrii Sulfas) and *hòu pò* (Magnoliae Officinalis Cortex). To treat damp-heat accumulation with stuffiness and fullness in the stomach and abdomen, or diarrhea and dysentery with tenesmus, it is often combined with *huáng qín* (Scutellariae Radix), *huáng lián* (Coptidis Rhizoma) and *dà huáng* (Rhei Radix et Rhizoma). To treat weakness of the spleen and stomach with stuffiness and fullness, distension and oppression in the stomach and abdomen, it is often combined with *bái zhú* (Atractylodis Macrocephalae Rhizoma). To treat qi stagnation due to spleen deficiency, coexistence of cold and heat, stuffiness and fullness below the heart, it is often combined with *hòu pò* (Magnoliae Officinalis Cortex), *huáng lián* (Coptidis Rhizoma) and *bàn xià* (Pinelliae Rhizoma).

2. 痰阻气滞，胸痹，结胸　本品辛散苦泄，善能化痰消痞，破气除满。用治痰浊痹阻，胸阳不振，胸痹心痛，常与薤白、桂枝、瓜蒌等同用。用治痰热结胸，胸脘痞闷疼痛，可与黄连、瓜蒌、半夏同用。用治痰涎壅盛，胸痛痞塞，咳嗽痰多，可与半夏、陈皮等同用。

(2) Phlegm obstruction and qi stagnation, thoracic obstruction, chest binding syndrome *Zhǐ shí* is acrid with dispersing effect and bitter in taste with descending effect. It is good at dissolving phlegm and dispersing stuffiness, breaking stagnant qi and removing fullness. To treat phlegm-turbidity obstruction and hypofunction of yang qi in the chest with pectoral stuffiness pain or pectoral pain, it is often combined with *xiè bái* (Allii Macrostemi Bulbus), *guì zhī* (Cinnamomi Ramulus) and *guā lóu* (Trichosanthis Fructus). To treat thoracic accumulation due to phlegm-heat with stuffiness, oppression and pain in the stomach cavity and chest, it is often combined with *huáng lián* (Coptidis Rhizoma), *guā lóu* (Trichosanthis Fructus) and *bàn xià* (Pinelliae Rhizoma). To treat obstruction and exuberance of phlegm-drool with cough and excessive phlegm, it can be combined with *bàn xià* (Pinelliae Rhizoma) and *chén pí* (Citri Reticulatae Pericarpium).

此外，本品尚可用治胃扩张及胃下垂、子宫脱垂、脱肛等脏器下垂，常配伍黄芪、升麻、柴胡等，以增强升提之效。

In addition, it can also be used for the treatment of gasterectasis and visceral prolapse, such as gastroptosis, hysteroptosis and proctoptosis. It is often combined with *huáng qí* (Astragali Radix), *shēng má* (Cimicifugae Rhizoma) and *chái hú* (Bupleuri Radix) to strengthen its raising and lifting effects.

【用法用量 / Usage and dosage】

煎服，3~10g。

Decoction, 3-10g.

【使用注意 / Precaution】

孕妇慎用。

It should be used with caution for pregnant women.

【现代研究 / Modern research】

本品主要含橙皮苷、新橙皮苷、柚皮苷、挥发油、辛弗林、去甲肾上腺素等。具有调节胃肠平滑肌、抗溃疡、利胆、升血压、强心、调节子宫收缩、镇痛等作用。

The main contents of *Zhǐ shí* are hesperidin, neohesperidin, naringin, volatile oil, synephrine and norepinephrine. It can regulate gastric and intestinal smooth muscle, inhibit ulcer, promote the function of gallbladder, raise blood pressure, inhibit uterus *in vitro*, relieve pain and also has cardiotonic action.

木香　*Mù xiāng* (Aucklandiae Radix)
《神农本草经》
Shen Nong's Classic of the Materia Medica (Shén Nóng Běn Cǎo Jīng)

【来源 / Origin】

为菊科植物木香 *Aucklandia lappa* Decne. 的干燥根。原产于印度、巴基斯坦、缅甸，称为"广木香"；我国现已栽培成功，主产于我国云南、广西，称为"云木香"。秋、冬二季采挖，干燥，切厚片，生用或煨用。本品气香特异，味微苦。《中国药典》规定，含木香烃内酯（$C_{15}H_{20}O_2$）和去氢木香内酯（$C_{15}H_{18}O_2$）的总量不得少于 1.80%，饮片不得少于 1.50%。

Mù xiāng is the dry root of *Aucklandia lappa* Decne., pertaining to Compositae. It is originally produced in India, Pakistan and Myanmar, which is called *guǎng mù xiāng*. Now it has been successfully cultivated in China. It is mainly produced in Yunnan Province, Guangxi Zhuang Autonomous Region of China, which is called *yún mù xiāng*. It is collected in autumn and winter, dried in the sun, cut into thick pieces, and used raw or roasted. It has peculiar fragrance, and is slightly bitter in taste. According to *Chinese Pharmacopoeia*, the total content of costunolide ($C_{15}H_{20}O_2$) and dehydrocostus lactone ($C_{15}H_{18}O_2$) should be no less than 1.80% and no less than 1.50% in decoction pieces.

【性味归经 / Medicinal properties】

辛、苦，温。归脾、胃、大肠、胆、三焦经。

Acrid, bitter and warm in nature; act on the spleen, stomach, large intestine, gallbladder and triple energizer meridians.

【主要功效 / Medicinal efficacies】

行气止痛，健脾消食。

Move qi and relieve pain, strengthen the spleen and promote digestion.

【临床应用 / Clinical application】

1. 脾胃气滞，脘腹胀痛　本品辛行苦泄温通，气味芳香，善行脾胃气滞而止痛，健运脾胃而消食化积。为治脾胃气滞，脘腹胀痛之要药，常与厚朴、陈皮、枳壳等同用。若治食积气滞，脘腹胀痛，嗳腐吞酸者，常与山楂、麦芽、神曲等同用。若治脾虚气滞，脘腹胀痛，食少便溏者，常与党参、白术、陈皮等同用。

(1) Qi stagnation in the spleen and stomach, distending pain in the stomach cavity and abdomen　*Mù xiāng* is acrid with moving effect and bitter in taste with function of descending. It is warm in nature with action of descending and discharging. It has fragrance and is good at moving qi stagnation in the spleen and stomach to relieve pain, strengthening spleen and stomach to promote digestion. To treat qi stagnation of spleen and stomach with distending pain in the stomach cavity and abdomen, it is often combined with *hòu pò* (Magnoliae Officinalis Cortex), *chén pí* (Citri Reticulatae Pericarpium) and *zhǐ qiào* (Aurantii Fructus). To treat qi stagnation due to food accumulation, manifested as distending pain in the stomach cavity and abdomen, fetid eructation and acid regurgitation, it is often combined with *shān zhā* (Crataegi Fructus), *mài yá* (Hordei Germinatus Fructus) and *shén qū* (Medicata Fermentata Massa). To treat qi stagnation due to spleen deficiency with distending pain in the stomach cavity and abdomen, poor appetite and loose stool, it is often combined with *dǎng shēn* (Codonopsis Radix), *bái zhú* (Atractylodis Macrocephalae Rhizoma) and *chén pí* (Citri Reticulatae Pericarpium).

2. 大肠气滞，泻痢后重　本品辛行苦降，亦善行大肠之气滞，使肠道气机通畅，大便通调，后重自除。用治湿热泻痢，里急后重，常与黄连配伍。若治食积气滞，脘腹胀满，大便秘结或泻而不爽，常与槟榔、青皮、大黄等同用。

(2) Qi stagnation in the large intestine, diarrhea and dysentery tenesmus　*Mù xiāng* is acrid with moving effect and bitter in taste with descending function. It is also good at treating qi stagnation in the large intestine, which smooth qi movement of intestines to promote defecation and relieve tenesmus. To treat damp-heat diarrhea and dysentery accompanied by tenesmus, it is often combined with *huáng lián*. To treat qi stagnation due to food accumulation with distension and fullness in the stomach and abdomen, constipation or incomplete diarrhea, it is often combined with *bīng láng* (Arecae Semen), *qīng pí* (Citri Reticulatae Viride Pericarpium) and *dà huáng* (Rhei Radix et Rhizoma).

3. 肝胆气滞，胁痛，黄疸　本品既能行气健脾，又能疏肝利胆。用治湿热郁蒸、气机不畅之脘腹胀痛、胁痛，可与柴胡、郁金、枳实等配伍。若治湿热黄疸，常与茵陈、大黄、金钱草等同用。

(3) Qi stagnation in the liver and gallbladder, hypochondriac pain and jaundice　*Mù xiāng* can not only move qi and invigorate spleen, but also soothe the liver and promote the function of gallbladder. To treat distending pain in the stomach cavity and abdomen as well as hypochondriac pain caused by retention and fumigation of damp-heat as well as unsmooth qi movement, it is often combined with *chái hú* (Bupleuri Radix), *yù jīn* (Curcumae Radix) and *zhǐ shí* (Aurantii Immaturus Fructus). To treat jaundice due to damp-heat, it is often combined with *yīn chén* (Artemisiae Scopariae Herba), *dà huáng* (Rhei Radix et Rhizoma) and *jīn qián cǎo* (Lysimachiae Herba).

此外，本品气芳香能醒脾开胃，故于滋补剂中少许加之，能健运脾胃，调畅气机，以免滋腻碍胃。

In addition, *mù xiāng* is fragrant and can invigorate spleen and stimulate appetite. Therefore, adding an appropriate amount to nourish-tonifying formula can reinforce spleen and stomach as well as regulate qi movement to avoid dysfunction of stomach due to overnutrition.

【用法用量 / Usage and dosage 】

煎服，3~6g。本品行气宜生用，实肠止泻宜煨用。

Decoction, 3-6g. The raw form has a strong effect of moving qi, and the roasted form is suitable for arresting diarrhea.

【现代研究 / Modern research 】

本品主要含木香烃内酯、去氢木香内酯、愈创内酯等挥发油，尚含较多的烯类成分、氨基酸及胆胺、木香碱、树脂等。具有促进胃肠运动、促进消化液分泌、抗溃疡、抗腹泻、松弛气管平滑肌、利尿、抑菌、抗炎等作用。

Mù xiāng mainly contains volatile oil, such as costunolide, dehydrocostus lactone and zaluzanin. It also contains alkenes, amino acid, cholamine, caryophyllene and resin. It has the functions of promoting bowel movement, promoting the secretion of digestive juice, inhibiting ulcer, antagonizing diarrhea, relaxing spasms of tracheal smooth muscle, promoting urination, inhibiting bacterium typhosum and antagonizing inflammation.

香附 *Xiāng fù* (Cyperi Rhizoma)
《名医别录》
Miscellaneous Records of Famous Physicians (Míng Yī Bié Lù)

【来源 / Origin】

为莎草科植物莎草 *Cyperus rotundus* L. 的干燥根茎。全国大部分地区均产，主产于广东、河南、四川等地。秋季采挖，晒干，生用或醋炙用，用时捣碎。本品气香，味微苦。《中国药典》规定，含挥发油不得少于 1.0%（ml/g）；饮片不得少于 0.8%（ml/g）。

Xiāng fù is the dried rhizome of *Cyperus rotundus* L., pertaining to Cyperaceae. It is produced in the most area of China, mainly in Guangdong, Henan and Sichuan Province. It is collected in autumn, dried in the sun, and used raw or stir-fried with vinegar, and pound into pieces. It has fragrance and is slightly bitter in taste. According to *Chinese Pharmacopoeia*, the content of volatile oil should be no less than 1.0% (ml/g), and no less than 0.8% (ml/g) in decoction pieces.

【性味归经 / Medicinal properties】

辛、微苦、微甘，平。归肝、脾、三焦经。

Acrid, slightly bitter, slightly sweet and neutral; act on the liver, spleen and triple energizer meridians.

【主要功效 / Medicinal efficacies】

疏肝解郁，调经止痛，理气调中。

Soothe the liver and resolve constraint, regulate menstruation and relieve pain, rectify qi and regulate the center.

【临床应用 / Clinical application】

1. 肝郁气滞证 本品主入肝经，辛香行散，善解肝气之郁结，味苦降泄以平肝气之横逆，味甘能缓肝气之急，为疏肝解郁、行气止痛之要药。用治肝气郁结，胁肋胀痛，常与柴胡、川芎、枳壳等同用。用治寒凝气滞、肝气犯胃之胃脘疼痛，常与高良姜同用。用治寒疝腹痛，多与小茴香、乌药、吴茱萸等同用。

(1) Liver constraint and qi stagnation *Xiāng fù* acts on the liver meridian. It is acrid and fragrant for dispersing and moving, so it is effective in soothing the liver and rectifying qi. It is bitter for descending and discharging so as to be used to rectify transverse flow of liver qi. It is sweet for relieving hyperactivity of liver qi, so it is an essential medicinal that can soothe the liver and resolve restraint, move qi and relieve pain. To treat distending pain in the hypochondrium due to constraint of liver qi, it is combined with *chái hú* (Bupleuri Radix), *chuān xiōng* (Chuanxiong Rhizoma) and *zhǐ qiào* (Aurantii Fructus). To treat pain in the stomach cavity due to cold congealing and qi stagnation and liver qi attacking stomach, it is often combined with *gāo liáng jiāng*. To treat abdominal pain from hernia, it is often combined with *xiǎo huí xiāng* (Foeniculi Fructus), *wū yào* (Linderae Radix) and *wú zhū yú* (Evodiae Fructus).

2. 月经不调，痛经，乳房胀痛 本品性平辛散，善于疏肝理气，调经止痛，为妇科调经止痛之要药。用治肝郁气滞之月经不调、痛经，常与柴胡、川芎、当归等同用。用治肝郁气滞，乳房胀痛或结块，多与柴胡、青皮、瓜蒌等同用。若治肝郁血滞，经闭腹痛，可与桃仁、红花、五灵脂等同用。

(2) Irregular menstruation, painful menstruation, distending pain in the chest *Xiāng fù* is neutral in nature and acrid in taste for dispersing, it is good at soothing the liver and rectifying qi, regulating menstruation and relieving pain, so it serves as a main medicinal to regulate menstruation and relieve pain in gynecology. To treat irregular menstruation and painful menstruation caused by liver constraint and qi stagnation, it is often combined with *chái hú* (Bupleuri Radix), *chuān xiōng* (Chuanxiong Rhizoma) and *dāng guī* (Angelicae Sinensis Radix). To treat distending pain in the breast or breast lumps due to liver constraint and qi stagnation, it is often combined with *chái hú* (Bupleuri Radix), *qīng pí* (Citri Reticulatae Viride Pericarpium) and *guā lóu* (Trichosanthis Fructus). To treat amenorrhea and abdominal pain due to liver constraint and blood stasis, it is often combined with *táo rén* (Persicae Semen), *hóng huā* (Carthami Flos) and *wǔ líng zhī* (Trogopterori Faeces).

3. **脾胃气滞证** 本品味辛入脾经，能理气宽中，和胃止痛。用治脾胃气滞，脘腹痞闷，胀满疼痛，可与木香、砂仁等同用。若治脾虚气滞，胃脘不舒，胀满疼痛，嗳气食少等，可与黄芪、党参、陈皮等同用。

(3) Qi stagnation of spleen and stomach *Xiāng fù* is acrid in flavor and acts on the spleen meridian. It can rectify qi, loosen middle energizer, harmonize stomach and relieve pain. To treat *pǐ* and oppression in the chest and abdomen with distension, fullness and pain due to qi stagnation of spleen and stomach, it is usually combined with *mù xiāng* (Aucklandiae Radix) and *shā rén* (Amomi Fructus). To treat oppression, distension, fullness and pain in the stomach cavity, belching and poor appetite due to qi stagnation caused by spleen deficiency, it is often combined with *huáng qí* (Astragali Radix), *dǎng shēn* (Codonopsis Radix) and *chén pí* (Citri Reticulatae Pericarpium).

【用法用量 / Usage and dosage】

煎服，6~10g。醋炙止痛力增强。

Decoction, 6-10g. When processed with vinegar, its effect in relieving pain would be increased.

【现代研究 / Modern research】

本品主要含香附子烯、香附醇、异香附醇、β-蒎烯、β-香附酮等挥发油，尚含黄酮类、三萜类、酚类、生物碱等。具有镇痛、抑制子宫平滑肌收缩、抑制肠管收缩、促进胆汁分泌、解热、抗炎、保肝、强心、降压等作用。

Xiāng fù mainly contains volatile oil such as cyperene, cyperyl alcohol, isocyperol, β-pinene and β-carotene. It also contains flavonoid, phenol and alkaloids. It has the functions of relieving pain, inhibiting contraction of uterus smooth muscle and intestinal canal, promoting secretion of bile, relieving heat, antagonizing inflammation, protecting the liver, cardiotonic and bring down blood pressure.

川楝子 *Chuān liàn zǐ* (Toosendan Fructus)
《神农本草经》
Shen Nong's Classic of the Materia Medica (Shén Nóng Běn Cǎo Jīng)

【来源 / Origin】

为楝科植物川楝树 *Melia toosendan* Sieb. et Zucc. 的干燥成熟果实。我国南方各地均产，以四川产者为佳。冬季果实成熟时采收，干燥，生用或炒用，用时打碎。本品气特异，味酸、苦。《中国药典》规定，含川楝素（$C_{30}H_{38}O_{11}$）应为 0.060%~0.20%，炒川楝子应为 0.040%~0.20%。

Chuān liàn zǐ is the dried fruit of *Melia toosendan* Sieb. et Zucc., pertaining to Meliaceae. It is mainly produced in the south China, but the medicinal produced in Sichuan Province is superior. It is collected in winter, dried, and used raw or stir-fried with bran and ground into pieces. It has a peculiar odor and is sour and bitter in taste. According to *Chinese Pharmacopoeia*, the content of toosendanin ($C_{30}H_{38}O_{11}$) should be 0.060%~0.20%, and that in fried *Chuān liàn zǐ* should be 0.040%~0.20%.

【性味归经 / Medicinal properties】

苦，寒；有小毒。归肝、小肠、膀胱经。

Bitter, cold and slightly toxic; act on the liver, small intestine, and bladder meridians.

【主要功效 / Medicinal efficacies】

疏肝泄热，行气止痛，杀虫。

Soothe the liver and discharge heat, move qi and relieve pain, kill worms.

【临床应用 / Clinical application】

1. 肝郁化火所致诸痛　本品苦寒清泄，既能清肝泻火，又能行气止痛。为治肝郁气滞诸痛之良药，尤善治肝郁化火诸痛。用治肝郁气滞或肝郁化火，胸胁脘腹疼痛，每与延胡索配伍。用治疝气痛因热所致者，可与延胡索、香附、橘核等同用；若治寒疝腹痛，则与小茴香、木香、吴茱萸等同用。

(1) **Pains due to qi constraint transforming into fire**　*Chuān liàn zǐ* is bitter and cold with discharging and descending effects, can clear liver-fire and reduce accumulated heat, move qi and relieve pain. It is a most effective medicinal to treat various pains due to liver constraint and qi stagnation, especially pains caused by liver constraint transforming into fire. To treat pain in the chest, hypochondrium, stomach cavity and abdomen due to liver constraint and qi stagnation or liver constraint transforming into fire, it is often combined with *yán hú suǒ* (Corydalis Rhizoma). To treat pain from hernia caused by heat accumulation, it can be combined with *yán hú suǒ* (Corydalis Rhizoma), *xiāng fù* (Cyperi Rhizoma) and *jú hé* (Citri Reticulatae Semen). To treat abdominal pain from cold *shàn*, it can be combined with *xiǎo huí xiāng* (Foeniculi Fructus), *mù xiāng* (Aucklandiae Radix) and *wú zhū yú* (Evodiae Fructus).

2. 虫积腹痛　本品苦寒有小毒，既能驱杀肠道寄生虫，又能行气止痛。用治蛔虫等引起的虫积腹痛，可与槟榔、使君子等同用。

(2) **Abdominal pain due to worm accumulation**　*Chuān liàn zǐ* is bitter, cold and slightly toxic with functions of eliminating and killing parasites, moving qi and relieving pain. To treat abdominal pain due to roundworms, it can be combined with *bīng láng* (Arecae Semen) and *shǐ jūn zǐ* (Quisqualis Fructus).

【用法用量 / Usage and dosage】

煎服，5~10g。外用适量，研末调涂。

Decoction, 5-10g. An appropriate amount is ground into powder for mixing and applying externally.

【使用注意 / Precaution】

脾胃虚寒者慎用，不宜过量或持续服用。

It should be used with caution for patients with deficiency-cold of spleen and stomach, and it is not proper for overdose and long-term taking.

【现代研究 / Modern research】

本品主要含川楝素、楝树碱、黄酮、多糖及脂肪油等。具有松弛奥迪括约肌、收缩胆囊、促进胆汁排泄、兴奋肠管平滑肌、驱虫、镇痛、抑菌、抗炎等作用。

Chuān liàn zǐ mainly contains toosendanin, margosin, kaempferol alcohol and fatty oil. It has the functions of relaxing sphincter of Oddi, contracting gallbladder, promoting the secretion of bile, exciting smooth muscle of the intestinal canal, killing worms, relieving pain, antagonizing bacteria and inflammation.

薤白　*Xiè bái* (Allii Macrostemonis Bulbus)
《神农本草经》
Shen Nong's Classic of the Materia Medica (Shén Nóng Běn Cǎo Jīng)

【来源 / Origin】

为百合科植物小根蒜 *Allium macrostemon* Bge. 或薤 *Allium chinense* G.Don 的地下鳞茎。全国各地均有分布，主产于东北、河北、江苏等地。夏、秋二季采挖，晒干，生用。本品有蒜臭，味微辣。

Xiè bái is the squamous bulb of *Allium macrostemon* Bge. or *Allium chinense* G.Don, pertaining to Liliaceae. It is distributed in various areas in China, and mainly produced in northeastern China, Hebei and Jiangsu Province. It is collected in summer and autumn, dried in the sun, and used raw. It has an alliaceous odor and is slightly acrid in taste.

【性味归经 / Medicinal properties】

辛、苦，温。归心、肺、胃、大肠经。

Acrid, bitter and warm; act on the heart, lung, stomach and large intestine meridians.

【主要功效 / Medicinal efficacies】

通阳散结，行气导滞。

Unblock yang and dissipate masses, move qi and remove stagnation.

【临床应用 / Clinical application】

1. 胸痹心痛　本品辛散苦降，温通滑利，上入心肺经，善通胸中之阳，散阴寒之凝滞，为治胸痹之要药。用治胸阳不振，寒湿痰浊凝滞于胸中之胸痹心痛，常与瓜蒌、半夏、枳实等配伍。若治痰瘀胸痹，可与丹参、川芎等同用。

(1) Chest impediment (pectoral stuffiness pain)　*Xiè bái* is acrid for dispersing and bitter for descending. It is warm in nature for unblocking and smoothing. It moves upward to the heart and lung meridian and is effective at unblocking the obstruction of thoracic yang and dissipating the congealing of yin-cold. It is an essential medicinal to treat chest impediment. To treat chest oppression and pain due to cold-phlegm obstruction and inactivation of thoracic yang, it is often combined with *guā lóu* (Trichosanthis Fructus), *bàn xià* (Pinelliae Rhizoma) and *zhǐ shí* (Aurantii Immaturus Fructus). To treat chest impediment due to phlegm accumulation, it is often combined with *dān shēn* (Salviae Miltiorrhizae Radix et Rhizoma) and *chuān xiōng* (Chuanxiong Rhizoma).

2. 脘腹胀痛，泻痢后重　本品辛行苦降，下入胃肠经，有行气导滞、消胀止痛之功。用治胃寒气滞，脘腹痞满胀痛，可与高良姜、砂仁、木香等同用。若治湿热内蕴，胃肠气滞，泻痢后重，可与黄连、木香、枳实等同用。

(2) Distending pain in the stomach and abdomen, diarrhea and dysentery with tenesmus　*Xiè bái* is acrid for moving and bitter for descending, it moves downward to the stomach and intestines meridians. It has efficacies of moving qi and guiding out food stagnation, eliminating distension and relieving pain. To treat *pǐ*, fullness, distension and pain in the stomach and abdomen due to stomach cold and qi stagnation, it can be combined with *gāo liáng jiāng* (Alpiniae Officinarum Rhizoma), *shā rén*

(Amomi Fructus) and *mù xiāng* (Aucklandiae Radix). To treat diarrhea and dysentery with tenesmus due to internal accumulation of damp-heat and qi stagnation in the stomach and intestines, it can be combined with *huáng lián* (Coptidis Rhizoma), *mù xiāng* (Aucklandiae Radix) and *zhǐ shí* (Aurantii Immaturus Fructus).

【用法用量 / Usage and dosage】

煎服，5~10g。

Decoction, 5-10g.

【现代研究 / Modern research】

本品主要含甾体皂苷 A~K 等，尚含大蒜氨酸、甲基大蒜氨酸、大蒜素、前列腺素、生物碱等。具有扩张血管、抗心肌缺血、降血脂、抗血小板聚集、抗动脉粥样硬化、止泻、镇痛、抑菌、抗炎等作用。

Xiè bái mainly contains sterol saponins A-K, alliin, methiin, allicin, prostaglandin and alkaloids. It has the functions of dilating blood vessels, antagonizing myocardial ischemia, reducing blood fat, and inhibiting platelet aggregation, antagonizing arteriosclerosis, reliving diarrhea, relieving pain, antagonizing inflammation, antagonizing bacteria.

其他理气药功用介绍见表 13-1。

The efficacies of qi-rectifying medicinals are shown in table 13-1.

表 13-1 其他理气药功用介绍

类别	药物	药性	功效	应用	用法用量
理气药	枳壳	苦、辛、酸，微寒。归脾、胃经	理气宽中，行滞消胀	胸胁气滞，胀满疼痛，食积不化，痰饮内停，脏器下垂	煎服，3~10g
	沉香	辛、苦，微温。归脾、胃、肾经	行气止痛，温中止呕，纳气平喘	寒凝气滞，胸腹胀闷疼痛，胃寒呕吐呃逆，肾虚气喘	煎服，1~5g，宜后下
	乌药	辛，温。归肺、脾、肾、膀胱经	行气止痛，温肾散寒	寒凝气滞，胸腹胀痛，肾阳不足，遗尿尿频	煎服，3~10g
	化橘红	辛、苦，温。归肺、脾经	理气宽中，燥湿化痰	咳嗽痰多，食积伤酒，呕恶痞闷	煎服，3~6g
	甘松	辛、甘，温。归脾、胃经	理气止痛，开郁醒脾；外用祛湿消肿	脘腹胀满，食欲不振，呕吐；外用治牙痛，脚气肿毒	煎服，3~6g。外用适量
	佛手	辛、苦、酸，温。归肝、脾、胃、肺经	疏肝理气，和胃止痛，燥湿化痰	肝胃气滞，胸胁胀痛，胃脘痞满，食少呕吐，咳嗽痰多	煎服，3~10g
	香橼	辛、苦、酸，温。归肝、脾、肺经	疏肝理气，宽中，化痰	肝胃气滞，胸胁胀痛，脘腹痞满，呕吐噫气，痰多咳嗽	煎服，3~10g

续表

类别	药物	药性	功效	应用	用法用量
理气药	玫瑰花	甘、微苦，温。归肝、脾经	行气解郁，和血，止痛	肝胃气痛，食少呕恶，月经不调，跌仆伤痛	煎服，3~6g
	大腹皮	辛，温。归脾、胃、大肠、小肠经	行气宽中，利水消肿	湿阻气滞，脘腹胀闷，大便不爽；水肿胀满，脚气浮肿，小便不利	煎服，5~10g
	檀香	辛，温。归脾、胃、心、肺经	行气止痛，散寒调中	寒凝气滞，胸膈不舒，胸痹心痛，脘腹疼痛，呕吐食少	煎服，2~5g，后下
	柿蒂	苦、涩，平。归胃经	降气止呃	呃逆证	煎服，5~10g

（管家齐）

题库

第十四章 消食药
Chapter 14　Digestion-promoting medicinals

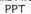

PPT

微课

学习目标｜Learning goals

1. **掌握** 消食药在性能、功效、主治、配伍及使用注意方面的共性；山楂、六神曲、麦芽的性能、功效、应用以及特殊的用法用量和特殊的使用注意。

2. **熟悉** 莱菔子、鸡内金的功效、主治以及特殊的用法用量和特殊的使用注意。

3. **了解** 消食药及相关功效术语的含义；稻芽的功效。

1. Master the commonness of digestion-promoting medicinals in efficacy, indications, property, compatibility and precautions; as well as the property, efficacy, application, special usage and dosage, and special precautions of *shān zhā*, *liù shén qǔ*, and *mài yá*.

2. Familiar with the efficacy, indications, special usage, dosage and precautions of *lái fú zǐ* and *jī nèi jīn*.

3. Understand the definitions of digestion-promoting medicinals and related efficacy terms; and the efficacy of *dào yá*.

凡以消食化积为主要功效，常用于治疗食滞胃脘证的药物，称为消食药。

With promoting digestion and eliminating accumulation as major efficacies, drugs that are used to treat the syndrome of food stagnation in the stomach cavity are called digestion-promoting medicinals.

消食药多性味甘平，主入脾、胃二经。以消食化积为主要功效，主治食滞胃脘证，症见脘腹胀满疼痛，厌食，嗳腐吞酸，或呕吐酸馊食物，大便臭秽，舌苔厚腻等。

Mostly sweet and neutral, digestion-promoting medicinals, mainly entering the spleen and stomach channels and with promoting digestion and eliminating accumulation as the primary efficacies, are mainly applied to treat the syndrome of food stagnation in the stomach cavity, with the symptoms of abdominal distention, fullness and pain, food sickness, belching with fetid odor and swallowing acid, or vomiting sour and spoiled food, stinking defecation, thick and greasy coating and so on.

消食药各有所长，饮食积滞的性质也不同，兼证也较多，病情又有寒热虚实之分，故应根据不同的病证选择本类药物并适当配伍。食积内停，多有气机阻滞，因此消食药常配伍理气药，使气行积消。若积滞化热，应配伍苦寒清热或轻下之品；若寒湿困脾，应配伍化湿药；兼有表证者，应配伍解表药；若脾胃虚弱，食积内停，当配伍补气健脾之品，以标本兼顾，不可单用消食药取效。

Each digestion-promoting medicinal has characteristics to their own advantages, the nature of food stagnation varies with many concurrent symptoms, and the disease also differs in cold and heat, or deficiency and excess. Thus, in the application of this kind of drugs, suitable medicinals should be chosen and combined according to different symptoms. For internal food accumulation, mostly with obstruction and stagnation of the qi mechanism, digestion-promoting medicinals often should be compatible with qi-rectifying medicinals to flow qi and eliminate accumulation. For those with accumulation and stagnation transforming into heat, bitter, cold and heat-clearing medicinals or those of mild purgation should be added; for those with cold-dampness encumbering the spleen, dampness-resolving medicinals should be combined; for those with concurrent exterior pattern, exterior-releasing medicinals should be used together; and for those with spleen-stomach weakness and internal food accumulation, they should be compatible with medicinals that can supplement qi and fortify the spleen. Giving consideration to both the incidental and fundamental, digestion-promoting medicinals should not be used alone to take effect.

本类药物虽多数效缓，但仍不乏有耗气之弊，故气虚而无积滞者慎用。

Although most of these medicinals work slowly, there is still a lot of qi consumption, so those with qi deficiency but without accumulation and stagnation should use them with caution.

山楂　*Shān zhā* (Crataegi Fructus)
《本草经集注》
Collective Commentaries on the Classic of Materia Medica (Běn Căo Jīng Jí Zhù)

【来源 / Origin 】

本品为蔷薇科植物山里红 *Crataegus pinnatifida* Bge.var.*major* N.E.Br. 或山楂 *Crataegus pinnatifida* Bge. 的干燥成熟果实。主产于河南、山东、河北等地。秋季果实成熟时采收。切片，干燥，生用或炒用。本品气微香，味酸、微甜。《中国药典》规定，含有机酸以枸橼酸（$C_6H_8O_7$）计，不得少于 5.0%；饮品不得少于 4.0%。

Shān zhā is the mature dry fruits of *Crataegus pinnatifida* Bge. var. *major* N. E. Br. or *Crataegus pinnatifida* Bge., pertaining to Rosaceae. Mainly distributed in Henan, Shandong, Hebei and some other places, it is collected in autumn when the fruits ripen, sliced into pieces, dried and used in raw or stir-fried form. It is slightly fragrant, sour and a little sweet. According to *Chinese Pharmacopoeia*, the content of organic acid, calculated as citric acid ($C_6H_8O_7$), should be no less than 5.0%, and no less than 4.0% in decoction pieces.

【性味归经 / Medicinal properties 】

酸、甘，微温。归脾、胃、肝经。

Sour, sweet and slightly warm; act on the spleen, stomach and liver meridians.

【主要功效 / Medicinal efficacies 】

消食健胃，行气散瘀，化浊降脂。

Fortify the stomach and promote digestion, move qi to dissipate stasis, remove turbidity and reduce lipid.

【临床应用 / Clinical application 】

1. 食滞胃脘证　本品酸甘，微温不热，功善消食化积，尤为消化油腻肉食积滞之要药，对于肉食积滞之脘腹胀满、嗳腐吞酸、腹痛便溏者，单用即可奏效。临床常用本品配伍麦芽、神曲等，用治一切饮食积滞病证。若治食积气滞脘腹胀痛，常与木香、青皮等同用。

(1) Food stagnation in the stomach cavity　Sour and sweet, slightly warm but not hot, *shān zhā* does well in promoting digestion and eliminating accumulation, and is an important drug especially for digesting the accumulation and stagnation of fatty meat, which can take effect alone for abdominal distention and fullness, belching with fetid odor and acid swallowing as well as abdominal pain with loose stool due to the accumulation and stagnation of meat. Clinically, it is often compatible with *mài yá* and *shén qū* (Medicata Fermentata Massa) to treat all syndromes of dietary accumulation and stagnation. For those with food accumulation and qi stagnation, as well as distending abdominal pain, it is often used together with *mù xiāng* (Aucklandiae Radix), *qīng pí* (Citri Reticulatae Viride Pericarpium), etc.

2. 泻痢腹痛，疝气疼痛 本品能行气散瘀，化滞止痛，炒用兼能止泻痢。用治泻痢腹痛，可单用本品，生用、炒用均有效，或与木香、黄连等同用。用治疝气疼痛，常与橘核、荔枝核等同用。

(2) Diarrhea, dysentery and abdominal pain, and hernia pain Moving qi to dissipate stasis, resolving stagnation and relieving pain, *shān zhā* can concurrently arrest diarrhea and dysentery if stir-fried. To treat diarrhea, dysentery and abdominal pain, it can be used alone, either for raw or stir-fried use, or used together with *mù xiāng*, *huáng lián* (Coptidis Rhizoma), etc. To treat hernia pain, it is often combined with *jú hé* (Citri Reticulatae Semen), *lì zhī hé*(Litchi Semen), etc.

3. 血瘀胸腹痛，经闭痛经 本品性温，兼入肝经血分，有活血祛瘀止痛之功。用治瘀滞胸痹心痛，常与川芎、丹参、红花等同用。用治妇女产后瘀阻腹痛以及痛经、经闭，多与当归、香附、红花等同用。

(3) Blood stasis and thoracoabdominal pain, menstrual block and dysmenorrhea *shān zhā* is warm and concurrently enter the liver channel and invade the blood level, which has the actions of invigorating blood and dispelling stasis. To treat chest impediment and heart pain due to stasis, it is often used together with *chuān xiōng* (Chuanxiong Rhizoma), *dān shēn* (Salviae Miltiorrhizae Radix et Rhizoma), *hóng huā* (Carthami Flos), etc. To treat abdominal pain, dysmenorrhea and menstrual block due to postpartum stasis, it is often combined with *dāng guī* (Angelicae Sinensis Radix), *xiāng fù* (Cyperi Rhizoma), *hóng huā*, etc.

4. 高脂血症 本品有良好的化浊降脂功效。用治高脂血症、冠心病、高血压等，可单用制成各种剂型，亦常与丹参、三七、葛根等配伍。

(4) Hyperlipidemia With good efficacies of removing turbidity and lowering lipid, to treat hyperlipidemia, coronary artery disease, hypertension and some other diseases, *shān zhā* can be used alone to process various preparations, or be compatible with *dān shēn*, *sān qī* (Notoginseng Radix et Rhizoma), *gé gēn* (Puerariae Lobatae Radix), etc.

【用法用量 / Usage and dosage】

煎服，9~12g。生山楂、炒山楂偏于消食散瘀，焦山楂消食导滞作用较强，山楂炭多用于止泻痢。

Decocted, 9~12g. While *shēng shān zhā* and *chǎo shān zhā* tend to promote digestion and dissipate stasis and *jiāo shān zhā* has a strong efficacy of promoting digestion and removing stagnation, *shān zhā tàn* is frequently used to arrest diarrhea and dysentery.

【使用注意 / Precaution】

脾胃虚弱而无积滞者或胃酸分泌过多者均慎用。

It should be used with caution for those with spleen-stomach weakness but without accumulation and stagnation, or those with excessive gastric acid secretion.

【现代研究 / Modern research】

本品主要含黄酮类、三萜皂苷类、游离酸、脂肪酸、维生素C及有机盐等。具有促进脂肪消化、增加消化酶分泌、降血压、降血脂、抗动脉粥样硬化、抗心律失常、抗心肌缺血、降血糖、保肝等作用。

Shān zhā mainly contains flavonoids, triterpene saponins, free acids, fatty acids, vitamin C, organic salt, etc. It has the functions of promoting fat digestion, increasing digestive enzyme secretion, lowering blood pressure and blood fat, resisting atherosclerosis, arrhythmia and myocardial ischemia, decreasing blood sugar, protecting the liver, and so on.

六神曲 · *Liù shén qǔ* (Medicata Fermentata Massa)
《药性论》
Treatise on Medicinal Properties (*Yào Xìng Lùn*)

【来源 / Origin】

为辣蓼、青蒿、杏仁等加入面粉混合后经发酵而成的加工品，全国各地均有生产，但规格、工艺略有差异。具体制法：取较大量面粉或麸皮与杏仁泥、赤小豆粉以及鲜青蒿、鲜苍耳、鲜辣蓼自然汁混合拌匀，使干湿适宜，放入筐内，覆以麻叶或楮叶，保温发酵一周，长出黄菌丝时取出，切成小块，晒干即成。生用或炒用。本品有特异的发酵香气，味微苦辛。

Liù shén qǔ is a processed product of *là liào* (Polygoni Hydropiperis Herba), *qīng hāo* (Artemisiae Annuae Herba), and *xìng rén* (Armeniacae Amarum Semen), which are mixed with flour and then fermented. It is produced throughout the country, with slightly different specifications and crafts. The specific method is: take a comparatively large amount of flour or wheat bran, mix it well with *xìng rén* mud, *chì xiǎo dòu* (Phaseoli Semen) flour, as well as the natural juice of fresh *qīng hāo*, fresh *cāng ěr* (Xanthii) and fresh *là liào* to make it neither dry nor damp, put it into the basket, cover it with *luó bù má yè* (Apocyni Veneti Folium) or *chǔ yè* (Broussonetia Papyrifera L.), insulated ferment for one week, take out the yellow hyphae upon appearing, cut them into small pieces and dry for raw or stir-fried use. It has a special fermented aroma, and slightly bitter taste.

【性味归经 / Medicinal properties】

甘、辛，温。归脾、胃经。

Sweet, acrid and warm; act on the spleen and stomach meridians.

【主要功效 / Medicinal efficacies】

消食和胃。

Promote digestion and harmonize the stomach.

【临床应用 / Clinical application】

食滞胃脘证 本品味甘而辛，气香性温，有消食化积、开胃和中之效，尤善消化谷麦酒食积滞。用治食滞不化，脘腹胀满，食少纳呆，肠鸣腹泻，常与山楂、麦芽、木香等同用。治食积日久，脘腹胀痛而有气滞者，多与木香、厚朴、莪术等同用。本品略兼解表之功，对外感兼食滞者，尤为适宜。

Syndromes of food stagnation in the stomach cavity Sweet and acrid, fragrant and warm, *liù shén qǔ* has the efficacies of promoting digestion and eliminating accumulation as well as promoting appetite and harmonizing the center, and is especially good at digesting the accumulation and stagnation of grains and alcohol. To treat undigested food stagnation, abdominal distention and fullness, poor appetite and digestion as well as rumbling intestines and diarrhea, it is often used together with *shān zhā, mài yá, mù xiāng*, etc. For those with long-time food accumulation and distending abdominal pain together with qi stagnation, it is often combined with *mù xiāng, hòu pò* (Magnoliae Officinalis Cortex), *é zhú* (Curcumae Rhizoma), etc. Since *liù shén qǔ* has a slight concurrent action of resolving the exterior, it is especially suitable for those with external contraction and concurrent food stagnation.

本品炒焦后又具止泻之功，对食积腹泻可发挥消食和止泻双重作用，常与焦山楂、焦麦芽同用。

If stir-fried until scorched, *liù shén qǔ* also with the action of arresting diarrhea, has a dual function of promoting digestion and arresting diarrhea for food accumulation and diarrhea, where it is often used together with *jiāo shān zhā* and *jiāo mài yá*.

【用法用量 / Usage and dosage】

煎服，6~15g。消食宜炒焦用。

Decocted, 6~15g; suitable to stir-fry until scorched to promote digestion.

【现代研究 / Modern research】

本品主要含酵母菌、淀粉酶、维生素 B 复合体、麦角甾醇、蛋白质及脂肪、挥发油等。具有增进食欲、维持正常消化功能等作用。

Liù shén qǔ mainly contains yeast, amylase, vitamin B complex, ergosterol, protein, fat, volatile oil, etc. It has the functions of increasing appetite and maintaining normal digestion.

麦芽 *Mài yá* (Hordei Fructus Germinatus)
《药性论》
Treatise on Medicinal Properties (*Yào Xìng Lùn*)

【来源 / Origin】

为禾本科植物大麦 *Hordeum vulgare* L. 的成熟果实经发芽干燥而成。全国各地均可生产。将麦粒用水浸泡后，保持适宜的温度和湿度，待幼芽长至约 0.5cm 时，晒干或低温干燥。生用、炒黄或炒焦用。本品气微，味微甘；炒麦芽有香气，味微苦。

Mài yá is the sprouted and dried mature fruit of *Hordeum vulgare* L., pertaining to the Poaceae. It is produced all over the country. After soaking the wheat grain in water, keep appropriate temperature and humidity, and when the buds grow to about 0.5cm, dry them in the sun or at low temperature for raw use, or stir-fry until yellow or scorched for use later. It has a slight odor and is slightly sweet in taste. *Chǎo mài yá* is fragrant and slightly bitter.

【性味归经 / Medicinal properties】

甘，平。归脾、胃经。

Sweet and neutral; act on the spleen and stomach meridians.

【主要功效 / Medicinal efficacies】

行气消食，健脾开胃，回乳消胀。

Move qi to promote digestion, fortify the spleen and promote appetite, terminate lactation and disperse distention.

【临床应用 / Clinical application】

1. 食滞胃脘证 本品甘平，有较好的消食化积、健脾开胃作用，能促进淀粉性食物的消化，主治米面薯芋等食滞证，常配伍山楂、神曲等。用治小儿乳食积滞，可单用本品煎服或研末服。用治脾胃虚弱而食滞不消、食后饱胀者，常与党参、白术、陈皮等同用。

(1) Syndromes of food stagnation in the stomach cavity Sweet and neutral, *mài yá*, with comparatively good efficacies of promoting digestion and eliminating accumulation as well as fortifying the spleen and promoting appetite, is good at promoting the digestion of starchy foods and thus is mainly applied to treat food stagnation of rice, flour, potatoes and taros, where it is often compatible with *shān zhā*, *shén qū*, etc. To treat infantile feeding accumulation, it can be decocted alone or powdered; to treat those with undigested food stagnation and bloating after eating due to spleen-stomach weakness, it is often used together with *dǎng shēn* (Codonopsis Radix), *bái zhú* (Atractylodis Macrocephalae Rhizoma), *chén pí* (Citri Reticulatae Pericarpium), etc.

2. **断乳，乳房胀痛** 本品有回乳消胀之功。治妇女断乳或乳汁郁积导致的乳房胀痛，可单用炒麦芽水煎服。

(2) Lactation termination and distending pain of the breast With the actions of terminating lactation and dispersing distention, *mài yá* can be used to terminate lactation or treat distending pain of the breast due to lactation stasis, where stir-fried *mài yá* can be decocted alone in water.

3. **肝郁气滞证** 本品兼能疏肝行气解郁，治肝郁气滞或肝胃不和之胁痛、脘腹胀痛，可作为辅助药使用，常与柴胡、香附等同用。

(3) Liver constraint and qi stagnation Entering the liver channel and with the concurrent functions of soothing the liver, moving qi and resolving constraint, *mài yá* can be applied to treat rib-side pain and distending abdominal pain caused by liver constraint and qi stagnation as well as liver-stomach disharmony. As an adjuvant medicinal, it is often used together with *chái hú* (Bupleuri Radix), *xiāng fù*, etc.

【用法用量 / Usage and dosage】

煎服，10~15g。回乳炒用60g。

Decocted, 10~15g; to terminate lactation, stir-fried, 60g.

【使用注意 / Precaution】

授乳期妇女不宜使用。

It should be avoided for women during lactation.

【现代研究 / Modern research】

本品主要含α-淀粉酶及β-淀粉酶、催化酶、麦芽糖及大麦芽碱、腺嘌呤、胆碱、氨基酸、蛋白质、B族维生素、维生素D、维生素E以及细胞色素C等。具有帮助消化、促进胃酸和胃蛋白酶分泌、降血糖以及催乳和回乳的双向作用（小剂量催乳，大剂量回乳）。

Mài yá mainly contains α-amylase and β-amylase, catalytic enzyme, maltose and hordenine, adenine, choline, amino acid, protein, vitamin B, vitamin D, vitamin E, cytochrome C, etc. It can help digestion, promote the secretion of gastric acid and pepsin, reduce blood sugar, mutually promote and terminate lactation (low-dose lactation promotion and high dose termination).

莱菔子 *Lái fú zǐ* (Raphani Semen)
《日华子本草》
Ri Huazi's Materia Medica (Rì Huá Zǐ Běn Cǎo)

【来源 / Origin】

为十字花科植物萝卜 *Raphanus sativus* L. 的干燥成熟种子。全国各地均有栽培。夏季果实成熟时采收，晒干，生用或炒用，用时捣碎。本品气微，味淡、微苦辛。《中国药典》规定，含芥子碱以芥子碱硫氰酸盐（$C_{16}H_{24}NO_5 \cdot SCN$）计，不得少于0.40%。

Lái fú zǐ is the mature dry seed of *Raphanus sativus* L., pertaining to Cruciferae. Cultivated all over the country, it is collected in autumn when the fruits ripen, dried, and used raw or stir-fried, which needs to be crushed for application. It has a slight odor, and tastes bland, slightly bitter and acrid. According to *Chinese Pharmacopoeia*, the content of sinapine, calculated in that of sinapine thiocyanate ($C_{16}H_{24}NO_5 \cdot SCN$), should be no less than 0.40%.

【性味归经 / Medicinal properties】

辛、甘，平。归肺、脾、胃经。

Acrid, sweet and neutral; act on the lung, spleen and stomach meridians.

【主要功效 / Medicinal efficacies】

消食除胀，降气化痰。

Promote digestion and eliminate fullness, direct qi downward and dissolve phlegm.

【临床应用 / Clinical application】

1. 食积气滞证　本品味辛行散，既能消食化积，又善行气消胀。宜用治食积气滞所致的脘腹胀满或疼痛，嗳气吞酸，大便秘结等，常与山楂、神曲、陈皮等同用。若治食积兼脾虚者，常与白术配伍，以攻补兼施。

(1) The syndrome of food accumulation and qi stagnation　Acrid and dispersing, *lái fú zǐ* can not only promote digestion and eliminate accumulation, but also move qi to disperse distention, and thus is suitable for abdominal distention and fullness or pain, belching and acid swallowing as well as constipation due to food accumulation and qi stagnation, where it is often used together with *shān zhā*, *shén qū*, *chén pí*, etc. To treat those with food accumulation with concurrent spleen deficiency, it is often compatible with *bái zhú* so as to treat with both attack and supplementation.

2. 咳喘痰多，胸闷食少　本品入肺经，能降气祛痰，止咳平喘。用治痰壅气逆，咳喘痰多，胸闷不舒而兼食积者，可单用本品研末服，或与白芥子、苏子等同用。

(2) Cough and panting with profuse phlegm and chest oppression with decreased food intake　Entering the lung channel, *lái fú zǐ* can direct qi downward to dispel phlegm, and relieve cough and panting as well. To treat phlegm congestion and qi counterflow, cough and panting with profuse phlegm, uncomfortable chest oppression and concurrent food accumulation, it can be powdered and used alone, or used together with *bái jiè zǐ* (Sinapis Semen), *sū zǐ* (Fructus Perillae), etc.

【用法用量 / Usage and dosage】

煎服，5~12g。炒用消食、化痰；生用涌吐风痰。

Decocted, 5~12g; promote digestion and dissolve phlegm if stir-fried; emit wind-phlegm for raw use.

【使用注意 / Precaution】

气虚而无食积、痰滞者慎用。

It should be used with caution for those with qi deficiency but without food accumulation and phlegm stagnation.

【现代研究 / Modern research】

本品主要含芥子碱、莱菔素、芥酸、亚油酸、亚麻酸、挥发油、β- 谷甾醇、蛋白质、氨基酸等。具有祛痰、镇咳、平喘、降血压、降血脂、抗菌、调节胃肠道运动、促进胃肠蠕动等作用。

Lái fú zǐ mainly contains sinapine, raphani, erucic acid, linoleic acid, linolenic acid, essential oil, β-sitosterol, protein, amino acids, etc. It has the functions of dispelling phlegm, relieving cough and panting, lowering blood pressure and blood fat, resisting bacteria, regulating gastrointestinal motility, promoting gastrointestinal peristalsis and so on.

鸡内金 *Jī nèi jīn* (Galli Gigerii Endothelium Corneum)
《神农本草经》
Shen Nong's Classic of the Materia Medica (Shén Nóng Běn Cǎo Jīng)

【来源 / Origin 】

为雉科动物家鸡 *Gallus gallus domesticus* Brisson 的干燥沙囊内壁。全国各地均产。干燥,生用、炒用或醋制用。本品气微腥,味微苦。

Jī nèi jīn is the dry endotheca of the gizzard of *Gallus gallus domesticus* Brisson, pertaining to the Phasianidae. Produced all through the country, it is dried for raw use. It also can be stir-fried or processed with vinegar. It is slightly fishy and bitter.

【性味归经 / Medicinal properties 】

甘,平。归脾、胃、小肠、膀胱经。

Sweet and neutral; act on the spleen, stomach, small intestine or bladder meridians.

【主要功效 / Medicinal efficacies 】

健胃消食,涩精止遗,通淋化石。

Fortify the stomach and promote digestion, arrest enuresis and emission with astringents, relieve strangury and expel stones.

【临床应用 / Clinical application 】

1. 食滞胃脘,小儿疳积 本品有较强的消食化积作用,并可健运脾胃,故广泛用于各种饮食积滞病证,若病情较轻,单用研末服即有效;若食滞较重,常与六神曲、山楂、麦芽等同用。若治小儿脾虚疳积,可与白术、山药、使君子等同用。

(1) Food stagnation in the stomach cavity and infantile malnutrition with accumulation *Jī nèi jīn* has a comparatively strong efficacy of promoting digestion and eliminating accumulation, and fortifying and activating the spleen and stomach as well. Therefore, it is widely applied to treat dietary accumulation of various kinds. In milder cases, it can take effect after being powdered and taken alone; for those with more serious food stagnation, it is often used together with *liù shén qǔ*, *shān zhā* and *mài yá*. To treat infantile malnutrition with accumulation due to spleen deficiency, it can be combined with *bái zhú*, *shān yào* (Dioscoreae Rhizoma), *shǐ jūn zǐ* (Quisqualis Fructus), etc.

2. 遗精、遗尿 本品有固精缩尿止遗之功。用治遗精、遗尿,可单用炒焦研末,温酒送服;或配伍菟丝子、桑螵蛸等。

(2) Seminal emission and enuresis With the actions of consolidating essence, reducing urination and arresting enuresis, *jī nèi jīn* can be used to treat seminal emission and enuresis, where it alone can be dry-fried until scorched, powdered and taken with warm wine; or it can be compatible with *tù sī zǐ* (Cuscutae Semen), *sāng piāo xiāo* (Mantidis Oötheca), etc.

3. 砂石淋证 本品入膀胱经,有化坚消石和通淋之功。用治砂淋、石淋,小便淋沥涩痛,常与金钱草、海金沙等同用。若治胆结石,常与金钱草、郁金、木香等同用。

(3) The syndrome of sandy stone strangury Entering the bladder channel, *jī nèi jīn* has the actions of resolving hard masses and eliminating stones as well as relieving strangury. To treat sand strangury, stony strangury, as well as difficult, painful and dribbling urination, it is often used together with *jīn qián cǎo* (Lysimachiae Herba), *hǎi jīn shā* (Lygodii Spora), etc. To treat gallstone, it is often combined with *jīn qián cǎo*, *yù jīn* (Curcumae Radix), *mù xiāng* and so on.

【用法用量 / Usage and dosage】

煎服，3~10g；研末服，每次 1.5~3g。研末服效果优于煎剂。

Decocted, 3~10g; powdered, 1.5~3g per time. Powder has a better effect than decoction.

【使用注意 / Precaution】

脾虚无积滞者慎用。

It should be used with caution for those with spleen deficiency and no accumulation and stagnation.

【现代研究 / Modern research】

本品主要含胃激素、角蛋白、淀粉酶、多种维生素和微量元素，以及 18 种氨基酸等。具有调节胃肠运动、增强胃运功能、增加胃排空速率、提高胃液分泌量和酸度、降血糖、降血脂、加强膀胱括约肌收缩等作用。

Jī nèi jīn mainly contains stomach hormone, keratin, amylase, various vitamins and trace elements, as well as 18 kinds of amino acids. It has the functions of regulating gastrointestinal motility, enhancing gastric motility, speeding up gastric emptying rate, increasing gastric juice secretion and acidity, lowering blood glucose and blood fat, strengthening sphincter contraction of bladder, and so on.

其他消食药功用介绍见表 14-1。

The efficacies of digestion-promoting medicinals are shown in table 14-1.

表 14-1　其他消食药功用介绍

分类	药物	药性	功效	应用	用法用量
消食药	稻芽	甘，温。归脾、胃经	消食和中，健脾开胃	食积不消，腹胀口臭，脾胃虚弱，不饥食少	煎服，9~15g

（柳海艳）

题库

第十五章　驱　虫　药
Chapter 15　Worm-expelling medicinals

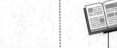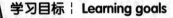
学习目标｜Learning goals

　　1. 掌握　驱虫药在性能、功效、主治、配伍及使用注意方面的共性；使君子、苦楝皮、槟榔的性能、功效、应用以及特殊的用法用量和特殊的使用注意。

　　2. 熟悉　贯众、南瓜子的功效、主治以及特殊的用法用量和特殊的使用注意。

　　3. 了解　雷丸、鹤草芽、鹤虱、榧子的功效以及特殊的用法用量和特殊的使用注意。

　　1. Master the commonness of worm-expelling medicinals in efficacy, indications, property, compatibility and cautions; as well as the property, efficacy, application, special usage and dosage and special precautions of *shǐ jūn zǐ*, *kǔ liàn pí* and *bīng láng*.

　　2. Familiar with the efficacy, indications, special usage, dosage and special precautions of *guàn zhòng* and *nán guā zǐ*.

　　3. Understand the efficacy, special usage and dosage and special precautions of *léi wán*, *hè cǎo yá*, *hè shī* and *fěi zǐ*.

　　凡以驱除或杀灭人体内寄生虫为主要功效，常用于治疗虫病的药物，称为驱虫药。

　　Medicinals with efficacies of expelling or killing parasites in the human body are known as worm-expelling medicinals, which are often used in the treatment of worm syndromes.

　　本类药物多入脾、胃、大肠经，部分药物具有毒性，对人体内的寄生虫，特别是肠道寄生虫具有麻痹或杀灭作用，促使其排出体外。主治肠道寄生虫病，如蛔虫病、蛲虫病、绦虫病、钩虫病、姜片虫病等。患有肠道寄生虫病的患者，常表现为绕脐腹痛，不思饮食或善饥多食，嗜食异物，肛门、耳、鼻瘙痒，迁延日久则见面色萎黄，形体消瘦，腹大胀满，青筋暴露，浮肿等，也有部分患者症状较轻，只在查验大便时才发现患有虫病。部分药物还可用治食积气滞、小儿疳积、便秘、疥癣等。

　　Mostly entering the spleen, stomach, and large intestine meridian, these medicinals, some being toxic, have the paralytic or killing effect on the parasite in the human body, especially the intestinal parasite, urging their excretion out of the body. They are mainly used to treat intestinal parasitic diseases, such as roundworm disease, pinworm disease, tapeworm disease, hookworm disease, fasciolopsiasis and so on. Patients suffering from intestinal parasitic diseases often show abdominal pain around the umbilicus, do not want to eat or eat more, have excessive appetite for foreign bodies, and bear itchy anus, ears and nose. If delayed for a long time, they may have sallow complexion, emaciated body, big and bulgy abdomen, exposed blue tendon, edema and so on. There are also some patients with mild symptoms, who were found to have insect diseases only in the examination of stool. Some drugs can also be used to treat food retention and qi stagnation, infantile malnutrition, constipation, scabies and so on.

使用驱虫药时，应根据寄生虫的种类及患者身体状况、病证缓急，选用适宜的驱虫药物，并根据兼证进行配伍。大便秘结者，当配伍泻下药。兼有积滞者，可与消积导滞药同用。脾胃虚弱者，应配伍补气健脾之品。体质虚弱者，须先补后攻或攻补兼施。对于肠道寄生虫病，多与泻下药配伍使用。使用无泻下作用的驱虫药时，亦常配伍泻下药以促进虫体的排出。

In the application, appropriate worm-expelling agents should be selected according to the type of parasite, the patient's physical condition and the urgency of the disease pattern, and compatibility should be conducted according to accompanying symptoms. For example, if with constipation, cathartic drugs should be used at the same time. If there is retention, it can be used together with the anti-accumulation and anti-hysteresis medicinals. Patients with weak spleen and stomach should be provided with tonic that could nourish qi and invigorate the spleen. For patients with weak constitution, it is necessary to make up first and then attack or both. Intestinal parasitic diseases often go together with laxative drugs. When applying the worm-expelling drugs without cathartic effect, cathartic drugs are often used together to promote the excretion of insect body.

驱虫药一般在空腹时服用，使药物充分作用于虫体而保证疗效。驱虫药属攻伐类药物，对人体正气多有损伤，且多有毒，因此使用时要注意用量、用法，以免中毒或伤及正气。年老体弱者、孕妇当慎用；发热或腹痛剧烈者，不宜急于驱虫，待症状缓解后，再使用驱虫药。

Worm-expelling medicinals should be generally taken in an empty stomach, so that the medicinal can fully acts on the insect body to ensure the curative effect. Belonging to the kind of attacking drugs, worm-expelling medicinals, often toxic, damage the vital qi somewhat, so in application, the dosage and usage should be paid attention to, so as to avoid poisoning or injury to the vital qi. They should be used with caution for the elderly and infirm, and pregnant women as well. For those with fever or acute abdominal pain, it is not advisable to drive the insect in a hurry. Instead, worm-expelling medicinals should be used after the symptoms are alleviated.

使君子　*Shǐ jūn zǐ* (Quisqualis Fructus)
《开宝本草》
Materia Medica of the Kaibao Era (*Kāi Bǎo Běn Cǎo*)

【来源 / Origin 】

为使君子科植物使君子 *Quisqualis indica* L. 的干燥成熟果实。产于广东、广西、四川等地。9~10 月果皮变紫黑时采收，晒干，去壳，取种仁，生用或炒香用。本品气微香，味微甜。《中国药典》规定，含胡芦巴碱（$C_7H_7NO_2$）不得少于 0.20%。

Shǐ jūn zǐ is the dry ripe fruit of *Quisqualis indica* L., pertaining to the Junaceae. It is mainly produced in Guangdong, Guangxi Zhuang Autonomous Region, Sichuan and other places. Collected from September to October when the peel turns purple-black, it is dried in the sun. Then the shell is removed, and the seed kernels are taken for raw or stir-fried use. This product is slightly fragrant in smell and a little sweet in taste. According to *Chinese Pharmacopoeia*, the content of fenugreek alkali ($C_7H_7NO_2$) should be no less than 0.20%.

【性味归经 / Medicinal properties 】

甘，温。归脾、胃经。

Sweet, warm; act on spleen and stomach meridians.

【主要功效 / Medicinal efficacies】

杀虫消积。

Kill worms and alleviate retention.

【临床应用 / Clinical application】

1．蛔虫病，蛲虫病　本品味甘甜气香，易于服用，有良好的驱杀蛔虫作用，兼有滑利通便之效，为驱蛔要药，尤宜于小儿。治蛔虫病，轻证可单用本品炒香嚼服；重证可与苦楝皮、芜荑等同用。用治蛲虫病，可与百部、槟榔、大黄等同用。

(1) Roundworm disease and pinworm disease　With sweet taste and fragrance, *shǐ jūn zǐ*, which is easy to take, has a good effect of repelling roundworms, and that of moistening and loosening the bowel as well. As a result, it is regarded as an important drug for repelling roundworms and is especially suitable for children. In the treatment of roundworm disease, patients with light syndrome can solely stir-fry and chew this product. Patients with severe syndrome can use it together with *kǔ liàn pí*, *wú yí* (Ulmi Macrocarpae Fructus Praeparata), etc. In the treatment of pinworm disease, it can be used together with *bǎi bù* (Stemonae Radix), *bīng láng* and *dà huáng* (Rhei Radix et Rhizoma).

2．小儿疳积　本品甘温，入脾、胃经，既能驱虫，又能健脾消积。用治小儿疳积，面色萎黄，形瘦腹大、腹痛有虫者，常与人参、白术、神曲等同用。

(2) Infantile malnutrition　Being sweet and warm, *shǐ jūn zǐ*, which goes into the spleen and stomach meridian, can not only expel worms but also strengthen the spleen and remove food retention. While being used to treat patients with infantile malnutrition, for those with impotent yellow complexion, thin shape but big abdomen, and worm-caused abdominal pain, it can be combined in application with *rén shēn* (Ginseng Radix et Rhizoma), *bái zhú* (Atractylodis Macrocephalae Rhizoma), *liù shén qū* (Medicata Fermentata Massa), etc.

【用法用量 / Usage and dosage】

煎服，使君子 9~12g，捣碎；使君子仁 6~9g，多入丸、散或单用，分 1~2 次服。小儿每岁 1~1.5 粒，炒香嚼服，1 日总量不超过 20 粒。

Decoction, *shǐ jūn zǐ* 9~12g, crushed; *shǐ jūn zǐ* seeds 6 ~ 9g, often in the form of pills and powder or used alone, taken separately for 1 ~ 2 times. 1 ~ 1.5 tablets per year for children, stir-fry and chew, do not exceed 20 tablets per day in total.

【使用注意 / Precaution】

用量不宜过大，服药时忌饮浓茶。

Dosage should not be too large, and strong tea should be avoided while taking the medicine.

【现代研究 / Modern research】

本品主要含使君子酸、苹果酸、柠檬酸、棕榈酸、亚油酸、硬脂酸、花生酸、胡芦巴碱及氨基酸等。具有麻痹蛔虫及蛲虫虫体、抑制皮肤真菌、抗滴虫等作用。

Shǐ jūn zǐ mainly contains quisqualic acid, malic acid, citric acid, palmitic acid, linoleic acid, stearic acid, arachidonic acid, fenugreek acid, amino acids, etc. It has the functions of paralyzing the body of roundworm and pinworm, inhibiting skin fungus, resisting trichomonas and so on.

苦楝皮　*Kǔ liàn pí* (Meliae Cortex)
《名医别录》
Miscellaneous Records of Famous Physicians (Míng Yī Bié Lù)

【来源 / Origin】

为楝科植物楝 *Melia azedarach* L. 或川楝 *Melia toosendan* Sieb. et Zucc. 的干燥树皮及根皮。主产于四川、湖北、贵州等地。四时可采，但以春、秋两季为宜。剥取根皮或干皮，刮去栓皮，洗净，鲜用或切片生用。本品气微，味苦。《中国药典》规定，含川楝素（$C_{30}H_{38}O_{11}$）应为 0.010%~0.20%。

Kǔ liàn pí is the dry bark and root bark of *Melia azedarach* L. or *Melia toosendan* Sieb. et Zucc., pertaining to the Meliaceae. It is mainly produced in Sichuan, Hubei, Guizhou and other places, collected in all of the four seasons, with the spring and autumn being the most advisable. Peel off the root or dry skin, scrape off the cork, and rinse. Fresh herb is used or sliced for raw use. It has a slight flavor and bitter taste. According to *Chinese Pharmacopoeia*, the content of azadirachtin ($C_{30}H_{38}O_{11}$) should be 0.010%-0.20%.

【性味归经 / Medicinal properties】

苦，寒；有毒。归肝、脾、胃经。

Bitter, cold; toxic; act on liver, spleen and stomach meridians.

【主要功效 / Medicinal efficacies】

杀虫，疗癣。

Kill worms and cure ringworm.

【临床应用 / Clinical application】

1. 蛔虫病，蛲虫病，钩虫病　本品苦寒有毒，杀虫力强，可驱杀多种肠道寄生虫。用治蛔虫病，可单用本品水煎、熬膏服用，或配伍使君子、槟榔等。用治蛲虫病，可与百部、乌梅同煎，取浓汁，每晚保留灌肠，连用 2~4 天。用治钩虫病，常与槟榔、石榴皮等同用。

(1) Roundworm disease, pinworm disease, and hookworm disease　*Kǔ liàn pí* is bitter, cold and toxic. With strong insecticidal force, it can expel and kill a variety of intestinal parasites. To treat roundworm disease, it can be used alone, decocted with water or boiled to a paste. It also can be compatible with *shǐ jūn zǐ*, *bīng láng*, etc. To treat pinworm disease, it can be decocted with *bǎi bù* and *wū méi* (Mume Fructus). Then the thick juice will be extracted to do retention enema every night, consecutively for 2 to 4 days. To treat hookworm disease, it is often used together with *bīng láng*, *shí liú pí* (Granati Pericarpium), etc.

2. 疥癣，湿疮　本品外用能清热燥湿，杀虫止痒。用治疥疮、头癣、湿疮、湿疹瘙痒等，可单用研末，用醋或猪脂调涂患处。

(2) Scabies and eczema　While used exteriorly, *kǔ liàn pí* can clear heat and dry dampness, kill parasites and relieve itching. It can be applied to treat scabies, head tinea, eczema, pruritus due to eczema, etc. Used alone, it can be powdered, dissolved in vinegar or porcine fat and then applied to the affected part.

【用法用量 / Usage and dosage】

煎服，3~6g。外用适量，研末，用猪脂调敷患处。

Decoction, 3~6g. For external use, powdered and applied to the affected part with porcine fat.

【使用注意 / Precaution】

孕妇及肝肾功能不全者慎用。

Pregnant women and patients with liver and kidney insufficiency should use it with caution.

【现代研究 / Modern research】

本品主要含川楝素、异川楝素、苦楝萜酮内酯、苦楝萜醇内酯、苦楝皮萜酮，尚含香豆素、酚酸和甾体等。具有麻痹蛔虫、蛲虫及钩虫虫体，以及抗血吸虫、镇痛、抗炎、止泻、利胆、抑菌、抗胃溃疡、抗病毒等作用。

It mainly contains azadirachtin, isoazadirachtin, azadirachterpene ketone, azadirachterpene olactone, azadirachterpene ketone, and also contains coumarin, phenolic acid and steroid. It has the functions of paralyzing roundworm, pinworm and hookworm, resisting schistosomiasis, analgesia, anti-inflammation, antidiarrheal, choleresis, bacteriostasis, anti-gastric ulcer, anti-virus and so on.

槟榔 *Bīng láng* (Arecae Semen)
《名医别录》
Miscellaneous Records of Famous Physicians (Míng Yī Bié Lù)

【来源 / Origin】

为棕榈科植物槟榔 *Areca catechu* L. 的干燥成熟种子。主产于海南、福建、云南等地。春末至秋初采收成熟果实，干燥，切薄片，生用、炒黄或炒焦用。本品气微，味涩、微苦。《中国药典》规定，含槟榔碱（$C_8H_{13}NO_2$）不得少于 0.20%，焦槟榔不得少于 0.10%。

Bīng láng is the dry ripe seed of *Areca catechu* L., pertaining to the Arecaceae. It is mainly produced in Hainan, Fujian, Yunnan and other places. Ripe fruits are collected from late spring to early autumn, dried, and cut into thin slices and used raw, or stir-fried until yellow or scorched. It has a mild odor, astringent taste, and is slightly bitter. According to *Chinese pharmacopoeia*, the content of arecoline ($C_8H_{13}NO_2$) should not be less than 0.20%, and not be less than 0.10% in *jiāo bīng láng* (Arecae Semen Praepareta).

【性味归经 / Medicinal properties】

苦、辛，温。归胃、大肠经。

Bitter, acrid and warm; act on stomach and large intestine meridians.

【主要功效 / Medicinal efficacies】

杀虫，消积，行气，利水，截疟。

Kill worms, disperse accumulation, move qi, promote urination, and prevent malaria.

【临床应用 / Clinical application】

1. 多种肠道寄生虫病　本品驱虫范围广泛，兼能泻下，能促进虫体排出，对绦虫、蛔虫、蛲虫、钩虫、姜片虫等多种肠道寄生虫都有驱杀作用，对绦虫病疗效最佳。用治绦虫病，常与南瓜子同用。用治蛔虫、蛲虫病，常与使君子、苦楝皮同用。用治姜片虫病，常与乌梅、甘草同用。用治钩虫病，可与贯众、榧子等同用。

(1) A variety of intestinal parasitic diseases　With an extensive worm-expelling range, *bīng láng* also has a draining effect, promoting the expulsion of worms. It has a worm-expelling effect for many intestinal parasites, such as tapeworm, roundworm, pinworm, hookworm and fasciolopsis buski, with the best efficacy for tapeworm disease. To treat tapeworm disease, it is often combined with *nán guā zǐ* (Cucurbitae Semen). To treat roundworm and pinworm disease, it is often used with *shǐ jūn zǐ* and *kǔ liàn pí*. To treat fasciolopsiasis, it often goes with *wū méi* and *gān cǎo* (Glycyrrhizae Radix et Rhizoma). To treat hookworm disease, it can be used with *guàn zhòng*, *fěi zǐ*, etc.

2. 食积气滞，泻痢后重　本品辛散苦泄，入胃、大肠经，既行胃肠气滞，消食化积，又缓泻通便以导滞。用治食积气滞、腹胀便秘等，常与木香、青皮、大黄等同用。用治湿热泻痢，里急后重，常与木香、黄连、大黄等同用。

(2) Food accumulation and qi stagnation, diarrhea with rectal heaviness　Entering stomach and large intestine meridians, *bīng láng*, acrid, dispersive, bitter and purgative, flows gastrointestinal qi stagnation, promotes digestion, removes accumulation, relieves diarrhea and promotes defecation so as to remove stagnation. To treat food accumulation and qi stagnation, abdomen distension and constipation, it is used together with *mù xiāng* (Aucklandiae Radix), *qīng pí* (Citri Reticulatae Viride Pericarpium), *dà huáng*, etc. To treat damp-heat diarrhea, abdominal urgency with rectal heaviness, it is combined with *mù xiāng*, *huáng lián* (Coptidis Rhizoma), *dà huáng*, etc.

3. 水肿，脚气肿痛　本品既能利水，又能行气。用治水肿实证，二便不利，可与商陆、泽泻、木通等同用。用治寒湿脚气肿痛，常与木瓜、吴茱萸、陈皮等同用。

(3) Edema, swelling and pain of foot　*Bīng láng* promotes urination, and moves qi as well. To treat excess pattern of edema and difficulty in urination and defecation, it can be combined with *shāng lù* (Phytolaccae Radix), *zé xiè* (Alismatis Rhizoma), *mù tōng* (Akebiae Caulis), etc. To treat cold-damp swelling and pain of foot, it can be used together with *mù guā* (Chaenomelis Fructus), *wú zhū yú* (Evodiae Fructus), *chén pí* (Citri Reticulatae Pericarpium), etc.

4. 疟疾　本品有截疟之功，用治疟疾，常配伍常山、草果、陈皮等。

(4) Malaria　*Bīng láng* has the action of preventing attack of malaria. To treat malaria, it is often compatible with *cháng shān* (Dichroae Radix), *cǎo guǒ* (Tsaoko Fructus), *chén pí*, etc.

【用法用量 / Usage and dosage】

煎服，3~10g。驱杀绦虫、姜片虫 30~60g。生用力佳，炒用力缓。焦槟榔功能消食导滞，用于食积不消，泻痢后重。

Decoction, 3~10g; for expelling and killing tapeworms and fasciolopsis buski, 30~60g; efficacy is good for raw use, and slow for dry-fried use; *jiāo bīng láng* (Arecae Semen Praepareta), with the actions of promoting digestion and removing stagnation, is used to treat food accumulation with insufficient digestion, and diarrhea with rectal heaviness.

【使用注意 / Precaution】

脾虚便溏、气虚下陷者忌用；孕妇慎用。

Patients with weak spleen and thin, loose stool as well as those with qi deficiency and sinking should be avoided; pregnant women should use it with caution.

【现代研究 / Modern research】

本品主要含槟榔碱、槟榔次碱、去甲基槟榔碱、去甲基槟榔次碱、月桂酸、肉豆蔻酸、棕榈酸、油酸，尚含鞣质、脂肪酸、萜类和甾体等。具有麻痹和驱杀绦虫、蛔虫、蛲虫、钩虫、血吸虫以及抑制皮肤真菌、抗流感病毒、抗炎、促进腺体分泌、增强肠蠕动、减慢心率、降血压、兴奋子宫平滑肌、抗过敏等作用。

Bīng láng mainly contains arecoline, arecaine, demethyl-arecoline, demethyl-arecaine, lauric acid, myristic acid, palmitic acid, oleic acid, etc., and also contain tannins, fatty acids, terpenes and steroids. It can paralyze and kill tapeworms, roundworms, pinworms, hookworms, and schistosoma, inhibit skin fungus, resist influenza virus and inflammation, promote gland secretion and intestinal peristalsis, slow heart rate, lower blood pressure, stimulate uterine smooth muscle, resist allergy, etc.

贯众 *Guàn zhòng* (Cyrtomii Rhizoma)
《神农本草经》
Shen Nong's Classic of the Materia Medica (Shén Nóng Běn Cǎo Jīng)

【来源 / Origin】

为鳞毛蕨科植物粗茎鳞毛蕨 *Dryopteris crassirhizoma* Nakai 的干燥根茎和叶柄残基。产于黑龙江、吉林、辽宁三省山区，习称"东北贯众"或"绵马贯众"。秋季采挖，晒干，切片，生用或炒炭用。本品气特异，味初淡，后渐苦辛。

Guàn zhòng is the dry root and petiole residues of *Dryopteris crassirhizoma* Nakai, pertaining to Dryopteridaceae. Mainly produced in Heilongjiang, Jilin and Liaoning, it is commonly known as *northeastern guàn zhòng* or *mián mǎ guàn zhòng* (Dryopteridis Crassirhizomatis Rhizoma). It is collected in autumn, dried, cut into slices and then used raw or dry-fried until scorched. It has a special odor, and tastes bland at first, bitter and acrid later.

【性味归经 / Medicinal properties】

苦，微寒；有小毒。归肝、胃经。

Bitter, slightly cold; slightly toxic; act on liver and stomach meridians.

【主要功效 / Medicinal efficacies】

杀虫，清热解毒，凉血止血。

Kill worms, clear heat and resolve toxins, cool the blood and stanch bleeding.

【临床应用 / Clinical application】

1. 多种肠道寄生虫病　本品有杀虫之功，可用于驱杀绦虫、钩虫、蛲虫、蛔虫等多种肠道寄生虫，但须用较大剂量才能取效，因其有毒，不宜单味重用。用治绦虫病，可与槟榔、雷丸等同用。用治蛔虫病，可与使君子、苦楝皮等同用。用治蛲虫病，可单用本品浓煎取汁，于睡前浸洗或搽于肛门。用治钩虫病，多与苦楝皮、槟榔等同用。

(1) A variety of intestinal parasitic diseases　With the action of killing worms, *guàn zhòng* can be used to kill many kinds of intestinal parasites such as tapeworms, hookworms, pinworms and roundworms. But only a comparatively large dose can take effect, and because of its toxicity, it is not advisable to use it alone and in large dose. To treat tapeworm disease, it can be used with *bīng láng*, *léi wán*, etc. To treat roundworm disease, it can be combined with *shǐ jūn zǐ*, *kǔ liàn pí*, etc. To treat pinworm disease, it can be used alone to be decocted and extract juice, which then can be used to embathe or rub on the anus before going to bed. To treat hookworm disease, it is often compatible with *kǔ liàn pí*, *bīng láng*, etc.

2. 温热病，外感风热，痄腮　本品苦寒，有清热解毒、凉血之功。用治温热病初起，或外感风热之发热、微恶风寒、头痛、咽痛等，多与金银花、牛蒡子等同用。用治温热病热入营血，或温毒发斑，常与水牛角、玄参、大青叶等同用。用治痄腮，常与板蓝根、连翘、金银花等同用。

(2) Warm febrile disease, wind-heat external contraction, mumps　Bitter and cold, *guàn zhòng* has the actions of clearing heat and resoling toxins as well as cooling the blood and stanching bleeding. To treat the early stage of warm febrile disease, or external contraction with wind-heat syndrome, fever, slight aversion to wind-cold, headache, sore throat, etc., it is often used together with *jīn yín huā* (Lonicerae Japonicae Flos), *niú bàng zǐ* (Arctii Fructus), etc. To treat warm febrile disease such as heat entering ying-blood or warm toxin with eruption, it is often combined with *shuǐ niú jiǎo* (Bubali Cornu), *xuán shēn* (Scrophulariae Radix), *dà qīng yè* (Isatidis Folium), etc. To treat mumps, it is usually compatible with *bǎn lán gēn* (Isatidis Radix), *lián qiáo* (Forsythiae Fructus), *jīn yín huā* (Lonicerae Japonicae Flos), etc.

3. 血热出血 本品味苦性寒，有清热凉血之功，可用治血热妄行的多种出血，尤善治崩漏下血。用治血热崩漏下血，可单用研末调服，或与五灵脂、乌贼骨等同用。用治血热吐血、衄血、便血，可与侧柏叶、白茅根、血余炭等同用。

(3) Blood-heat bleeding Being bitter and cold, *guàn zhòng* has the actions of clearing heat and cooling blood, and thus can be used to treat a variety of bleeding due to blood heat, especially good for the treatment of flooding and spotting. To treat blood-heat flooding and spotting, it can be powdered and taken alone after the mixture with liquid. It also can be used together with *wǔ líng zhī* (Trogopterori Faeces), *wū zéi gǔ* (Cleistocactus sepium), etc. To treat blood-heat hematemesis, epistaxis, and bloody stool, it can be compatible with *cè bǎi yè* (Platycladi Cacumen), *bái máo gēn* (Imperatae Rhizoma), *xuè yú tàn* (Crinis Carbonisatus), etc.

【用法用量 / Usage and dosage】

煎服，5~10g。清热解毒、驱虫宜生用；止血宜炒炭用。外用适量。

Decoction, 5~10g; advisable to clear heat and resolve toxins in raw form, and to stanch bleeding when stir-fried until scorched; moderate for external use.

【使用注意 / Precaution】

用量不宜过大；忌油腻；脾胃虚寒及孕妇慎用。

The dosage should not be too large; avoid greasy; patients with deficiency-cold of the spleen and stomach and pregnant women should use with caution.

【现代研究 / Modern research】

本品主要含绵马酸类、黄绵马酸类、绵马酚、绵马次酸、白绵马素类、去甲绵马素类、粗蕨素等间苯三酚类化合物，尚含三萜类、鞣质、挥发油、树脂等。具有麻痹绦虫、蛔虫、钩虫以及抗病毒、抑菌、抗疟原虫、收缩子宫平滑肌、抗早孕、抗肿瘤、止血、保肝等作用。

It mainly contains phloroglucinol compounds such as filicins, flavaspidic acids, aspidinol, filicinic acid, albaspidins, desaspidins, dryocrassin, etc., and also contains triterpenes, tannins, volatile oils, resins, etc. It has the functions of paralyzing tapeworm, roundworm and hookworm, resisting virus, bacteria and plasmodium, contracting uterine smooth muscle, resisting early pregnancy and tumor, stanching bleeding and protecting liver as well.

其他驱虫药功用介绍见表15-1。

The efficacies of worm-expelling medicinals are shown in table 15-1.

表 15-1 其他驱虫药功用介绍

分类	药物	药性	功效	应用	用法用量
驱虫药	南瓜子	甘，平。归胃、大肠经	杀虫	绦虫病	研粉，60~120g，冷开水调服
	雷丸	微苦，寒。归胃、大肠经	杀虫消积	绦虫病，钩虫病，蛔虫病，虫积腹痛，小儿疳积	15~21g，不宜入煎剂，一般研粉服，一次5~7g，饭后用温开水调服，1日3次，连服3天
	鹤草芽	苦、涩、凉。归肝、小肠、大肠经	杀虫	绦虫病	研粉吞服，每日30~45g，小儿0.7~0.8g/kg，每日1次，早起空腹服

续表

分类	药物	药性	功效	应用	用法用量
驱虫药	榧子	甘，平。归肺、胃、大肠经	杀虫消积，润肺止咳，润燥通便	钩虫病，蛔虫病，绦虫病，虫积腹痛，小儿疳积，肺燥咳嗽，肠燥便秘	煎服，9~15g
	鹤虱	苦、辛，平；有小毒。归脾、胃经	杀虫消积	蛔虫病，蛲虫病，绦虫病，虫积腹痛，小儿疳积	煎服，3~9g
	芜荑	辛、苦，温。归脾、胃经	杀虫消积	蛔虫病，蛲虫病，绦虫病，虫积腹痛，小儿疳积	煎服，3~10g；入丸散，每次2~3g。外用适量，研末调敷

（柳海艳）

第十六章 止血药
Chapter 16　Blood-stanching medicinals

 学习目标 | Learning goals

1. **掌握** 止血药在性能、功效、主治、配伍及使用注意方面的共性；小蓟、地榆、白茅根、三七、茜草、白及、仙鹤草、艾叶的性能、功效、应用以及特殊的用法用量和特殊的使用注意。

2. **熟悉** 止血药的分类；大蓟、槐花、蒲黄、炮姜的功效、主治以及特殊的用法用量和特殊的使用注意。

3. **了解** 止血药、凉血止血药、化瘀止血药、收敛止血药、温经止血药及相关功效术语的含义；侧柏叶、苎麻根、花蕊石、景天三七、紫珠叶、鸡冠花、棕榈炭、血余炭、藕节的功效以及特殊的用法用量和特殊的使用注意。

1. Master the commonness of blood-stanching medicinals in efficacy, indications, property, compatibility and cautions; as well as the property, efficacy, application, special usage and dosage and special precautions of *xiǎo jì*, *dì yú*, *bái máo gēn*, *sān qī*, *qiàn cǎo*, *bái jí*, *xiān hè cǎo* and *ài yè*.

2. Familiar with the classification of blood-stanching medicinals; and the efficacy, indications, special usage, dosage and special precautions of *dà jì*, *huái huā*, *pú huáng* and *páo jiāng*.

3. Understand the definitions of blood-stanching medicinals, blood-cooling and bleeding-stanching medicinals, stasis-resolving and bleeding-stanching medicinals, astringent bleeding-stanching medicinals, channel-warming and bleeding-stanching medicinals and other related efficacy terms; and the efficacy, special usage and dosage and special precautions of *cè bǎi yè*, *zhù má gēn*, *huā ruǐ shí*, *jīng tiān sān qī*, *zǐ zhū yè*, *jī guān huā*, *zōng lǘ tàn*, *xuè yú tàn* and *ǒu jié*.

凡以制止体内外出血为主要功效，常用以治疗出血证的药物，称为止血药。
Medicinals that have the ability to stop various forms of bleeding, internal or external, are called blood-stanching medicinals.

止血药多归心、肝经，入血分，均具有止血作用，因其药性有寒、温、散、敛之不同，故本类药物有凉血止血、温经止血、化瘀止血和收敛止血的区别，主治咯血、衄血、吐血、便血、尿血、崩漏及外伤出血等体内外各种出血。

Most blood-stanching medicinals are bitter, sour and astringent in flavor and they mainly act on the heart and liver meridians. They can prevent the blood from escaping out of the meridians and have an inward directed astringent effect. Their main efficacy is to stanch bleeding, and some also have the function of clearing away heat, resolving stasis, relieving pain and dispersing cold. They can be used to treat various internal or external bleedings, such as expectoration of blood, coughing of blood, nosebleed, spitting of blood, bloody stool, blood urine, metrorrhagia, metrostaxis and bleeding due to external injuries.

根据止血药的药性及功效主治差异，可分为凉血止血药、化瘀止血药、收敛止血药与温经止血药四类。

Blood-stanching medicinals can be classified into four categories based on their properties and efficacies as well as their different clinical applications: blood-cooling and bleeding-stanching medicinals, stasis-resolving and bleeding-stanching medicinals, astringent bleeding-stanching medicinals, channel-warming and bleeding-stanching medicinals.

出血病证，病因不同，病情有异，部位有别，因此，在使用止血药时，必须根据出血的不同原因、病情和部位，选用相应的药物，并进行必要的配伍。如血热妄行而出血者，宜选用凉血止血药，并配伍清热泻火、清热凉血药；瘀血内阻，血不循经而出血者，宜选用化瘀止血药，并配伍行气活血药；虚寒性出血者，宜选用温经止血药或收敛止血药，并配伍益气健脾、温阳药。根据前贤"下血必升举，吐衄必降气"之论，对于下部出血，如便血、崩漏等，应适当配伍升举之品；对于上部出血，如衄血、吐血等，可适当配伍降气之品。

Bleeding diseases have different etiology, different condition and manifested in different body parts. So different bleeding-stanching medicinals should be selected and combined with other medicinals according to the causes and mechanisms. For bleeding due to blood heat, blood-cooling and bleeding-stanching medicinals should be selected and combined with those that can clear heat and cool blood; for bleeding due to blood stasis, or bleeding with stasis, stasis-resolving and bleeding-stanching medicinals should be selected and combined with those that can circulate qi and blood; in cases of bleeding due to deficiency and cold, it is better to use channel-warming and bleeding-stanching medicinals and astringent bleeding-stanching medicinals, usually in combination with those that can replenish qi, strengthen the spleen and warm yang. In addition, there is an ancient saying that "to treat bleeding, qi should be raised; to treat epistaxis, qi should be lowered". Thus, for bleeding in the lower part of the body such as bloody stool and purpura, medicinals that can raise yang should be combined, while for bleeding in the upper part of the body such as nosebleed and spitting of blood, those that can direct qi downward should be utilized together.

使用止血药时还应注意止血不留瘀，尤其是凉血止血药和收敛止血药，易凉遏而留瘀，故出血兼有瘀滞者不宜单独使用，大剂量使用凉血止血药和收敛止血药时，可适当加入活血之品以防留瘀之弊。若出血过多，气随血脱，当急投大补元气之药，益气固脱以救其急。

It is required that no stasis should be created when blood-stanching medicinals are utilized to stanch bleeding. It is especially true for astringent and blood-cooling and bleeding-stanching medicinals, which tend to cause lingering pathogen and stasis. For bleeding accompanied with stasis, astringent and blood-cooling medicinals are not advised to use alone, but used in combination with blood-activating medicinals. When using large doses of blood cooling and astringent bleeding-stanching medicinals, appropriate blood-activating medicinals can be added to prevent the disadvantages of retention of blood stasis. If the bleeding is too much and qi is removed with the blood, the medicine of invigorating vital energy should be given urgently to replenish and firm the qi to save the emergency.

前人经验认为止血药多炒炭用，一般而言，炒炭后其味苦、涩，可加强止血之效，但也有少数药物以生品止血效果更好。故止血药是否炒炭用应视具体药物而定，不可一概而论，总以提高疗效为原则。

Blood-stanching medicinals stir-fried to scorch can increase the effect of stanching bleeding, so it is advised to be dry-fried to scorch. However, some may have a better effect in stanching bleeding when used in the raw form. Therefore, whether they are used by stir-frying to scorch or not depends on the specific medicinals and always with the principle of improving the curative effect.

第一节　凉血止血药
Section 1　Blood-cooling and bleeding-stanching medicinals

本类药物药性寒凉，味多甘苦，入血分，既能止血，又能清泄血分之热，主治血热妄行所致的各种出血。

Most of the blood-cooling and bleeding-stanching medicinals are cool and cold in property, sweet an bitter in taste. They can stanch bleeding through cooling blood and are mainly used to treat various forms of bleeding caused by blood-heat.

小蓟　*Xiǎo jì* (Cirsii Herba)
《名医别录》
Miscellaneous Records of Famous Physicians (Míng Yī Bié Lù)

【来源 / Origin】

为菊科植物刺儿菜 *Cirsium setosum*（Willd.）MB. 的干燥地上部分。全国大部分地区均产。夏、秋季花开时采割，晒干，切段，生用或炒炭用。本品气弱，味微苦而甘。《中国药典》规定，含蒙花苷（$C_{28}H_{32}O_{14}$）不得少于 0.70%。

Xiǎo jì is the dry aboveground part of *Cirsium setosum* (Willd.) MB., pertaining to Asteraceae. It is produced in most parts of China and collected in summer and autumn when flowers bloom. It is dried, and cut into segments, used raw or dry-fried to scorch. It has slight odor and is slightly bitter and sweet in taste. According to *Chinese Pharmacopoeia*, the content of smectin ($C_{28}H_{32}O_{14}$) should be no less than 0.70%.

【性味归经 / Medicinal properties】

甘、苦，凉。归心、肝经。

Sweet, bitter and cool; act on the heart and liver meridians.

【主要功效 / Medicinal efficacies】

凉血止血，散瘀解毒消痈。

Cool blood and stanch bleeding, disperse blood stasis and resolve toxins to eliminate carbuncle.

【临床应用 / Clinical application】

1. 血热出血　本品性凉入血分，能凉血止血，兼能散瘀，凉血止血而无留瘀之弊，凡血热妄行之衄血、吐血、尿血、便血、崩漏等出血，皆可选用，常与大蓟、侧柏叶、白茅根等同用。因其兼能利尿通淋，故以治尿血、血淋最为适宜，常配伍生地黄、栀子、木通等。

(1) Bleeding caused by blood-heat It can cool the blood, stanch bleeding and disperse blood stasis. To treat nosebleed, spitting of blood, bloody stool, blood urine, metrorrhagia and metrostaxis, it is usually combined with *dà jì* (Cirsii Japonici Herba), *cè bǎi yè* (Platycladi Cacumen) and *bái máo gēn* (Imperatae Rhizoma); due to its action of promoting urination to treat strangury, it is often used to treat hematuria and blood strangury and is often combined with *shēng dì huáng* (Rehmanniae Radix), *zhī zǐ* (Gardeniae Fructus) and *mù tōng* (Akebiae Caulis).

2. 痈肿疮毒　本品能清热解毒，散瘀消肿。用治热毒疮疡初起肿痛者，可单用鲜品捣烂外敷，或配伍乳香、没药等。

(2) Sores and carbuncles caused by toxic-heat It can clear away heat, resolve toxin and disperse blood stasis and eliminate swelling. It can be used alone to treat sores and carbuncles due to toxic-heat, applied to the affected part after being smashed, or combined with *rǔ xiāng* and *mò yào*.

【用法用量 / Usage and dosage】

煎服，5~12g，鲜品加倍。外用适量，捣敷患处。

Decoction, 5~12g, when it is used fresh, the dosage can be doubled. An appropriate amount is used externally to apply directly on the affected area.

【现代研究 / Modern research】

本品主要含蒙花苷、芸香苷、原儿茶酸、绿原酸、咖啡酸、蒲公英甾醇、蒲公英甾醇乙酸乙酯、β-谷甾醇等。具有止血、抑菌、降脂、利胆、强心、利尿、抗肿瘤等作用。

It mainly contains smectin, rutin, protocatechuic acid, chlorogenic acid, caffeic acid, dandelion sterol, dandelion sterol ethyl acetate and β-sitosterol, etc. It has hemostasis, bacteriostasis, lipid-lowering, cholagogic, cardiotonic, diuretic, antitumor and other functions.

大蓟　*Dà jì* (Cirsii Japonici Herba)
《名医别录》
Miscellaneous Records of Famous Physicians (*Míng Yī Bié Lù*)

【来源 / Origin】

为菊科植物蓟 *Cirsium japonicum* Fisch. ex DC. 的干燥地上部分。全国大部分地区均产。夏、秋季花开时采割地上部分，晒干，切段，生用或炒炭用。本品气微，味淡。《中国药典》规定，含柳穿鱼叶苷（$C_{28}H_{34}O_{15}$）不得少于0.20%。

Dà jì is the dry aboveground part of *Cirsium japonicum* Fisch. ex DC., pertaining to Asteraceae. It is produced in most parts of China and collected in summer and autumn when the flowers bloom. It is dried, and cut into segments, used raw or dry-fried to scorch. It has a slight odor and tastes bland. According to *Chinese Pharmacopoeia*, the content of salidroside($C_{28}H_{34}O_{15}$) should be no less than 0.20%.

【性味归经 / Medicinal properties】

甘、苦，凉。归心、肝经。

Sweet, bitter and cool; act on the heart and liver meridians.

【主要功效 / Medicinal efficacies】

凉血止血，散瘀解毒消痈。

Cool blood and stanch bleeding; resolve toxins to eliminate carbuncles.

【临床应用 / Clinical application】

1. 血热出血　本品性凉入血分，功似小蓟，但凉血止血之功较小蓟为优，可用治血热妄行所致的各种出血，尤多用于吐血、咯血、崩漏等，常与小蓟、侧柏叶等同用。

(1) **Bleeding caused by blood-heat**　It can cool the blood and has similar functions with *xiǎo jì*, which has stronger actions. To treat hematemesis, hemoptysis, metrorrhagia and metrostaxis due to toxic-heat, it is usually combined with *xiǎo jì* and *cè bǎi yè* (Platycladi Cacumen).

2. 痈肿疮毒　本品苦凉清泄，能清热解毒，散瘀消肿，功似小蓟而力胜，内外痈肿皆可用之。若治热毒疮疡初起肿痛之证，常单用鲜品内服或捣烂外敷。若治肠痈腹痛，可与金银花、大血藤、地榆等同用。若治肺痈，以鲜品煎汤内服。

(2) **Sores and carbuncles caused by toxic-heat**　With the nature of bitter and cool, it can clear heat and resolve toxins to eliminate carbuncles. It has similar but stronger function than *xiǎo jì*. It can be used alone to treat sores and carbuncles due to toxic-heat, applied to the affected part after being smashed; to treat abdominal pain due to intestinal carbuncle, it is often combined with *jīn yín huā*, *dà xuè téng* (Sargentodoxae Caulis) and *dì yú* (Sanguisorbae Radix); to treat lung carbuncle, it is decocted for oral administration.

【用法用量 / Usage and dosage】

煎服，9~15g，鲜品加倍。外用适量，捣敷患处。

Decoction, 9-15g, when it is used fresh, the dosage can be doubled. An appropriate amount is used externally to apply directly to the affected area.

【现代研究 / Modern research】

本品主要含柳穿鱼叶苷、蒙花苷、蒲公英甾醇乙酸酯、豆甾醇及三萜类、挥发油等。具有止血、抑菌、降压、抑制结核分枝杆菌、抑制疱疹病毒等作用。

It mainly contains salidroside, monksin, dandelion sterol acetate, stigmasterol, triterpenoids and volatile oil etc. It has the functions of hemostasis, bacteriostasis, hypotension, inhibiting tubercle bacilli, and inhibiting herpes virus, etc.

地榆　*Dì yú* (Sanguisorbae Radix)
《神农本草经》
Shen Nong's Classic of the Materia Medica (Shén Nóng Běn Cǎo Jīng)

【来源 / Origin】

为蔷薇科植物地榆 *Sanguisorba officinalis* L. 或长叶地榆 *Sanguisorba officinalis* L.var.*longifolia*（Bert.）Yü et Li 的干燥根。前者产于全国各地，后者产于安徽、浙江、江苏等地，习称"绵地榆"。春季将发芽时或秋季植株枯萎后采挖。晒干，切片，生用或炒炭用。本品气微，味微苦涩。《中国药典》规定，含鞣质不得少于 8.0%，没食子酸（$C_7H_6O_5$）不得少于 1.0%。

Dì yú is the dry root of S*anguisorba officinalis* L. or *Sanguisorba officinalis* L. var. *longifolia* (Bert.) Yü et Li, pertaining to Rosaceae. The former is produced in most regions in China while the latter is produced in Anhui, Zhejiang and Jiangsu Province, which is called *mián dì yú*. It is collected in spring before it is going to sprout or in autumn after the plant has withered. It is dried and sliced, used in raw or dry-fried to scorch. It has a slight odor and is bitter and astringent in taste. According to *Chinese Pharmacopoeia*, the content of tannin should be no less than 8.0%, and gallic acid ($C_7H_6O_5$) should be no less than 1.0%.

【性味归经 / Medicinal properties】

苦、酸、涩，微寒。归肝、大肠经。

Bitter, sour, astringent and slightly cold; act on the liver and large intestine meridians.

【主要功效 / Medicinal efficacies】

凉血止血，解毒敛疮。

Cool blood and stanch bleeding; resolve toxins and heal up sores.

【临床应用 / Clinical application】

1. **血热出血** 本品苦寒入血分，长于泄热而凉血止血；其味酸涩，又能收敛止血，为清热凉血、收敛止血之良药，可用治多种血热出血。又因其沉降下行，故尤宜于下焦血热之便血、痔血、血痢、崩漏等。如治血热便血，常与黄芩、生地黄等同用。如治痔疮出血，血色鲜红者，常与槐花、防风等同用。如治崩漏下血，量多色红者，常配伍生地黄、黄芩、蒲黄等。如治血痢不止，常与甘草同用。

(1) Bleeding caused by blood-heat With the nature of bitter and cold, it is good at cooling the blood and stanching bleeding; with the nature of sour and astringent, it is a good medicine for clearing heat, cooling blood and astringing hemostasis. It can be used to treat many kinds of bleeding caused by blood heat. It is also suitable for treating bloody stool, hemorrhoid blood, dysentery, metrorrhagia and metrostaxis. To treat bloody stool due to blood heat, it is often combined with *huáng qín* and *shēng dì huáng*; to treat bleeding due to hemorrhoids, it is usually combined with *huái huā* and *fáng fēng*; for metrorrhagia with polychromatic and red blood, it is often used with *shēng dì huáng*, *huáng qín* and *pú huáng*; to treat chronic dysentery with bloody stool, it is often combined with *gān cǎo*.

2. **水火烫伤，湿疹，痈肿疮毒** 本品苦寒能泻火解毒，味酸涩能敛疮生肌，为治水火烫伤之要药，可单味研末麻油调敷，或与大黄粉、冰片同用。用治湿疹及皮肤溃烂，可单用本品浓煎外洗，或以纱布浸药外敷。用治热毒疮痈，无论成脓与否均可使用，既可内服，又可外敷，以鲜品为佳，或与蒲公英、连翘等同用。

(2) Scald, eczema, sores and ulcers, swollen pains with the nature of bitter and cold, it can drain fire and resolve toxin; with the nature of sour and astringent, it can heal up sores and promote granulation, so it is an important medicinal to treat scald caused by hot liquid or fire. It can be used alone by grinding into powder and mixed with sesame oil or combined with powder of *dà huáng* (Rhei Radix et Rhizoma) and *bīng piàn* (Borneolum Syntheticum); to treat eczema and skin ulceration, thick decoction can be used for external washing or apply it with gauze after soaking in decoction; to treat sores and carbuncles due to heat-toxin, whether they are purulent or not, it can be taken internally or applied externally and the fresh one is preferred, or in combination with *pú gōng yīng* and *lián qiáo*.

【用法用量 / Usage and dosage】

煎服，9~15g。外用适量，研末涂敷患处。止血多炒炭用，解毒敛疮多生用。

Decoction, 9-15g. An appropriate amount is used externally by grinding into powder and apply directly on the affected area. It is stir-fried to scorch for stanching bleeding and the raw one for resolving toxin and healing up sores.

【使用注意 / Precaution】

治疗烧烫伤，忌大面积外用。

External application is not suitable for extensive burns or scalds.

【现代研究 / Modern research】

本品主要含鞣质、右旋儿茶素、地榆糖苷、地榆皂苷 A~E 等。具有止血、抑菌、抗烫伤、抗炎、促进造血等作用。

It mainly contains tannin, d-catechin, sanguinoside and sanguinoside A-E, etc. It has the functions of arresting bleeding, bacteriostasis, anti scald, anti inflammation and promoting hematopoiesis, etc.

槐花　*Huái huā* (Sophorae Flos)
《日华子本草》
Ri Huazi's Materia Medica (Rì Huá Zǐ Běn Cǎo)

【来源 / Origin】

为豆科植物槐 *Sophora japonica* L. 的干燥花及花蕾。产于河北、山东、河南等地。夏季花开放或花蕾形成时采收，前者习称"槐花"，后者习称"槐米"，生用、炒黄或炒炭用。本品气微，味微苦。《中国药典》规定，含总黄酮以芦丁（$C_{27}H_{30}O_{16}$）计，槐花不得少于 8.0%，槐米不得少于 20.0%；含芦丁，槐花不得少于 6.0%，槐米不得少于 15.0%。

Huái huā is the dry flower or flower bud of *Sophora japonica* L., pertaining to Leguminosae. It is produced in Hebei, Shandong and Henan Province in China. It is collected in summer before or when the flowers bloom. The former is often called *huái huā*, while the latter is often called *huái mǐ* (Sophorae Immaturus Flos). It can be used raw, stir-fried or dry-fried until charred. It has a slight odor and is slightly bitter in taste. According to *Chinese Pharmacopoeia*, the content of total flavonoids in terms of rutin ($C_{27}H_{30}O_{16}$) in *huái huā* should be no less than 8.0% and that in *huái mǐ* should be no less than 20.0%; the content of rutin in *huái huā* should be no less than 6.0% while that in *huái mǐ* should be no less than 15.0%.

【性味归经 / Medicinal properties】

苦，微寒。归肝、大肠经。

Bitter and slightly cold; act on the liver and large intestine meridians.

【主要功效 / Medicinal efficacies】

凉血止血，清肝泻火。

Cool blood and stanch bleeding, clear liver heat and drain liver fire.

【临床应用 / Clinical application】

1. **血热出血**　本品味苦性寒，能清血分之热而凉血止血，凡血热所致的各种出血，均可应用。因其沉降下行，归大肠经，善清泄大肠之火热而止血，故善治便血、痔血等下部出血，常与地榆炭、荆芥穗、侧柏炭等同用。

(1) Bleeding due to blood-heat　With the nature of bitter and cold, it can clear the heat of blood and cool the blood to stanch bleeding. It can be used to treat all kinds of bleeding caused by blood heat. Because of its descending sedimentation, it acts on the large intestine meridian and is effective in stanching bleeding through clearing and discharging pathogenic heat in large intestine, and is really good at treating bleeding in the lower part of the body, such as hemorrhoids and bloody stool. It is often combined with *dì yú* (stir-fried to scorch), *jīng jiè suì* (Schizonepetae Spica) and *cè bǎi* (stir-fried to scorch).

2. **肝热目赤，头痛眩晕**　本品苦凉入肝经，长于清泻肝火，用治肝火上炎之目赤肿痛、头痛、眩晕，可单用本品煎汤代茶饮，或与夏枯草、菊花、黄芩等同用。

(2) Red eyes, headache and dizziness due to liver heat　With the nature of bitter and cool and acting on the liver meridian, it is good at clearing liver heat. To treat red eyes, headache and dizziness due to liver heat, it can be decocted alone and taken as tea, or can be combined with *xià kū cǎo* (Prunellae

Spica), *jú huā* (Chrysanthemi Flos) and *huáng qín*.

【用法用量 / Usage and dosage】

煎服，5~10g。止血炒炭用，清热泻火生用。

Decoction, 5-10g. It is stir-fried to scorch for stanching bleeding while the raw form for clearing heat and fire.

【现代研究 / Modern research】

本品主要含芦丁、槲皮素、异鼠李素、赤豆皂苷Ⅰ~Ⅴ及槐花皂苷Ⅰ~Ⅲ等。具有止血、抗炎、抑菌、扩张冠状动脉、降血压等作用。

It mainly contains rutin, quercetin, isorhamnetin, red bean saponin Ⅰ-Ⅴ and sophora saponin Ⅰ, Ⅱ, Ⅲ, etc. It has the functions of stanching bleeding, anti-inflammatory, bacteriostasis, coronary artery dilation and blood pressure reduction.

白茅根　*Bái máo gēn* (Imperatae Rhizoma)
《神农本草经》
Shen Nong's Classic of the Materia Medica (Shén Nóng Běn Cǎo Jīng)

【来源 / Origin】

为禾本科植物白茅 *Imperata cylindrica* Beauv.var. *major*（Nees）C.E. Hubb. 的根茎。全国各地均产。春、秋二季采挖，晒干，切段，生用或炒炭用。本品气微，味微甜。

Bái máo gēn is the rhizome of *Imperata cylindrica* Beauv.var. *major* (Nees) C.E. Hubb., pertaining to Gramineae. It's produced in all regions in China. It is collected in spring and autumn and dried in the sun and cut into segments. It is used raw or stir-fried to scorch. It has a slight odor and is slightly sweet in taste.

【性味归经 / Medicinal properties】

甘，寒。归肺、胃、膀胱经。

Sweet and cold; act on the lung, stomach and bladder meridians.

【主要功效 / Medicinal efficacies】

凉血止血，清热利尿。

Cool blood and stanch bleeding, clear heat and promote urination.

【临床应用 / Clinical application】

1. **血热出血**　本品性寒入血分，能清血分之热而凉血止血，可用于吐血、衄血、尿血等多种血热出血。因其入膀胱经，兼能利尿，故对尿血、血淋最为适宜，可单用煎服，或配伍小蓟、黄芩、血余炭等。

(1) Bleeding due to blood-heat　With the nature of cold, it can clear the heat of blood and cool the blood to stanch bleeding. It can be used to treat many kinds of bleeding caused by blood heat such as hematemesis, nosebleed and hematuria. Because it can enter bladder meridian and promote urination, it is most suitable for hematuria and blood drenching. It can be taken by decocting alone or combined with *xiǎo jì*, *huáng qín* and *xuè yú tàn*.

2. **热淋，水肿，黄疸**　本品能清热利尿以通淋消肿、除湿退黄。用治热淋、水肿尿少，可单用本品煎服，或与车前子、金钱草等同用。用治湿热黄疸，常配伍茵陈、栀子等。

(2) Heat strangury, edema and jaundice　It can clear heat and promote urination to relieve swelling, dampness and jaundice. To treat heat strangury and edema with little urine, it can be taken orally in decoction alone or used in combination with *chē qián zǐ* (Plantaginis Semen) and *jīn qián cǎo* (Lysimachiae Herba); to treat damp-heat jaundice, it is often combined with *yīn chén* (Artemisiae

Scopariae Herba) and *zhī zǐ* (Gardeniae Fructus).

3. **热病烦渴，胃热呕吐，肺热咳喘**　本品甘寒，归肺、胃经，善清肺胃之热，既能清胃热以生津、止呕，又能清肺热而止咳。用治热病烦渴，可与芦根、天花粉等同用。用治胃热呕吐，常与黄连、竹茹等同用。用治肺热咳喘，常与桑白皮、地骨皮等同用。

(3) Thirst due to heat pathogen, vomiting due to stomach heat, cough and asthma due to lung heat　With the nature of sweet and cold and acting on the stomach meridian, it is good at clearing the heat of the lung and stomach. It can not only clear the heat of the stomach to promote body fluid production and stop vomiting, but also clear the heat of the lung to stop coughing. To treat thirst due to heat pathogen, it can be used in combination with *lú gēn* (Phragmitis Rhizoma) and *tiān huā fěn* (Trichosanthis Radix); to treat vomiting due to stomach heat, it is usually combined with *huáng lián* (Coptidis Rhizoma) and *zhú rú* (Bambusae Caulis in Taenia); to treat cough and asthma due to lung heat, it is often combined with *sāng bái pí* (Mori Cortex) and *dì gǔ pí* (Lycii Cortex).

【用法用量 / Usage and dosage】

煎服，15~30g，鲜品加倍。

Decoction, 15-30g. When it is used fresh, the dosage can be doubled.

【现代研究 / Modern research】

本品主要含芦竹素、白茅素、印白茅素、薏苡素、白头翁素，以及5-羟色胺、有机酸、甾醇、糖类等。具有止血、利尿、抑菌、抗炎、增强免疫等作用。

It mainly contains asparagus, citronella, citronella, coix, anemone, 5-hydroxytryptamine, organic acid, sterol and sugar, etc. It has the functions of stanch bleeding, promoting urination, bacteriostasis, anti inflammation and immunity enhancement.

第二节　化瘀止血药

Section 2　Stasis-resolving and bleeding-stanching medicinals

本类药物性味多辛温，既能止血，又能化瘀，具有止血而不留瘀的特点。主治瘀血内阻，血不循经之各种出血。若随证配伍，也可用于其他各种出血。

Stasis-resolving and bleeding-stanching medicinals are pungent and warm, which can not only stanch bleeding but also remove blood stasis. It has the characteristics of stanching blood without leaving blood stasis. It is mainly used to treat all kinds of bleeding due to blood stasis and internal obstruction and the failure of blood circulating in the vessels. If combined with other medicinals, it can also be used for other kinds of bleeding.

三七　*Sān qī* (Notoginseng Radix et Rhizoma)
《本草纲目》
The Grand Compendium of Materia Medica (Běn Cǎo Gāng Mù)

【来源 / Origin】

为五加科植物三七 *Panax notoginseng*（Burk.）F. H. Chen 的干燥根。主产于云南、广西等

微课

地。夏末秋初开花前或冬季种子成熟后采挖。晒干，生用，碾细粉为三七粉。本品气微，味苦回甜。《中国药典》规定，含人参皂苷 Rg_1（$C_{42}H_{72}O_{14}$）、人参皂苷 Rb_1（$C_{54}H_{92}O_{23}$）及三七皂苷 R_1（$C_{47}H_{80}O_{18}$）的总量不得少于 5.0%。

Sān qī is the dry root of *Panax notoginseng* (Burk.) F. H. Chen, pertaining to Araliaceae, and is mainly produced in Yunnan Province and Guangxi Zhuang Autonomous Region. It is collected in late summer and early autumn before it blooms or in winter after the seeds are ripe. It is dried and used raw or ground into powder. It has a slight odor and tastes bitter at first but becomes sweet after a while. According to *Chinese Pharmacopoeia*, the total content of Ginsenoside Rg_1 ($C_{42}H_{72}O_{14}$), ginsenoside Rb_1 ($C_{54}H_{92}O_{23}$) and Notoginsenoside R_1 ($C_{47}H_{80}O_{18}$) should be no less than 5.0%.

【性味归经 / Medicinal properties】

甘、微苦，温。归肝、胃经。

Sweet and slightly bitter; act on the liver and stomach meridians.

【主要功效 / Medicinal efficacies】

化瘀止血，活血定痛。

Remove blood stasis to stanch bleeding, activate blood circulation and alleviate pain.

【临床应用 / Clinical application】

1. 体内外各种出血　本品入肝经血分，功善止血，又能化瘀，有止血不留瘀、化瘀不伤正的特点，为止血之良药。对体内外各种出血，无论有无瘀滞，均可应用，尤以有瘀滞者为宜。单味内服外用，或配伍使用均有良效。用治吐血、衄血，可单用本品，米汤调服。用治咯血、吐血、衄血、尿血、便血，可与花蕊石、血余炭等同用。用治外伤出血，可单用本品研末外掺，或配伍龙骨、血竭等。

(1) **Internal and external bleeding**　Acting on blood aspect of the liver meridian, it is good at stanching bleeding and removing blood stasis. It has the characteristics of stanching bleeding without causing stasis and removing blood stasis without hurting the body. It can be applied to all kinds of internal and external bleeding, whether there is stasis or not, especially for those with stasis. It has good effect for internal and external usage, alone or in combination with other medicinals. To treat hematemesis and nosebleed it can be used alone and taken with rice soup; to treat hemoptysis, hematemesis, nosebleed, bloody urination and stool, it is used in combination with *huā ruǐ shí* (Ophicalcitum) and *xuè yú tàn* (Crinis Carbonisatus); to treat bleeding due to external injuries, it can be used alone by grinding into powder for externally application, or in combination with *lóng gǔ* (Draconis Os) and *xuè jié* (Draconis Sanguis).

2. 跌仆肿痛，胸腹刺痛　本品活血化瘀，消肿定痛，为治瘀血诸痛之佳品，伤科之要药。用治跌打损伤，骨折筋伤，瘀血肿痛，可单味研末，黄酒或白开水送服；或配伍红花、当归、土鳖虫等。用治胸痹刺痛，常与丹参、川芎、瓜蒌等同用。用治血瘀经闭、痛经、产后瘀阻腹痛，可与当归、红花、桃仁等配伍。用治痈疽肿痛或破烂，多与乳香、没药、儿茶等同用。

(2) **Trauma and painful swelling with blood stasis, stabbing pain in the chest and stomach**　It can promote blood circulation and remove blood stasis, reduce swelling and relieve pain. It is a primary medicinal for treating pain due to blood stasis and an important medicine for the department of injury. To treat bruises, broken tendons, blood stasis, swelling and pain, it can be used alone by grinding into powder and served with rice wine or boiled water; or combined with *hóng huā*, *dāng guī* and *tǔ biē chóng*; to treat stabbing pain in the chest and stomach, it is often combined with *dān shēn*, *chuān xiōng* and *guā lóu* (Trichosanthis Fructus); to treat menorrhea due to blood stasis, dysmenorrhea, postpartum stasis

and abdominal pain, it is used in combination with *dāng guī*, *hóng huā* and *táo rén*; to treat carbuncle, swelling, pain or festering, it is often combined with *rǔ xiāng*, *mò yào* and *ér chá*.

【用法用量 / Usage and dosage】

煎服，3~9g。研末吞服，1 次 1~3g。外用适量。

Decoction, 3-9g. It should be ground into powder for oral taking, 1-3g every time; appropriate amount for external application.

【使用注意 / Precaution】

孕妇慎用。

It should be used with caution for pregnant women.

【现代研究 / Modern research】

本品主要含人参皂苷 Rb$_1$、人参皂苷 Rb、人参皂苷 Re、人参皂苷 Rg$_1$、人参皂苷 Rg$_2$、人参皂苷 Rh$_1$，三七皂苷 R$_1$~R$_7$，三七皂苷 A~J，尚含三七素、槲皮素、氨基酸、多糖等。具有促凝血和抗凝血双向调节、抗血小板聚集、抗血栓形成、镇痛、改善心肌缺血、扩张脑血管、降血脂、降血压、抗纤维化、抗炎、抗衰老、增强免疫、抗疲劳等作用。

It mainly contains ginsenoside Rb$_1$, Rb, Re, Rg$_1$, Rg$_2$, Rh$_1$, notoginsenoside R$_1$-R$_7$, notoginsenoside A-J and notoginsenoside, quercetin, amino acid, and polysaccharide, etc. It has the functions of promoting coagulation and anticoagulant dual-directional regulation, anti platelet aggregation, anti thrombosis, analgesia, improving myocardial ischemia, expanding cerebral vessels, reducing blood fat and blood pressure, anti fibrosis, anti-inflammatory, anti-aging, enhancing immunity and anti fatigue, etc.

茜草　*Qiàn cǎo* (Rubiae Radix et Rhizoma)
《神农本草经》
Shen Nong's Classic of the Materia Medica (Shén Nóng Běn Cǎo Jīng)

【来源 / Origin】

为茜草科植物茜草 *Rubia cordifolia* L. 的干燥根和根茎。产于安徽、江苏、山东等地。春、秋二季采挖。切厚片或段，生用或炒炭用。本品气微，味微苦，久嚼刺舌。《中国药典》规定，含大叶茜草素（C$_{17}$H$_{15}$O$_4$）不得少于 0.40%，羟基茜草素（C$_{14}$H$_8$O$_5$）不得少于 0.10%。

Qiàn cǎo is the dry root and rhizome of *Rubia cordifolia* L., pertaining to Rubiaceae, mainly produced in Anhui, Jiangsu and Shandong Province in China. It is collected in spring and autumn, cut into thick slices or segments, and used raw or stir-fried to scorch. It has a slight odor and tastes a little bitter. Chewing it for a long time may bring a stinging feeling on the tongue. According to *Chinese Pharmacopoeia*, the content of alizarin (C$_{17}$H$_{15}$O$_4$) should be no less than 0.40%, and that of hydroxyalizarin (C$_{14}$H$_8$O$_5$) should be no less than 0.10%.

【性味归经 / Medicinal properties】

苦，寒。归肝经。

Bitter and cold; act on the liver meridian.

【主要功效 / Medicinal efficacies】

凉血，祛瘀，止血，通经。

Cool blood and dispel stasis, stanch bleeding and unblock the channels.

【临床应用 / Clinical application】

1. **血热夹瘀出血**　本品苦寒，入肝经血分，既能凉血止血，又能化瘀止血，适用于血热妄行或瘀血所致的各种出血，对于血热夹瘀之出血尤为适宜。用治吐血、衄血，常与大蓟、侧柏叶等同用。用治崩漏，常配伍生地黄、蒲黄、侧柏叶等。用治尿血，可与小蓟、白茅根等同用。用治外伤出血，可单味研末外掺。

(1) Bleeding due to combination of blood heat and blood stasis   With the nature of bitter, cold and acting on the liver meridian, it can not only cool the blood and stanch bleeding but also dispel stasis. It is suitable for all kinds of bleeding caused by blood heat or blood stasis, especially for bleeding due to combination of blood heat and blood stasis. To treat hematemesis and nosebleed, it is often combined with *dà jì* and *cè bǎi yè*; to treat metrorrhagia and metrostaxis, it is usually used in combination with *shēng dì huáng, pú huáng and cè bǎi yè*; to treat bloody urination, it is often combined with *xiǎo jì* and *bái máo gēn*; to treat bleeding due to external injury, it is often used alone by grinding into powder for externally application.

2. 瘀阻经闭，关节痹痛，跌仆肿痛   本品能行瘀滞，通经脉，利关节，尤多用于妇科。用治血瘀经闭，常配伍桃仁、红花、当归等。用治痹证，关节痹痛，可单用浸酒服，或与独活、海风藤等同用。用治跌仆肿痛，常与三七、乳香、没药等同用。

(2) Amenorrhea due to blood stasis, arthralgia (*bì* syndrome) and trauma   It can remove stasis, unblock channels and collaterals, and benefit joints so it is especially used for gynecology. To treat amenorrhea due to blood stasis, it is often combined with *táo rén, hóng huā* and *dāng guī*; to treat *bì* syndrome and arthralgia, it can be taken orally after soaking in wine, or used in combination with *dú huó* and *hǎi fēng téng* (Piperis Kadsurae Caulis); to treat trauma, it is often combined with *sān qī, rǔ xiāng* and *mò yào*.

【用法用量 / Usage and dosage】

煎服，6~10g。止血炒炭用，祛瘀通经生用或酒炒用。

Decoction, 6-10g. It is stir-fried to scorch for stanching bleeding while the raw or wine-roasted form for dispelling stasis to unblock the channels.

【现代研究 / Modern research】

本品主要含大叶茜草素、茜草双酯、茜草萘酸、羟基茜草素、异羟基茜草素、茜草素、茜黄素，尚含萜类、多糖等。具有促进血液凝固、抗炎、抑菌、抗肿瘤、升高白细胞等作用。

It mainly contains alizarin, alizarin diester, alizarinic acid, hydroxyalizarin, isohydroxyalizarin, alizarin, qianflavin, terpenes and polysaccharides, etc. It has the functions of promoting blood coagulation, anti-inflammatory, bacteriostatic, anti-tumor and increasing leukocyte, etc.

蒲黄   *Pú huáng* (Typhae Pollen)
《神农本草经》
Shen Nong's Classic of the Materia Medica (Shén Nóng Běn Cǎo Jīng)

【来源 / Origin】

为香蒲科植物水烛香蒲 *Typha angustifolia* L.、东方香蒲 *Typha orientalis* Presl 或同属植物的干燥花粉。产于浙江、江苏、安徽等地。夏季采收蒲棒上部的黄色雄花序，晒干后碾轧，筛取细粉，生用或炒炭用。本品气微，味淡。《中国药典》规定，含异鼠李素-3-O-新橙皮苷（$C_{28}H_{32}O_{16}$）和香蒲新苷（$C_{34}H_{42}O_{20}$）的总量不得少于 0.50%。

Pú huáng is the dry pollen of *Typha angustifolia* L., *Typha Orientalis* Presl or other species of the same genus, pertaining to Typhaceae. It is mainly produced in Zhejiang, Jiangsu and Anhui Province in China. The yellow male inflorescence on the top of cattail's spike is collected in summer. After it is dried in the sun and ground, the fine powder is sieved. It is used raw or stir-fried to scorch. It has slight odor and is bland in taste. According to *Chinese Pharmacopoeia*, the total content of isorhamnetin-3-O-neohesperidin ($C_{28}H_{32}O_{16}$) and typhoside($C_{34}H_{42}O_{20}$) should be no less than 0.50%.

【性味归经 / Medicinal properties 】

甘，平。归肝、心包经。

Sweet and neutral; act on the liver and pericardium meridian.

【主要功效 / Medicinal efficacies 】

止血，化瘀，利尿通淋。

Stanch bleeding and dissolve stasis; promote urination and relieve strangury.

【临床应用 / Clinical application 】

1. **体内外各种出血**　本品甘平，长于收敛止血，兼有化瘀之功，可广泛用于体内外各种出血，且无论寒热，有无瘀滞皆可应用。用治吐血、衄血、咯血、尿血、便血、崩漏等，可单用冲服，或配伍白及、地榆、大蓟等。用治月经过多、漏下不止，可与艾叶、山茱萸等同用。用治外伤出血，可单用外掺伤口。

(1) **Various bleeding interior and exterior**　With the nature of sweet and neutral, it is good at stanching bleeding and relieving stasis, therefore, it can be used to treat all interior and exterior bleeding conditions, whether the syndrome are due to cold or heat, with or without blood-stasis. To treat hematemesis nosebleed, spitting of blood, bloody stool, blood urine, metrorrhagia and metrostaxis, it can be taken alone after mixing with water or combined with *bái jí*, *dì yú* and *dà jì*; to treat menorrhagia and leakage, it is often combined with *ài yè* (Artemisiae Argyi Folium), and *shān zhū yú*; to treat traumatic bleeding, it can be used alone for external application.

2. **瘀血诸痛**　本品能活血通经，祛瘀止痛，可用于瘀血诸痛，尤为妇科所常用。若治瘀血阻滞，经闭痛经、产后瘀痛以及心腹刺痛等，常与五灵脂相须为用。若治跌打损伤，瘀肿疼痛，可单用蒲黄粉，温酒调服。

(2) **Pain caused by blood stasis**　It can activate blood, dredge channels, remove blood stasis and relieve pain. It can be used in all kinds of pain, especially in gynecology. To treat dysmenorrhea due to stasis block, postpartum stasis pain and pain in the heart and abdomen, it is often combined with *wǔ líng zhī*; to treat injuries from falling, bruise and pain, the powder can be used alone by mixing with wine for oral taking.

3. **血淋涩痛**　本品既能止血，又能利尿通淋，用治血淋涩痛，常与生地黄、石韦等同用。

(3) **Bloody strangury**　It can not only stop bleeding, but also promote urination and relieve gonorrhea. To treat bloody strangury, it is usually combined with *shēng dì huáng* and *shí wéi* (Pyrrosiae Folium).

【用法用量 / Usage and dosage 】

5~10g，包煎。外用适量，敷患处。止血多炒用，化瘀、利尿多生用。

Decoction in cloth bags, 5-10g. Appropriate amount for external application. The stir-fried form is usually used for stanching bleeding while the raw form for dissolving stasis and promoting urination.

【使用注意 / Precaution 】

孕妇慎用。

It should be used with caution for pregnant women.

【现代研究 / Modern research 】

本品主要含柚皮素、异鼠李素 –3-O- 新橙皮苷、香蒲新苷、槲皮素、山奈素、异鼠李素，尚含甾类、多糖、挥发油、酸类及烷类等。具有止血、抗血栓形成、抗心肌缺血、抗脑缺血、镇痛、利尿、抗炎、收缩子宫、降血压、降血脂等作用。

It mainly contains naringin, isorhamnetin-3-*O*-neohesperidin, typhoside, quercetin, kaempferol, isorhamnetin, steroids, polysaccharides, volatile oil, acids and alkanes. It has the functions of stanching bleeding, antithrombotic, anti myocardial ischemia, anti cerebral ischemia, analgesia, diuresis, anti-inflammatory, contraction of uterus, lowering blood pressure and blood lipid.

第三节　收敛止血药

Section 3　Astringent bleeding-stanching medicinals

本类药物多味涩，或为炭类，或质黏，药性平和，或凉而不寒，功善收敛止血，广泛用于各种出血而无瘀滞和实邪者。

Most medicinals of this category are astringent in taste, and some are in the carbonized form or sticky with a mild and neutral property. They can stanch bleeding with their astringent actions, so they are mainly used to treat bleeding syndromes without stasis and excess pathogens.

白及　*Bái jí* (Bletillae Rhizoma)
《神农本草经》
Shen Nong's Classic of the Materia Medica (Shén Nóng Běn Cǎo Jīng)

【来源 / Origin】

为兰科植物白及 *Bletilla striata*（Thunb.）Reichb.f. 的干燥块茎。主产于贵州、四川、湖南。夏、秋二季采挖，晒干，切薄片，生用。本品气微，味苦，嚼之有黏性。

Bái jí is the dry tuber of *Bletilla striata* (Thunb.) Reichb.f., pertaining to Orchidaceae, mainly produced in Guizhou, Sichuan and Hunan Province in China. It is collected in summer and fall, dried in the sun and then cut into thin slices. It is used raw. *Bái jí* has a slight odor and tastes bitter. Chewing it may bring a sticky feeling in the mouth.

【性味归经 / Medicinal properties】

苦、甘、涩，微寒。归肺、肝、胃经。

Bitter, sweet, astringent and mildly cold; act on the lung, liver and stomach meridians.

【主要功效 / Medicinal efficacies】

收敛止血，消肿生肌。

Stanch bleeding by astringing, relieve swelling and promote granulation.

【临床应用 / Clinical application】

1. **体内外各种出血**　本品味涩质黏，止血作用较强，为收敛止血之要药，可用于体内外多种出血。因其主入肺、胃经，故尤宜于咯血、吐血等肺、胃出血。用治咯血，可单用为末，与蔗糖粉混匀服。用治吐血、便血，可与乌贼骨等分研末内服。用治外伤出血，单味研末或与煅石膏研末外敷。

(1) **Internal and external bleeding**　It is astringent in taste and sticky in property with strong effect of stanching bleeding, and is an essential medicinal to stanch bleeding by astringing. It can be used

for various internal and external bleedings. It mainly acts on the lung and stomach meridians, so it is especially effective in treating bleeding in the lung and stomach, such as hematemesis and hemoptysis. It can be ground into powder and mixed with sucrose powder for oral taking to treat hematemesis and hemoptysis. To treat expectoration of blood and hematochezia, it is combined with *wū zéi gǔ* (Cleistocactus Sepium) in equal amount and ground into powder for oral taking. To treat bleeding due to traumatic injury, it is singly ground into powder or together ground with *duàn shí gāo* (Gypsum Fibrosum Praeparatum) for applying on the injured parts.

2. **疮疡肿毒，皮肤皲裂，水火烫伤**　本品寒凉苦泄，能消散痈肿；味涩质黏，又能敛疮生肌，为外疡消肿生肌之要药。用治疮疡肿毒初起，多与金银花、皂角刺、乳香等同用。若治疮疡已溃，久不收口者，可单用本品研末外敷，或与黄连、贝母、轻粉等同用。若治皮肤皲裂，水火烫伤，可将本品研末，麻油调敷，或与煅石膏、凡士林调膏外用。

(2) Sores, ulcers, swelling and toxin, rhagadia of hand and foot, burns and scalds by hot water and fire　It is cold, cool and bitter for draining fire to dispel carbuncle and swelling; it is astringent and sticky for healing sores and engender flesh, and an important medicinal to heal sores, remove swelling and generating flesh. To treat early stage of sores, ulcers, swelling and toxin, it is often combined with *jīn yín huā* (Lonicerae Japonicae Flos), *zào jiǎo cì* (Gleditsiae Spina) and *rǔ xiāng* (Olibanum). To treat erupted and unclosed sores and ulcers, it can be used alone and ground into powder for external application, or combined with *huáng lián* (Coptidis Rhizoma), *bèi mǔ* (Fritillaria Bulbus) and *qīng fěn* (Calomelas). To treat rhagadia of hand and foot, burns and scalds by hot water and fire, it is ground into powder and mixed with *má yóu* (Sesami Oleum) for external use, or combined with *duàn shí gāo* (Gypsum Fibrosum Praeparatum) and vaseline, made into paste for applying on the affected areas.

【用法用量 / Usage and dosage】

煎服，6~15g；研末吞服，3~6g。外用适量。

Decoction, 6-15g; it can be ground into powder for swallow, 3-6g, each time. A proper amount for external application.

【使用注意 / Precaution】

不宜与川乌、制川乌、草乌、制草乌、附子同用。

It is not proper to be used with *chuān wū* (Aconiti Radix), *zhì chuān wū* (Aconiti Radix Praeparata), *cǎo wū* (Aconiti Kusnezoffii Radix), *zhì cǎo wū* (Aconiti Kusnezoffii Radix Praeparata) and *fù zǐ* (Aconiti Lateralis Radix Praeparata).

【现代研究 / Modern research】

本品主要含联苄类、菲类、蒽醌类、芬酸类、双菲醚类、胶质、淀粉等。具有止血、抗胃溃疡、促进肉芽生长和创面愈合、抑菌、抗肿瘤等作用。

It mainly contains bibenzyl, phenanthrene, anthraquinones, fenoic acid, diphenanthrene ether, pectin and starch. It has the functions of stanching bleeding, anti-gastric ulcer, promoting granulation and skin wound healing, inhibiting bacteria and anti-tumor.

仙鹤草　*Xiān hè cǎo* (Agrimoniae Herba)

《本草图经》

Illustrated Classic of Materia Medica (Běn Cǎo Tú Jīng)

【来源 / Origin】

为蔷薇科植物龙芽草 *Agrimonia pilosa* Ledeb. 的干燥地上部分。产于浙江、江苏、湖南等地。

夏、秋二季采割。晒干，切段，生用。本品气微，味微苦。

Xiān hè cǎo is the above-ground part of *Agrimonia pilosa* Ledeb., pertaining to Rosaceae, mainly produced in Zhejiang, Jiangsu and Hunan Province in China. It is collected in summer and autumn. It is dried in the sun, cut into segments and used raw. *Xiān hè cǎo* has a slight odor and tastes slightly bitter.

【性味归经 / Medicinal properties】

苦、涩，平。归心、肝经。

Bitter, astringent and neutral; act on the heart and liver meridians.

【主要功效 / Medicinal efficacies】

收敛止血，止痢，截疟，解毒，补虚。

Stanch bleeding by astringing, arrest dysentery, prevent attack of malaria, resolve toxin, and supplement deficiency.

【临床应用 / Clinical application】

1. **各种出血** 本品味涩收敛，功能收敛止血，可用治全身各部位的出血。因其性平，故凡是出血，无论寒热虚实，皆可应用。用治血热妄行之出血，可配伍生地黄、侧柏叶、牡丹皮等。用治虚寒性出血，可与党参、炮姜、艾叶等同用。

(1) **Bleeding** It is astringent in taste with effect of stanching bleeding, which can be used to treat bleeding of all parts of human body. It is neutral in nature, so it can be used for bleeding due to both cold and heat syndrome. To treat bleeding caused by blood heat accelerating blood circulation, it is combined with *dì huáng* (Rehmanniae Radix), *cè bǎi yè* (Platycladi Cacumen) and *mǔ dān pí* (Moutan Cortex). To treat bleeding due to deficient cold, it is used with *dǎng shēn* (Codonopsis Radix), *páo jiāng* (Zingiberis Praeparatum Rhizoma) and *ài yè* (Artemisiae Argyi Folium).

2. **血痢，久泻久痢** 本品味涩，能涩肠止泻止痢，因其兼能补血，又能止血，故对于血痢及久泻久痢尤为适宜，可单用本品水煎服，或配伍地榆、肉豆蔻等。

(2) **Blood dysentery, chronic diarrhea and dysentery** It is astringent in flavor with efficacies of astringing the intestines, checking diarrhea and dysentery. It can also nourish blood and stanch bleeding, so it is especially effective in treating blood dysentery and chronic diarrhea and dysentery. For this condition, it can be decocted alone for oral taking, or combined with *dì yú* (Sanguisorbae Radix) and *ròu dòu kòu* (Myristicae Semen).

3. **疟疾** 本品有截疟之功，用治疟疾寒热，每日发作，可单用本品研末，于疟发前2小时吞服。

(3) **Malaria** It has the function of preventing attack of malaria. To treat daily attack of malaria with chills and fever, it can be ground into powder for swallow 2 hours before attack.

4. **痈肿疮毒，阴痒带下** 本品有解毒消肿、杀虫止痒之功。用治痈肿疮疖，可单用本品熬膏调蜜外涂，或同时内服。用治阴痒带下，可单用煎汤熏洗。

(4) **Carbuncle, swelling, sores and toxin, pruritus vulvae and leukorrhea** It has efficacies of resolving toxin and removing swelling, as well as killing worms and relieving itching. To treat carbuncle, swelling, sores and furuncle, it can be mixed with honey and made into paste for applying on the affected areas, or for oral taking. To treat pruritus vulvae and leukorrhea, it is decocted alone for fumigating and washing.

5. **脱力劳伤** 本品有补虚强壮作用，用治脱力劳伤，症见神倦乏力、面色萎黄而纳食正常者，常与大枣同煎服。治气血亏虚，神疲乏力，头晕目眩者，可与党参、熟地黄、龙眼肉等同用。

(5) Exhaustion and internal lesion due to overexertion   It has the function of supplementing deficiency. To treat exhaustion and internal lesion due to overexertion, manifested as spiritual lassitude, fatigue, and sallow complexion with normal appetite, it is often combined with *dà zǎo* (Jujubae Fructus). To treat spiritual lassitude, fatigue, dizziness and vertigo due to deficiency of qi and blood, it is used with *dǎng shēn* (Codonopsis Radix), *shú dì huáng* (Rehmanniae Radix Praeparata) and *lóng yǎn ròu* (Longan Arillus).

【用法用量 / Usage and dosage 】

煎服，6~12g。外用适量。

Decoction, 6-12g. A proper amount for external application.

【现代研究 / Modern research 】

本品主要含仙鹤草素、仙鹤草酚、仙鹤草内酯、木犀草素 –7– 葡萄糖苷、芹菜素 –7– 葡萄糖苷、槲皮素、芸香苷、鞣质等。具有止血、抗炎、镇痛、加强心肌收缩、抑制和杀灭疟原虫及阴道滴虫、抑菌、抗肿瘤等作用。

It mainly contains agrimonine, agrimol, agrimonolide, luteolin-7-glucoside, apigenin-7-glucoside, quercetin, rutin and tannins. It has the functions of stanching bleeding, anti-inflammation, relieving pain, strengthening myocardial contraction, inhibiting and killing malarial parasites and trichomoniasis, inhibiting bacteria and anti-tumor.

第四节　温经止血药

Section 4   Channel-warming and bleeding-stanching medicinals

PPT

本类药物性温热，能温脾阳，固冲脉而统摄血液，具有温经止血之功。主治脾不统血，冲脉失固之虚寒性出血。

Medicinals of this category are warm and heat in nature with effects of warming spleen yang and consolidating thoroughfare vessel to control blood. They have efficacies of warming channels and stanching bleeding, and are mainly indicated to treat bleeding due to deficient cold resulting from spleen failing to control blood and insecurity of thoroughfare vessel.

艾叶　*Ài yè* (Artemisiae Argyi Folium)
《名医别录》
Miscellaneous Records of Famous Physicians (Míng Yī Bié Lù)

【来源 / Origin 】

为菊科植物艾 *Artemisia argyi* Lévl.et Vant. 的干燥叶。全国大部分地区均产，以湖北蕲州产者为佳，称"蕲艾"。夏季花未开时采摘，晒干，生用或炒炭用。本品气清香，味苦。《中国药典》规定，含桉油精（$C_{10}H_8O$）不得少于 0.050%，含龙脑（$C_{10}H_{18}O$）不得少于 0.020%。

Ài yè is the leaf of *Artemisia argyi* Lévl.et Vant., pertaining to Compositae, produced in most areas of China. Those produced in Qizhou, Hubei Province are of superior quality, so it is called *qí ài*. *Ài*

医药大学堂
WWW.YIYAODXT.COM

yè is collected in summer when the flower is to bloom, dried in the sun. It is used raw or stir-fried to scorch. It has a delicate fragrance and tastes bitter. According to *Chinese Pharmacopeia*, the content of eucalyptol ($C_{10}H_8O$) should be no less than 0.050%, the content of borneol ($C_{10}H_{18}O$) should not be less than 0.020%.

【性味归经 / Medicinal properties】

辛、苦，温；有小毒。归肝、脾、肾经。

Acrid, bitter, warm and slightly toxic; act on the liver, spleen and kidney meridians.

【主要功效 / Medicinal efficacies】

温经止血，散寒止痛，调经，安胎；外用祛湿止痒。

Warm channels and stanch bleeding, dissipate cold to relieve pain, regulate menstruation, calm the fetus, dispel dampness and relieve itching for external use.

【临床应用 / Clinical application】

1. 虚寒性出血 本品气香味辛，性温散寒，能温气血而暖经脉，为温经止血之要药，适用于虚寒性出血。因其主入肝、肾经，故尤宜于下元虚冷，冲任不固所致的崩漏、月经过多，为妇科止血之要药，常与阿胶、当归、干地黄等同用。

(1) Bleeding due to deficiency-cold It is acrid with aroma and warm in nature for eliminating cold. It can warm qi and blood to warm channels, which is an essential medicinal to warm channels and stanch bleeding, and is often applied to treat bleeding due to deficiency-cold. *Ài yè* also serves as a vital medicinal to stanch bleeding in gynecology. Since it acts on the liver and kidney meridians, it is especially effective in treating metrorrhagia and hypermenorrhea caused by deficiency-cold of kidney and insecurity of thoroughfare and conception vessels in combination with *ē jiāo* (Corii Asini Colla), *dāng guī* (Angelicae Sinensis Radix) and *gān dì huáng* (Rehmanniae Recens Radix).

2. 月经不调，痛经，胎动不安 本品性温，入三阴经而走下焦，能温经散寒，调经止痛，止血安胎，为治下焦虚寒或寒客胞宫之要药。用治下焦虚寒，月经不调、痛经、宫冷不孕等，常配伍香附、吴茱萸、当归等。用治下焦虚寒，冲任不固之胎漏下血、胎动不安，常配伍阿胶、当归、桑寄生等。

(2) Irregular menstruation, painful menstruation and threatened miscarriage It is warm in nature and acts on the three yin meridians as well as lower energizer. It has the functions of warming channels to dispel cold, regulating menstruation to relieve pain, as well as stanching bleeding to calm the fetus. It is considered an important medicinal to treat deficiency-cold of lower energizer or attack of uterus by cold. To treat deficiency-cold of lower energizer, manifested as irregular menstruation, painful menstruation and sterility due to cold uterus, it is often combined with *xiāng fù* (Cyperi Rhizoma), *wú zhū yú* (Evodiae Fructus) and *dāng guī* (Angelicae Sinensis Radix). To treat vaginal bleeding during pregnancy and threatened miscarriage caused by deficiency-cold of lower energizer and insecurity of thoroughfare and conception vessels, it is often combined with *ē jiāo* (Corii Asini Colla), *dāng guī* (Angelicae Sinensis Radix) and *sāng jì shēng* (Taxilli Herba).

3. 皮肤瘙痒 本品外用能祛湿杀虫止痒，用治湿疹、阴痒、疥癣等皮肤瘙痒，单用或配伍黄柏、花椒等煎汤外洗。

(3) Itchy skin It can eliminate wind, kill worms and relieve itching for external application. To treat itchy skin caused by eczema, pruritus vulvae and scabies, it is used alone or decocted with *huáng bó* (Phellodendri Chinensis Cortex) and *huā jiāo* (Zanthoxyli Pericarpium) for external washing.

此外，将本品捣绒，制成艾条、艾炷等，用以熏灸体表穴位，能温煦气血，透达经络，为温灸的主要原料。

In addition, it can be pounded into floss and made into moxa sticks or moxa cones which are used to fume and ignite over the acupoints to warm qi and blood so as to make them move smoothly in the channels. It is a primary raw material for needle warming moxibustion.

【用法用量 / Usage and dosage】

煎服，3~9g。外用适量，供灸治或熏洗。温经止血宜炒炭用，余则生用。

Decoction, 3-9g. A proper amount for moxibustion or external fumigation and washing. It is mostly used in the raw. When used to warm the channel and stanch bleeding, it is stir-fried to scorch.

【现代研究 / Modern research】

本品主要含桉油精、香叶烯、α-蒎烯芳樟醇、β-蒎烯芳樟醇、樟脑、异龙脑、喹诺酸、β-石竹烯、异泽兰黄素等。具有止血、镇痛、抑菌、抗炎、镇咳、平喘、祛痰、抗过敏等作用。

It mainly contains eucalyptol, myrcene, α-pinene and β-pinene linalool, camphor, isoborneol, quinolinic acid, β-caryophyllene and eupatilin. It has effects of stanching bleeding, relieving pain, inhibiting bacteria, anti-inflammation, relieving cough and panting, eliminating sputum and anti-allergy.

炮姜　*Páo jiāng* (Zingiberis Praeparatum Rhizoma)
《珍珠囊》
Pouch of Pearls (*Zhēn Zhū Náng*)

【来源 / Origin】

为姜科植物姜 *Zingiber officinale* Rosc. 的干燥根茎的炮制品。产于四川、贵州、湖北等地。以干姜砂烫至鼓起，表面呈棕褐色，或炒炭至外表色黑，内至棕褐色入药。本品气香特异，味微辛辣。《中国药典》规定，含6-姜辣素（$C_{17}H_{26}O_4$）不得少于0.30%。

Páo jiāng is the rhizome of *Zingiber officinale* Rosc., pertaining to Zingiberaceae, and is mainly produced in Sichuan, Guizhou and Hubei Province in China. The dried ginger can be utilized after it is heated with sand until it knobs and the surface turns brown. Or it is dry-fried until the surface turns black and the interior is dark-brown. It has a unique fragrance and tastes slightly acrid and hot. According to *Chinese Pharmacopeia*, the content of 6-gingerol ($C_{17}H_{26}O_4$) should be no less than 0.30%.

【性味归经 / Medicinal properties】

苦、涩，温。归脾、肝经。

Bitter, astringent and warm; act on the spleen and liver meridians.

【主要功效 / Medicinal efficacies】

温经止血，温中止痛。

Warm channels and stanch bleeding, warm middle to relieve pain.

【临床应用 / Clinical application】

1. **虚寒性出血**　本品性温，主入脾经，能温暖中焦而止血，尤宜于脾胃虚寒，脾不统血之虚寒性出血。用治虚寒性吐血、便血，常与人参、黄芪、附子等同用。用治冲任虚寒，崩漏下血，可与乌梅、艾叶、棕榈炭等同用。

(1) **Bleeding due to deficiency-cold**　It is warm and acts on the spleen meridian with effect of warming the middle energizer to stanch bleeding, which is especially effective in treating deficiency-cold bleeding due to deficiency-cold of spleen and stomach failing to control blood. To treat hematemesis

and hematochezia due to deficiency cold, it is often used with *rén shēn* (Ginseng Radix et Rhizoma), *huáng qí* (Astragali Radix) and *fù zǐ* (Aconiti Lateralis Radix Praeparata). To treat uterus bleeding due to deficiency-cold of thoroughfare and conception vessels, it is often combined with *wū méi* (Mume Fructus), *ài yè* (Artemisiae Argyi Folium) and *zōng lǔ tàn* (Trachycarpi Petiolus Carbonisatus).

2. **腹痛，腹泻** 本品能温中止痛、止泻，善治虚寒性腹痛、腹泻。用治中焦受寒之腹痛，常与高良姜同用。用治产后血虚寒凝，小腹疼痛，常配伍当归、川芎、桃仁等。用治脾肾阳虚，腹痛久泻，多与附子、肉豆蔻等同用。

(2) Abdominal pain, diarrhea It has the functions of warming middle and relieving pain, as well as arrest diarrhea, which is effective in treating abdominal pain and diarrhea due to deficiency-cold. To treat abdominal pain caused by attack of middle energizer by cold, it is used with *gāo liáng jiāng* (Alpiniae Officinarum Rhizoma). To treat postpartum blood deficiency and cold congealing, manifested as pain in the lower abdomen, it is often combined with *dāng guī* (Angelicae Sinensis Radix), *chuān xiōng* (Chuanxiong Rhizoma) and *táo rén* (Persicae Semen). To treat yang deficiency of spleen and kidney, manifested as abdominal pain and chronic diarrhea, it is often combined with *fù zǐ* (Aconiti Lateralis Radix Praeparata) and *ròu dòu kòu* (Myristicae Semen).

【用法用量 / Usage and dosage】

煎服，3~10g。

Decoction, 3-10g.

【现代研究 / Modern research】

本品主要含 6-姜辣素、姜烯、水芹烯、莰烯、姜酮、姜醇，尚含树脂、淀粉等。具有止血、抗胃溃疡等作用。

It mainly contains 6-gingerol, zingiberene, cyclohexadiene, camphene, zingerone, gingerol, resin and starch. It has functions of stanching bleeding and anti-gastric ulcer.

其他止血药功用介绍见表 16-1。

The efficacies of other blood-stanching medicinals are shown in table 16-1.

表 16-1 其他止血药功用介绍

分类	药物	药性	功效	应用	用法用量
凉血止血药	侧柏叶	苦、涩、寒。归肺、肝、脾经	凉血止血，化痰止咳，生发乌发	血热出血；肺热咳嗽，痰黄黏稠；血热脱发，须发早白	煎服，6~12g。外用适量
	苎麻根	甘，寒。归心、肝经	凉血止血，安胎，清热解毒	血热出血，热盛胎动不安，胎漏下血；痈肿疮毒	煎服，10~30g。外用适量，煎汤外洗，或捣敷
化瘀止血药	花蕊石	酸、涩，平。归肝经	化瘀止血	咯血、吐血、外伤性出血等兼有瘀滞者，跌仆肿痛	煎服，4.5~9g；多研末内服。外用适量，研末外掺或调敷
	景天三七	甘、微酸，平。归肝、心经	散瘀止血，养血安神，解毒消肿	多种出血；跌打伤痛；心悸失眠，烦躁不安；蝎蜂螫伤	煎服，15~30g。外用适量

续表

分类	药物	药性	功效	应用	用法用量
收敛止血药	紫珠叶	苦、涩，凉。归肝、肺、胃经	凉血收敛止血，散瘀解毒消肿	多种出血；热毒疮疡，水火烫伤	煎服，3~15g；研末吞服，1.5~3g。外用适量
	鸡冠花	甘、涩，凉。归肝、大肠经	收敛止血，止带，止痢	多种出血，赤白带下，久痢不止	煎服，6~12g
	棕榈炭	苦、涩，平。归肝、肺、大肠经	收敛止血	多种出血	煎服，3~9g
收敛止血药	血余炭	苦、涩，平。归肝、胃经	收敛止血，化瘀，利尿	多种出血，小便不利	煎服，5~10g。外用适量
	藕节	甘、涩，平。归肝、肺、胃经	收敛止血，化瘀	多种出血	煎服，9~15g
温经止血药	灶心土	辛，温。归脾、胃经	温中止血，止泻，止呕	虚寒性出血，胃寒呕吐，脾虚久泻	煎服，15~30g，布包先煎；或60~120g，煎汤代水

题库

（胡晨霞）

第十七章　活血化瘀药
Chapter 17　Blood-invigorating and stasis-dissolving medicinals

 学习目标 | Learning goals

1. **掌握**　活血化瘀药在性能、功效、主治、配伍及使用注意方面的共性；川芎、延胡索、郁金、丹参、红花、桃仁、益母草、牛膝、虎杖、土鳖虫、水蛭、莪术的性能、功效、应用以及特殊的用法用量和特殊的使用注意。

2. **熟悉**　活血化瘀药的分类；姜黄、乳香、没药、五灵脂、鸡血藤、马钱子、自然铜、苏木、血竭、三棱的功效、主治以及特殊的用法用量和特殊的使用注意。

3. **了解**　活血化瘀药、活血止痛药、活血调经药、活血疗伤药、破血消癥药以及相关功效术语的含义；西红花、川牛膝、泽兰、王不留行、月季花、刘寄奴、穿山甲的功效以及特殊的用法用量和特殊的使用注意。

1. Master the commonness of blood-invigorating and stasis-dissolving medicinals in efficacy, indications, property, compatibility and cautions; as well as the property, efficacy, application, special usage and dosage and special precautions of *chuān xiōng, yán hú suǒ, yù jīn, dān shēn, hóng huā, táo rén, yì mǔ cǎo, niú xī, hǔ zhàng, tǔ biē chóng, shuǐ zhì* and *é zhú*.

2. Familiar with the classification of blood-invigorating and stasis-dissolving medicinals in efficacy, indications, special usage, dosage and special precautions of *jiāng huáng, rǔ xiāng, mò yào, wǔ líng zhī, jī xuè téng, mǎ qián zǐ, zì rán tóng, sū mù, xuè jié* and *sān léng*.

3. Understand the definitions of blood-invigorating and stasis-dissolving medicinals, blood-invigorating and pain-reliving medicinals, blood-invigorating and menstruation-regulating medicinals, blood-invigorating and wound-healing medicinals, blood-stasis breaking and mass-resolving medicinals and other related efficacy terms; and the efficacy, special usage and dosage and special precautions of *xī hóng huā, chuān niú xī, zé lán, wáng bù liú xíng, yuè jì huā, liú jì nú* and *chuān shān jiǎ*.

凡以通利血脉、促进血行、消散瘀血为主要功效，常用以治疗瘀血证的药物，称为活血化瘀药，又称活血祛瘀药。其中活血化瘀功效强者，又称破血药或逐瘀药。

Medicinals with the main efficacy of facilitating blood vessels, promoting blood circulation and removing blood stasis are known as blood-invigorating and stasis-dissolving medicinals, which are commonly used to treat blood stasis syndrome. Among them, those with powerful actions are also called blood-stasis breaking or blood stasis removing medicinals.

活血化瘀药多具有辛、苦味，药性偏温，主归心、肝经，入血分，善能通行血脉，消散瘀血而具有活血化瘀作用，通过活血化瘀这一基本作用，又可达到止痛、调经、疗伤、消癥、通痹、消痈等多种不同的功效，主治瘀血证。由于瘀血病证涉及内、外、伤、妇等临床各科，故其应用范围十分广泛，如内科的胸痹心痛、胁肋胀痛、脘腹疼痛、头痛、中风半身不遂、肢体麻木、关节痹痛、癥瘕积聚；外科的疮痈肿痛；伤科的跌打损伤；妇科的月经不调、闭经、痛经、产后瘀阻腹痛等。

Blood-invigorating and stasis-dissolving medicinals are mostly acrid, bitter and relatively warm, and act on heart and liver meridians in blood aspect. With the basic function of promoting blood circulation and removing blood stasis, it can achieve many different effects, such as relieving pain, regulating meridians, healing wounds, eliminating abdominal mass, clearing arthralgia and eliminating carbuncle, etc., and it mainly treats blood stasis syndrome. Because the syndrome of blood stasis involves internal, external, trauma, gynecology and other clinical departments, its application ranges widely, such as chest pain, costal pain, epigastric pain, headache, hemiplegia after stroke, limb numbness, arthralgia, syndrome accumulation; menstruation disorder, amenorrhea, dysmenorrhea, postpartum stasis and abdominal pain in gynecology; sores, carbuncle and swelling pains; injuries and bruise caused by falling and fracture, etc.

根据活血化瘀药的功效特点和主治差异，可分为活血止痛药、活血调经药、活血疗伤药、破血消癥药四类。

According to the difference of efficacies, properties and clinical applications, the blood-invigorating and stasis-dissolving medicinals can be classified into four categories:blood-invigorating and pain-relieving medicinals, blood-invigorating and menstruation-regulating medicinals, blood-invigorating and wound-healing medicinals, blood-stasis breaking and lump-resolving medicinals.

使用活血化瘀药时，应根据各类药物的不同特点随证选用，尚需针对瘀血的不同成因进行配伍。如寒凝瘀血，宜配伍温经散寒药；瘀热互结者，宜配伍清热凉血药；痰湿阻滞者，宜配伍化痰祛湿药；风湿痹阻者，宜配伍祛风除湿药；因虚致瘀或久瘀致虚者，宜配伍补虚药；若癥瘕积聚，应配伍软坚散结药。因"气为血帅""气行则血行"，故本类药物常与行气药同用，以增强活血化瘀的功效。

When using blood-invigorating and stasis-dissolving medicinals, doctors should make proper compatibility according to different symptoms and different characteristics of each kind and the different causes of blood stasis. In order to treat blood-stasis caused by cold-obstruction, they are usually combined with medicinals that can warm meridians and disperse cold. To treat blood stasis combined with heat, it is suitable to be combined with those that can clear heat and cool blood. To treat phlegm dampness block, it should be combined with those that can remove phlegm and dampness. To treat rheumatism block, it should be combined with those that can remove wind and dampness. To treat deficiency caused by long-term stasis, it should be combined with medicinals that can supplement deficiency. To treat abdominal mass, it should be combined with those that can resolve hard lump. Because qi is the commander of blood, and replenishing qi is to activate blood circulation, so this kind of medicinal is often used together with medicinal that can invigorate qi to enhance the effect of promoting blood circulation and removing blood stasis.

本类药物易耗血动血，出血而无瘀血阻滞及妇女月经过多者均当慎用。孕妇当慎用或忌用。破血逐瘀之品更易伤人正气，体虚者应慎用。

This kind of medicinal is easy to consume and move blood. It should be used with caution in patients with bleeding without blood stasis and women with menorrhagia. Pregnant women should use it with caution or avoid using it. The stasis-breaking or removing medicinal is more likely to hurt people's health qi, and it should be used with caution for those with weak constitutions.

第一节　活血止痛药
Section 1　Blood-invigorating and pain-relieving medicinals

PPT

本类药物味多辛、苦，归肝、心经，既能活血祛瘀，又有良好的止痛作用，而且多兼能行气。主治血瘀或血瘀气滞所致的头痛、胸胁痛、心腹痛、痛经、产后腹痛、痹痛、跌仆伤痛等各种痛证，也可用治其他血瘀证。

This kind of medicine has an acrid and bitter taste and act on the heart and liver meridians. It can not only promote blood circulation and remove blood stasis, but also has a good analgesic effect, and can also move qi. It mainly deals with headache, pain in the chest and rib side, pain in heart and stomach, dysmenorrhea, postpartum abdominal pain, *bì* syndrome (impediment), falling servant pain and other syndromes caused by blood stasis or qi stagnation. It can also be used to treat other blood stasis syndrome.

微课

川芎　*Chuān xiōng* (Chuanxiong Rhizoma)
《神农本草经》
Shen Nong's Classic of the Materia Medica (Shén Nóng Běn Cǎo Jīng)

【来源 / Origin】
为伞形科植物川芎 *Ligusticum chuanxiong* Hort. 的干燥根茎。主产于四川。夏季采收，切片，生用或酒炙用。本品气浓香，味苦、辛，稍有麻舌感，微回甜。《中国药典》规定，含阿魏酸（$C_{10}H_{10}O_4$）不得少于 0.10%。

Chuān xiōng is the dried rhizome of *Ligusticum chuanxiong* Hort., mainly produced in Sichuan Province, collected in summer, sliced, and used raw or wine roasted. It has a strong fragrance, and is bitter and pungent, with slightly tingling and sweet in taste. According to *Chinese Pharmacopoeia*, the content of ferulic acid ($C_{10}H_{10}O_4$) should be no less than 0.10%.

【性味归经 / Medicinal properties】
辛，温。归肝、胆、心包经。
Acrid and warm; act on the live, gallbladder and pericardium meridian.

【主要功效 / Medicinal efficacies】
活血行气，祛风止痛。
Invigorate blood and move qi, dispel wind and alleviate pain.

【临床应用 / Clinical application】
1. **血瘀气滞诸痛**　本品辛香行散，温通血脉，既能活血，又能行气，为"血中气药"，并善止痛，凡血瘀气滞诸证，皆为常用，尤为治血瘀气滞诸痛之要药。用治心脉瘀阻，胸痹心痛，常

医药大学堂
WWW.YIYAODXT.COM

与丹参、红花、三七等同用。用治肝郁气滞，胁肋作痛，常与柴胡、香附等同用。用治跌仆损伤，瘀肿疼痛，可与三七、乳香、没药等同用。用治中风偏瘫，肢体麻木，多与黄芪、地龙等同用。因其下行血海，长于"下调经水，中开郁结"，故为妇科活血调经常用药。用治血瘀闭经、痛经，常配伍当归、桃仁、红花等。用治产后恶露不下，瘀阻腹痛，常与当归、桃仁、炮姜等同用。用治冲任虚寒，瘀血阻滞的月经不调、痛经，常配伍吴茱萸、桂枝、当归等。

(1) Pains due to qi stagnation and blood stasis　With acrid and fragrant nature, *chuān xiōng* can not only invigorate blood, but also promote qi circulation. It is good at relieving pain and commonly used to treat all the syndromes (especially pains) due to qi stagnation and blood stasis. It can be used to treat heart stasis, chest arthralgia and heartache, and often combined with *dān shēn* (Salviae Miltiorrhizae Radix et Rhizoma), *hóng huā* (Carthami Flos) and *sān qī* (Notoginseng Radix et Rhizoma); to treat liver depression, qi stagnation and hypochondriac pain, it is often combined with *chái hú* (Bupleuri Radix), *xiāng fù* (Cyperi Rhizoma); to treat bruise and pain, it is often combined with *sān qī* (Notoginseng Radix et Rhizoma), *rǔ xiāng* (Olibanum), *mò yào* (Myrrha); to treat stroke hemiplegia and numbness, it is often combined with *huáng qí* (Astragali Radix) and *dì lóng* (Pheretima).It is often used for promoting and regulating blood circulation in gynecology with its nature of descending the blood sea and "lowering menstrual flow and opening stasis in the middle". It can be used to treat blood stasis amenorrhea and dysmenorrhea, and is often combined with *dāng guī* (Angelicae Sinensis Radix), *táo rén* (Persicae Semen) and *hóng huā* (Carthami Flos); to treat postpartum lochia, stasis and abdominal obstruction, it is often combined with *dāng guī* (Angelicae Sinensis Radix), *táo rén* (Persicae Semen) and *páo jiāng* (Zingiberis Praeparatum Rhizoma);to treat irregular menstruation and dysmenorrhea due to deficiency of thoroughfare and conception vessels and stagnation of blood stasis, it is often combined with *wú zhū yú* (Evodiae Fructus), *guì zhī* (Cinnamomi Ramulus) *and dāng guī* (Angelicae Sinensis Radix).

2. 头痛　本品药性升散，能"上行头目"，通畅气血，祛风止痛，为治头痛要药，可随证配伍治疗多种头痛。用治风寒头痛，常配伍羌活、白芷等。用治风热头痛，常配伍菊花、石膏等。用治风湿头痛，常配伍羌活、防风等。用治血瘀头痛，常与赤芍、麝香等同用。用治血虚头痛，可与当归、熟地黄等同用。

(2) Headache　With its upward-dispersion and outward penetration nature, the effect of *chuān xiōng* can go up to the head and eyes, and invigorate blood and move qi, thus has the function of dispelling wind and relieving pain, so it is an important medicinal for treating headache and can be combined with other medicinals to treat many kinds of headache. To treat headache contraction of wind-cold, it is often combined with *qiāng huó* (Notopterygii Rhizoma et Radix) and *bái zhǐ* (Angelicae Dahuricae Radix) etc; if the headache is due to wind-heat, it should be combined with *jú huā* (Chrysanthemi Flos) and *shí gāo* (Gypsum Fibrosum) etc.; if the headache is due to wind-dampness, it is often combined with *qiāng huó* (Notopterygii Rhizoma et Radix) and *fáng fēng* (Saposhnikoviae Radix), etc.; to treat headache due to blood stasis, it is often combined with *chì sháo* (Paeoniae Rubra Radix) and *shè xiāng* (Moschus); to treat headache caused by blood deficiency, it is often combined with *dāng guī* (Angelicae Sinensis Radix) and *shú dì huáng* (Rehmanniae Radix Praeparata).

3. 痹证　本品辛散温通，能"旁通络脉"，祛风通络止痛，亦为痹证所常用。用治风寒湿痹，肢体麻木，关节疼痛，常与羌活、独活、桂枝等同用。

(3) *Bì* syndrome (arthralgic)　It is arid and warm, ascending and dispering, so it can warm and promote blood circulation, which can remove wind, dredge collaterals and relieve pain by bypassing collaterals. *Chuān xiōng* can be used to treat *bì*-syndrome (arthralgic) pain. To treat coldness and dampness, numbness of limbs, joint pain, it is often combined with *qiāng huó* (Notopterygii Rhizoma et Radix), *dú huó* (Angelicae Pubescentis Radix) and *guì zhī* (Cinnamomi Ramulus).

【用法用量 / Usage and dosage】

煎服，3~10g。

Decoction, 3-10g.

【使用注意 / Precaution】

阴虚火旺、月经过多及出血性疾病而无瘀滞者，不宜使用。孕妇慎用。

It is not suitable for those suffering deficiency of yin and hyperactivity of fire, menorrhagia and hemorrhagic diseases without stasis. Caution for pregnant women.

【现代研究 / Modern research】

本品主要含川芎嗪、阿魏酸、藁本内酯、川芎内酯以及维生素 A、叶酸、甾醇、脂肪油等。具有扩张冠状动脉、增加冠脉血流量、降低心肌耗氧量、扩张脑血管、增加脑血流量、改善微循环、抑制血小板聚集、抗血栓形成、降血压、镇静、镇痛、利胆等作用。

It mainly contains ligustrazine, ferulic acid, ligustilide, ligustilide, vitamin A, folic acid, sterol and fat oil, etc. It has the functions of dilating coronary artery, increasing coronary blood flow, reducing myocardial oxygen consumption, dilating cerebral vessels, increasing cerebral blood flow, improving microcirculation, inhibiting platelet aggregation, antithrombotic, lowering blood pressure, sedation, analgesia, cholagogue and so on.

延胡索 *Yán hú suǒ* (Corydalis Rhizoma)
《雷公炮炙论》
Master Lei's Discourse on Medicinal Processing (Léi Gōng Páo Zhì Lùn)

【来源 / Origin】

为罂粟科多年生植物延胡索 *Corydalis yanhusuo* W. T.Wang 的干燥块茎。主产于浙江、江苏、湖北等地。夏初采收，切厚片或捣碎，生用或醋炙用。本品气微，味苦。《中国药典》规定，含四氢帕马丁（延胡索乙素）（$C_{21}H_{25}NO_4$）不得少于 0.050%，饮片不得少于 0.040%。

Yán hú suǒ is the dried tuber of *Corydalis yanhusuo* W. T. Wang, pertaining to Papaveraceae. It is mainly produced in Zhejiang, Jiangsu and Hubei Province in China, collected in early summer and sliced or mashed, and used raw or prepared with vinegar. It has a slight odor and bitter taste. According to *Chinese Pharmacopoeia*, the content of tetrahydropalmatine ($C_{21}H_{25}NO_4$) should be no less than 0.050%, and no less than 0.040% in decoction pieces.

【性味归经 / Medicinal properties】

辛、苦，温。归肝、脾、心经。

Acrid, bitter and warm; act on the liver, spleen and heart meridians.

【主要功效 / Medicinal efficacies】

活血，行气，止痛。

Invigorate blood circulation, activate qi and relieve pain.

【临床应用 / Clinical application】

血瘀气滞诸痛　本品辛散温通，既能活血，又能行气，尤长于止痛，故专治一身上下诸痛，为止痛良药，无论何种痛证，均可选用。用治心脉瘀阻，胸痹心痛，常与川芎、三七等同用。用治肝郁化火，气滞血瘀之胸胁脘腹疼痛，常与川楝子同用。用治肝郁气滞，胁肋胀痛，多与柴胡、香附等同用。用治寒滞胃痛，常与香附、高良姜等同用。用治妇女痛经，产后瘀阻腹痛，可与当归、川芎、香附等同用。用治跌打损伤，瘀肿疼痛，常与乳香、没药等同用。用治寒疝腹痛，多配伍吴茱萸、小茴香等。用治风湿痹痛，可与秦艽、桂枝等同用。

Pains due to blood stasis and qi stagnation　*Yán hú suǒ* is good at promoting blood circulation and qi activation, especially for pain relief. It can be used for any kind of pains. To treat heart blood stasis, chest obstruction and heartache, it is often combined with *chuān xiōng* and *sān qī*; for the pain in the chest, stomach or rib side, it is often combined with *chuān liàn zǐ* (Toosendan Fructus); to treat liver depression, qi stagnation, costal distention and pain, often combined with *chái hú* (Bupleuri Radix) and *xiāng fù* (Cyperi Rhizoma); to treat cold stagnation and stomachache, it is often combined with *xiāng fù* (Cyperi Rhizoma) and *gāo liáng jiāng* (Alpiniae Officinarum Rhizoma) etc.; to treat dysmenorrhea, postpartum stasis and abdominal pain, often combined with *dāng guī*, *chuān xiōng* and *xiāng fù*; to treat bruise and pain, it is often combined with *rǔ xiāng* (Olibanum)and *mò yào* (Myrrha); to treat cold hernia and abdominal pain, it is often combined with *wú zhū yú* (*Evodiae Fructus*) and *xiǎo huí xiāng* (Foeniculi Fructus); to treat rheumatic arthralgia, it is often combined with *qín jiāo* (Gentianae Macrophyllae Radix) and *guì zhī* (Cinnamomi Ramulus).

【用法用量 / Usage and dosage 】

煎服，3~10g；研末吞服，1 次 1.5~3g。醋制可增强止痛之功。

Decoction, 3-10g; grind into powder, 1.5-3g for each administration. Processing with vinegar can enhance the function of pain relief.

【现代研究 / Modern research 】

本品主要含延胡索甲素、乙素、丙素、丁素、庚素、辛素、壬素、寅素、丑素、子素等20余种生物碱。具有镇痛、镇静、催眠、抗心肌缺血、抗心律失常、提高耐缺氧能力、降血压、抗溃疡、抗炎等作用。

It mainly contains more than 20 kinds of alkaloids, such as corydalis A, B, C, D, G, etc. It has the functions of analgesia, sedation, hypnosis, anti myocardial ischemia, anti arrhythmia, improving hypoxia tolerance, lowering blood pressure, anti ulcer, and anti-inflammatory, etc.

郁金　*Yù jīn* (Curcumae Radix)

《药性论》

Treatise on Medicinal Properties (*Yào Xìng Lùn*)

【来源 / Origin 】

为姜科植物温郁金 *Curcuma wenyujin* Y.H.Chen et C.Ling、姜黄 *Curcuma longa* L.、广西莪术 *Curcuma kwangsiensis* S.G.Lee et C.F.Liang 或蓬莪术 *Curcuma phaeocaulis* Val. 的干燥块根。分别习称 "温郁金" "黄丝郁金" "桂郁金" "绿丝郁金"。主产于四川、浙江、广西等地。冬季采收，切薄片，生用或醋炙用。温郁金气微香，味微苦；黄丝郁金气芳香，味辛辣；桂郁金气微，味微辛苦；绿丝郁金气微，味淡。

Yù jīn is the tuberous root of *Curcuma wenyujin* Y.H.Chen et C.Ling, *Curcuma longa* L., *Curcuma kwangsiensis* S.G.Lee et C.F.Liang or *Curcuma phaeocaulis* Val., pertaining to Zingiberaceae. They are known as *wēn yù jīn*, *huáng sī yù jīn*, *guì yù jīn* and *lǜ sī yù jīn* respectively in Chinese, mainly produced in Sichuan, Zhejiang Province, and Guangxi Zhuang Autonomous Region. It is collected in winter, cut into thin slices, and used raw or prepared with vinegar. *Wēn yù jīn* is slightly fragrant and bitter in taste; *huáng sī yù jīn* is fragrant and spicy in taste; *guì yù jīn* is slightly fragrant, acrid and bitter in taste; *lǜ sī yù*

jīn is slightly fragrant with a slight odor.

【性味归经 / Medicinal properties】

辛、苦，寒。归肝、胆、心、肺经。

Acrid, bitter and cold; act on the liver, gallbladder and lung meridian.

【主要功效 / Medicinal efficacies】

活血止痛，行气解郁，清心凉血，利胆退黄。

Invigorate blood circulation to relieve pain, promote qi to relieve depression, clear heart and cool blood, benefit gallbladder and eliminate jaundice.

【临床应用 / Clinical application】

1. **血瘀气滞诸痛** 本品辛散苦泄，既能活血祛瘀止痛，又能疏肝行气解郁，善治肝郁气滞血瘀诸证。因其药性寒凉，故对血瘀气滞而有郁热者最为适宜。用治气血瘀滞之胸腹胁肋胀痛、刺痛，常与柴胡、香附等同用。用治肝郁有热，气滞血瘀之痛经、乳房胀痛，常与柴胡、栀子等同用。用治心脉瘀阻，胸痹心痛，可与丹参、赤芍等配伍。用治癥瘕痞块（各种肿瘤），可与五灵脂、马钱子等同用。

(1) **Pains due to blood stasis and qi stagnation** With the nature of acrid and fragrant and being good at dispersing bitterness, *yù jīn* can not only promote blood circulation, remove blood stasis and relieve pain, but also dredge liver and more qi to relieve depression, so it is good at treating liver depression, qi stagnation and blood stasis. Because of its cold property, it is most suitable for those with stagnation of blood and qi stasis with stagnant heat. To treat pain in chest, stomach and rib side due to stagnation of qi and blood, it is often combined with *chái hú* (Bupleuri Radix) and *xiāng fù* (Cyperi Rhizoma); to treat dysmenorrhea and breast distention caused by stagnation of liver qi and blood stasis, it is often combined with *chái hú* and *zhī zǐ* (Gardeniae Fructus); for heart stasis, chest obstruction and heartache, it is often combined with *dān shēn* (Salviae Miltiorrhizae Radix et Rhizoma) and *chì sháo* (Paeoniae Rubra Radix);to treat the symptoms and masses (various tumors), it is often combined with *wǔ líng zhī* (Trogopterori Faeces) and *mǎ qián zǐ* (Strychni Semen Pulveratum).

2. **热病神昏，癫痫发狂** 本品苦寒入心经，能清心解郁开窍。用治湿温病，湿浊蒙蔽清窍之神志不清，常配伍石菖蒲、竹沥、栀子等。用治痰浊蒙蔽心窍之癫痫发狂，常与白矾、牛黄同用。

(2) **Febrile disease, epilepsy and mania** With bitter and cold nature, acting on the heart meridian, *yù jīn* can clear the heart, relieve depression and open the mind. To treat damp-warm diseases which blind the consciousness, it is often combined with *shí chāng pú* (Acori Tatarinowii Rhizoma), *zhú lì* (Bambusae Succus) and *zhī zǐ* (Gardeniae Fructus); to treat epilepsy and mania with phlegm turbid which blinds the mind, it is often combined with *bái fán* (Alumen) and *niú huáng* (Calculus Bovis).

3. **血热吐衄** 本品苦寒清降，既能清肝经血分之热而凉血，又能顺气降火，气降则火降，火降则血不妄行，可因凉血降气而达止血之效。用治肝郁化火，气火上逆，迫血妄行之吐血、衄血、妇女倒经等，常与生地黄、栀子、牛膝等同用。用治热伤血络之尿血、血淋，可与小蓟、白茅根等同用。

(3) **Hematemesis due to blood heat** With the nature of cold and clear, *yù jīn* can not only clear the heat and cool the blood of liver meridians, but also reduce the fire with qi. Qi descending promotes fire descending, and fire descending causes abnormal circulation of blood. It can achieve the effect of hemostasis by cooling blood and descending qi. It can be used to treat hematemesis and reverse menstruation of women due to stagnation of liver-qi and transforming into fire counterflowing upward and forcing blood to flourish, often combined with raw *dì huáng* (Rehmanniae Radix), *zhī zǐ* and *niú xī*

(Achyranthis Bidentatae Radix); to treat urine blood and blood drench due to blood collaterals after heat injury, it is often combined with *xiǎo jì* (Cirsii Herba) and *bái máo gēn* (Imperatae Rhizoma).

4. 湿热黄疸，胆胀胁痛　本品苦寒清泄，入肝胆经，能清利肝胆湿热以退黄、排石。用治湿热黄疸，常配伍茵陈、栀子等。用治胆石症，胁肋胀痛，常与金钱草、木香、鸡内金等同用。

(4) Dampness-heat jaundice, gall distention and hypochondriac pain　With the nature of bitter and cold and act on liver and gallbladder meridian, *yù jīn* can clear the liver and gall to eliminate jaundice and remove calculus. To treat jaundice due to dampness and heat, it is often combined with *yīn chén* (Artemisiae Scopariae Herba) and *zhī zǐ*; to treat cholelithiasis and costal pain, it is often combined with *jīn qián cǎo* (Lysimachiae Herba), *mù xiāng* (Aucklandiae Radix) and *jī nèi jīn* (Corneum Gigeriae Galli Endothelium).

【用法用量 / Usage and dosage】

煎服，3~10g。

Decoction, 3-10g.

【使用注意 / Precaution】

不宜与丁香、母丁香同用。孕妇慎用。

Yù jīn is not suitable to combine with *dīng xiāng* (Caryophylli Flos) and *mǔ dīng xiāng* (Caryophylli Fructus). Pregnant women should use it with caution.

【现代研究 / Modern research】

本品主要含姜黄素、脱甲氧基姜黄素、双脱甲氧基姜黄素、姜黄酮、莪术醇、倍半萜烯醇、茨烯，尚含生物碱、多糖、木脂素、脂肪酸等。具有保肝、促进胆汁分泌和排泄、降低血黏度、抑制血小板聚集、抗炎、镇痛、抑菌、刺激胃酸及十二指肠液分泌等作用。

It mainly contains curcumin, demethoxycurcumin, double demethoxycurcumin, curcumin, curcumol, sesquiterpenol, camphene, alkaloid, polysaccharide, lignan and fatty acid, etc. It has the functions of protecting liver, promoting bile secretion and excretion, reducing blood viscosity, inhibiting platelet aggregation, anti-inflammatory, analgesic, bacteriostatic, stimulating gastric acid and duodenal secretion, etc.

姜黄　*Jiāng huáng* (Curcumae Longae Rhizoma)

《新修本草》

Newly Revised Materia Medica (Xīn Xiū Běn Cǎo)

【来源 / Origin】

为姜科植物姜黄 *Curcuma longa* L. 的干燥根茎。主产于四川。冬季采收，切厚片，生用。本品气香特异，味苦、辛。《中国药典》规定，含挥发油不得少于 7.0%（ml/g），含姜黄素（$C_{21}H_{20}O_6$）不得少于 1.0%；饮片含挥发油不得少于 5.0%（ml/g），含姜黄素不得少于 0.90%。

Jiāng huáng is the dried rhizome of *Curcuma longa* L., pertaining to Zingiberaceae. It is mainly produced in Sichuan and collected in winter, often cut into thick slices and used raw. It has a special fragrance, bitter and pungent in taste. According to *Chinese Pharmacopoeia*, the content of volatile oil should be no less than 7.0% (ml/g), curcumin ($C_{21}H_{20}O_6$) no less than 1.0%; the content of volatile oil in decoction pieces should be no less than 5.0% (ml/g), curcumin no less than 0.90%.

【性味归经 / Medicinal properties】

辛、苦，温。归肝、脾经。

Acrid, bitter and warm; act on the liver and spleen meridians.

【主要功效 / Medicinal efficacies】

活血行气，通经止痛。

Invigorate blood circulation and move qi, promote menstruation and relieve pain.

【临床应用 / Clinical application】

1. **血瘀气滞诸痛** 本品辛散温通，能活血行气，并长于止痛，善治血瘀气滞诸痛。用治血瘀气滞，胸胁刺痛，常与当归、乌药等同用。用治肝胃寒凝气滞之胸胁疼痛，常与桂心、枳壳、甘草等同用。用治血瘀气滞之痛经、闭经、产后腹痛，常配伍川芎、红花等。用治跌打损伤，瘀肿疼痛，常配伍乳香、没药等。

(1) All pains due to blood stasis and qi stagnation With acrid, fragrant and warm nature, *jiāng huáng* can not only activate blood, but also activate qi. It is good at relieving pain especially pains due to blood stasis and qi stagnation. To treat prickling in chest and hypochondrium caused by blood stasis and qi stagnation, it is often combined with *dāng guī* (Angelicae Sinensis Radix) and *wū yào* (Linderae Radix); to treat chest and hypochondriac pain caused by liver and stomach cold and stagnation of qi, it is often combined with *guì xīn*, *zhi qiào* (Aurantii Fructus) and *gān cǎo* (Glycyrrhizae Radix et Rhizoma); to treat dysmenorrhea, amenorrhea and postpartum abdominal pain due to blood stasis and qi stagnation, it is often combined with *chuān xiōng* and *hóng huā* (Carthami Flos);to treat bruise and pain, it is often combined with *rǔ xiāng* and *mò yào*.

2. **痹证** 本品辛散苦燥温通，能外散风寒湿邪，内行气血，通经止痛，尤长于行肢臂而除痹痛。用治风寒湿痹，肩臂疼痛，常与羌活、当归、防风等同用。

(2) *Bì*-syndrome (arthralgic) With the nature of acrid, bitter, dry and warm, *jiāng huáng* can disperse wind, cold and dampness. It can promote qi and blood, relieve pain, especially in limbs and arms. To treat pains due to wind, cold and dampness, shoulder and arm pain, it is often combined with *qiāng huó*, *dāng guī* and *fáng fēng*.

【用法用量 / Usage and dosage】

煎服，3~10g。外用适量。

Decoction, 3-10g. Proper amount for external use.

【使用注意 / Precaution】

孕妇慎用。

Pregnant women should use it with caution.

【现代研究 / Modern research】

本品主要含姜黄酮、芳姜黄酮、莪术酮、莪术醇、姜烯、水芹烯、龙脑、樟脑等挥发油以及姜黄素等。具有抑制血小板聚集、降低血黏度、降血脂、降压、抗炎、保肝、利胆、保护胃黏膜、兴奋子宫、抗肿瘤等作用。

It mainly contains ginger flavone, aromatic ginger flavone, curcumone, curcumol, curcumene, carvone, borneol, camphor and other volatile oil as well as curcumin. It has the functions of inhibiting platelet aggregation, reducing blood viscosity, reducing blood fat and blood pressure, anti inflammation, protecting liver, cholagogue, protecting gastric mucosa, stimulating uterus and anti-tumor.

乳香　*Rǔ xiāng* (Olibanum)

《名医别录》

Miscellaneous Records of Famous Physicians (Míng Yī Bié Lù)

【来源 / Origin】

为橄榄科植物乳香树 *Boswellia carterii* Birdw. 及同属植物 *Boswellia bhaw-dajiana* Birdw. 树皮渗出的树脂。主产于索马里、埃塞俄比亚等地，分为索马里乳香和埃塞俄比亚乳香。春、夏季采收，打碎，醋炙用。本品有特异香气，味微苦。《中国药典》规定，索马里乳香含挥发油不得少于 6.0%（ml/g），埃塞俄比亚乳香含挥发油不得少于 2.0%（ml/g）。

Rǔ xiāng is the resin exuded from the bark of *Boswellia carterii* Birdw. and *Boswellia bhaw-dajiana* Birdw., pertaining to Burseraceae. It is mainly produced in Somalia, and Ethiopia and classified into Somalian frankincense and Ethiopian frankincense. It is collected in spring and summer, smashed and used with vinegar. It has a special fragrance and a slightly bitter taste. According to *Chinese Pharmacopoeia*, Somalian frankincense should contain at least 6.0% (ml/g) of volatile oil, and Ethiopian frankincense should contain at least 2.0% (ml/g) of volatile oil.

【性味归经 / Medicinal properties】

辛、苦，温。归心、肝、脾经。

Acrid, bitter and warm; act on the heart, liver and spleen meridians.

【主要功效 / Medicinal efficacies】

活血定痛，消肿生肌。

Invigorate blood circulation, alleviate pain, reduce swelling and promote tissue regeneration.

【临床应用 / Clinical application】

1. **跌打损伤，痈肿疮疡**　本品辛香走窜，苦泄温通，既能散瘀止痛，又能活血消痈，祛腐生肌，为外伤科要药。用治跌打损伤，瘀滞肿痛，常配伍没药、血竭等。用治疮疡肿毒初起，红肿热痛，常与金银花、白芷、没药等同用。用治疮疡破溃，久不收口，可与没药研末外敷，或配伍儿茶、血竭等。用治痰疽、瘰疬、痰核坚硬不消，常与麝香、雄黄等同用。

(1) **Bruise and injuries, carbuncle and sore**　With the nature of spicy, fragrant, bitter, and warm, *rǔ xiāng* is not only good at dispersing blood stasis and relieving pain, but also can promote blood circulation and eliminate carbuncle, eliminate putrefaction and generate muscle. It is an important medicinal for trauma department. To treat bruise, stasis, swelling and pain, it is often combined with *mò yào* and *xuè jié* (Draconis Sanguis); to treat sore swelling, fever and pain, it is often combined with *jīn yín huā* (Lonicerae Japonicae Flos), *bái zhǐ* (Angelicae Dahuricae Radix) and *mò yào*; to treat swelling and ulcer on the body surface, it can be applied externally with *mò yào* (both ground into powder), or combined with *ér chá* (Catechu) and *xuè jié* (Draconis Sanguis); to treat carbuncle, scrofula and hard phlegm, it is often combined with *shè xiāng* (Moschus) and *xióng huáng* (Realgar).

2. **血瘀气滞诸痛**　本品辛散温通，能活血行气止痛。用治血瘀气滞之胃脘疼痛、胸痹心痛、痛经经闭、产后瘀阻、癥瘕腹痛等，常与没药相须为用。本品又能活血舒筋，用治风寒湿痹，筋脉拘挛，可与没药、威灵仙、姜黄等同用。

(2) **Pains due to blood stasis and qi stagnation**　With the nature of spicy and warm, *rǔ xiāng* can promote blood circulation, activate qi and relieve pain. It can be used to treat epigastralgia, chest pain, dysmenorrhea, amenorrhea, postpartum stasis, and abdominal pain, etc, often combined with *mò yào*; it can also activate blood and relax tendons. It can be used to treat wind, cold, dampness arthralgia, often

289

combined with *mò yào*, *wēi líng xiān* (Potentillae Chinensis Herba) and *jiāng huáng*.

【用法用量 / Usage and dosage】

煎汤或入丸、散，3~5g。外用适量，研末调敷。

Decoction or made into pill or powder, 3-5g; proper amount for external use by grinding.

【使用注意 / Precaution】

孕妇及胃弱者慎用。

Pregnant women and those with weak stomach should use it with caution.

【现代研究 / Modern research】

本品主要含乙酸辛酯、α-蒎烯、榄香烯、桉树脑、游离 α 和 β 乳香脂酸、香树脂酮、乳香树脂烃以及树胶等。具有镇痛、抗炎、保护胃黏膜、抗溃疡、祛痰、抑制血小板聚集等作用。

It mainly contains octyl acetate, α-pinene, elemene, Eucalyptus brain, free α and β lacteal fatty acid, rosin ketone, rosin hydrocarbon and gum. It has the functions of analgesia, anti-inflammatory, protecting gastric mucosa, anti ulcer, eliminating phlegm, inhibiting platelet aggregation and so on.

没药 *Mò yào* (Myrrha)
《开宝本草》
Materia Medica of the Kaibao Era (Kāi Bǎo Běn Cǎo)

【来源 / Origin】

为橄榄科植物地丁树 *Commiphora myrrha* Engl. 或哈地丁树 *Comniphora molmol* Engl. 的干燥树脂。分为天然没药和胶质没药。主产于索马里、埃塞俄比亚等地。11 月至次年 2 月采收，打碎，醋炙用。本品有特异香气，天然没药味苦而微辛，胶质没药味苦而有黏性。《中国药典》规定，天然没药含挥发油不得少于 4.0%（ml/g），胶质没药不得少于 2.0%（ml/g），饮片不得少于 2.0%（ml/g）。

Mò yào is the drying resin of *Commiphora myrrha* Engl. or *Comniphora molmol* Engl., pertaining to Burseraceae. It can be classified into natural myrrh and colloid myrrh, which mainly produced in Somalia, Ethiopia and other places. It is collected from November to February of the next year, and used in the broken form and roasted with vinegar. *Mò yào* has a special fragrance and a bitter and slightly pungent taste in nature, and the colloid myrrh is sticky with bitter taste. According to *Chinese Pharmacopoeia*, natural myrrh should contain volatile oil no less than 4.0% (ml/g), colloid myrrh no less than 2.0% (ml/g), and decoction pieces no less than 2.0% (ml/g).

【性味归经 / Medicinal properties】

辛、苦，平。归心、肝、脾经。

Acrid, bitter and neutral; act on the heart, liver and spleen meridians.

【主要功效 / Medicinal efficacies】

散瘀定痛，消肿生肌。

Disperse stasis and alleviate pain, eliminate swelling and promote tissue regeneration.

【临床应用 / Clinical application】

瘀血阻滞诸痛　本品功似乳香，治疗血瘀之心腹诸痛、跌仆伤痛、风湿痹痛、痈肿疼痛以及疮疡不敛等，常与乳香相须用。二者区别在于乳香偏于行气，伸筋；没药偏于散血化瘀。

Blood stasis or block pains　The efficacies of *mò yào* and *rǔ xiāng* are similar. *Mò yào* can treat pains of heart and abdomen, pains of falling and flapping, pains of rheumatism and arthralgia, carbuncle and swelling, and the non convergence of sores, often combined with *rǔ xiāng*. The difference between them is that *rǔ xiāng* tends to move qi and stretch muscles while *mò yào* tends to disperse blood and remove stasis.

【用法用量 / Usage and dosage】

煎服，3~5g，炮制去油，多入丸、散用。外用适量。

Decoction, 3-5g; processed and degreased, often used in pill and powder. Proper amount for external use.

【使用注意 / Precaution】

孕妇及胃弱者慎用。

Pregnant women and those with weak stomach should use it with caution.

【现代研究 / Modern research】

本品主要含挥发油、树脂类、树胶、少量苦味质，尚含没药酸、甲酸、乙酸及氧化酶等。具有镇痛、抗血栓形成、抗炎、降血脂、抗肿瘤等作用。

It mainly contains volatile oil, resins, gum, with a small amount of bitterness, and also contains myrrh acid, formic acid, acetic acid and oxidase. It has the functions of analgesic, antithrombotic, anti-inflammatory, hypolipidemic and antitumor.

第二节　活血调经药

Section 2　Blood-invigorating and menstruation-regulating medicinals

PPT

本类药物辛行苦泄，入肝经血分，具有活血化瘀之功，尤善于通畅血脉而调经。主治瘀血阻滞所致的月经不调、痛经、闭经、产后瘀滞腹痛等，亦可用于其他瘀血证。

With the nature of bitter and acrid, this kind of medicine has the functions of promoting blood circulation and removing blood stasis. It is especially good at regulating menstruation. It mainly treats irregular menstruation, dysmenorrhea, amenorrhea and postpartum abdominal pain caused by blood stasis and block. It can also be used for other blood stasis syndromes.

丹参　*Dān shēn* (Salviae Miltiorrhizae Radix et Rhizoma)
《神农本草经》
Shen Nong's Classic of the Materia Medica (Shén Nóng Běn Cǎo Jīng)

微课

【来源 / Origin】

为唇形科植物丹参 *Salvia miltiorrhiza* Bge. 的干燥根及根茎。主产于四川、山东、河北。春、秋二季采收，切厚片，生用或酒炙用。本品气微，味微苦涩。《中国药典》规定，含丹参酮ⅡA（$C_{19}H_{18}O_3$）、隐丹参酮（$C_{19}H_{20}O_3$）和丹参酮Ⅰ（$C_{18}H_{12}O_3$）的总量不得少于0.25%，丹酚酸B（$C_{36}H_{30}O_{16}$）不得少于3.0%。

Dān shēn is the dry root and rhizome of *Salvia miltiorrhiza* Bge., pertaining to Labiatae. It is mainly produced in Sichuan, Shandong and Hebei Province, collected in spring and autumn, used raw cut into thick slices, or roasted with wine. It has a slight odor and tastes bitter. According to *Chinese Pharmacopoeia*, the total content of tanshinone ⅡA ($C_{19}H_{18}O_3$), cryptotanshinone ($C_{19}H_{20}O_3$) and tanshinone I ($C_{18}H_{12}O_3$) should be no less than 0.25%, and salvianolic acid B ($C_{36}H_{30}O_{16}$) should be no less than 3.0%.

【性味归经 / Medicinal properties】

苦，微寒。归心、肝经。

Bitter and slightly cold; act on the heart and liver meridians.

【主要功效 / Medicinal efficacies】

活血祛瘀，通经止痛，清心除烦，凉血消痈。

Promote blood circulation to remove blood stasis; relieve pain by stimulating menstrual; clear heart to eliminate fidgety; cool blood to eliminate carbuncle.

【临床应用 / Clinical application】

1. 血瘀证　本品苦泄，主入心肝血分，性善通行，功能活血化瘀，善调妇女经水，且作用平和，活血祛瘀而不伤正，为妇科调经要药。因其性偏微寒，故宜于血热瘀滞者。其临床应用广泛，若治瘀血阻滞之月经不调、痛经、经闭、产后瘀阻腹痛，可单味研末酒调服，或配伍当归、红花、益母草等。若治血瘀气滞，胸痹心痛，常与三七、冰片合用。若治血瘀气滞，心胃疼痛，常配伍檀香、砂仁等。若治癥瘕积聚，常与三棱、莪术等同用。若治跌打损伤，瘀滞肿痛，常配伍乳香、没药等。若用治风湿热痹，关节红肿热痛，常与秦艽、忍冬藤、桑枝等同用。

(1) **Blood-stasis syndrome**　With the nature of bitter and property of reliving, *dān shēn* is mainly into blood aspect of heart and liver meridians. It is good at clearing, promoting blood circulation, removing stasis and regulating women's menstrual flow, and has a mild effect without hurting the body. It is an essential medicine for regulating menstrual flow in gynecology. Because of its mild cold nature, it is suitable for those with blood heat stagnation. It is widely used in clinical treatment, such as irregular menstruation, dysmenorrhea, amenorrhea, postpartum stasis and abdominal pain. It can be used alone with wine in the form of levigating, or combined with *dāng guī*, *hóng huā* (Carthami Flos) and *yì mǔ cǎo*; to treat blood stasis and qi stagnation, chest arthralgia and heartache, it is often combined with *sān qī* and *bīng piàn* (Borneolum Syntheticum); to treat blood stasis and qi stagnation, heart and stomach pain, often combined with *tán xiāng* (Santali Albi Lignum) and *shā rén* (Amomi Fructus); to treat symptoms of abdominal mass, often combined with *sān léng* (Sparganii Rhizoma) and *é zhú* (Curcumae Rhizoma); to treat injuries from falls, fractures, contusions and strains, bruise, stasis, swelling and pain, often combined with *mò yào* and *rǔ xiāng*; to treat rheumatism and arthralgia, it is often combined with *qín jiāo* (Gentianae Macrophyllae Radix), *rěn dōng téng* (Lonicerae Japonicae Caulis) and *sāng zhī* (Mori Ramulus).

2. 疮痈肿痛　本品性寒，既能凉血活血，又能清热消痈。用治热毒瘀阻所致的疮痈肿痛，常与金银花、连翘、紫花地丁等同用。

(2) **Sores, carbuncle, swelling and pain**　With the cold nature, *dān shēn* can cool and activate blood, clear heat and eliminate carbuncle. To treat sore, carbuncle, swelling and pain caused by heat, toxin and stasis, it is often combined with *jīn yín huā* (Lonicerae Japonicae Flos), *lián qiáo* (Forsythiae Fructus) and *zǐ huā dì dīng* (Violae Herba).

3. 热病烦躁，心悸失眠　本品性寒入心经，能清心凉血、除烦安神。用治温热病热入营血，高热神昏，烦躁不寐，常配伍生地黄、玄参等。若治心血不足之心悸失眠，常配伍酸枣仁、柏子仁、五味子等。

(3) **Restlessness and insomnia**　With cold nature and act on the heart meridian, *dān shēn* can clear the heart and cool the blood, eliminate fidgety and calm the nerves. It is used to treat febrile fever, heat, dizziness and restlessness by being combined with raw *dì huáng* (Rehmanniae Radix) and *xuán*

shēn (Scrophulariae Radix); to treat palpitation and insomnia caused by deficiency of heart blood, often combined with *suān zǎo rén* (Ziziphi Spinosae Semen), *bǎi zǐ rén* (Platycladi Semen) and *wǔ wèi zi* (Schisandrae Chinensis Fructus).

【用法用量 / Usage and dosage】

煎服，10~15g。活血化瘀宜酒炙用。

Decoction, 10-15g. Roasting with wine to promote blood circulation and remove blood stasis.

【使用注意 / Precaution】

不宜与藜芦同用。

Not suitable for use with *lí lú* (Veratri Nigri Radix et Rhizoma).

【现代研究 / Modern research】

本品主要含丹参酮Ⅰ、丹参酮ⅡA、丹参酮ⅡB、丹参酮Ⅲ、隐丹参酮、丹酚酸A、丹酚酸B、丹参素、原儿茶醛、原儿茶酸等。具有扩张冠脉及外周血管、增加冠脉血流量、改善微循环、提高耐缺氧能力、降血压、降低血黏度、抗血栓形成、抗动脉粥样硬化、调节血脂、镇静、镇痛、保肝、抗炎、抗菌、抗过敏等作用。

Dān shēn mainly contains tanshinone Ⅰ, tanshinone ⅡA, tanshinone ⅡB, tanshinone Ⅲ, cryptotanshinone, salvianolic acid A, salvianolic acid B, tanshinone, protocatechuic aldehyde, and protocatechuic acid, etc. It has the functions of expanding coronary artery and peripheral blood vessels, increasing coronary blood flow, improving microcirculation and hypoxia tolerance, lowering blood pressure, reducing blood volume, anti thrombosis, anti atherosclerosis, regulating blood lipid, sedation, analgesia, liver protection, anti-inflammatory, antibacterial and anti allergy, etc.

红花　*Hóng huā* (Carthami Flos)
《新修本草》
Newly Revised Materia Medica (Xīn Xīu Běn Cǎo)

【来源 / Origin】

为菊科植物红花 *Carthamus tinctorius* L. 的干燥花。主产于河南、新疆、四川。夏季采收，生用。本品气微香，味微苦。《中国药典》规定，含羟基红花黄色素 A（$C_{27}H_{32}O_{16}$）不得少于 1.0%，山奈素（$C_{15}H_{10}O_6$）不得少于 0.050%。

Hóng huā is the dried flower of *Carthamus tinctorius* L., pertaining to Composite. It is mainly produced in Henan Province, Xinjiang Uygur Autonomous Region and Sichuan Province, collected in summer and used raw. It has a slight odor and bitter taste. According to *Chinese Pharmacopoeia*, the content of hydroxysafflor yellow A ($C_{27}H_{32}O_{16}$) should be no less than 1.0%, and kaempferol ($C_{15}H_{10}O_6$) should be no less than 0.050%.

【性味归经 / Medicinal properties】

辛，温。归心、肝经。

Acrid and warm; act on the heart and liver meridians.

【主要功效 / Medicinal efficacies】

活血通经，散瘀止痛。

Invigorate blood and promote menstruation, remove blood stasis and alleviate pain.

【临床应用 / Clinical application】

血瘀证　本品辛散温通，入心肝血分，功能活血化瘀，通经止痛，消癥散结，为活血祛瘀之要药，广泛用于临床各科血瘀证，尤善治妇科经产瘀滞病证。用治血瘀经闭、痛经，常与桃仁、当归、川芎等同用。用治产后瘀滞腹痛，常与当归、蒲黄、牡丹皮等同用。用治跌打损伤、瘀滞肿痛，可用红花油或红华酊涂搽，或与乳香、没药等同用。用治心脉瘀阻，胸痹心痛，常配伍三七、丹参等。用治血瘀气滞，胁肋刺痛，常配伍柴胡、桃仁、大黄等。用治癥瘕积聚，多与莪术、三棱等同用。用治疮疡肿痛，常与金银花、连翘等同用。

Blood stasis syndrome With the nature of acrid and warm, acting on blood aspect of heart and liver, *hóng huā* has the functions of promoting blood circulation and removing blood stasis, promoting menstruation, relieving pain, eliminating masses and resolving stasis. It is an essential medicinal for promoting blood circulation and removing blood stasis. It is widely used in various clinical blood stasis syndromes, especially good at treating gynecology syndrome of stagnation of energy, production and stasis. To treat blood stasis, amenorrhea and dysmenorrhea, it is often combined with *dāng guī* (Angelicae Sinensis Radix), *pú huáng* (Typhae Pollen) and *mǔ dān pí* (Moutan Cortex); to treat bruise, stasis, swelling, pain and injuries from falls, fractures, contusions and strains, safflower oil or Honghua tincture is often used, or *hóng huā* is combined with *mò yào* and *rǔ xiāng*; to treat heart stasis, chest obstruction and heartache, often combined with *sān qī* and *dān shēn* (Salviae Miltiorrhizae Radix et Rhizoma); to treat blood stasis, qi stagnation and costal stabbing pain, often combined with *chái hú* (Bupleuri Radix), *táo rén* (Persicae Semen) and *dà huáng* (Rhei Radix et Rhizoma); to treat abdominal mass, often combined with *é zhú* (Curcumae Rhizoma) and *sān léng* (Sparganii Rhizoma); to treat sore, swelling and pain, often combined with *jīn yín huā* (Lonicerae Japonicae Flos) and *lián qiáo* (Forsythiae Fructus).

此外，本品能活血散瘀以消斑，可用治热郁血瘀之斑疹色暗，多与紫草、大青叶、当归等同用。

In addition, *hóng huā* can promote blood circulation and remove blood stasis to eliminate maculae. It can be used to treat the maculae with dark color of heat stagnation and blood stasis, and is often combined with *zǐ cǎo* (Arnebiae Radix), *dà qīng yè* (Isatidis Folium) and *dāng guī*.

【用法用量 / Usage and dosage】

煎服，3~10g。

Decoction, 3-10g.

【使用注意 / Precaution】

孕妇慎用；有出血倾向者不宜多用。

Pregnant women and those with bleeding tendency should use it with caution.

【现代研究 / Modern research】

本品主要含羟基红花黄色素A、山奈素、红花苷、前红花苷、绿原酸、咖啡酸、棕榈酸、月桂酸、马鞭烯酮、桂皮酸甲酯，尚含多糖、维生素、微量元素等。具有改善心肌缺血、抗血小板聚集、降低血黏度、兴奋子宫、降血压、镇痛、镇静、抗炎、抗惊厥等作用。

It mainly contains hydroxysafflor yellow A, kaempferol, anthocyanin, proanthocyanidins, chlorogenic acid, caffeic acid, palmitic acid, lauric acid, verbenone, methyl cinnamate, polysaccharide, vitamins, microelements, etc. It has the functions of improving myocardial ischemia, anti platelet aggregation, reducing blood viscosity, stimulating uterus, lowering blood pressure, analgesia, sedation, anti inflammation, and anti convulsion, etc.

桃仁 *Táo rén* (Persicae Semen)
《神农本草经》
Shen Nong's Classic of the Materia Medica (Shén Nóng Běn Cǎo Jīng)

【来源 / Origin】

为蔷薇科植物桃 *Prunus persica*（L.）Batsch 或山桃 *Prunus davidiana*（Carr.）Franch. 的干燥成熟种子。主产于山东、陕西、河南等地。果实成熟后采收，生用或去皮用、炒用。本品气微，味微苦。《中国药典》规定，含苦杏仁苷（$C_{20}H_{27}NO_{11}$）不得少于 2.0%，燀桃仁不得少于 1.50%，炒桃仁不得少于 1.60%。

Táo rén is the dry and mature seed of *Prunus persica* (L.) Batsch or *Prunus davidiana* (Carr.) Franch., pertaining to Rosaceae. It is mainly produced in Shandong, Shaanxi, Henan and other provinces in China. The fruit is collected after ripening, and used raw or peeled and fried. It has a slight odor and bitter taste. According to *Chinese Pharmacopoeia*, the content of amygdalin ($C_{20}H_{27}NO_{11}$) should be no less than 2.0%, no less than 1.50% in soaked *táo rén*, and no less than 1.60% in stir-fried *táo rén*.

【性味归经 / Medicinal properties】

苦、甘，平。归心、肝、大肠经。

Bitter, sweet and neutral; act on the heart, liver and large intestine meridians.

【主要功效 / Medicinal efficacies】

活血祛瘀，润肠通便，止咳平喘。

Invigorate blood and remove blood stasis, moisten intestines to promote defecation, relieve cough and asthma.

【临床应用 / Clinical application】

1. 血瘀证 本品味苦性平，入心肝血分，善泄血滞，活血祛瘀力强，临床应用广泛，为治疗各科血瘀证的常用药。用治血瘀经闭、痛经及产后瘀滞腹痛，常与红花、当归、川芎等同用。用治产后恶露不尽，小腹冷痛，常配伍炮姜、川芎等。用治癥瘕痞块，多与莪术、三棱等同用。用治跌打损伤，瘀血肿痛，常与当归、红花、大黄等同用。

(1) **Blood stasis syndrome** With the nature of bitter and neutral, *táo rén* is good at discharging blood stagnation, and is a kind of commonly used medicine for treating blood stasis syndrome in various departments. To treat blood stasis, dysmenorrhea and postpartum abdominal pain, it is often combined with *hóng huā*, *dāng guī* and *chuān xiōng*; to treat postpartum lochia, abdominal cold pain, often combined with *páo jiāng* and *chuān xiōng*; to treat bruise, stasis, swelling, pain and injuries from falls, fractures, contusions and strains, often combined with *hóng huā*, *dāng guī* and *dà huáng*.

2. 肺痈，肠痈 本品活血祛瘀，善泄血分之壅滞，为治疗热壅血瘀之肺痈、肠痈的常用药。用治肺痈，常配伍苇茎、冬瓜仁、鱼腥草等。用治肠痈，常与大黄、牡丹皮等同用。

(2) **Pulmonary and intestine abscesses** *Táo rén* can promote blood circulation and remove blood stasis. It is good at removing blood stasis and a common medicine for lung and intestinal abscesses with heat blocking. To treat lung abscesses, it is often combined with *wěi jìng*, *dōng guā rén* (Benincasae Semen) and *yú xīng cǎo* (Houttuyniae Herba); to treat intestinal abscesses, it is often combined with *dà huáng* and *mǔ dān pí* (Moutan Cortex).

3. 肠燥便秘 本品富含油脂，能润燥滑肠，用治肠燥便秘，常配伍当归、火麻仁、瓜蒌仁等。

(3) **Constipation due to dryness of intestines** *Táo rén* is rich in grease, and can moisten dryness

and smooth intestines, so it can be used to treat constipation due to dryness of intestines, and often combined with *dāng guī*, *huǒ má rén* (Cannabis Fructus) and *guā lóu rén* (Trichosanthis Semen).

4. 咳嗽气喘　本品味苦，能降泄肺气，有止咳平喘之效。用治咳嗽气喘，可单用煮粥食用，或与苦杏仁同用。

(4) Coughing and asthma *Táo rén* is bitter in taste, can reduce and relieve lung qi and have the effect of relieving coughing and asthma. To treat cough and asthma, it can be eaten with porridge alone, or combined with *kǔ xìng rén* (Armeniacae Amarum Semen).

【用法用量 / Usage and dosage 】

煎服，5~10g。

Decoction, 5-10g.

【使用注意 / Precaution 】

孕妇及脾虚便溏者慎用。

Pregnant women and those with spleen deficiency and loose stools should use it with caution.

【现代研究 / Modern research 】

本品主要含苦杏仁苷、野樱苷、甘油三酯、苦杏仁酶，尚含糖类、蛋白质、氨基酸、挥发油等。具有扩张血管、抗血小板聚集、增加脑血流量、收缩子宫、镇咳、平喘、镇痛、抗炎、抑菌、抗过敏、抗肝纤维化等作用。

It mainly contains amygdalin, wild cherry glycoside, triglyceride, amygdaline, sugar, protein, amino acid, volatile oil, etc. It has the functions of dilating blood vessels, anti platelet aggregation, increasing cerebral blood flow, contracting uterus, relieving cough and asthma, analgesia, anti inflammation, bacteriostasis, anti allergy and anti liver fibrosis, etc.

益母草　*Yì mǔ cǎo* (Leonuri Herba)
《神农本草经》
Shen Nong's Classic of the Materia Medica (Shén Nóng Běn Cǎo Jīng)

【来源 / Origin 】

为唇形科植物益母草 *Leonurus japonicus* Houtt. 的新鲜或干燥地上部分。我国大部分地区均产。鲜品春季至初夏采收，干品夏季采收，生用或熬膏用。本品气微，味微苦。《中国药典》规定，含盐酸水苏碱（$C_7H_{13}NO_2 \cdot HCl$）不得少于 0.50%，盐酸益母草碱（$C_{14}H_{21}O_5N_3 \cdot HCl$）不得少于 0.050%；饮片含盐酸水苏碱不得少于 0.40%，盐酸益母草碱不得少于 0.040%。

Yì mǔ cǎo is the fresh or dry aboveground part of *Leonurus japonicus* Houtt., pertaining to Labiatae. It is produced in most parts of China. Fresh ones shall be collected from spring to early summer and dry ones shall be collected in summer. It is used in raw form or decocted into paste. It has a slight odor and with bitter taste. According to *Chinese Pharmacopoeia*, the content of stachydrine hydrochloride ($C_7H_{13}NO_2 \cdot HCl$) should be no less than 0.50%, leonuri hydrochloride ($C_{14}H_{21}O_5N_3 \cdot HCl$) no less than 0.050%; the content of stachydrine hydrochloride in decoction pieces should be no less than 0.40%, leonuri hydrochloride should be no less than 0.040%.

【性味归经 / Medicinal properties 】

苦、辛，微寒。归肝、心包、膀胱经。

Bitter, acrid and slightly cold; act on the liver, pericardium, and bladder meridians.

【主要功效 / Medicinal efficacies 】

活血调经，利尿消肿，清热解毒。

Invigorate blood circulation and regulate menstruation, promote urination and alleviate edema, clear heat and remove toxin.

【临床应用 / Clinical application】

1. 血瘀证　本品苦泄辛散，主入血分，功善活血调经，祛瘀通经，为妇科经产要药，故有"益母"之称。用治血瘀痛经、经行不畅、经闭、月经不调、产后恶露不尽等，可单用熬膏服，如益母草膏，或与当归、川芎、丹参等同用。用治跌打损伤，瘀血肿痛，可与当归、乳香、没药等同用。

(1) **Blood stasis syndrome**　With the nature of bitter and acrid, *yì mǔ cǎo* has the greatest benefits for women's health. It is mainly used for promoting blood circulation and regulating menstruation, removing stasis and dredging meridians and it is an important medicinal for gynecology and multiparity. To treat blood stasis, dysmenorrhea, amenorrhea, irregular menstruation and endless postpartum lochia, it can be decocted alone into paste, called *yì mǔ cǎo gāo* (Motherwort Paste) to be taken orally, or be combined with *dāng guī*, *chuān xiōng* and *dān shēn*; to treat bruise, swelling, pain and injuries from falls, fractures, contusions and strains, often combined with *dāng guī*, *rǔ xiāng* and *mò yào*.

2. 水肿尿少　本品既能利水消肿，又能活血化瘀，对水瘀互阻的水肿较为适宜，可单用，或与白茅根、泽兰等同用。

(2) **Dysuria and edema**　*Yì mǔ cǎo* can not only promote water and detumescence, but also promote blood circulation and remove stasis. It is suitable for edema with mutual resistance of water and stasis. It can be used alone, or combined with *bái máo gēn* (Imperatae Rhizoma) and *zé lán* (Lycopi Herba).

3. 疮痈肿毒　本品苦寒清热解毒，味辛能散瘀消痈。用治疮痈肿毒，皮肤痒疹，可单用外洗或外敷，或配伍黄柏、苦参、蒲公英等。

(3) **Sores, carbuncle and swelling toxin**　With the nature of bitter and cold, *yì mǔ cǎo* has the functions of clearing heat and remove toxin, and has a pungent taste, which can disperse blood stasis and eliminate carbuncle. It can be used to treat sore, carbuncle, swelling and skin pruritus, and can be washed or applied externally alone, or combined with *huáng bó* (Phellodendri Chinensis Cortex), *kǔ shēn* (Sophorae Flavescentis Radix) and *pú gōng yīng* (Taraxaci Herba).

【用法用量 / Usage and dosage】

煎服，9~30g；鲜品12~40g。

Decoction, 9-30g; 12-40g for fresh products.

【使用注意 / Precaution】

孕妇慎用。

Pregnant women should use it with caution.

【现代研究 / Modern research】

本品主要含益母草碱、水苏碱、益母草定等生物碱，尚含二萜类及挥发油等。具有兴奋子宫、抗着床、抗早孕、强心、抗心肌缺血、抗血栓形成、降低血黏度、降压、利尿等作用。

It mainly contains alkaloids such as leonurus alkaloids, stachydrine, leonurus japonicus and diterpenoids and volatile oil. It has the functions of stimulating uterus, anti implantation, anti early pregnancy, strengthening heart, anti myocardial ischemia, anti thrombosis, reducing blood viscosity and blood pressure, diuresis, etc.

牛膝 *Niú xī* (Achyranthis Bidentatae Radix)
《神农本草经》
Shen Nong's Classic of the Materia Medica (Shén Nóng Běn Cǎo Jīng)

【来源 / Origin】

为苋科植物牛膝 *Achyranthes bidentata* Bl. 的干燥根。主产于河南。冬季茎叶枯萎时采挖，晒干，切段，生用或酒炙用。本品气微，味微甜而稍苦涩。《中国药典》规定，含 β- 蜕皮甾酮（$C_{27}H_{44}O_7$）不得少于 0.030%。

Niú xī is the dry root of *Achyranthes bidentata* Bl., pertaining to Amaranthaceae plant, mainly produced in Henan Province. They are collected when the stems and leaves wither in winter, and dried and cut sections, and used raw or stir-baked with liquor. *niú xī* is slightly sweet and bitter and astringent. According to *Chinese Pharmacopoeia*, β-ecdysterone ($C_{27}H_{44}O_7$) should be no less than 0.030%.

【性味归经 / Medicinal properties】

苦、甘、酸，平。归肝、肾经。

Bitter, sweet, sour and neutral; act on the liver and spleen meridians.

【主要功效 / Medicinal efficacies】

逐瘀通经，补肝肾，强筋骨，利尿通淋，引血下行。

Expel stasis and promote menstruation, supplement and boost the liver and kidney, strengthen muscles and bones, alleviate edema and relieve strangury, conduct blood fire to go downward.

【临床应用 / Clinical application】

1. 血瘀证　本品苦泄血滞，性善下行，长于活血通经，并能祛瘀止痛，常用于妇科血瘀经产诸疾及跌打损伤等。用治血瘀痛经、经闭、月经不调、产后腹痛，常配伍当归、桃仁、红花等。用治跌打损伤，腰膝瘀痛，常与续断、当归、红花等同用。

(1) Blood stasis syndrome　With the nature of bitter, *niú xī* is good at discharging stasis, descending and activating blood circulation. It can remove stasis and relieve pain and is commonly used in gynecology and other diseases of blood stasis and meridians and injuries caused by falling and striking. To treat dysmenorrhea, amenorrhea, irregular menstruation and postpartum abdominal pain, it is often combined with *dāng guī*, *táo rén* and *hóng huā*; to treat injuries caused by falling and striking, bruise and pain of waist and knee, it is often combined with *dāng guī*, *xù duàn* (Dipsaci Radix) and *hóng huā*.

2. 腰膝酸痛，筋骨无力　本品入肝、肾经，既能补益肝肾，强筋健骨，又能通血脉、利关节，为治腰膝酸痛、无力病证的常用药。用治肝肾不足，腰膝酸痛，筋骨无力，常与杜仲、续断、补骨脂等同用。用治痹痛日久，损及肝肾，腰膝酸痛，常配伍独活、桑寄生等。用治湿热成痿，足膝痿软，常与苍术、黄柏等同用。

(2) Pain in the waist and knees, weakness of muscles and bones　*Niú xī* can not only benefit the liver and kidney, strengthen the muscles and bones, but also promote blood circulation and benefit the joints. It is the common medicine to treat syndromes such as soreness and pain in the waist and knees and weakness of muscles and bones. To treat pain in the waist and knees caused by liver and kidney deficiency, weakness of muscles and bones, it is often combined with *dù zhòng* (Eucommiae Cortex), *xù duàn* (Dipsaci Radix) and *bǔ gǔ zhī* (Psoraleae Fructus); to treat damage to the liver and kidney due to arthralgia for a long time, lumbago and knee pain, it is often combined with *dú huó* (Angelicae Pubescentis Radix) and *sāng jì shēng* (Taxilli Herba); to treat impotence due to dampness and heat, it is often combined with *cāng zhú* (Atractylodis Rhizoma) and *huáng bó* (Phellodendri Chinensis Cortex).

3. 淋证，水肿，小便不利 本品性善下行，功能化瘀利尿通淋。用治热淋、血淋、砂淋，常配伍冬葵子、瞿麦、滑石等。用治水肿、小便不利，常与地黄、泽泻、车前子等同用。

(3) Gonorrhea, edema, dysuria *Niú xī* is good at descending and removing stasis, diuresis, and relieving stranguria. To treat heat, blood and urolithic stranguria, it is often combined with *dōng kuí zǐ* (Malvae Fructus), *qú mài* (Dianthi Herba) and *huá shí* (Talcum); to treat edema and dysuria, often combined with *dì huáng* (Rehmanniae Radix), *zé xiè* (Alismatis Rhizoma) and *chē qián zǐ* (Plantaginis Semen).

4. 气火上逆，血热出血，肝阳上亢 本品酸苦降泄，性善下行，能引上炎之火下降、上逆之血下行、上亢之阳下潜。用治胃火上炎之牙龈肿痛、口舌生疮，常配伍石膏、知母、生地黄等。用治气火上逆，血热妄行之吐血、衄血，常配伍白茅根、栀子、赭石等。用治肝阳上亢之头痛眩晕，常配伍赭石、生牡蛎、白芍等。

(4) Qi and fire ascending counterflow, bleeding due to heat and ascendant hyperactivity of liver yang With the nature of bitter and sour, *niú xī* can descend, discharge and move downward, leading up-flaming fire to descend, ascending counterflow blood to move downward, and live yang to sink. To treat toothache and aphthae, swelling and sore in mouth and tongue caused by stomachache fire, it is often combined with *shí gāo* (Gypsum Fibrosum), *zhī mǔ* (Anemarrhenae Rhizoma) and *shēng dì huáng* (Rehmanniae Radix); to treat blood vomiting and bleeding caused by the adverse reactions of qi and fire, often combined with *bái máo gēn* (Imperatae Rhizoma), *zhī zǐ* and *zhě shí* (Haematitum); to treat headache and vertigo caused by excess of liver yang, it is often combined with *zhě shí* (Haematitum), *mǔ lì* (Ostreae Concha) and *bái sháo* (Paeoniae Alba Radix).

【用法用量 / Usage and dosage】

煎服，5~12g。活血通经、利尿通淋、引血（火）下行宜生用，补肝肾、强筋骨宜酒炙用。

Decoction, 5-12g. It is suitable for using the raw form to invigorate blood and menstruation, alleviate edema and relieve strangury while being stirred with liquor to nourish liver and kidney and strengthen muscles and bones.

【使用注意 / Precaution】

孕妇慎用。

Pregnant women should use it with caution.

【现代研究 / Modern research】

本品主要含 β- 蜕皮甾酮、牛膝甾酮、人参皂苷 R_0、牛膝皂苷 Ⅰ、牛膝皂苷 Ⅱ、蜕皮甾酮、芦丁、异槲皮素，尚含多糖及氨基酸等。具有兴奋子宫、抗着床、抗早孕、降低血黏度、抗凝、降血脂、降血压、降血糖、抗炎、镇痛、提高免疫等作用。

It mainly contains *β*-ecdysterone, achyranthes bidentata sterone, ginsenoside R_0, achyranthes bidentata saponin Ⅰ, achyranthes bidentata saponin Ⅱ, ecdysterone, rutin, isoquercetin, polysaccharides and amino acids. It has the functions of stimulating uterus, anti implantation and early pregnancy, reducing blood viscosity, anticoagulation, lowering blood lipid and pressure, lowering blood sugar, anti inflammation, analgesia and improving immunity, etc.

虎杖 *Hǔ zhàng* (Polygoni Cuspidati Rhizoma ET Radix)
《名医别录》
Miscellaneous Records of Famous Physicians (Míng Yī Bié Lù)

【来源 / Origin 】

为蓼科植物虎杖 *Polygonum cuspidatum* Sieb.et Zucc. 的干燥根茎和根。主产于华东、西南。春、秋采收，切段或厚片，生用。本品气微，味微苦、涩。《中国药典》规定，含大黄素（$C_{15}H_{10}O_5$）不得少于 0.60%，含虎杖苷（$C_{20}H_{22}O_8$）不得少于 0.15%。

Hǔ zhàng is the dry rhizomes and roots of *Polygonum cuspidatum* Sieb.et Zucc. It is mainly produced in east and southwest China, collected in spring and autumn and used in the raw form of cut sections or thick slices. It is slightly bitter and astringent. According to the *Chinese Pharmacopoeia*, the content of emodin ($C_{15}H_{10}O_5$) should be no less than 0.60%, and that of polydatin ($C_{20}H_{22}O_8$) should be no less than 0.15%.

【性味归经 / Medicinal properties 】

微苦，微寒。归肝、胆、肺经。

Slightly bitter and cold; act on the liver, gallbladder and lung meridians.

【主要功效 / Medicinal efficacies 】

散瘀止痛，利湿退黄，清热解毒，化痰止咳。

Remove blood stasis and relieve pain, remove dampness and jaundice, clear heat and remove toxin, remove phlegm and stop cough.

【临床应用 / Clinical application 】

1. 血瘀证　本品苦泄入肝经血分，有活血散瘀止痛之功。用治瘀血阻滞之经闭、痛经，常与桃仁、红花等同用。用治癥瘕积聚，可与三棱、莪术等同用。用治风湿痹证，可与独活、威灵仙等同用。用治跌打伤痛，可与红花、乳香、没药等配伍。

(1) **Blood stasis syndrome**　With the nature of bitter, *hǔ zhàng* can discharge and act on blood aspect of the liver meridian and has the function of promoting blood circulation, removing blood stasis and relieving pain. To treat of amenorrhea and dysmenorrhea due to blood stasis, it is often combined with *táo rén* and *hóng huā*; to treat abdominal mass, often combined with *sān léng* and *é zhú*; to treat rheumatic arthralgia syndromes, often combined with *dú huó* (Angelicae Pubescentis Radix) and *wēi líng xiān* (Clematidis Radix et Rhizoma); to treat injuries and pains caused by falling and striking, it is often combined with *hóng huā*, *rǔ xiāng* (Olibanum) and *mò yào* (Myrrha).

2. 湿热黄疸，淋浊，带下　本品苦寒，有清热利湿之功，为治湿热黄疸常用药，常配伍茵陈、黄柏、栀子等。若治湿热淋证，可与车前子、泽泻、猪苓等同用。若治湿热带下，可与苍术、黄柏等同用。

(2) **Dampness-heat jaundice, turbid stranguria, leukorrhagia**　*Hǔ zhàng* is bitter and cold. It has the function of clearing heat and removing dampness. It is a common medicine for treating damp heat and jaundice and often combined with *yīn chén* (Artemisiae Scopariae Herba), *huáng bó* (Phellodendri Chinensis Cortex) and *zhī zǐ*; to treat drenching syndrome due to dampness and heat, often combined with *chē qián zǐ* (Plantaginis Semen), *zé xiè* (Alismatis Rhizoma) and *zhū líng* (Polyporus); to treat morbid leukorrhoea, it is often combined with *cāng zhú* (Atractylodis Rhizoma) and *huáng bó* (Phellodendri Chinensis Cortex).

3. 痈肿疮毒，水火烫伤，毒蛇咬伤　本品苦寒，有清热解毒之功。用治热毒痈疮，可用鲜品捣烂外敷，或配伍蒲公英、连翘等。用治水火烫伤，可单用研末，水调敷，或与地榆、冰片共研末，以香油调敷。若治毒蛇咬伤，可取鲜品捣烂敷患处，亦可煎浓汤内服。

(3) Carbuncle, swelling, sore, scald and snake bite *Hŭ zhàng* is bitter and cold. It can clear heat and remove toxin. It can treat carbuncle and sore caused by heat toxin by using the mashed fresh products to apply externally, or it can be combined with *pú gōng yīng* (Taraxaci Herba) and *lián qiáo* (Forsythiae Fructus); using the ground powder mixed with water and applying externally to treat water and fire burns, or combined with *dì yú* (Sanguisorbae Radix) and *bīng piàn* (Borneolum Syntheticum) mixed with sesame oil; for the treatment of snake bites, fresh products can be mashed to apply to the affected area, or decoction for internal use.

4. 肺热咳嗽 本品苦寒入肺经，能清肺化痰止咳，用治肺热咳嗽，可单用，或与黄芩、鱼腥草等同用。

(4) Cough due to lung heat With the nature of bitter and cold and act on lung meridian, *hŭ zhàng* can clear the lung, dissipate phlegm and stop coughing. It can be used alone to treat lung heat coughing, or combined with *huáng qín* (Scutellariae Radix) and *yú xīng căo* (Houttuyniae Herba).

此外，本品还有泻热通便作用，可用治热结便秘。

In addition, it has the effect of discharging heat and relaxing bowels, which can be used to treat constipation caused by heat.

【用法用量 / Usage and dosage】
煎服，9~15g。外用适量，制成煎液或油膏涂敷。

Decoction, 9-15g. Apply appropriate amount for external use, make into decoct or ointment for coating.

【使用注意 / Precaution】
孕妇慎用。

Pregnant women should use it with caution.

【现代研究 / Modern research】
本品主要含大黄素、大黄酚、大黄素甲醚、虎杖苷、白藜芦醇、白藜芦醇苷等，尚含多糖、氨基酸、鞣质等。具有改善微循环、降血压、止血、抑菌、抗炎、抗病毒、镇痛、祛痰、镇咳、平喘、泻下、抗肝损伤等作用。

It mainly contains emodin, chrysophanol, emodin methyl ether, polygonum cuspidatum glycoside, resveratrol, resveratrol glycoside, and polysaccharide, amino acid and tannin, etc. It has the functions of improving microcirculation, lowering blood pressure, hemostasis, bacteriostasis, anti-inflammatory, antiviral, analgesic, expectorant, antitussive, antiasthmatic, purgative and anti liver injury.

第三节 活血疗伤药

Section 3 Blood-invigorating and wound-healing medicinals

PPT

微课

本类药物功善活血化瘀而消肿止痛，又多兼续筋接骨或止血生肌等功效，主治跌打损伤、瘀肿疼痛、骨折筋损、金疮出血等伤科疾患，也可用于其他血瘀证。

This kind of medicinals are good at invigorating blood circulation, removing stasis, detumescence and pain relief, and it also has the effects of reinforcing muscles and bones, hemostasis and muscle regeneration, etc. It is mainly used for the treatment of injuries such as bruise injury, swelling pain, fracture and tendon damage, incised wound and bleeding, etc. It can also be used for other blood stasis syndromes.

土鳖虫 *Tǔ biē chóng* (Eupolyphaga Steleophaga)
《神农本草经》
Shen Nong's Classic of the Materia Medica (Shén Nóng Běn Cǎo Jīng)

【来源 / Origin】

为鳖蠊科昆虫地鳖 *Eupolyphaga sinensis* Walker. 或冀地鳖 *Steleophaga plancyi*（Boleny）雌虫的全体。主产于江苏、浙江、湖南等地。野生者夏季捕捉，饲养者全年可捕捉。用沸水烫死，晒干或烘干，生用。本品气腥臭，味微咸。

Tǔ biē chóng is the whole female body of *Eupolyphaga sinensis* Walker. or *Steleophaga plancy* (boleny), pertaining to Eupolyphaga. It is mainly produced in Jiangsu, Zhejiang, Hunan and other provinces in China. Wild ones are caught in summer and breeders are caught all year round. Scald with boiling water and dry it in the sun or roasted, use in the raw form. It has a stinking smell and with a slightly salty taste.

【性味归经 / Medicinal properties】

咸，寒；有小毒。归肝经。

Salty and cold and mildly toxic; act on the liver meridians.

【主要功效 / Medicinal efficacies】

破血逐瘀，续筋接骨。

Break and expel blood stasis, strengthen muscles and reconnect bones.

【临床应用 / Clinical application】

1. 跌打损伤　本品性善走窜，能活血消肿止痛，续筋接骨疗伤，为伤科常用药，尤多用于骨折筋伤，瘀血肿痛。用治跌打损伤，骨折伤痛，常与三七、红花等同用。用治骨折筋伤后筋骨软弱，常配伍续断、杜仲等。

(1) Injuries from falls, fractures, contusions and strains *Tǔ biē chóng* is good at promoting blood circulation, detumescence, relieving pain, strengthening muscles and connecting bones. It is a common medicine in the department of tramatic injury, especially for fracture and tendon injury, blood stasis and swelling pain. To treat injuries caused by falls and fractures, it is often combined with *sān qī* and *hóng huā*; to treat weakness of muscles and bones after fracture and tendon injury, it is often combined with *xù duàn* and *dù zhòng* (Eucommiae Cortex).

2. 血瘀经闭，产后瘀滞腹痛，癥瘕痞块　本品入肝经血分，能破血逐瘀而通经、消癥。用治血瘀经闭，产后瘀滞腹痛，常与大黄、桃仁等同用。用治癥瘕积聚，多与桃仁、鳖甲等同用。

(2) Blood stasis and amenorrhea, postpartum stasis and abdominal pain, abdominal mass and ruffles *Tǔ biē chóng* act on liver meridians and blood vessels, which can break and remove blood stasis to dredge meridians and eliminate symptoms. To treat blood stasis and amenorrhea, postpartum stasis and abdominal pain, it is often combined with *dà huáng* and *táo rén*; to treat abdominal mass, it is often combined with *táo rén* and *biē jiǎ* (Trionycis Carapax).

【用法用量 / Usage and dosage】

煎服，3~10g。

Decoction, 3-10g.

【使用注意 / Precaution】

孕妇忌服。

Pregnant women should use it with caution.

【现代研究 / Modern research】

本品主要含棕榈油酸、油酸、软脂酸、硬脂酸等脂肪酸，尚含尿嘧啶、尿囊素、生物碱、氨基酸、微量元素、甾醇等。具有抗血栓、提高心肌和脑对缺氧的耐受力、降低心和脑组织的耗氧量、促进骨折愈合、保肝等作用。

It mainly contains palmitoleic acid, oleic acid, palmitic acid, stearic acid and other fatty acids, and uracil, allantoin, alkaloid, amino acid, microelement, and sterol, etc. It has the functions of antithrombotic, improving the tolerance of heart and brain to hypoxia, reducing oxygen consumption of heart and brain, promoting fracture healing and protecting liver.

马钱子　*Mǎ qián zǐ* (Strychni Semen)

《本草纲目》

The Grand Compendium of Materia Medica (Běn Cǎo Gāng Mù)

【来源 / Origin】

为马钱科植物马钱 *Strychnos nux-vomica* L. 的干燥成熟种子。主产于印度、越南、缅甸等地，我国云南、广东、海南等地亦产。冬季果实成熟时采收。晒干，炮制后入药。《中国药典》规定，含士的宁（$C_{21}H_{22}N_2O_2$）应为 1.20%~2.20%，马钱子碱（$C_{23}H_{26}N_2O_4$）不得少于 0.80%。

Mǎ qián zǐ is the dry and mature seed of *Strychnos nux-vomica* L., pertaining to Strychnos. It is mainly produced in India, Vietnam and Myanmar. It is also produced in Yunnan, Guangdong, Hainan and other places in China. It is collected in winter when the fruits are ripe. It is dried in the sun and processed to use as medicine. According to *Chinese Pharmacopoeia*, the content of strychnine ($C_{21}H_{22}N_2O_2$) should be 1.20%-2.20% and brucine ($C_{23}H_{26}N_2O_4$) should be no less than 0.80%.

【性味归经 / Medicinal properties】

苦，温；大毒。归肝、脾经。

Bitter and warm;extremely toxic; act on the liver and spleen meridians.

【主要功效 / Medicinal efficacies】

通络止痛，散结消肿。

Unblock collaterals, relieve pain, disperse the nodes and eliminate swelling.

【临床应用 / Clinical application】

1. 跌打损伤，骨折肿痛　本品苦泄温通，功善活血通络，止痛之力颇强，为伤科疗伤止痛之要药。用治跌打损伤，骨折肿痛，可单用，或与土鳖虫、乳香、没药等同用。

(1) Bruise, swelling and pain caused by fracture, falling and injury　With the nature of bitter and warm, *mǎ qián zǐ* has the functions of relieving, warming and unblocking. It is good at invigorating blood circulation and unblocking collaterals and has a strong pain relieving effect. It is an essential medicine for the department of traumatology. It can be used alone to treat injuries swelling and pain caused by falls and fractures, or combined with *tǔ biē chóng*, *rǔ xiāng* and *mò yào*.

2. 风湿顽痹，麻木瘫痪　本品善祛筋骨间之风湿，开通经络，透达关节，并长于止痛，为治风湿顽痹，拘挛疼痛，麻木瘫痪的常用药，单用有效，或配伍麻黄、乳香、全蝎等。

(2) Arthralgia caused by wind-dampness and numbness and paralysis　*Mǎ qián zǐ* is good at removing rheumatism between muscles and bones, opening channels and collaterals, penetrating joints, and is good at pain relief. It is a common medicine for treating rheumatism, persistent arthralgia, contracture pain, numbness and paralysis, and is effective when used alone, or can be combined with *má*

huáng (Ephedrae Herba), *rǔ xiāng* and *quán xiē* (Scorpio).

3. **痈疽疮毒，咽喉肿痛** 本品有大毒，能散结消肿，攻毒止痛。用治痈疽疮毒，多作外用，单用即可。治喉痹肿痛，可与山豆根等分为末吹喉。

(3) Carbuncle, trauma, gangrene and sore throat *Mǎ qián zǐ* is extremely toxic, which can dispel the swelling, attack poison and relieve pain. It can be used for treating carbuncle, gangrene and sores and are often for external use alone. To treat larynx arthralgia and swelling pain, it can be combined with *shān dòu gēn* (Sophorae Tonkinensis Radix et Rhizoma), ground into powder to blow the throat.

【用法用量 / Usage and dosage】

炮制后入丸、散，日服 0.3~0.6g。

After processing, make into pills or powder, 0.3-0.6g per day.

【使用注意 / Precaution】

孕妇忌用。不宜多服、久服及生用。运动员慎用。外用不宜大面积涂敷。

Pregnant women should not take it. It is not suitable to take more for a long time and not suitable for using the raw form. Athletes should use it with caution. Large area coating is not suitable for external use.

【现代研究 / Modern research】

本品主要含士的宁、番木鳖次碱、伪番木鳖碱、马钱子碱、伪马钱子碱、奴伐新碱等生物碱，尚含脂肪油、蛋白质、绿原酸等。具有兴奋神经中枢、镇痛、镇咳、祛痰、抑菌、抗炎、抗血栓形成等作用，并能促进消化、增强食欲。

It mainly contains alkaloids such as strychnine, strychnine, pseudostrychnine, brucine, pseudobrucine and novartine, etc. It also contains fat oil, protein and chlorogenic acid, etc. It has the functions of stimulating nerve center, analgesia, antitussive, expectorant, bacteriostatic, anti-inflammation and antithrombotic. It also can promote digestion and appetite.

血竭 *Xuè jié* (Draconis Sanguis)
《雷公炮炙论》
Master Lei's Discourse on Medicinal Processing (Léi Gōng Páo Zhì Lùn)

【来源 / Origin】

为棕榈科植物麒麟竭 *Daemonorops draco* Bl. 果实渗出的树脂经加工制成。主产于印度尼西亚、马来西亚、印度等地，我国广东、台湾等地也有种植。秋季采收，打成碎粒或研成细末用。本品气微，味淡。《中国药典》规定，含血竭素（$C_{17}H_{14}O_3$）不得少于 1.0%。

Xuè jié is the resin exuded from the fruit and trunk of the palm plant *Daemonorops draco* Bl. It is mainly produced in Indonesia, Malaysia, India and other places. It is also planted in Guangdong, Taiwan and other places in China and often collected in autumn. To break into small pieces or grind into small pieces while using. It is mild in flavor and bland in taste. According to *Chinese Pharmacopoeia*, the content of draconis ($C_{17}H_{14}O_3$) should be no less than 1.0%.

【性味归经 / Medicinal properties】

甘、咸，平。归心、肝经。

Sweet, salty and neutral; act on the heart and liver meridian.

【主要功效 / Medicinal efficacies】

活血定痛，化瘀止血，敛疮生肌。

Promote blood circulation and relieve pain, remove blood stasis and hemostasis, astringe sores and promote granulation.

【临床应用 / Clinical application】

1. 跌打损伤，心腹瘀痛 本品入血分而散瘀止痛，为骨伤科及治疗其他瘀滞痛证之要药。用治跌打损伤，筋骨疼痛，常配伍乳香、没药、儿茶等。用治心腹瘀痛及血瘀痛经、经闭、产后腹痛等，可与当归、莪术、三棱等同用。

(1) Injuries from falls, fractures, bruise and pain of heart and abdomen *Xuè jié* can act into blood aspect and remove blood stasis to relieve pain, so it is the essential medicine for orthopedics and other syndrome of stasis pain. It can be used to treat injuries caused by falls, pains of muscles and bones and often combined with *rǔ xiāng*, *mò yào* and *ér chá*; to treat heart and abdomen stasis pain and blood stasis dysmenorrhea, amenorrhea and postpartum abdominal pain, it is often combined with *dāng guī*, *é zhú* and *sān léng* (Sparganii Rhizoma).

2. 外伤出血，疮疡不敛 本品有散瘀止血、生肌敛疮之功。适用于瘀血内阻，血不归经之出血，尤宜于外伤出血，既可单用研末外敷患处，亦可配伍儿茶、乳香、没药等。用治疮疡久溃不敛，可单用研末外敷，或配伍乳香、没药等。

(2) Bleeding due to trauma, unastringent sores *Xuè jié* has the function of dispersing blood stasis and hemostasis, generating muscle and astringent sores. It is suitable for treating the bleeding caused by blood stasis and internal obstruction, bleeding due to no blood returning to meridians, especially for the bleeding of trauma. It can be applied to the affected area alone by using the ground powder or combined with *ér chá*, *rǔ xiāng* and *mò yào*; to treat unastringent sores, it can be applied externally alone by using the ground powder or combined with *rǔ xiāng* and *mò yào*.

【用法用量 / Usage and dosage】

多入丸、散，或研末服，每次 1~2g。外用适量，研末外敷。

Mostly making into pills, powder or grinding form, 1-2g per administration. Appropriate amount for external application; applied externally by using the powder.

【使用注意 / Precaution】

孕妇及月经期妇女忌用。

Not for women in pregnant and menstruation.

【现代研究 / Modern research】

本品主要含血竭素、血竭红素、去甲基血竭素、去甲基血竭红素及黄烷醇、查耳酮、树脂酸等。具有抑制血小板聚集、防止血栓形成、抑菌、抗炎等作用。

It mainly contains dracorhodin, dracorubin, demethylation dracorhodin, demethylation dracorubin, and flavanol, chalcone and resin acid, etc. It has the functions of inhibiting platelet aggregation, preventing thrombosis, bacteriostasis and anti inflammation, etc.

第四节 破血消癥药

Section 4　Blood-stasis breaking and mass-resolving medicinals

PPT

本类药物药性峻猛，能破血逐瘀、消癥散积，主治瘀血时间长、程度重的癥瘕积聚，亦可用于血瘀经闭、瘀肿疼痛等。

This kind of medicine is fierce and can break blood stasis and eliminate abdominal mass. It is mainly used in severe cases caused by blood stasis, especially in treatment of concretion and abdominal masses. Besides, it can also be used to treat menstruation block due to blood-stasis, pain due to blood stasis.

莪术　*É zhú* (Curcumae Rhizoma)
《药性论》
Treatise on Medicinal Properties (Yào Xìng Lùn)

【来源 / Origin】

为姜科植物蓬莪术 *Curcuma phaeocaulis* Val.、广西莪术 *Curcuma kwangsiensis* S.G.Lee et C.F.Liang 或温郁金 *Curcuma wenyujin* Y.H.Chen et C.Ling 的干燥根茎。后者习称"温莪术"。依次主产于四川、广西、浙江。冬季茎叶枯萎后采挖，晒干，切厚片，生用或醋制用。本品气微香，味微苦而辛。《中国药典》规定，含挥发油不得少于 1.5%（ml/g）；饮片不得少于 1.0%（ml/g）。

É zhú is the dry rhizome of *Curcuma phaeocaulis* Val., *Curcuma kwangsiensis* S.G.Lee et C.F.Liang or *Curcuma wenyujin* Y.H.Chen et C.Ling, pertaining to Zingiberaceae, mainly produced in Sichuan, Guangxi Zhang Autonomous Region and Zhejiang respectively, and the latter one are known as *wēn é zhú*. After the stems and leaves wither in winter, they should be collected, dried, cut into thick slices, and used raw or with vinegar. It is slightly fragrant, bitter and pungent in taste. According to *Chinese Pharmacopoeia*, the content of volatile oil should be no less than 1.5%, ready-made pills should not be less than 1.0% (ml/g).

【性味归经 / Medicinal properties】

辛、苦，温。归肝、脾经。

Acrid, bitter and warm; act on the liver and spleen meridians.

【主要功效 / Medicinal efficacies】

破血行气，消积止痛。

Break blood and promote qi, eliminate abdominal mass and relieve pain.

【临床应用 / Clinical application】

1. 癥瘕积聚，瘀血经闭，心腹瘀痛　本品辛散苦泄温通，既能破血逐瘀，又能行气止痛，尤长于消癥瘕积聚。用治血瘀气滞，癥瘕积聚，常与三棱相须为用。用治血瘀痛经、经闭，常与三棱、当归、香附等同用。用治胸痹心痛，多与丹参、川芎等同用。此外，本品能破血祛瘀，消肿止痛，也可用治跌打伤痛，常与苏木、骨碎补等同用。

(1) Menstrual block and abdominal pain, concretion and abdominal mass　With the nature of arid, bitter and warm, *é zhú* can not only break and remove blood stasis, but also relieve pain and activate qi, it is especially good at treating abdominal mass accumulation. To treat abdominal mass caused by blood stasis and qi stagnation, it is often combined with *sān léng* (Sparganii Rhizoma); to treat blood stasis, dysmenorrhea and amenorrhea, often combined with *sān léng* (Sparganii Rhizoma), *dāng guī* and *xiāng fù*; to treat abdominal pain, often combined with *dān shēn* and *chuān xiōng*. In addition, it also can break and remove stasis, reduce swelling and relieve pain. It can be used to treat the injury caused by falling and beating and often combined with *sū mù* (Sappan Lignum) and *gǔ suì bǔ* (Drynariae Rhizoma).

2. 食积气滞，脘腹胀痛　本品能行气止痛，消食化积。用治食积气滞，脘腹胀痛，可与青皮、槟榔等同用。若治脾虚食积之脘腹胀痛，应配伍党参、茯苓、白术等。

(3) Food accumulation and qi stagnation, abdominal distention and pain　*É zhú* can move qi, relieve pain and eliminate food accumulation. It can be used to treat food accumulation, qi stagnation, abdominal distention and pain, and often combined with *qīng pí* (Citri Reticulatae Viride Pericarpium) and *bīng láng* (Arecae Semen); to treat abdominal distention and pain due to deficiency of spleen qi, it is often combined with *dǎng shēn* (Codonopsis Radix), *fú líng* (Poria) and *bái zhú* (Atractylodis Macrocephalae Rhizoma).

【用法用量 / Usage and dosage】

煎服，6~9g。醋制后可增强祛瘀止痛作用。

Decoction, 6-9g. Being prepared with vinegar can enhance the effect of removing blood stasis and relieving pain.

【使用注意 / Precaution】

孕妇及月经过多者忌用。

Women in pregnant and with excessive menstruation should not take it.

【现代研究 / Modern research】

本品主要含挥发油类成分，如 α－蒎烯、β－蒎烯、柠檬烯、姜烯、樟脑、1,8－桉叶醇、龙脑、莪术醇、异莪术烯醇、丁香酚、莪术酮、芳姜酮、姜黄酮、去水莪术酮等。具有抗癌、抗胃溃疡、抑制血小板聚集、抗血栓形成、抑菌、抗炎、镇痛、保肝、抗早孕等作用。

It mainly contains components of volatile oil, such as α-pinene, β-pinene, limonene, gingerene, camphor, 1,8-cineole, borneol, curcumol, isocurcumenol, eugenol, zedoary ketone, zingiberene, gingerone, zedoary turmeric ketone, etc. It has the functions of anticancer, anti gastric ulcer, inhibition of platelet aggregation, antithrombotic, bacteriostatic, anti-inflammatory, analgesic, liver protection and anti early pregnancy, etc.

三棱 *Sān léng* (Sparganii Rhizoma)
《本草拾遗》
Supplement to the Materia Medica (Běn Cǎo Shí Yí)

【来源 / Origin】

为黑三棱科植物黑三棱 *Sparganium stoloniferum* Buch. -Ham 的干燥块茎。主产于江苏、河南、山东等地。冬季至次年春季采挖，晒干，切片，生用或醋炙后用。本品气微，味淡，嚼之微有麻辣感。

Sān léng is the dry tuber of *Sparganium stoloniferum* Buch.-Ham, pertaining to Sparganiaceae, and mainly produced in Jiangsu, Henan, Shandong and other places. It is collected from winter to the next spring, dried and sliced and used raw or stir-fried with vinegar. It has a slight odor and tastes bland. Chewing it may bring a tingling sensation in the mouth.

【性味归经 / Medicinal properties】

辛、苦，平。归肝、脾经。

Acrid, bitter and neutral; act on the liver and spleen meridians.

【主要功效 / Medicinal efficacies】

破血行气，消积止痛。

Break up blood stasis and promote qi, eliminate accumulation and relieving pain.

【临床应用 / Clinical application】

本品功效和主治与莪术基本相同，然三棱偏于破血，莪术偏于破气，两者常相须为用。

The efficacy and actions of *sān léng* are basically the same as *é zhú*. The difference is that *sān léng* is efficacious in dissipating and removing blood stasis while *é zhú* is effective in breaking stagnant qi. They are often used together for mutual reinforcement.

【用法用量 / Usage and dosage】

煎服，5~10g。醋制后可增强祛瘀止痛作用。

Decoction, 5-10g. Being stir-fried with vinegar can enhance the effect of removing blood stasis and relieving pain.

【使用注意 / Precaution】

孕妇及月经过多者忌用。不宜与芒硝、玄明粉同用。

Women in pregnant and with profuse menstruation should not take it. It is not advisable to be used together with natrii sulfas and natrii sulfas exsiccatus.

【现代研究 / Modern research】

本品主要含苯乙醇、对苯二酚、十六酸、去茎木香内酯、山柰素以及脂肪酸、甾醇等。具有抗凝、抑制血小板聚集、降低血黏度、镇痛、抗癌、兴奋子宫等作用。

Sān léng mainly contains phenylethanol, hydroquinone, hexadecylic acid, stemless lignonolactone, kaempferol, fatty acid and sterol, etc. It has the functions of anticoagulation, inhibiting platelet aggregation, reducing blood viscosity, analgesia, anticancer, and stimulating uterus, etc.

水蛭　*Shuǐ zhì* (Hirudo)
《神农本草经》
Shen Nong's Classic of the Materia Medica (Shén Nóng Běn Cǎo Jīng)

【来源 / Origin】

为水蛭科动物蚂蟥 *Whitmania pigra* Whitman、水蛭 *Hirudo nipponica* Whitman 及柳叶蚂蟥 *W. acranulata* Whitman 的干燥体。全国大部分地区均有出产，夏、秋二季捕捉，晒干或低温干燥，生用，或用滑石粉烫后用。本品气微腥。《中国药典》规定，本品每1g含抗凝血酶活性水蛭应不低于 16.0U，蚂蟥、柳叶蚂蟥应不低于 3.0U。

Shuǐ zhì is the dry body of *Whitmania pigra* Whitman, *Hirudo nipponica* Whitman and *W. acranulata* Whitman, pertaining to Hirudinidae. It can be found in most regions of China. It can be caught in summer and autumn, dried in the sun or at low temperature, used raw or after scalding with talcum powder. It is slightly fishy. According to *Chinese Pharmacopoeia*, one gram of it should contain at least 16.0U of antithrombin activity leech, and the latter two should contain at least 3.0U.

【性味归经 / Medicinal properties】

咸、苦，平；有小毒。归肝经。

Salty, bitter, neutral and mildly toxic; act on the liver meridian.

【主要功效 / Medicinal efficacies】

破血通经，逐瘀消癥。

Break up blood stasis and promote menstruation; expel stasis and resolve masses.

【临床应用 / Clinical application】

1. 癥瘕积聚，血瘀经闭，跌打损伤　本品咸苦入血，破血逐瘀力强，有消癥、通经、疗伤之功。用治血滞经闭，癥瘕积聚，常与三棱、莪术、红花等同用；若兼体虚，应配伍人参、当归等。用治跌打损伤，筋伤骨折，瘀滞肿痛，多与乳香、没药等同用。

(1) Menstrual block caused by stagnation of blood, concretions and abdominal masses, and traumatic injuries　*Shuǐ zhì* has the functions of eliminating masses, promoting menstruation and curing wounds. To treat menorrhea due to blood stagnation and abdominal mass, it is often combined with *sān léng, é zhú* and *hóng huā*; for the patient with body deficiency, it should be combined with *rén shēn* (Ginseng Radix et Rhizoma) and *dāng guī*; to treat bruise, fracture, stasis, swelling and pain, it should be combined with *rǔ xiāng* and *mò yào*.

2. **中风偏瘫** 本品破血逐瘀，通经活络。用治气虚血瘀络阻型中风病，症见半身不遂或偏身麻木，口舌㖞斜，言语不利，可与人参、全蝎、蜈蚣等同用。

(2) Apoplectic and hemiplegia It can be used to treat apoplexy due to qi deficiency, blood stasis and collaterals obstruction. For symptoms as hemiplegia or partial numbness, askew mouth and tongue and slurred speech, it should combined with *rén shēn*, *quán xiē* (Scorpio) and *wú gōng* (Scolopendra).

【用法用量 / Usage and dosage】
煎服，1~3g。研末服，0.3~0.5g。以入丸、散或研末服为宜。
Decoction, 1-3g. 0.3-0.5g for grinding into powder. Suitable to make into pills or ground into powder.

【使用注意 / Precaution】
孕妇及月经过多者忌用。
Women in pregnant and with profuse menstruation should not take it.

【现代研究 / Modern research】
本品主要含蛋白质，唾液中含有水蛭素，尚含肝素、抗血栓素及组胺样物质。具有较强的抗凝血作用和改善血液流变学、抑制血小板聚集、抗血栓形成、促进脑血肿吸收、缓解颅内压升高、降血脂、抗动脉粥样硬化、终止妊娠等作用。

It mainly contains protein, hirudin in its saliva, and heparin, antithrombin and histamine. It has a strong anticoagulant effect and can improve hemorheology, inhibit platelet aggregation, antithrombotic, promote the absorption of hematoma, relieve the increase of intracranial pressure, reduce blood lipid, resist atherosclerosis, and terminate pregnancy.

其他活血化瘀药功用介绍见表 17-1。
The efficacies of other blood-invigorating and stasis-dissolving medicinals are shown in table 17-1.

表 17-1 其他活血化瘀药功用介绍

分类	药物	药性	功效	应用	用法用量
活血止痛药	五灵脂	苦、咸、甘，温。归肝经	活血止痛，化瘀止血	瘀血阻滞诸痛，瘀滞出血证	煎服，3~10g，包煎
活血调经药	鸡血藤	苦、甘，温。归肝、肾经	活血补血，调经止痛，舒筋活络	月经不调，痛经，闭经；风湿痹痛，肢体麻木，血虚萎黄	煎服，9~15g
	西红花	甘、微寒。归心、肝经	活血化瘀，凉血解毒，解郁安神	经闭癥瘕，产后瘀阻，温毒发斑，忧郁痞闷，惊悸发狂	1~3g，煎服或沸水泡服
	川牛膝	甘、微苦，平。归肝、肾经	逐瘀通经，通利关节，利尿通淋	经闭癥瘕，胞衣不下，跌仆损伤，风湿痹痛，足痿筋挛，尿血血淋	煎服，5~10g
	泽兰	苦、辛，微温。归肝、脾经	活血调经，祛瘀消痈，利水消肿	血瘀月经不调，经闭痛经，产后瘀阻腹痛，跌打伤痛，疮痈肿毒，水肿，腹水	煎服，6~12g

续表

分类	药物	药性	功效	应用	用法用量
活血调经药	王不留行	苦、平。归肝、胃经	活血通经，下乳消肿，利尿通淋	血瘀经闭，痛经，难产，产后乳汁不下，乳痈肿痛，淋证涩痛	煎服，5~10g
	月季花	甘，温。归肝经	活血调经，疏肝解郁	气滞血瘀，月经不调，痛经，闭经，胸胁胀痛	煎服，3~6g
活血疗伤药	苏木	甘、咸，平。归心、肝、脾经	活血祛瘀，消肿止痛	跌打损伤，筋伤骨折，瘀滞肿痛；血滞经闭，产后瘀阻，胸腹刺痛，痈肿疮毒	煎服，3~10g。外用适量
	自然铜	辛，平。归肝经	散瘀止痛，续筋接骨	跌打损伤，骨折筋伤，瘀肿疼痛	多入丸、散，每次0.3g。煎服，3~9g，宜先煎。外用适量
	刘寄奴	苦，温。归心、肝、脾经	散瘀止痛，疗伤止血，破血通经，消食化积	跌打肿痛，血瘀经闭腹痛，食积腹痛，赤白痢疾	煎服，3~10g
破血消癥药	穿山甲	咸，微寒。归肝、胃经	活血消癥，通经下乳，消肿排脓，搜风通络	血滞经闭，癥瘕，乳汁不通，疮痈肿痛，风湿痹痛	煎服，5~10g

（周 鹏 高峰）

题库

第十八章 化痰止咳平喘药
Chapter 18　Phlegm-dissolving, cough and panting-relieving medicinals

 学习目标 | Learning goals

　　1. 掌握　化痰止咳平喘药在性能、功效、主治、配伍及使用注意方面的共性；半夏、天南星、旋覆花、川贝母、浙贝母、瓜蒌、桔梗、苦杏仁、紫苏子、百部、桑白皮、葶苈子的性能、功效、应用以及特殊的用法用量和特殊的使用注意。

　　2. 熟悉　化痰止咳平喘药的分类；芥子、前胡、竹茹、紫菀、款冬花、白果的功效、主治以及特殊的用法用量和特殊的使用注意。

　　3. 了解　化痰止咳平喘药、温化寒痰药、清化热痰药和止咳平喘药及相关功效术语的含义；竹沥、皂荚、天竺黄、胖大海、海藻、昆布、黄药子、海蛤壳、海浮石、瓦楞子、礞石、白前、枇杷叶、洋金花的功效以及特殊的用法用量和特殊的使用注意。

　　1. Master the commonness of phlegm-dissolving, cough and panting-relieving medicinals in efficacy, indications, property, compatibility and cautions; as well as the property, efficacy, application, special usage and dosage and special precautions of *bàn xià, tiān nán xīng, xuán fù huā, chuān bèi mǔ, zhè bèi mǔ, guā lóu, jié gěng, kǔ xìng rén, zǐ sū zǐ, bǎi bù, sāng bái pí*, and *tíng lì zǐ*.

　　2. Familiar with the classification of phlegm-dissolving, cough and panting-relieving medicinals as well as the efficacy, indications, special usage, dosage and special precautions of *jiè zǐ, qián hú, zhú rú, zǐ wǎn, kuǎn dōng huā* and *bái guǒ*.

　　3. Understand the definition of phlegm-dissolving, cough and panting-relieving medicinals, cold-phlegm warming and dissolving medicinals, hot-phlegm clearing and dissolving medicinals, cough and panting relieving medicinals, and other terms referring to related efficacies; and the efficacy, special usage and dosage and special precautions of, *zhú lì, zào jiá, tiān zhú huáng, pàng dà hǎi, hǎi zǎo, kūn bù, huáng yào zǐ, hǎi gé qiào, hǎi fú shí, wǎ léng zǐ, méng shí, bái qián, pí pa yè* and *yáng jīn huā*.

微课

　　凡以祛痰或消痰为主要功效，常用于治疗痰证的药物，称为化痰药；以制止或减轻咳嗽和喘息为主要功效，常用于治疗咳嗽、喘证的药物，称为止咳平喘药。因在病证上，痰、咳、喘每多相互兼杂，且化痰药多兼止咳平喘作用，止咳平喘药又常兼化痰作用，故将化痰药与止咳平喘药合并一章介绍。

　　With dispelling or dispersing phlegm as major efficacies, the drugs which are often used to treat

医药大学堂
WWW.YIYAODXT.COM

phlegm syndromes are called phlegm-dissolving medicinals; and with relieving or alleviating cough and panting as primary efficacies, the drugs that are frequently used to treat cough and panting syndromes are called cough and panting relieving medicinals. Since phlegm, cough and panting are often interrelated with each other for certain diseases, and while phlegm-dissolving medicinals often have concurrent functions of relieving cough and panting, cough and panting relieving medicinals also frequently play concurrent role of dissolving phlegm, phlegm-dissolving medicinals and cough and panting relieving medicinals will be introduced together in this chapter.

根据化痰止咳平喘药的药性及功效主治差异，可分为温化寒痰药、清化热痰药和止咳平喘药三类。

According to the differences in the properties, efficacies and indications of phlegm-dissolving, cough and panting-relieving medicinals, they can be further divided into three categories, namely, cold-phlegm warming and dissolving medicinals, hot-phlegm clearing and dissolving medicinals and cough and panting-relieving medicinals.

化痰药味多苦、辛，药性或温或寒（凉），主入肺、脾经，功能祛痰、消痰，主治各种痰证。具体来说，痰证又分为寒痰、湿痰、热痰、燥痰证。痰既是病理产物，又是致病因素，它"随气升降，无处不到"，致病范围广泛，因此痰的病证甚多，如痰阻于肺之咳喘痰多；痰蒙心窍之昏厥、癫痫；痰蒙清阳之眩晕；痰扰心神之失眠多梦；肝风夹痰之中风、惊厥；痰阻经络之肢体麻木、半身不遂、口眼㖞斜；痰火互结之瘰疬、瘿瘤；痰凝肌肉，流注骨节之阴疽流注等。止咳平喘药味或苦或辛或甘，药性或温或寒，主归肺经，以止咳平喘为主要功效，主治各种原因所致的咳嗽和喘证。

Often bitter and acrid in taste and warm or cold (cool) in property, phlegm-dissolving medicinals, mainly entering lung and spleen channels, have the functions of dispelling and dissolving phlegm, and thus can be used to treat various phlegm syndromes, which, to be specific, can be further divided into the syndromes of cold phlegm, damp phlegm, heat phlegm and dryness phlegm. A pathological product and a pathogenic factor at the same time, phlegm "ascends and descends with qi, going to anywhere it wants to". It can cause diseases of a wide range, and thus there are many symptoms of phlegm, for example cough and panting with profuse phlegm due to phlegm obstructing the lung, fainting or epilepsy due to phlegm confounding the heart orifices, dizziness due to phlegm clouding clear yang, insomnia with profuse dreaming due to phlegm harassing the heart spirit, wind stroke and convulsion due to liver wind with phlegm, limb numbness, hemiplegia and obliquity of mouth and eyes due to phlegm obstructing channels and collaterals, scrofula, goiter and tumor due to binding of phlegm and fire, multiple yin abscesses due to phlegm coagulating muscles and joint abscess, etc. With relieving cough and panting as the major efficacy, cough and panting relieving medicinals, bitter, acrid or sweet in taste and warm or cold in property, mainly enter the lung channel, and are primarily used to treat cough and panting of various reasons.

应用本类药物时，应根据不同的病证，有针对性地选择不同的化痰药及止咳平喘药，还要根据病因病机和具体病情的不同予以配伍。如外感而致者，应配伍解表药；火热而致者，应配伍清热泻火药；里寒者，应配伍温里药；虚劳者，应配伍补虚药。若治癫痫、惊厥、眩晕、昏迷，当配伍平肝息风、开窍、安神药；若治痰核、瘰疬、瘿瘤，当配伍软坚散结药；若治阴疽流注，当配伍温阳通滞散结药。脾为生痰之源，故在应用化痰药时，常配伍健脾药，以治其生痰之源。因咳喘每多夹痰，痰多易发咳喘，故化痰药与止咳平喘药常配伍使用。又因痰易阻滞气机，"气滞则痰凝""气顺则痰消"，故化痰药常配伍行气药。

According to different syndromes, medicinals in this chapter, namely, phlegm-dissolving medicinals and cough and panting-relieving medicinals, should be targeted and meantime compatible with other drugs based on the differences in etiology, pathogenesis and specific conditions. For those caused by external contraction, they should be compatible with exterior-releasing medicinals; for those led by fire heat, heat-clearing and fire-draining medicinals should be added; for those with cold interior, interior-warming medicinals should be used together; and for those with deficiency consumption, deficiency-supplementing medicinals should be combined. To treat those with epilepsy, convulsion, dizziness and fainting, they should be used together with liver-calming and wind-extinguishing, orifice-opening or mind-calming medicinals; to treat those with phlegm nodule, scrofula, goiter and tumor, they can be combined with spleen-fortifying medicinals; to treat those with multiple yin abscesses, they can go together with yang-warming, stagnation-flowing and mass-dissipating medicinals. The spleen is the source of phlegm generation, and thus phlegm-dissolving medicinals are often compatible with spleen-fortifying medicinals in application, so that the source of phlegm can be eliminated. Since cough often goes together with phlegm and the latter is prone to lead to cough and panting, phlegm-dissolving medicinals and cough and panting-relieving medicinals are often used together. Moreover, since it is easy for the phlegm to obstruct qi movement, "qi stagnation may cause phlegm coagulation" and "qi flow may lead to phlegm elimination", phlegm-dissolving medicinals are often combined with qi-moving medicinals.

温燥之性较强的化痰药，不宜用于痰中带血或咳嗽咯血者，以免加重出血。麻疹初起兼有表邪之咳嗽，忌用收敛性强及性质温燥的化痰止咳平喘药。部分药物有毒，内服应注意用法，控制用量。

Phlegm-dissolving medicinals, with stronger warm dryness, are not suitable for those with blood in phlegm or hemoptysis, so as not to aggravate the bleeding. For those with measles at the early stages as well as concurrent cough due to exterior pathogen, it should be forbidden to use the phlegm-dissolving, cough and panting-relieving medicinals that are endowed with strong astringing power and warm dryness. Parts of the medicinals are toxic. Thus, for interior use, the usage should be paid attention to and the dosage should be controlled.

第一节　温化寒痰药

Section 1　Cold-phlegm warming and dissolving medicinals

PPT

本类药物味多辛苦，性偏温燥，主归肺、脾经。具有温肺祛寒、燥湿化痰之功，主治寒痰、湿痰证见咳嗽气喘、痰多色白清稀、苔腻等，以及寒痰、湿痰所致的眩晕、肢体麻木、阴疽流注等。

Mostly acrid and bitter in taste and warm and dry in property, medicinals in this chapter, mainly entering lung and spleen channels, have the actions of warming the lung and dispelling cold as well as drying dampness and dissolving phlegm. They are mainly used to treat cold-phlegm and damp-phlegm syndromes such as cough and panting, profuse watery and clear white phlegm, greasy furred tongue, etc. They also can be applied to dizziness, limb numbness and multiple yin abscesses caused by cold phlegm and damp phlegm.

半夏 *Bàn xià* (Pinelliae Rhizoma)
《神农本草经》
Shen Nong's Classic of the Materia Medica (Shén Nóng Běn Cǎo Jīng)

【来源 / Origin】

为天南星科植物半夏 *Pinellia ternata*（Thunb.）Breit. 的干燥块茎。主产于四川、湖北、河南等地。夏、秋二季采挖，晒干为生半夏；或用白矾制成清半夏；用生姜、白矾制成姜半夏；用生石灰、甘草制成法半夏。本品气微，味辛辣、麻舌而刺喉。《中国药典》规定，含白矾以含水硫酸铝钾〔KAl（SO$_4$）$_2$·12H$_2$O〕计，姜半夏不得过 8.5%，清半夏不得过 10.0%。

Bàn xià is the dried tuber of *Pinellia ternate* (Thunb.) Breit., pertaining to the Araceae. It is mainly produced in Sichuan, Hubei, Henan and some other places. Collected in summer and autumn, it can be dried to make *shēng bàn xià* (Pinelliae Rhizoma), processed with *bái fán* (Alumen) to make *qīng bàn xià* (Pinelliae Concisum Rhizoma), with *shēng jiāng* (Zingiberis Recens Rhizoma) and *bái fán* to make *jiāng bàn xià* (Pinelliae Rhizoma Praeparatum), and with *shēng shí huī* (Calx) and *gān cǎo* (Glycyrrhizae Radix et Rhizoma) to make *fǎ bàn xià* (Pinelliae Praeparatum Rhizoma). Light in smell, acrid and bitter in taste, *bàn xià* is tongue-tingling and throat-piercing. According to *Chinese Pharmacopoeia*, as for the content of alumbre, that of potassium aluminium sulfate〔KAl (SO$_4$)$_2$·12H$_2$O〕should be no more than 8.5% in *jiāng bàn xià*, and no more than 10% in *qīng bàn xià*.

【性味归经 / Medicinal properties】

辛，温；有毒。归脾、胃、肺经。

Acrid and warm; toxic; act on the spleen, stomach and lung meridians.

【主要功效 / Medicinal efficacies】

燥湿化痰，降逆止呕，消痞散结；外用消肿止痛。

Dry dampness and dissolve phlegm, direct counterflow downward and arrest vomiting, disperse *pǐ* and dissipate masses. For exterior use, diminish swelling and relieve pain.

【临床应用 / Clinical application】

1. 湿痰、寒痰证　本品辛温而燥，长于燥湿化痰，温化寒痰，兼能止咳，尤善治脏腑湿痰。用治痰湿壅肺之咳嗽痰多，色白易咳者，常与陈皮、茯苓等同用。用治寒饮咳喘，痰多清稀者，常配伍细辛、干姜、五味子等。用治风痰上扰之眩晕头痛，常与天麻、白术等同用。若配伍瓜蒌、黄芩等清热化痰药，也可用治热痰咳嗽。

(1) Damp-phlegm, cold-phlegm syndromes　Acrid, warm but dry, *bàn xià* is good at drying dampness and dissolving phlegm, warming and dissolving cold-phlegm, and relieving cough as well, especially good at treating damp phlegm accumulated in viscera and bowels. To treat cough with profuse phlegm and white phlegm with easy expectorations due to phlegm-damp obstructing the lung, it is often used together with *chén pí* (Citri Reticulatae Pericarpium), *fú líng* (Poria), etc. To treat those with cough and panting due to cold rheum as well as profuse clear and thin phlegm, it is often compatible with *xì xīn* (Asari Radix et Rhizoma), *gān jiāng* (Zingiberis Rhizoma), *wǔ wèi zǐ* (Schisandrae Chinensis Fructus), etc. To treat dizziness and headache caused by wind-phlegm harassing the upper body, it is often combined with *tiān má* (Gastrodiae Rhizoma), *bái zhú* (Atractylodis Macrocephalae Rhizoma), etc.

Together with heat-clearing and phlegm-dispelling medicinals such as *guā lóu* and *huáng qín* (Scutellariae Radix), it also can be used to treat heat-phlegm cough.

2. 呕吐　本品入胃经，既能燥湿化痰，又长于和胃降逆，为止呕要药。各种原因所致的呕吐，皆可随证配伍应用。对痰饮或胃寒呕吐者尤为适宜，常与生姜同用。若治胃热呕吐，可与黄连、竹茹等同用。若治胃阴虚呕吐，可与石斛、麦冬等同用。若治胃气虚呕吐，可配伍人参、白蜜等。若治妊娠呕吐，证属脾胃虚寒，痰湿内阻者，常与人参、干姜等同用。

(2) Vomitting　Entering the stomach channel, *bàn xià* is not only good at drying dampness and dispelling phlegm, but also at harmonizing the stomach and directing counterflow downward, and thus is an important drug to arrest vomiting, which can be combined with other drugs in accordance with specific symptoms to treat vomiting of various reasons. It is especially suitable for those with phlegm rheum or stomach cold vomiting, where *shēng jiāng* is often added. To treat stomach-heat vomiting, it can be used together with *huáng lián* (Coptidis Rhizoma), *zhú rú*, etc. To treat vomiting due to stomach yin deficiency, it can go with *shí hú* (Dendrobii Caulis), *mài dōng* (Ophiopogonis Radix), etc. To treat vomiting due to stomach qi deficiency, it can be combined with *rén shēn*, *bái mì* (Apis cerana Fabr), etc. To treat vomiting during pregnancy, whose symptoms are in accordance with deficiency-cold of the spleen and stomach as well as phlegm-damp internal obstruction, it can be used together with *rén shēn*, *gān jiāng*, etc.

3. 心下痞，结胸，梅核气　本品辛开散结，化痰消痞。用治痰热阻滞，心下痞满，常配伍干姜、黄连、黄芩等。用治痰热结胸，胸脘痞闷，按之则痛，常与瓜蒌、黄连等同用。用治气郁痰凝之梅核气，常与苏叶、厚朴、茯苓等同用。

(3) Epigastric stuffiness , chest bind syndrome, and plum-stone qi　*Bàn xià* can use acridity to open and dissipate masses, and dispel phlegm and disperse *pǐ* as well. To treat those with phlegm-heat obstruction and retentive epigastric stuffiness, it is often compatible with *gān jiāng*, *huáng lián*, *huáng qín*, etc. To treat phlegm-heat binding chest as well as stuffiness and oppression of chest cavity, which aches when pressed, it is often combined with *guā lóu*, *huáng lián*, etc. To treat plum-stone qi due to qi constraint and phlegm coagulation, it is often used together with *sū yè* (Perillae Folium), *hòu pò* (Magnoliae Officinalis Cortex), *fú líng*, etc.

4. 瘿瘤，痰核，痈疽肿毒及毒蛇咬伤　本品内服能消痰散结，外用能消肿止痛。用治瘿瘤痰核，常配伍昆布、海藻、贝母等。用治痈疽发背或乳疮初起，可单用本品研末，鸡子白调涂。用治毒蛇咬伤，可生品研末调敷或鲜品捣敷。

(4) Goiter and tumor, phlegm nodule, carbuncle-abscess, pyogenic infections, and poisonous snake bites　*Bàn xià* can disperse phlegm and dissipate masses while used interiorly, and diminish swelling and relieve pain while used exteriorly. To treat goiter, tumor and phlegm nodule, it is often compatible with *kūn bù*, *hǎi zǎo*, *bèi mǔ* (Fritillaria Bulbus), etc. To treat carbuncle-abscess invading the back or early stage of breast sores, *bàn xià*, used alone, can be powdered, mixed with *jī zǐ bái* (Gallus gallus domesticus Brisson) and applied to the affected area.

【 用法用量 / Usage and dosage 】

煎服，3~9g，内服宜炮制用。外用适量。

Decoction, 3~9g, preferable to be processed for interior use. Used externally with appropriate dosage.

【 使用注意 / Precaution 】

不宜与川乌、制川乌、草乌、制草乌、附子同用。阴虚燥咳、血证、热痰、燥痰应慎用。生品内服宜慎。

It is not suitable to combine *bàn xià* with *chuān wū* (Aconiti Radix), *zhì chuān wū* (Aconiti Radix Praeparata), *căo wū* (Aconiti Kusnezoffii Radix), *zhì căo wū* (Aconiti Kusnezoffii Radix Praeparata), and *fù zĭ* (Aconiti Lateralis Radix Praeparata). It should be used with caution for patients with dryness cough due to yin deficiency, bleeding, hot phlegm or dryness phlegm. Be cautious to take raw products for internal use.

【现代研究 / Modern research】

本品主要含挥发油、半夏蛋白、半夏淀粉、β-谷甾醇、葡萄糖苷、氨基酸、皂苷、生物碱、胆碱等。具有镇咳、祛痰、平喘、镇吐、抑制胃液分泌、促进胆汁分泌、抗心律失常、镇静、催眠、抗肿瘤、抗胃溃疡、抑菌、抗炎等作用。

It mainly contains volatile oil, pinellia protein, pinellia starch, β-sitosterol, glucosides, amino acids, saponins, alkaloids, choline and so on. It has the functions of relieving cough, dispelling phlegm, relieving asthma, suppressing vomiting, inhibiting gastric juice secretion, promoting bile secretion, resisting arrhythmia, calming the mind, helping to fall asleep, resisting tumor, gastric ulcer, bacteria, inflammation, and so on.

天南星　*Tiān nán xīng* (Arisaematis Rhizoma)
《神农本草经》
Shen Nong's Classic of the Materia Medica (Shén Nóng Běn Căo Jīng)

【来源 / Origin】

为天南星科植物天南星 *Arisaema erubescens*（Wall.）Schott、异叶天南星 *Arisaema heterophyllum* Bl. 或东北天南星 *Arisaema amurense* Maxim. 的干燥块茎。天南星主产于河南、河北、四川；异叶天南星主产于江苏、浙江；东北天南星主产于辽宁、吉林。秋、冬二季茎叶枯萎时采挖，生用，或用生姜、白矾制过用。本品气微辛，味麻辣。《中国药典》规定，含总黄酮以芹菜素（$C_{15}H_{10}O_5$）计不得少于 0.050%。

Tiān nán xīng is the dried tuber of *Arisaema erubescens* (Wall.) Schott, *Arisaema heterophyllum* Bl., or *Arisaema amurense* Maxim., pertaining to the Araceae. *Tiān nán xīng* is mainly produced in Henan, Hebei and Sichuan, while *yì yè tiān nán xīng* is mainly produced in Jiangsu and Zhejiang, *dōng běi tiān nán xīng* can mainly be found in Liaoning and Jilin. Collected in autumn and winter when the stem and leaf wither, it is used in raw form or processed with *shēng jiāng* and *bái fán* for use later. *Tiān nán xīng* is slightly acrid, spicy and hot. According to *Chinese Pharmacopoeia*, the content of general flavone, calculated as apigenin ($C_{15}H_{10}O_5$), should be no less than 0.050%.

【性味归经 / Medicinal properties】

苦、辛，温；有毒。归肺、肝、脾经。

Bitter, acrid and warm; toxic; enters the lung, liver and spleen channels.

【主要功效 / Medicinal efficacies】

燥湿化痰，祛风止痉，散结消肿。

Dry dampness and dissolve phlegm, dispel wind and arrest convulsion, dissipate masses and diminish swelling.

【临床应用 / Clinical application】

1. 湿痰，寒痰，顽痰证　本品苦辛而温燥，既能燥湿化痰，又能止咳，功似半夏而温燥毒烈之性更强，也可用治湿痰、寒痰证，但不如半夏常用。尤善治顽痰阻肺，咳喘胸闷，常与半夏、枳实、橘红等配伍。

(1) Damp-phlegm, cold-phlegm and stubborn-phlegm syndromes Bitter, acrid, warm and drying, *tiān nán xīng* can dry dampness and dissolve phlegm, and relieve cough as well. Having similar actions as *bàn xià* but with a stronger effect of warming dryness and toxicity, it also can be used to treat damp-phlegm and cold-phlegm syndromes, but is not so commonly used as the latter. It is especially good at treating obstinate phlegm obstructing the lung, cough, panting and chest oppression, where it is often compatible with *bàn xià*, *zhǐ shí* (Aurantii Immaturus Fructus), *jú hóng* (Citri Rubrum Exocarpium), etc.

2. 风痰证 本品入肝经，走经络，善祛风痰而止痉，为开涤风痰之专药。用治风痰上扰之眩晕头痛，可配伍半夏、天麻等。用治风痰留滞经络，半身不遂，手足顽麻，口眼㖞斜，常与半夏、川乌、白附子等同用。用治破伤风，角弓反张，痰涎壅盛，可与白附子、天麻、防风等同用。用治癫痫，可与半夏、全蝎、僵蚕等同用。

(2) Wind-phlegm syndrome Entering the liver channel and flowing through the channels and collaterals, *tiān nán xīng* is good at dispelling wind and arresting convulsion, and thus is a special medicinal of dispering and clearing up wind phlegm. To treat dizziness and headache due to wind-phlegm harassing the upper body, it can be compatible with *bàn xià*, *tiān má*, etc. To treat retention of wind-phlegm in channels and collaterals, half-body paralysis, stubborn numbness of limbs, or obliquity of mouth and eyes, it is often used together with *bàn xià*, *chuān wū*, *bái fù zǐ*, etc. To treat tetanus, opisthotonus as well as congestion and exuberance of phlegm-drool, it can be used together with *bái fù zǐ*, *tiān má*, *fáng fēng* (Saposhnikoviae Radix), etc. To treat epilepsy, it can be combined with *bàn xià*, *quán xiē* (Scorpio), *jiāng cán* (Batryticatus Bombyx), etc.

3. 痈疽肿痛，蛇虫咬伤 本品外用能解毒消肿，散结止痛。用治痈疽肿痛、瘰疬痰核，可研末醋调外敷，或配伍半夏、川乌、贝母等。用治毒蛇咬伤，可配伍雄黄外敷。

(3) Swelling and pain of carbuncle-abscess, poisonous snake bites To be used exteriorly, *tiān nán xīng* can resolve toxins, diminish swelling, dissipate masses and relieve pain. To treat swelling and pain of carbuncle-abscess, scrofula and phlegm nodule, it can be powdered and mixed with vinegar to be applied exteriorly, or to be compatible with *bàn xià*, *chuān wū*, *bèi mǔ*, etc. To treat poisonous snake bites, it can be combined with *xióng huáng* (Realgar) and used exteriorly.

【用法用量 / Usage and dosage】

煎服，3~9g，多制用。外用适量，研末以醋或酒调敷患处。

Decoction, 3-9g, mostly processed before use. Used externally with appropriate dosage, powdered and mixed with vinegar or alcohol, and apply to the affected area.

【使用注意 / Precaution】

孕妇慎用。生品内服宜慎。

It should be used with caution for pregnant women. Be cautious to take raw products for internal use.

【现代研究 / Modern research】

本品主要含夏佛托苷、异夏佛托苷、芹菜素 -6- 阿拉伯糖 -8-C- 半乳糖苷、芹菜素 -6- 半乳糖 -8-C- 阿拉伯糖苷、芹菜素 -6,8- 二 -C- 吡喃葡萄糖苷等黄酮类成分，尚含安息香酸、甘露醇、苯甲酸、D- 甘露醇、凝集素、多糖、秋水仙碱、氨基酸等。具有祛痰、抗惊厥、镇静、镇痛、抗心律失常、抗肿瘤等作用。

It mainly contains flavonoids such as schaftoside, isoschaftoside, apigenin-6-arabinose-8-C-galactoside, apigenin-6-galactosid-8-C-arabinosidase, apigenin-6, 8-two-C-glucopyranoside, etc. It also contains benzoic acid, mannitol, D-mannitol, lectin, polysaccharide, colchicine, amino acid, etc. It has the functions of dispelling phlegm, resisting convulsion, calming the mind, relieving pain, resisting arrhythmia and tumor, etc.

白附子　*Bái fù zǐ* (Typhonii Rhizoma)
《中药志》
Records of Chinese Medicinals (Zhōng Yào Zhì)

【来源 / Origin 】

为天南星科植物独角莲 *Typhonium giganteum* Engl. 的干燥块茎。主产于河南、甘肃、湖北。秋季采挖，生用，或用白矾、生姜炮制后用。本品气微，味淡，麻辣刺舌。

Bái fù zǐ is the dried tuber of *Typhonium giganteum* Engl., pertaining to the Araceae. It is mainly produced in Henan, Gansu and Hubei. Collected in autumn, it is used raw, or processed with *bái fán* and *shēng jiāng* for use later. Light in smell and bland in flavor, *bái fù zǐ* is spicy and tongue-tingling.

【性味归经 / Medicinal properties 】

辛，温；有毒。归胃、肝经。

Acrid and warm; toxic; act on the stomach and liver meridians.

【主要功效 / Medicinal efficacies 】

燥湿化痰，祛风止痉，止痛，解毒散结。

Dry dampness and dissolve phlegm, dispel wind and arrest convulsion, relieve pain, resolve toxins and dissipate masses.

【临床应用 / Clinical application 】

1. 风痰证　本品辛温燥烈，既能燥湿化痰，更善祛风痰，定惊搐而解痉止痛，功似天南星，亦为治风痰之常用药。然其性上行，长于祛头面风痰，多用于头面部风痰诸证。用治风痰留滞经络，中风口眼㖞斜，语言謇涩，常与全蝎、僵蚕同用。用治痫证抽搐，可与牛黄、石菖蒲等同用。用治破伤风，常与防风、天麻、天南星等同用。用治痰厥头痛、眩晕，可与半夏、天南星等同用。用治偏正头痛，多配伍川芎、白芷等。

(1) Wind-phlegm syndromes　Acrid, warm and drying, *bái fù zǐ* not only can dry dampness and dissolve phlegm, but is even better at dispelling wind phlegm, calming frightening and convulsion to resolve convulsion and relieve pain. Having similar functions as *tiān nán xīng*, it is a common drug to treat wind phlegm. However, because of its ascending nature, it is good at dispelling wind-phlegm of head and face, and thus is frequently used in a variety of head-face wind-phlegm syndromes. To treat the retention of wind-phlegm in channels and collaterals as well as obliquity of mouth and eyes due to wind stroke and dysphasia, it is often used together with *quán xiē* and *jiāng cán*. To treat eclampsia and convulsion, it can be combined with *niú huáng* (Calculus Bovis), *shí chāng pú* (Acori Tatarinowii Rhizoma), etc. To treat tetanus, it often goes with *fáng fēng*, *tiān má*, *tiān nán xīng*, etc. To treat phlegm syncope, headache and dizziness, it can be used with *bàn xià*, *tiān nán xīng*, etc. To treat hemilateral or over-all headache, it is often compatible with *chuān xiōng* (Chuanxiong Rhizoma), *bái zhǐ* (Angelicae Dahuricae Radix), etc.

2. 瘰疬痰核，痈疽肿毒，毒蛇咬伤　本品有攻毒散结、消肿止痛之功。用治瘰疬痰核，可用鲜品捣烂外敷。用治痈疽肿毒，可配伍天南星外敷。用治毒蛇咬伤，可单用捣汁内服并外敷，或配伍雄黄共研细末，用水或白酒调涂患处。

**(2) Scrofula and phlegm nodule, carbuncle-abscess, pyogenic infections and poisonous snake

bites *Bái fù zǐ* has the actions of attacking toxins, dissipating masses, diminishing swelling and relieving pain. To treat scrofula and phlegm nodule, fresh *bái fù zǐ* can be crushed for exterior application. To treat carbuncle-abscess and pyogenic infections, it can be combined with *tiān nán xīng* to be applied exteriorly. To treat poisonous snake bites, it can be crushed alone to extract juice to be taken interiorly and applied exteriorly as well, or it also can be compatible with *xióng huáng* to be powdered finely and then mixed with water or alcohol to be applied to the affected area.

【用法用量 / Usage and dosage】

煎服，3~6g，一般炮制后用。外用适量，生品捣烂，或研末以酒调敷患处。

Decoction, 3-6g, usually processed before use. Used externally with appropriate dosage, fresh *bái fù zǐ* can be crushed or powdered, and mixed with alcohol for exterior application.

【使用注意 / Precaution】

孕妇慎用。生品内服宜慎。

It should be used with caution for pregnant women. Be cautious to take raw products for internal use.

【现代研究 / Modern research】

本品主要含有油酸、亚油酸、琥珀酸、棕榈酸、β-谷甾醇、氨基酸、胆碱、尿嘧啶、黏液质等。具有祛痰、镇静、催眠、镇痛、抗惊厥、抑菌、抗炎、抗肿瘤、抑制结核分枝杆菌等作用。

It mainly contains oleic acid, linoleic acid, succinic acid, palmitic acid, β-sitoserol, amino acid, choline, uracil, mucilage and so on. It has the functions of expectoration, sedation, hypnosis, analgesia, anti-convulsion, bacteriostasis, anti-inflammation, anti-tumor and anti-tuberculosis bacillus, etc.

芥子 *Jiè zǐ* (Sinapis Semen)
《新修本草》
Newly Revised Materia Medica (Xīn Xīu Běn Cǎo)

【来源 / Origin】

为十字花科植物白芥 *Sinapis alba* L. 或芥 *Brassica juncea*（L.）Czern.et Coss. 的干燥成熟种子。主产于河南、安徽。夏末秋初采收，晒干，生用或炒用。本品气微，味辛辣。《中国药典》规定，含芥子碱以芥子碱硫氰酸盐（$C_{16}H_{24}NO_5 \cdot SCN$）计不得少于 0.50%；炒芥子不得少于 0.40%。

Jiè zǐ is the dried mature seed of *Sinapis alba* L., or *Brassica juncea* (L.) Czern. et Coss., pertaining to the Cruciferae. Mainly produced in Henan and Anhui, it is collected in later summer and early autumn, and dried for raw or stir-fried use. *Jiè zǐ* is light in smell, and acrid and spicy in flavor. According to *Chinese Pharmacopoeia*, the content of sinapine, calculated as sinapine thiocyanate ($C_{16}H_{24}NO_5 \cdot SCN$), should be no less than 0.50%, and for stir-fried *jiè zǐ*, that should be no less than 0.40%.

【性味归经 / Medicinal properties】

辛，温。归肺经。

Acrid and warm; act on the lung meridian.

【主要功效 / Medicinal efficacies】

温肺豁痰利气，散结通络止痛。

Warm lung, eliminate phlegm and reinforce qi, dissipate masses, unblock the collaterals and relieve pain.

【临床应用 / Clinical application】

1. 寒痰证，悬饮 本品辛散温通，专入肺经，既能温肺祛痰，又能利气宽胸。用治寒痰壅肺，咳喘胸闷，痰多清稀者，常配伍紫苏子、莱菔子等。若治悬饮咳喘，胸满胁痛者，常与甘遂、大戟等同用。

(1) Cold-phlegm syndromes and pleural rheum   Acrid, dispersing, warm and flowing, *jiè zǐ* particularly entering the lung meridian, can warm the lung and dispel phlegm as well as reinforce qi and relieve chest stiffness. To treat those with cold-phlegm obstructing the lung, cough, panting and chest oppression, as well as profuse clear and thin phlegm, it is often compatible with *zǐ sū zǐ*, *lái fú zǐ* (Raphani Semen), etc. To treat those with cough and panting due to pleural rheum, fullness sensation in chest and rib-side pain, it is often used together with *gān suí* (Kansui Radix), *dà jǐ* (Euphorbia pekinensis Rupr.), etc.

2. 肢体麻木，关节肿痛，阴疽流注   本品辛温走窜，能祛经络之痰，又能消肿散结，通络止痛。用治痰湿阻滞经络之肢体麻木或关节肿痛，常配伍马钱子、没药、肉桂等。用治痰湿流注，阴疽肿毒，常与鹿角胶、肉桂、熟地黄等同用。

(2) Limb numbness, joint pain and swelling, multiple yin abscesses   Acrid, warm and channeling, *jiè zǐ* can dispel phlegm of channels and collaterals, diminish swelling and dissipate masses, and unblock the collaterals and relieve pain as well. To treat limb numbness or joint pain and swelling due to phlegm-damp obstructing channels and collaterals, it is often compatible with *mǎ qián zǐ* (Strychni Semen), *mò yào* (Myrrha), *ròu guì* (Cinnamomi Cortex), etc. To treat multiple phlegm dampness, yin abscesses and pyogenic infections, it is often used together with *lù jiǎo jiāo* (Cervi Cornus Colla), *ròu guì*, *shú dì huáng* (Rehmanniae Radix Praeparata), etc.

【用法用量 / Usage and dosage】
煎服，3~9g。外用适量。
Decoction, 3-9g. Used externally with appropriate dosage.

【使用注意 / Precaution】
久咳肺虚及阴虚火旺、消化道溃疡、出血及皮肤过敏者忌用。

It should be avoided for those with chronic cough and lung deficiency, and yin deficiency resulting in vigorous fire; and those with peptic ulcer, bleeding and skin allergy as well.

【现代研究 / Modern research】
本品主要含芥子苷、芥子碱、芥子酶、胡萝卜苷、脂肪油、蛋白质及黏液质等。具有镇咳、祛痰、平喘、抗炎、镇痛、催吐、抑制皮肤真菌、抗衰老等作用。

It mainly contains sinigrin, sinapine, myrosinase, daucosterol, fatty oil, protein, mucilage, etc. It has the functions of relieving cough, dispelling phlegm, relieving panting, resisting inflammation, easing pain, promoting emesis, inhibiting skin fungal, resisting aging and so on.

旋覆花 *Xuán fù huā* (Inulae Flos)
《神农本草经》
Shen Nong's Classic of the Materia Medica (Shén Nóng Běn Cǎo Jīng)

【来源 / Origin】
为菊科植物旋覆花 *Inula japonica* Thunb. 或欧亚旋覆花 *Inula britannica* L. 的干燥头状花序。主产于河南、河北、江苏等地。夏、秋二季采收，晒干，生用或蜜炙用。本品气微，味微苦。

Xuán fù huā is the dried flower head of *Inula japonica* Thunb. or *Inula britannica* L., pertaining to the Compositae. Mainly produced in Henan, Hebei and Jiangsu, it is collected in summer and autumn, dried in the sun, and then used in raw or honey-fried form. *Xuán fù huā* is light and slightly and bitter.

【性味归经 / Medicinal properties】

苦、辛、咸，微温。归肺、脾、胃、大肠经。

Bitter, acrid, salty, and slightly warm; act on the lung, spleen, stomach and large intestine meridians.

【主要功效 / Medicinal efficacies】

降气，消痰，行水，止呕。

Descend qi, disperse phlegm, move water and arrest vomiting.

【临床应用 / Clinical application】

1. 咳喘痰多，胸膈痞满 本品苦降辛开，咸能软坚，微温不燥，入肺经，能降肺气、消痰水、平喘咳、除痞满，凡是痰浊阻肺，咳喘痰黏，胸闷不舒者，不论寒热，皆可配伍应用。若治寒痰咳喘，胸闷痰多者，常与紫苏子、半夏、细辛等同用。若治痰热咳喘，胸闷气短者，多与桑白皮、川贝母、紫菀等同用。若治外感风寒，痰湿内蕴，咳嗽痰多者，常与麻黄、半夏、前胡等同用。若治顽痰胶结，难以咳出，胸中满闷者，常配伍海浮石、海蛤壳等。

(1) Cough and panting with profuse phlegm, stuffiness and fullness in chest diaphragm With bitterness to descend, acridity to open and saltiness to soften hard masses, *xuán fù huā*, slightly warm but not drying at all, enters the lung channel, and can descend lung qi, disperse phlegm, relieve cough and panting, and eliminate stuffiness and fullness. As for those with turbid phlegm obstructing the lung, cough with sticky phlegm, chest oppression and discomfort, no matter cold or hot, it all can be compatible in application. To treat those with cold-phlegm cough and panting, chest oppression and profuse phlegm, it is often used together with *zǐ sū zǐ*, *bàn xià*, *xì xīn*, etc. To treat those with phlegm-heat cough and panting, chest oppression and shortness of breath, it is often combined with *sāng bái pí*, *chuān bèi mǔ*, *zǐ wǎn*, etc. To treat exogenous wind-cold, phlegm-damp retention, and cough with profuse phlegm, it often goes together with *má huáng* (Ephedrae Herba), *bàn xià*, *qián hú*, etc. To treat stubborn phlegm coagulation, difficulty in expectoration, as well as fullness and oppression in chest, it is often compatible with *hǎi fú shí*, *hǎi gé qiào*, etc.

2. 噫气，呕吐 本品苦降胃气，善止呕噫。用治痰浊中阻，胃气上逆而噫气呕吐，胃脘痞硬，常与赭石、半夏、生姜等同用。若治胃热呕逆，可与黄连、竹茹等同用。

(2) Belching, vomiting Being bitter and descending stomach qi, *xuán fù huā* is good at arresting vomiting and belching. To treat randomized stagnation of turbid phlegm, belching and vomiting due to ascending counterflow of stomach qi, and *pǐ* hardness in the stomach cavity, it is often used together with *zhě shí* (Haematitum), *bàn xià*, *shēng jiāng*, etc. To treat vomiting and counterflowing due to stomach heat, it can be combined with *huáng lián*, *zhú rú*, etc.

【用法用量 / Usage and dosage】

煎服，3~9g，包煎。

Decoction, 3~9g, decocted while wrapped.

【使用注意 / Precaution】

阴虚劳嗽、津伤燥咳者慎用。

It should be used with caution for those with taxation cough due to yin deficiency and dryness cough caused by fluid consumption.

【现代研究 / Modern research】

本品主要含旋覆花素、大花旋覆花素、旋覆花内酯、槲皮素、异槲皮素、咖啡酸、绿原酸等。具有镇咳、祛痰、抗支气管痉挛、抑菌、增加胃酸分泌、提高胃肠平滑肌张力、促进胆汁分泌、抗炎等作用。

It mainly contains inulicin, brevicornin britanin, spiralolactone, dendrobium, isodendrobium, caffeic acid, chlorogenic acid, etc. It has the functions of relieving cough, dispelling phlegm, resisting bronchospasm and bacteria, increasing the secretion of gastric acid, improving the tension of gastrointestinal smooth muscle, promoting bile secretion and resisting inflammation, etc.

第二节　清化热痰药

Section 2　Hot-phlegm clearing and dissolving medicinals

PPT

本类药物味多苦，性多寒凉，具有清化热痰之功，部分药物味甘质润，又兼能润燥化痰，主治热痰、燥痰证，症见咳嗽气喘、痰黄质稠，或干咳少痰、咳痰不爽、唇舌干燥；以及痰火所致的癫痫、中风、惊厥、瘿瘤、瘰疬等。

Mostly bitter in taste, cold and cool in property, medicinals in this chapter have the actions of clearing and dissolving hot phlegm, and since parts of the medicinals are sweet and moistening, they have the concurrent functions of moistening dryness and dissolving phlegm. They are mainly used to treat heat or dryness-phlegm symdromes, with the symptoms of cough and panting, thick yellow phlegm, or dry cough with little phlegm, expectoration with sensation of incompletion, dry lip and tongue; or to treat phlegm-fire-caused epilepsy, wind stroke, convulsion, goiter and tumor as well as scrofula.

川贝母　*Chuān bèi mǔ* (Fritillariae Cirrhosae Bulbus)
《神农本草经》
Shen Nong's Classic of the Materia Medica (Shén Nóng Běn Cǎo Jīng)

【来源 / Origin】

为百合科植物川贝母 *Fritillaria cirrhosa* D.Don、暗紫贝母 *Fritillaria unibracteata* Hsiao et K.C.Hsia、甘肃贝母 *Fritillaria przewalskii* Maxim.、梭砂贝母 *Fritillaria delavayi* Franch.、太白贝母 *Fritillaria taipaiensis* P. Y. Li 或瓦布贝母 *Fritillaria unibracteata* Hsiao et K.C. Hsia var. *wabuensis*（S. Y. Tang et S. C. Yue）Z. D. Liu，S. Wang et S.C. Chen 的干燥鳞茎。按性状不同分别习称"松贝""青贝""炉贝"和"栽培品"。主产于四川、青海、甘肃等地。夏秋采挖，干燥，生用。本品气微，味微苦。《中国药典》规定，含总生物碱以西贝母碱（$C_{27}H_{43}NO_3$）计，不得少于 0.050%。

Chuān bèi mǔ is the dried bulb of *Fritillaria cirrhosa* D.Don, *Fritillaria unibracteata* Hsiao et K.C.Hsia, *Fritillaria przewalskii* Maxim., *Fritillaria delavayi* Franch., *Fritillaria taipaiensis* P. Y. Li or *Fritillaria unibracteata* Hsiao et K.C. Hsia var. *wabuensis* (S. Y. Tang et S. C. Yue) Z. D. Liu, S. Wang et S.C. Chen, pertaining to the Liliaceae. According the differences in characters, *chuān bèi mǔ* is also known as *sōng bèi*, *qīng bèi*, *lú bèi* and *zāi péi pǐn*. Mainly produced in Sichuan, Qinghai, and Gansu, it is collected in summer and autumn, and dried for raw use. It is light and slightly bitter. According to *Chinese Pharmacopoeia*, the content of alkaloid, calculated as sipeimine ($C_{27}H_{43}NO_3$), should be no less

医药大学堂
WWW.YIYAODXT.COM

than 0.050%.

【性味归经 / Medicinal properties 】

苦、甘，微寒。归肺、心经。

Bitter, sweet, and slightly cold; act on the lung and heart meridians.

【主要功效 / Medicinal efficacies 】

清热润肺，化痰止咳，散结消痈。

Clear heat to moisten the lung, dissolve phlegm and relieve cough, dissipate masses and eliminate abscesses.

【临床应用 / Clinical application 】

1. **热痰、燥痰证** 本品苦寒清热，味甘质润，能清肺化痰，润肺止咳，尤宜于内伤久咳，燥痰、热痰之证。用治燥痰证，干咳痰少，咳痰不爽，咽干口燥等，常与知母相须配用。用治阴虚劳嗽，久咳有痰，常配伍沙参、麦冬、知母等。用治热痰证，咳嗽痰多色黄者，可与黄芩、桔梗、枇杷叶等同用。

(1) Heat and dryness-phlegm syndromes Bitter, cold, clear and hot, *chuān bèi mǔ*, sweet and moistening at the same time, can clear lung heat to dissolve phlegm, moisten the lung to relieve cough, and thus is especially suitable for chronic cough due to internal damage, dryness-phlegm and heat-phlegm syndromes. To treat dryness-phlegm syndromes, with the symptoms such as dry cough with scant phlegm, expectoration with sensation of incompletion, dry throat and parched mouth, etc, it should be compatible with *zhī mǔ* (Anemarrhenae Rhizoma). To treat taxation cough due to yin deficiency and chronic cough with phlegm, it is often combined with *shā shēn* (Adenophorae seu Glehniae Radix), *mài dōng, zhī mǔ*, etc. To treat heat-phlegm syndromes, for example, cough with profuse yellow phlegm, it can be used together with *huáng qín, jié gěng, pí pá yè*, etc.

2. **瘰疬、乳痈、肺痈** 本品苦寒，能清热化痰，散结消痈。用治瘰疬，常配伍玄参、牡蛎等。用治乳痈、肺痈、疮痈，常与蒲公英、天花粉、鱼腥草等同用。

(2) Scrofula, breast and lung abscesses Bitter and cold, *chuān bèi mǔ* can clear heat and dissolve phlegm, dissipate masses and eliminate abscesses. To treat scrofula, it is often compatible with *xuán shēn* (Scrophulariae Radix), *mǔ lì* (Ostreae Concha), etc. To treat breast and lung abscesses, sores and abscesses, it is often used together with *pú gōng yīng* (Taraxaci Herba), *tiān huā fěn* (Trichosanthis Radix), *yú xīng cǎo* (Houttuyniae Herba), etc.

【用法用量 / Usage and dosage 】

煎服，3~10g；研粉冲服，1 次 1~2g。

Decoction, 3-10g; powdered and infused, 1-2g per time.

【使用注意 / Precaution 】

不宜与川乌、制川乌、草乌、制草乌、附子同用。

It is not suitable to be used together with *chuān wū, zhì chuān wū, cǎo wū, zhì cǎo wū* and *fù zǐ*.

【现代研究 / Modern research 】

本品主要含川贝碱、西贝母碱、青贝碱、松贝碱、松贝甲素、梭砂贝母碱、贝母素乙、川贝酮碱、岷山碱甲、岷山碱乙等，尚含无机元素等。具有镇咳、祛痰、解痉、降压、抑菌、抗炎、兴奋子宫、镇痛等作用。

It mainly contains fritimine, sipeimine, chinpeimine, sonpeimine, songbeinine, hupehenine, peiminine, chuanbeinone, minshanmine, minshanminine, and other inorganic elements. It has the functions of relieving cough, dispelling phlegm, resolving convulsion, reducing hypertension, resisting bacteria and inflammation, exciting uterus, suppressing pain, etc.

浙贝母 *Zhè bèi mǔ* (Fritillariae Thunbergii Bulbus)
《轩岐救正论》
Treatise on Correcting Mistakes by Xuanyuan and Qibo (Xuān Qí Jiù Zhèng Lùn)

【来源 / Origin】

为百合科植物浙贝母 *Fritillaria thunbergii* Miq. 的干燥鳞茎。主产于浙江。初夏采挖，切厚片或打成碎块，生用。本品气微，味微苦。《中国药典》规定，含贝母素甲（$C_{27}H_{45}NO_3$）和贝母素乙（$C_{27}H_{43}NO_3$）的总量不得少于 0.080%。

Zhè bèi mǔ is the dried bulb of *Fritillaria thunbergii* Miq., pertaining to the Liliaceae. Mainly produced in Zhejiang, it is collected in early summer, cut into thick slices or crushed for raw use. *Zhè bèi mǔ* is light and slightly bitter. According to *Chinese Pharmacopoeia*, the total content of peimine ($C_{27}H_{45}NO_3$) and peiminine ($C_{27}H_{43}NO_3$) should be no less than 0.080%.

【性味归经 / Medicinal properties】

苦，寒。归肺、心经。

Bitter and cold; act on the lung and heart meridians.

【主要功效 / Medicinal efficacies】

清热化痰止咳，解毒散结消痈。

Clear heat, dissolve phlegm and relieve cough; resolve toxins, dissipate masses and eliminate abscesses.

【临床应用 / Clinical application】

1. **风热咳嗽，痰热咳嗽**　本品功似川贝母，但其苦寒之性较甚，善于清热化痰，降泄肺气，适宜于风热咳嗽及痰热郁肺之咳嗽，前者常与桑叶、牛蒡子、前胡等同用，后者多配伍瓜蒌、桔梗、知母等。

(1) Wind-heat cough and phlegm-heat cough　With similar actions as those of *chuān bèi mǔ*, *zhè bèi mǔ* is much bitterer and colder. It is adept in clearing heat and dissolving phlegm as well as descending and discharging lung qi, and thus is suitable for wind-heat cough and cough due to phlegm-heat constraining the lung. For the former, it is often used together with *sāng yè* (Mori Folium), *niú bàng zǐ* (Arctii Fructus), *qián hú*, etc. For the latter, it is often compatible with *guā lóu*, *jié gěng*, *zhī mǔ*, etc.

2. **瘰疬，瘿瘤，肺痈，乳痈，疮痈**　本品类似于川贝母而解毒散结消痈之力更强，用治瘰疬结核，常与玄参、牡蛎等同用。用治瘿瘤，多与海藻、昆布等同用。用治肺痈，常与鱼腥草、芦根、桃仁等同用。用治疮痈、乳痈，常配伍连翘、蒲公英等。

(2) Scrofula, goiter and tumor, lung abscesses, breast abscesses, sores and abscesses　With functions similar to those of *chuān bèi mǔ*, *zhè bèi mǔ* has a stronger force of resolving toxins, dissipating masses and eliminating abscesses. To treat scrofula and nodule, it is often used together with *xuán shēn* and *mǔ lì*. To treat goiter and tumor, it is often combined with *hǎi zǎo*, *kūn bù*, etc. To treat lung abscesses, it often goes with *yú xīng cǎo*, *lú gēn* (Phragmitis Rhizoma), *táo rén* (Persicae Semen), etc. To treat sores and abscesses, breast abscesses, it is often compatible with *lián qiáo* (Forsythiae Fructus), *pú gōng yīng*, etc.

【用法用量 / Usage and dosage】

煎服，5~10g。

Decoction, 5~10g.

【使用注意 / Precaution】

同川贝母。

The same as *chuān bèi mǔ*.

【现代研究 / Modern research】

本品主要含贝母素甲、贝母素乙、贝母辛、浙贝母碱、异浙贝母碱、浙贝宁、浙贝母酮、浙贝母碱苷等生物碱，尚含胆酸、脂肪酸、β-谷甾醇等。具有镇咳、祛痰、平喘、镇静、镇痛、抑菌、抗炎、抗肿瘤、降压、扩瞳、兴奋子宫等作用。

It mainly contains alkaloids such as peimine, peiminine, peimisine, verticine, isoverticine, zhebeinine, zhebeinone and zhebeirine glucoside, and also contains cholic acid, fatty acid, β-sitosterol, etc. It has the functions of relieving cough, dispelling phlegm, relieving panting, calming the mind, suppressing pain, resisting bacteria, inflammation and tumor, reducing hypertension, enlarging pupil, exciting uterus, etc.

瓜蒌　*Guā lóu* (Trichosanthis Fructus)
《神农本草经》
Shen Nong's Classic of the Materia Medica (Shén Nóng Běn Cǎo Jīng)

【来源 / Origin】

为葫芦科植物栝楼 *Trichosanthes kirilowii* Maxim. 或双边栝楼 *Trichosanthes rosthornii* Harms 的干燥成熟果实。主产于山东、浙江、河北等地。秋季采收，生用。本品具焦糖气，味微酸、甜。

Guā lóu is the dried mature fruit of *Trichosanthes kirilowii* Maxim. or *Trichosanthes rosthornii* Harms. Mainly produced in Shandong, Zhejiang, Hebei and other places, it is collected in autumn for raw use. With the smell of caramel, *guā lóu* is slightly sour and sweet.

【性味归经 / Medicinal properties】

甘、微苦，寒。归肺、胃、大肠经。

Sweet, slightly bitter, and cold; act on the lung, stomach and large intestine meridians.

【主要功效 / Medicinal efficacies】

清热涤痰，宽胸散结，润燥滑肠。

Clear heat and clear up phlegm, relieve chest stiffness to dissipate mass, moisten dryness to loosen bowel.

【临床应用 / Clinical application】

1. 痰热咳嗽，肺热燥咳　本品苦寒清泄，甘寒润燥，入肺经，善清肺热，润肺燥，涤痰浊。用治痰热阻肺，咳嗽痰黄，质稠难咳，胸膈痞满，常配伍黄芩、胆南星、枳实等。用治燥热伤肺，干咳无痰或痰少质黏，咳吐不利，多与川贝母、天花粉、桔梗等同用。

(1) **Phlegm-heat cough, dryness cough due to lung heat**　With bitterness and coldness clearing and discharging heat, and sweetness and coldness moistening dryness, *guā lóu*, entering the lung channel, is good at clearing lung heat, moistening lung dryness and clearing up phlegm turbidity. To treat phlegm-heat obstructing the lung, cough with yellow phlegm, difficult expectoration of thick phlegm, as well as *pǐ* and fullness in chest diaphragm, it is often compatible with *huáng qín*, *dǎn nán xīng* (Arisaema cum Bile), *zhǐ shí*, etc. To treat dryness heat damaging the lung, dry cough without phlegm or scanty sticky and thick phlegm, as well as difficulty in expectoration, it is often used together with *chuān bèi mǔ*, *tiān*

huā fěn, *jié gěng*, etc.

2. **胸痹，结胸** 本品能清肺胃之热而化痰，利气散结以宽胸，善于通利胸膈之痹塞。用治痰浊痹阻，胸阳不振之胸痹心痛，常与薤白、半夏同用。用治痰热结胸，胸膈痞满，按之则痛，常配伍黄连、半夏等。

(2) Chest impediment and chest bind *Guā lóu* is able to clear lung and stomach heat to dissolve phlegm, reinforce qi and dissipate masses to relieve chest stiffness, and is adept at breaking through blockage in chest and diaphragm as well. To treat phlegm turbidity obstruction, chest impediment and heartache due to hypofunction of chest yang, it is often used together with *xiè bái* (Allii Macrostemi Bulbus) and *bàn xià*. To treat phlegm-heat binding the chest, stuffiness and fullness in chest and diaphragm, and pains on pressing, it is often compatible with *huáng lián*, *bàn xià*, etc.

3. **肺痈，肠痈，乳痈** 本品清热散结消痈。用治肺痈咳吐脓血，常配伍鱼腥草、芦根、桃仁等。用治肠痈腹痛，可与败酱草、大血藤、薏苡仁等同用。用治乳痈初起，红肿热痛，可与牛蒡子、金银花、青皮等同用。

(3) Lung, intestine and breast abscess *Guā lóu* clear heat, dissipate masses and eliminate abscesses. To treat expectoration of pus and blood due to lung abscesses, it is often compatible with *yú xīng cǎo*, *lú gēn*, *táo rén*, etc. To treat abdominal pain caused by intestine abscesses, it can be used together with *bài jiàng cǎo* (Patriniae Herba), *dà xuè téng* (Sargentodoxae Caulis), *yì yǐ rén* (Coicis Semen), etc. To treat the early stage of breast abscesses, it can be combined with *niú bàng zǐ*, *jīn yín huā* (Lonicerae Japonicae Flos), *qīng pí* (Citri Reticulatae Viride Pericarpium), etc.

4. **肠燥便秘** 本品质润多脂，能润燥滑肠。用治肠燥便秘，常与火麻仁、郁李仁等同用。

(4) Constipation due to intestinal dryness Moistening and fatty, *guā lóu* can moisten dryness to loosen bowel. To treat constipation due to intestinal dryness, it is often used together with *huǒ má rén* (Cannabis Fructus), *yù lǐ rén* (Pruni Semen), etc.

【用法用量 / Usage and dosage】
煎服，9~15g。
Decoction, 9-15g.

【使用注意 / Precaution】
脾虚便溏者忌用。不宜与川乌、制川乌、草乌、制草乌、附子同用。

It should be avoided for those with loose stool due to spleen deficiency. It is not suitable to be used together with *chuān wū, zhì chuān wū, cǎo wū, zhì cǎo wū* and *fù zǐ*.

【现代研究 / Modern research】
本品主要含有正三十四烷酸、富马酸、琥珀酸、栝楼萜二醇、丝氨酸蛋白酶A、丝氨酸蛋白酶B及甾醇等。具有祛痰、抗炎、抑菌、降血压、扩张冠状动脉、增加冠脉流量、抗血小板聚集、抗癌等作用。

It mainly contains tetratriacontarioic acid, fumaric acid, succinic acid, karounidiol, terpene diol, serine protease A, serine protease B and sterol, etc. It has the functions of dispelling phlegm, resisting inflammation and bacteria, lowering blood pressure, expanding coronary arteries, increasing coronary flow, resisting platelet aggregation and cancer.

竹茹 *Zhú rú* (Bambusae Caulis in Taenias)
《本草经集注》
Collective Commentaries on the Classic of Materia Medica (Běn Cǎo Jīng Jí Zhù)

【来源 / Origin 】

为禾本科植物青秆竹 *Bambusa tuldoides* Munro、大头典竹 *Sinocalamus beecheyanus*（Munro）McClure var. *pubescens* P. F. Li 或淡竹 *Phyllostachy nigra*（Lodd.）Munro var. *henonis*（Mitf.）Stapf ex Rendle 的茎秆的干燥中间层。主产于江苏、浙江、江西等地。全年均可采制，阴干，生用或姜汁炙用。本品气微，味淡。

Zhú rú is the dry middle layer of the stem of *Bambusa tuldoides* Munro, *Sinocalamus beecheyanus* (Munro) McClure var. *pubescens* P. F. Li or *Phyllostachy nigra* (Lodd.) Munro var. *henonis* (Mitf.) Stapf ex Rendle, pertaining to the Poaceae. Mainly produced in Jiangsu, Zhejiang and Jiangxi, it can be collected all the year around, dried in the shadow for raw use or fried use with *jiāng zhī* (Rhizomatis Zingiberis Succus). *Zhú rú* is light in flavor and bland in taste.

【性味归经 / Medicinal properties 】

甘，微寒。归肺、胃、心、胆经。

Sweet, and slight cold; act on the lung, stomach, heart and gallbladder meridians.

【主要功效 / Medicinal efficacies 】

清热化痰，除烦，止呕。

Clear heat and dissolve phlegm, eliminate vexation, and arrest vomiting.

【临床应用 / Clinical application 】

1. 痰热咳嗽，心烦不寐 本品性微寒，入肺经，善于清热化痰，并可清心热以除烦。用治肺热咳嗽，痰黄黏稠，常配伍瓜蒌、黄芩等。用治痰火内扰，胸闷痰多，心烦不寐，常与枳实、半夏等同用。若治中风痰迷，舌强不语，可与牛黄、胆南星、生姜汁等同用。

(1) Phlegm-heat cough, vexation and sleeplessness Slightly cold, *zhú rú*, entering the lung channel, is good at clearing heat and dissolving phlegm, and clearing heart heat to eliminate vexation as well. To treat lung-heat cough and sticky thick yellow sputum, it is often compatible with *guā lóu*, *huáng qín*, etc. To treat phlegm-fire harassing the interior, chest oppression with profuse phlegm, as well as vexation and sleeplessness, it is often used together with *zhǐ shí*, *bàn xià*, etc. To treat wind stroke due to phlegm confusion and stiff tongue impeding speech, it can be combined with *niú huáng*, *dǎn nán xīng*, *shēng jiāng zhī* (Zingiberis Rhizomatis Succus), etc.

2. 胃热呕吐、妊娠恶阻 本品入胃经，能清胃热止呕，为治胃热呕逆常用药。用治胃热呕吐，常与黄连、芦根等同用。用治胃虚有热之呕吐，可与人参、陈皮、生姜等同用。用治怀胎蕴热，恶阻呕逆，可与枇杷叶、陈皮等同用。

(2) Stomach-heat vomiting, pernicious vomiting during pregnancy Entering the stomach channel, *zhú rú* can clear stomach heat and arrest vomiting, and thus is a common drug for vomiting and counterflowing due to stomach heat. To treat stomach-heat vomiting, it is often used together with *huáng lián*, *lú gēn*, etc. To treat vomiting due to stomach deficiency with heat, it can be used together with *rén shēn* (Ginseng Radix et Rhizoma), *chén pí*, *shēng jiāng*, etc. To treat heat accumulation during pregnancy, pernicious vomiting and counterflowing, it can be combined with *pí pá yè*, *chén pí*, etc.

【用法用量 / Usage and dosage 】

煎服，5~10g。生用清热化痰，姜汁炙用则和胃止呕。

Decoction, 5-10g. Clear heat and dissolve phlegm for raw use, harmonize the stomach and arrest vomiting if fried with *jiāng zhī*.

【现代研究 / Modern research】

本品主要含 2,5– 二甲氧基 – 对苯醌、对羟基苯甲醛、丁香醛、松柏醛、香荚兰酸、阿魏酸、氨基酸、多糖等。具有祛痰、镇咳、抑菌、镇吐、抗氧化等作用。

It mainly contains 2,5-dimethoxyl-*p*-benzoquinone, *p*-hydroxybenzaldehyde, syringaldehyde, coniferyl aldehyde, vanilla acid, ferulic acid, amino acid, polysaccharide and so on. It has the functions of dispelling phlegm, relieving cough, resisting bacteria, arresting vomiting, resisting oxidation, etc.

前胡　*Qián hú* (Peucedani Radix)
《雷公炮炙论》
Master Lei's Discourse on Medicinal Processing (Léi Gōng Páo Zhì Lùn)

【来源 / Origin】

为伞形科植物白花前胡 *Peucedanum praeruptorum* Dunn 的干燥根。主产于浙江、湖南、四川等地。冬季至次春采挖，切薄片，生用或蜜炙用。本品气芳香，味微苦、辛。《中国药典》规定，含白花前胡甲素（$C_{21}H_{22}O_7$）不得少于 0.90%，含白花前胡乙素（$C_{24}H_{26}O_7$）不得少于 0.24%。

Qián hú is the dry root of *Peucedanum praeruptorum* Dunn, pertaining to the Umbelliferae. Mainly produced in Zhejiang, Hunan and Sichuan, it is collected from winter to the next spring, and cut into slices for raw or honey-fried use. It is aromatic, a little bitter, and acrid. According to *Chinese Pharmacopoeia*, the content of praeruptorin A ($C_{21}H_{22}O_7$) should be no less than 0.90%, and that of praeruptorin B ($C_{24}H_{26}O_7$) should be no less than 0.24%.

【性味归经 / Medicinal properties】

苦、辛，微寒。归肺经。

Bitter, acrid, and slightly cold; act on the lung meridian.

【主要功效 / Medicinal efficacies】

降气化痰，散风清热。

Descend qi and dissolve phlegm, dissipate wind and clear heat.

【临床应用 / Clinical application】

1. 痰热咳喘　本品苦泄辛散，性寒清热，具有清肺降气化痰之效。用治痰热壅肺，肺失宣降之咳喘胸满，咳痰黄稠，常与苦杏仁、桑白皮、浙贝母等同用。因本品寒性不著，若配伍半夏、白前等，亦可用治寒痰、湿痰证。

(1) **Cough and panting due to phlegm heat**　With bitterness to discharge and acridity to open, *qián hú*, cold and heat-clearing, has the efficacies of clearing lung heat, directing qi downward and dissolving phlegm. To treat phlegm-heat obstructing the lung, fullness sensation in chest caused by lung failing to diffuse and govern descent and expectoration of thick yellow phlegm, it is often used together with *kǔ xìng rén*, *sāng bái pí*, *zhè bèi mǔ*, etc. Since *qián hú* is not cold enough in property, if compatible with *bàn xià* and *bái qián*, it also can be used to treat the syndromes of cold and damp phlegm.

2. 风热咳嗽　本品味辛性微寒，能疏散风热，降气化痰。用治外感风热，咳嗽痰多，常与桑叶、牛蒡子、桔梗等同用。若治风寒咳嗽，可与苦杏仁、紫苏叶等同用。

(2) **Wind-heat cough**　Acrid and slightly cold, *qián hú* can dissipate wind heat, direct qi downward and dissolve phlegm. To treat exogenous wind heat, cough with profuse phlegm, it is often used together with *sāng yè*, *niú bàng zǐ*, *jié gěng*, etc. To treat wind-cold cough, it can be combined with *kǔ xìng rén* and

zǐ sū yè (Perillae Folium).

【用法用量 / Usage and dosage】

煎服，3~10g。

Decoction, 3-10g.

【现代研究 / Modern research】

本品主要含白花前胡甲素、白花前胡乙素、白花前胡丙素、白花前胡丁素等香豆素类，尚含皂苷、挥发油等。具有祛痰、镇咳、平喘、抑菌、抗炎、镇静、镇痛、抗血小板聚集、抗溃疡、降血压、降血脂等作用。

It mainly contains coumarins such as praeruptorin A, praeruptorin B, praeruptorin C and praeruptorin D, and also contains saponins and volatile oils. It has the functions of dispelling phlegm, relieving cough, calming panting, resisting bacteria and inflammation, calming the mind, alleviating pain, resisting platelet aggregation and ulcer, reducing blood pressure and blood lipid, etc.

桔梗　*Jié gěng* (Platycodonis Radix)
《神农本草经》
Shen Nong's Classic of the Materia Medica (*Shén Nóng Běn Cǎo Jīng*)

【来源 / Origin】

为桔梗科植物桔梗 *Platycodon grandiflorum*（Jacq.）A. DC. 的干燥根。全国大部分地区均产。春、秋二季采挖，干燥，切厚片，生用。本品气微，味微甜后苦。《中国药典》规定，含桔梗皂苷 D（$C_{57}H_{92}O_{28}$）不得少于 0.10%。

Jié gěng is the dry root of *Platycodon grandiflorum* (Jacq.) A. DC., pertaining to the Campanulaceae. Produced in most parts of China, it is collected in spring and autumn, dried, cut into thick slices and used raw. *Jié gěng* is light, slightly sweet and then bitter. According to *Chinese Pharmacopoeia*, the content of platycodin D ($C_{57}H_{92}O_{28}$) should be no less than 0.10%.

【性味归经 / Medicinal properties】

苦、辛，平。归肺经。

Bitter, acrid and neutral; act on the lung meridian.

【主要功效 / Medicinal efficacies】

宣肺，祛痰，利咽，排脓。

Diffuse the lung, dispel phlegm, relieve sore throat and evacuate pus.

【临床应用 / Clinical application】

1. 咳嗽痰多，胸闷不畅　本品辛散苦泄，善于开宣肺气而利胸膈咽喉，并能稀释稠痰而有较好的祛痰作用。因其性平，故凡咳嗽痰多，胸闷不畅，无论寒热皆可应用。若治风寒咳嗽，常与紫苏叶、苦杏仁等同用。若治风热咳嗽，多与桑叶、菊花、苦杏仁等同用。若治肺热咳嗽，痰稠色黄，常与浙贝母、黄芩、枇杷叶等同用。

(1) Cough with profuse phlegm, inhibited chest oppression　With acridity to disperse and bitterness to discharge, *jié gěng* is adept at dispersing lung qi so as to benefit chest diaphragm and throat, and diluting thick phlegm so as to have a better efficacy of dispelling phlegm as well. Since it is neutral, it can be applied to cough with profuse phlegm and inhibited chest oppression, no matter cold or hot. To treat wind-cold cough, it is often used together with *zǐ sū yè*, *kǔ xìng rén*, etc. To treat wind-heat cough, it is often combined with *sāng yè*, *jú huā* (Chrysanthemi Flos), *kǔ xìng rén*, etc. To treat lung-heat cough with thick yellow phlegm, it is often compatible with *zhè bèi mǔ*, *huáng qín* and *pí pá yè*.

2. **咽痛音哑** 本品辛散入肺，能宣肺利咽开音。为治咽喉肿痛、声音嘶哑的常用药。用治风热犯肺，咽痛失音，常与甘草、牛蒡子等同用。用治热毒内盛，咽喉肿痛、失音，多与射干、板蓝根等同用。

(2) Sore throat and dumbness Acrid and dispersing, *jié gěng*, entering the lung, can diffuse the lung, relieve sore throat, and ease-up the voice. It is a common drug to treat sore and swollen throat and hoarseness. To treat wind-heat invading the lung, sore throat and loss of voice, it is often used together with *gān cǎo*, *niú bàng zǐ*, etc. To treat exuberance of internal heat toxin, sore and swollen throat, and loss of voice, it is often combined with *shè gān* (Belamcandae Rhizoma), *bǎn lán gēn* (Isatidis Radix), etc.

3. **肺痈吐脓** 本品能宣肺排脓。用治肺痈之胸痛、咯吐脓血、痰黄腥臭，常与甘草、鱼腥草、芦根等同用。

(3) Lung abscesses with pus *Jié gěng* can diffuse the lung and evacuate pus. To treat lung abscesses, chest pain, expectoration of pus and blood as well as stinking yellow phlegm, it is often used together with *gān cǎo*, *yú xīng cǎo*, *lú gēn*, etc.

此外，本品可开宣肺气而通二便，用治癃闭、便秘。

In addition, *jié gěng* is able to disperse lung qi so as to promote defecation and urination, and thus can be applied to treat dribbling urinary block and constipation.

【用法用量 / Usage and dosage】

煎服，3~10g。

Decoction, 3-10g.

【使用注意 / Precaution】

凡气机上逆，呕吐、呛咳、眩晕、阴虚火旺咯血等不宜用。用量不宜过大。

It is not suitable for those with ascending counterflow of qi movement, vomiting, bucking, dizziness, coughing of blood due to yin deficiency resulting in vigorous fire, etc. The dosage should not be too large.

【现代研究 / Modern research】

本品主要含桔梗皂苷A和D、远志皂苷、多糖、脂肪酸、微量元素、维生素等。具有祛痰、镇咳、平喘、抑菌、抗炎、镇静、镇痛、解热、降血压、降血脂、降血糖、抗肿瘤、免疫调节等作用。

It mainly contains platycodin A and D, onjisapomin, polysaccharides, fatty acids, trace elements, vitamins, etc. It has the functions of dispelling phlegm, relieving cough, calming panting, resisting bacteria and inflammation, calming the mind, alleviating pain, allaying fever, reducing blood pressure, blood lipid and blood glucose, resisting tumor, regulating immune system, etc.

第三节 止咳平喘药

Section 3 Cough and panting-relieving medicinals

本类药物味或辛或苦或甘，药性或温或寒，主归肺经，有的偏于止咳，有的偏于平喘，有的则兼而有之。概而言之，以止咳平喘为主要功效，主治各种原因所致的咳嗽、喘证。

Acrid or bitter or sweet in taste, warm or cold in property, medicinals of this group are mainly distributed to the lung meridian, while some of them in relieving cough and some in calming panting, some are specialized in both. In a word, with relieving cough and panting as the main efficacy, they are mainly used to treat cough and panting of various reasons.

苦杏仁 *Kǔ xìng rén* (Armeniacae Semen Amarum)
《神农本草经》
Shen Nong's Classic of the Materia Medica (Shén Nóng Běn Cǎo Jīng)

【来源 / Origin】

为蔷薇科植物山杏 *Prunus armeniaca* L. var. *ansu* Maxim.、西伯利亚杏 *Prunus sibirica* L.、东北杏 *Prunus mandshurica*（Maxim.）Koehne 或杏 *Prunus armeniaca* L. 的干燥成熟种子。主产山西、河北、内蒙古等地。夏季采收，生用或用燀法去皮用，或炒用。本品气微，味苦。《中国药典》规定，含苦杏仁苷（$C_{20}H_{27}NO_{11}$）不得少于 3.0%，燀苦杏仁不得少于 2.4%，炒苦杏仁不得少于 2.4%。

Kǔ xìng rén is the dry or ripe seed of *Prunus armeniaca* L. var. *ansu* Maxim., *Prunus sibirica* L., *Prunus mandshurica* (Maxim.) Koehne, or *Prunus armeniaca* L., pertaining to the Rosaceae. Mainly produced in Shanxi, Hebei Province, Inner Mongolia Autonomous Region and other places, it is collected in summer, used raw or processed with fire and water to remove the peel for use later, or applied in dry-fried form. *Kǔ xìng rén* is light and bitter. According to *Chinese Pharmacopoeia*, the content of amygdalin ($C_{20}H_{27}NO_{11}$) should be no less than 3.0%, no less than 2.4% in roasted *kǔ xìng rén* and no less than 2.4% in stir-fried *kǔ xìng rén*.

【性味归经 / Medicinal properties】

苦，微温；有小毒。归肺、大肠经。

Bitter, slightly warm; a little toxic; act on the lung and large intestine meridians.

【主要功效 / Medicinal efficacies】

降气止咳平喘，润肠通便。

Descend qi, relieve cough and panting, moisten the intestines to promote defecation.

【临床应用 / Clinical application】

1. 咳嗽气喘　本品味苦降泄，主入肺经，长于降泄肺气，略有宣肺之效，可使肺的宣发肃降功能复常而咳喘自平，故为止咳平喘之要药，随证配伍可用治多种原因所致的咳喘病证。若治风寒咳喘，常配伍麻黄、甘草。若治风热咳嗽，常与桑叶、菊花、薄荷等同用。若治肺热咳喘，常与石膏、麻黄、甘草同用。若治燥热咳嗽，痰少难咳，多与桑叶、贝母、沙参等同用。若治寒痰咳喘，可与干姜、半夏、茯苓等同用。

(1) **Cough and panting** Bitter, descending and discharging, *kǔ xìng rén*, mainly entering the lung channel, is good at descending and discharging lung qi. With a slight efficacy of diffusing the lung, *kǔ xìng rén* can recover the lung's functions of diffusion, dispersion, purification and descent so as to let the cough and panting recover on its own, and thus is an important medicinal to relieve cough and panting, which can be combined with other medicinals to treat cough and panting of various reasons. To treat wind-cold cough and panting, it is often compatible with *má huáng* and *gān cǎo*. To treat wind-heat cough, it is often used together with *sāng yè*, *jú huā*, *bò he* (Menthae Herba), etc. To treat lung-heat cough and panting, it is often combined with *shí gāo* (Gypsum Fibrosum), *má huáng*, *gān cǎo*, etc. To treat dryness-heat cough and panting as well as difficult expectoration of scant phlegm, it often goes with *sāng yè*, *bèi mǔ*, *shā shēn*, etc. To treat cold-phlegm cough and panting, it can be combined with *gān jiāng*, *bàn*

xià, fú líng, etc.

2. 肠燥便秘 本品质润多脂，能润肠通便。用治肠燥便秘，每与柏子仁、郁李仁、桃仁等同用。若治血虚便秘，可与当归、熟地黄等同用。

(2) Constipation due to intestinal dryness Moistening and fatty, *kǔ xìng rén* can moisten the intestines to promote defecation. To treat constipation due to intestinal dryness, it is always used together with *bǎi zǐ rén* (Platycladi Semen), *yù lǐ rén*, *táo rén*, etc. To treat blood-deficiency constipation, it can be combined with *dāng guī* (Angelicae Sinensis Radix), *shú dì huáng*, etc.

【用法用量 / Usage and dosage】

煎服，5~10g，打碎入煎，生品入煎剂宜后下。

Decoction, 5-10g, pounded before decoction, and suitable to be added later as a fresh medicinal.

【使用注意 / Precaution】

内服不宜过量。婴儿慎用。

Avoid excessive internal administration. It should be taken with caution for infants.

【现代研究 / Modern research】

本品主要含有苦杏仁苷、苦杏仁酶、脂肪油、蛋白质等。具有镇咳、平喘、祛痰、润滑性通便、抗炎、镇痛、增强免疫、抗肿瘤、抗消化性溃疡等作用。

It mainly contains amygdalin, amygdalase, fat oil, protein and so on. It has the functions of relieving cough, calming panting, dispelling phlegm, promoting lubricating defecation, resisting inflammation, alleviating pain, boosting immunization, resisting tumor and peptic ulcer, etc.

紫苏子 *Zǐ sū zǐ* (Perillae Fructus)

《本草经集注》

Collective Commentaries on the Classic of Materia Medica (Běn Cǎo Jīng Jí Zhù)

【来源 / Origin】

为唇形科植物紫苏 *Perilla frutescens*（L.）Britt. 的干燥成熟果实。主产于湖北、江苏、河南等地。秋季采收，晒干，生用或炒用。本品压碎有香气，味微辛。《中国药典》规定，含迷迭香酸（$C_{18}H_{16}O_8$）不得少于 0.25%，药材不得少于 0.20%。

Zǐ sū zǐ is the dry ripe fruit of *Perilla frutescens* (L.) Britt., pertaining to the Labiatae. Mainly produced in Hubei, Jiangsu, Henan and other places, it is collected in autumn, dried in the sun, and used raw or dry-fried for use later. *Zǐ sū zǐ* is aromatic if crushed, and a little acrid. According to *Chinese Pharmacopoeia*, the content of rosmarinic acid ($C_{18}H_{16}O_8$) should be no less than 0.25%, and no less than 0.20% in decoction pieces.

【性味归经 / Medicinal properties】

辛，温。归肺经。

Acrid and warm; act on the lung meridian.

【主要功效 / Medicinal efficacies】

降气化痰，止咳平喘，润肠通便。

Descend qi and dissolve phlegm, relieve cough and panting, moisten intestines to promote defecation.

【临床应用 / Clinical application】

1. 咳喘痰多 本品质润主降，温而不燥，既可化痰，又可止咳平喘，故宜于咳喘痰多、胸闷食少者，常与芥子、莱菔子同用。治上盛下虚之久咳痰喘，胸膈满闷，常配伍肉桂、当归、厚朴等。治风寒外束，痰热内蕴之哮喘咳嗽，痰多色黄，多与麻黄、桑白皮、半夏等同用。

(1) Cough and panting with profuse phlegm Moistening and descending, *zǐ sū zǐ*, warm but not dry, can dissolve phlegm, and relieve cough and panting as well. Thus it is suitable for those with cough and panting with plentiful phlegm, chest oppression and deficiency of food, where it is often used together with *jiè zǐ* and *lái fú zǐ*. To treat chronic cough with phlegm panting due to upper excess and lower deficiency as well as fullness and oppression of chest diaphragm, it is often compatible with *ròu guì*, *dāng guī*, *hòu pò*, etc. To treat the exterior tightened by pathogenic wind-cold, cough and panting due to accumulation of phlegm-heat in the interior, and profuse yellow phlegm, it is often combined with *má huáng*, *sāng bái pí*, *bàn xià*, etc.

2. 肠燥便秘 本品富含油脂，能润燥滑肠，且可降肺气以助大肠传导。用治肠燥便秘，常配伍苦杏仁、火麻仁、瓜蒌仁等。

(2) Constipation due to intestinal dryness Rich in oil, *zǐ sū zǐ* can moisten dryness to loosen bowel, and descend lung qi to help the large intestine to conduct and transmit as well. To treat constipation due to intestinal dryness, it is often compatible with *kǔ xìng rén*, *huǒ má rén*, *guā lóu rén* (Trichosanthis Semen), etc.

【用法用量 / Usage and dosage】

煎服，3~10g。

Decoction, 3~10g.

【使用注意 / Precaution】

脾虚便溏者慎用。

It should be used with caution for those with loose stool due to spleen deficiency.

【现代研究 / Modern research】

本品主要含油酸、亚油酸、亚麻酸、迷迭香酸及氨基酸、维生素、微量元素等。具有镇咳、祛痰、平喘、抗炎、抗过敏、增强免疫、降血脂、降血压、提高记忆力等作用。

It mainly contains oleic acid, linoleic acid, linolenic acid, rosmarinic acid and amino acids, vitamins, trace elements, etc. It has the functions of relieving cough, dispelling phlegm, calming panting, resisting inflammation and allergy, boosting immunization, reducing blood lipid and blood pressure, enhancing memory, etc.

百部 *Bǎi bù* (Stemonae Radix)
《名医别录》
Miscellaneous Records of Famous Physicians (Míng Yī Bié Lù)

【来源 / Origin】

为百部科植物直立百部 *Stemona sessilifolia*（Miq.）Miq.、蔓生百部 *Stemona japonica*（Bl.）Miq. 或对叶百部 *Stemona tuberosa* Lour. 的干燥块根。主产于安徽、山东、江苏等地。春、秋二季采挖，切厚片，生用或蜜炙用。本品气微，味甘、苦。

Bǎi bù is the dry root tuber of *Stemona sessilifolia* (Miq.) Miq., *Stemona japonica* (Bl.) Miq., or *Stemona tuberosa* Lour., pertaining to the Stemonaceae. Mainly produced in Anhui, Shandong, Jiangsu and some other places, it is collected in spring and autumn, and cut into thick pieces for raw or honey-fried use. *Bǎi bù* is light, sweet and bitter.

【性味归经 / Medicinal properties】

甘、苦，微温。归肺经。

Sweet, bitter and slightly warm; act on the lung meridian.

【主要功效 / Medicinal efficacies】

润肺下气止咳，杀虫灭虱。

Moisten lung, lower qi and relieve cough, kill worms and louses.

【临床应用 / Clinical application】

1. 新久咳嗽，肺痨咳嗽，顿咳　本品甘润苦降，微温不燥，功善润肺下气止咳。凡是咳嗽，无论外感内伤、病程新久、属寒属热皆可配伍应用，尤宜于阴虚痨嗽、小儿顿咳。若治肺痨咳嗽，痰中带血，应配伍阿胶、川贝母、沙参等。若治小儿顿咳，多配伍川贝母、白前、紫菀等。若治风寒咳嗽，常与荆芥、桔梗、陈皮等同用。若治风热咳嗽，可与桑叶、菊花、桔梗等同用。若治气阴两虚之久咳不已，多与黄芪、沙参、麦冬等同用。

(1) New and chronic cough, cough due to lung consumption and whooping cough　Sweet, moistening, bitter and descending, slightly warm but not dry, *bǎi bù* has good actions of moistening the lung, lowering qi and relieving cough. It can be added to treat all coughs, no matter exterior or interior, new or chronic, cold or hot, and it is especially suitable for comsumption cough due to yin deficiency and whooping cough in children. To treat cough due to lung consumption and phlegm with blood, it should be compatible with *ē jiāo* (Corii Asini Colla), *chuān bèi mǔ*, *shā shēn*, etc. To treat whooping cough in children, it is often combined with *chuān bèi mǔ*, *bái qián*, *zǐ wǎn*, etc. To treat wind-cold cough, it often goes with *jīng jiè* (Schizonepetae Herba), *jié gěng*, *chén pí*, etc. To treat wind-heat cough, it can be used together with *sāng yè*, *jú huā*, *jié gěng*, etc. To treat endless chronic cough due to deficiency of both qi and yin, it is frequently combined with *huáng qí* (Astragali Radix), *shā shēn*, *mài dōng*, etc.

2. 头虱体虱，蛲虫病，阴痒　本品有杀虫灭虱之功。用治头虱、体虱及疥癣，可制成20%乙醇液，或50%水煎剂外搽。用治蛲虫病，可单用本品浓煎，睡前保留灌肠。用治阴道滴虫，外阴瘙痒，常配伍蛇床子、苦参等煎汤坐浴外洗。

(2) Head louses, body louses, pinworms and vaginal itching　*Bǎi bù* has the actions of killing worms and louses. To treat head louses, body louses and acariasis, it can be processed into 20% ethanol solution, or 50% water decoction to be applied exteriorly. To treat pinworm diseases, it alone can be processed into thick decoction for retention enema before going to bed. To treat trichomonas vaginalis and pruritus of the genital, it is often compatible with *shé chuáng zǐ* (Cnidii Fructus) and *kǔ shēn* (Sophorae Flavescentis Radix) to be decocted for sitz bath and exterior wash.

【用法用量 / Usage and dosage】

煎服，3~9g。外用适量，水煎或酒浸。润肺止咳宜蜜炙用，杀虫灭虱宜生用。

Decoction, 3~9g. Used externally with appropriate dosage, decocted with water or soaked in water. Suitable for honey-fried use to moisten the lung to relieve cough, and suitable for raw use to kill worms and louses.

【现代研究 / Modern research】

本品主要含百部碱、原百部碱、百部定碱、直立百部碱、对叶百部碱、蔓生百部碱等生物碱，尚含糖类、脂类、蛋白质、有机酸等。具有镇咳、平喘、抑菌、抗病毒、抗真菌、杀蛲虫、灭虱等作用。

Bǎi bù mainly contains alkaloids such as stemonine, protostemonine, stemonidine, sessilistemonine, tuberostemonine and stemonamine, and also contains sugars, lipids, proteins, organic acids and so on. It has the functions of relieving cough, calming panting, resisting bacteria, virus and fungus, killing pinworm and louses, etc.

紫菀　*Zǐ wǎn* (Asteris Radix et Rhizoma)
《神农本草经》
Shen Nong's Classic of the Materia Medica (Shén Nóng Běn Cǎo Jīng)

【来源 / Origin】

为菊科植物紫菀 *Aster tataricus* L.f. 的干燥根和根茎。主产于河南、安徽、黑龙江等地。春、秋二季采挖，切厚片，生用或蜜炙用。本品气微香，味甜、微苦。《中国药典》规定，含紫菀酮（C₃₀H₅₀O）不得少于 0.15%，蜜紫菀不得少于 0.10%。

Zǐ wǎn is the dry root and tuber of *Aster tataricus* L.f., pertainint to the Compositae. Mainly produced in Henan, Anhui and Heilongjiang, it is collected in spring and autumn and cut into thick pieces for raw or honey-fried use. *Zǐ wǎn* is slightly fragrant, sweet and a little bitter. According to *Chinese Pharmacopoeia*, the content of shionone ($C_{30}H_{50}O$) should be no less than 0.15%, and that of stir-fried shionone with honey no less than 0.10%.

【性味归经 / Medicinal properties】

辛、苦，温。归肺经。

Acrid, bitter, and warm; act on the lung meridian.

【主要功效 / Medicinal efficacies】

润肺下气，化痰止咳。

Moisten lung and lower qi, dissolve phlegm and relieve cough.

【临床应用 / Clinical application】

咳嗽有痰　本品辛散苦降，温而不热，主入肺经，善降肺气，开肺郁，化痰浊而止咳。凡是咳嗽，不论外感内伤，寒热虚实，病程长短，皆可用之，尤宜于肺气壅塞，咳嗽痰多，咳痰不爽者。若治风寒咳嗽，咳痰不爽，常配伍荆芥、桔梗、百部等。若治肺热咳嗽，痰多色黄，常与浙贝母、桑白皮、黄芩等同用。若治阴虚久咳，痰中带血，可与阿胶、川贝母等同用。

Cough with phlegm　Acrid, dispering, bitter and descending, warm but not hot, *zǐ wǎn*, mainly entering the lung channel, is good at descending lung qi, opening up lung constraint, and dissolving phlegm turbidity to relieve cough. It can be applied to treat all coughs, no matter exterior or interior, cold or hot, deficient or excess, with a long or short course of disease, and is especially suitable for those with lung qi congestion, cough with profuse phlegm and expectoration with sensation of incompletion. To treat wind-cold cough and expectoration with sensation of incompletion, it is often compatible with *jīng jiè, jié gěng, bǎi bù*, etc. To treat lung-heat cough and profuse yellow phlegm, it is often used together with *zhè bèi mǔ, sāng bái pí, huáng qín*, etc. To treat chronic cough due to yin deficiency and phlegm with blood, it can be combined with *ē jiāo, chuān bèi mǔ*, etc.

【用法用量 / Usage and dosage】

煎服，5~10g。外感暴咳生用，肺虚久咳蜜炙用。

Decoction, 5-10g. Raw use for exogenous sudden cough, and honey-fried use for chronic cough due to lung deficiency.

【现代研究 / Modern research】

本品主要含紫菀皂苷 A~G、紫菀苷、紫菀酮、丁基 –D– 核酮糖苷、槲皮素、无羁萜、表无羁萜醇、紫菀五肽、大黄素、大黄酚以及甾醇、有机酸、挥发油等。具有祛痰、镇咳、平喘、抑菌、抗病毒、抗肿瘤、利尿等作用。

Zǐ wǎn mainly contains astersaponin A-G, asterin, shionone, butyl-D-ribuloside, quercetin, friedelin, epifriedelinol, aster pentapeptide, emodin, chrysophanol and sterol, organic acid, volatile oil, etc. It has the functions of dispelling phlegm, relieving cough, calming panting, resisting bacteria, virus and tumor, promoting urination, etc.

款冬花 *Kuǎn dōng huā* (Farfarae Flos)
《神农本草经》
Shen Nong's Classic of the Materia Medica (Shén Nóng Běn Cǎo Jīng)

【来源 / Origin】

为菊科植物款冬 *Tussilago farfara* L. 的干燥花蕾。主产于内蒙古、甘肃、山西等地。12 月或地冻前花尚未出土时采挖，生用或蜜炙用。本品气香，味微苦而辛。《中国药典》规定，含款冬酮（$C_{23}H_{34}O_5$）不得少于 0.070%。

Kuǎn dōng huā is the dry flower bud of *Tussilago farfara* L., pertaining to the Compositae. Mainly produced in Inner Mongolia Autonomous Region, Gansu, Shanxi and other places, it is excavated in December or before the time when the land is frozen but the flowers are not unearthed yet. Aromatic, slightly bitter but acrid, *kuǎn dōng huā* can be used in the raw or honey-fried form. According to *Chinese Pharmacopoeia*, the content of tussilagone ($C_{23}H_{34}O_5$) should be no less than 0.070%.

【性味归经 / Medicinal properties】

辛、微苦，温。归肺经。

Acrid, slightly bitter and warm; act on the lung meridian.

【主要功效 / Medicinal efficacies】

润肺下气，止咳化痰。

Moisten lung and descend qi, relieve cough and dissolve phlegm.

【临床应用 / Clinical application】

多种咳嗽　本品辛散而润，温而不燥，能润肺降气止咳，兼能化痰，功似紫菀，可广泛用于各种咳嗽，尤宜于肺寒咳嗽。然款冬花长于止咳，紫菀长于化痰，二者配用则止咳化痰之力俱佳。若治寒邪伤肺，久咳不止，常与紫菀相须配用。若治外感风寒，痰饮内停，咳喘痰多，常与麻黄、半夏、细辛等同用。若治肺热咳喘，可与桑白皮、黄芩等同用。若治阴虚燥咳，多与沙参、麦冬等同用。若治肺痈咳吐脓痰，可与鱼腥草、薏苡仁、芦根等同用。

Various kinds of cough　Acrid, dispersing and moistening, warm but not dry, *kuǎn dōng huā* can not only moisten the lung and direct qi downward to relieve cough, but also dissolve phlegm. With similar actions as *zǐ wǎn*, it can be widely applied to treat a variety of coughs, and is especially suitable for lung-cold cough. While *kuǎn dōng huā* is good at relieving cough, *zǐ wǎn* does well in dissolving phlegm. If combined together, the two have a good efficacy of relieving cough and dissolving phlegm. To treat cold pathogen damaging the lung and endless chronic cough, it is often compatible with *zǐ wǎn*. To treat exogenous wind-cold, congestion of fluid-retention and cough and panting with plentiful phlegm, it is often used together with *má huáng*, *bàn xià*, *xì xīn*, etc. To treat lung-heat cough and panting, it can be combined with *sāng bái pí* and *huáng qín*. To treat dryness cough due to yin deficiency, it is frequently used with *shā shēn*, *mài dōng*, etc. To treat lung abscesses and expectoration of thick phlegm, it can go with *yú xīng cǎo*, *yì yǐ rén*, *lú gēn*, etc.

【用法用量 / Usage and dosage】

煎服，5~10g。外感暴咳宜生用，内伤久咳宜蜜炙用。

Decoction, 5-10g. Raw use for exogenous sudden cough, and honey-fried use for chronic cough due to internal damage.

【现代研究 / Modern research】

本品主要含款冬花碱、千里碱、款冬花素、款冬二醇、款冬酮、芸香苷、金丝桃苷、槲皮素以及有机酸、挥发油等。具有镇咳、祛痰、平喘、抗炎、升血压、抗血小板聚集、抗肿瘤等作用。

Kuǎn dōng huā mainly contains tussilagine, senecionine, farfaratine, faradiol, tussilagone, butin, hyperin, quercetin, and organic acid, volatile oil, etc. It has the functions of relieving cough, dispelling phlegm, calming panting, resisting inflammation, raising blood pressure, resisting platelet aggregation and tumor.

桑白皮 *Sāng bái pí* (Mori Cortex)
《神农本草经》
Shen Nong's Classic of the Materia Medica (Shén Nóng Běn Cǎo Jīng)

【来源 / Origin】

为桑科植物桑 *Morus alba* L. 的干燥根皮。主产于安徽、河南、浙江等地。秋末叶落至次春发芽前采挖，切丝，干燥，生用或蜜炙用。本品气微，味微甘。

Sāng bái pí is the dry root-bark of *Morus alba* L., pertaining to the Moraceae. Mainly produced in Anhui, Henan, Zhejiang and other places, it is collected from late autumn when the leaves begin to fall to the next spring before germination, cut into shreds, dried and used raw or honey-fried. It is light and slightly sweet.

【性味归经 / Medicinal properties】

甘，寒。归肺经。

Sweet and cold; act on the lung meridian.

【主要功效 / Medicinal efficacies】

泻肺平喘，利水消肿。

Drain the lung and calming panting, promote urination and diminish swelling.

【临床应用 / Clinical application】

1. **肺热咳喘** 本品性寒入肺经，长于清泻肺火以平喘咳，兼能泻肺中水气。用治肺热咳喘，常与地骨皮、甘草等同用。用治肺虚有热而咳喘气短、潮热盗汗，可与人参、五味子、熟地黄等同用。用治水饮停肺，胀满喘息，多与麻黄、苦杏仁、葶苈子等配伍。

(1) **Lung-heat cough and panting** Entering the lung channel, *sāng bái pí*, cold, is good at draining the lung fire to relieve cough and panting, and draining water pathogen in the lung concurrently. To treat lung-heat cough and panting, it is often combined with *dì gǔ pí* (Lycii Cortex), *gān cǎo*, etc. To treat lung deficiency with heat, cough with shortage of breath, as well as tidal fever and night sweat, it can be used together with *rén shēn*, *wǔ wèi zǐ*, *shú dì huáng*, etc. To treat fluid retention stagnating in the lung, distention and fullness with cough and dyspnea, it is often compatible with *má huáng*, *kǔ xìng rén* (rmeniacae Amarum Semen), *tíng lì zǐ*, etc.

2. **水肿尿少** 本品能泻肺降气，通调水道而利水消肿。用治全身面目肌肤浮肿，胀满喘急，小便不利者，常与茯苓皮、大腹皮、陈皮等同用。

(2) **Edema with little urine** *Sāng bái pí* can drain the lung and dissolve phlegm, as well as free and regulate the waterways to promote urination and diminish swelling. To treat those with general edema, distention and fullness with dyspnea, as well as disturbance of urination, it is often used together

with *fú líng pí* (Poriae Cutis), *dà fù pí* (Arecae Pericarpium), *chén pí*, etc.

【用法用量 / Usage and dosage】

煎服，6~12g。肺虚咳喘宜蜜炙用，其他宜生用。

Decoction, 6-12g. Suitable for honey-fried use for cough and panting due to lung deficiency, and suitable for raw use for other aspects.

【现代研究 / Modern research】

本品主要含桑根皮素、环桑根皮素、桑皮素、桑皮色烯素、伞形花内酯、东莨菪素、东莨菪内酯等，尚含多糖、鞣质、挥发油等。具有镇咳、平喘、祛痰、利尿、降血压、降血糖、镇静、抗惊厥、镇痛、抑菌、抗肿瘤等作用。

Sāng bái pí mainly contains morusin, cy-omorusin, mulberrin, mulberrochromene, umbelliferone, scopoletin, scopoletin, etc. It also contains polysaccharide, tannin and essential oil. It has the functions of relieving cough and panting, dispelling phlegm, promoting urination, lowering blood pressure and blood sugar, calming the mind, resisting convulsion, relieving pain, resisting bacteria and tumor, etc.

葶苈子　*Tíng lì zǐ* (Descurainiae Semen; Lepidii Semen)
《神农本草经》
Shen Nong's Classic of the Materia Medica (Shén Nóng Běn Cǎo Jīng)

【来源 / Origin】

为十字花科植物播娘蒿 *Descurainia sophia*（L.）Webb. ex Prantl. 或独行菜 *Lepidium apetalum* Willd. 的干燥成熟种子。前者习称"南葶苈"，主产于江苏、山东、安徽等地；后者习称"北葶苈"，主产于河北、辽宁、内蒙古等地。夏季果实成熟时采收，晒干，生用或炒用。《中国药典》规定，本品含槲皮素–O–β–D–葡萄糖–7–O–β–D–龙胆双糖苷（$C_{33}H_{40}O_{22}$）不得少于 0.075%。

Tíng lì zǐ is the dry ripe seed of *Descurainia sophia* (L.) Webb. ex Prantl. or *Lepidium apetalum* Willd., pertaining to the Cruciferae. The former, also known as *nán tíng lì*, is mainly produced in Jiangsu, Shandong, and Anhui; while the latter, commonly known as *běi tíng lì*, is mainly produced in Hebei, Liaoning, and Inner Mongolia Autonomous Region and other places. It is collected in summer when the fruit ripens, dried in the sun, and used in raw or dry-fried form. According to *Chinese Pharmacopoeia*, the content of quercetin-3-O-β-D-glucose-7-O-β-D-gentiobioside ($C_{33}H_{40}O_{22}$) should be no less than 0.075%.

【性味归经 / Medicinal properties】

辛、苦，大寒。归肺、膀胱经。

Acrid, bitter and extremely cold; act on the lung and bladder meridians.

【主要功效 / Medicinal efficacies】

泻肺平喘，行水消肿。

Drain the lung and relieve panting, move water and diminish swelling.

【临床应用 / Clinical application】

1. 痰涎壅盛，喘咳痰多，不得平卧　本品苦泄辛散，性寒清热，善泻肺中水饮及痰火而平喘咳，适用于痰涎壅盛，喘咳痰多，胸胁胀满，不得平卧，常佐大枣以缓其性，临床常与苏子、桑白皮、苦杏仁等同用。若治痰热壅肺之咳嗽咳痰、喘息胸闷，常与石膏、蜜麻黄、白果等同用。

(1) Congestion and exuberance of phlegm-drool, cough and panting with profuse phlegm, and inability to lie flat　With bitterness to discharge and acridity to disperse, *tíng lì zǐ*, cold and heat-clearing, is good at draining fluid retention and phlegm fire in the lung so as to relieve cough and panting, and thus is suitable for congestion and exuberance of phlegm-drool, cough and panting with profuse phlegm, distention and fullness in the chest and rib-side, and inability to lie flat. In such a case, it is often assistant by *dà zǎo* (Jujubae Fructus) to make it milder, and clinically is often used together with *sū zǐ*, *sāng bái pí*, *kǔ xìng rén*, etc. To treat cough and expectoration due to phlegm-heat obstructing the lung, cough, dyspnea and chest oppression, it is often combined with *shí gāo*, *mì má huáng* (Herba Ephedrae Emllita), *bái guǒ*, etc.

2. 水肿，胸腹积水　本品善泄肺气之壅闭而通调水道，利水消肿。用治肺气壅闭，水饮停聚，水肿胀满，小便不利，常配伍牵牛子、茯苓皮、大腹皮等。用治湿热内阻之腹水肿满，常与防己、椒目、大黄等同用。用治痰热结胸之胸胁积水，多与苦杏仁、大黄、芒硝等同用。

(2) Edema and thoracoabdominal fluid accumulation　Being good at discharging congestion and blockage of lung qi, *tíng lì zǐ* can free and regulate the waterways, promote urination and diminish swelling. To teat congestion and blockage of lung qi, fluid retention and accumation, edema, distention and fullness, as well as disturbance of urination, it is often compatible with *qiān niú zǐ* (Pharbitidis Semen), *fú líng pí*, *dà fù pí*, etc. To treat abdominal dropsy as well as swelling and fullness due to internal obstruction of dampness-heat, it is often used together with *fáng jǐ* (Stephaniae Tetrandrae Radix), *jiāo mù* (Zanthoxyli Semen), *dà huáng* (Rhei Radix et Rhizoma), etc. To treat fluid accumulation in the chest and rib-side due to phlegm-heat binding chest, it is often combined with *kǔ xìng rén*, *dà huáng*, *máng xiāo* (Natrii Sulfas), etc.

【用法用量 / Usage and dosage】

煎服，3~10g，包煎。

Decoction, 3-10g, decocted while wrapped.

【现代研究 / Modern research】

本品主要含槲皮素 –3–*O*–β–D– 葡萄糖 –7–*O*–β–D– 龙胆双糖苷、槲皮素、强心苷、挥发油、脂肪油、芥子苷、蛋白质、糖类等。具有强心、利尿、抑菌、抗癌等作用。

It mainly contains quercetin-3-*O*-β-D-glucose-7-*O*-β-D-gentiobioside, quercetin, cardiac glycosides, essential oil, fat oil, glucosinolate, protein, carbohydrate, and so on. It has the functions of tonifying the heart, promoting urination, resisting bacteria and cancer, etc.

白果　*Bái guǒ* (Ginkgo Semen)

《日用本草》

Household Materia Medica (Rì Yòng Běn Cǎo)

【来源 / Origin】

为银杏科植物银杏 *Ginkgo biloba* L. 的干燥成熟种子。主产于河南、四川、广西等地。秋季采收，生用或炒用，用时捣碎。本品气微，味甘、微苦。

Bái guǒ is the dry ripen seed of *Ginkgo biloba* L., pertaining to the Ginkgoaceae. Mainly produced in Henan, Sichuan Province, Guangxi Zhuang Autonomous Region and other places, it is collected in autumn, and used in raw or dry-fried form, crushed for use. It is light, sweet and slightly bitter.

【性味归经 / Medicinal properties】

甘、苦、涩，平；有毒。归肺、肾经。

Sweet, bitter, acrid and neutral; toxic; act on the lung and kidney meridians.

【主要功效 / Medicinal efficacies】

敛肺定喘，止带缩尿。

Astringe lung and relieve panting, arrest vaginal discharge and reduce urination.

【临床应用 / Clinical application】

1. 哮喘痰嗽　本品涩敛苦降，入肺经，善敛肺降气而定喘，兼可化痰，为治哮喘痰嗽常用之品。用治外感风寒引发的哮喘痰嗽，常配伍麻黄、甘草等。用治内有蕴热、复感风寒之喘咳痰多黄稠，常与麻黄、黄芩、桑白皮等同用。用治肺肾两虚之虚喘，常与五味子、胡桃肉等同用。用治肺热燥咳，喘咳无痰，多与天冬、麦冬、款冬花等同用。

(1) **Asthma and cough with phlegm**　Astringent, bitter and descending, *bái guǒ*, entering the lung channel, is adept at astringing the lung and directing qi downward so as to relieve panting, with the concurrent function of dissolving phlegm as well, and thus a common drug to treat asthma and cough with phlegm. To treat asthma and cough with phlegm due to exogenous wind-cold, it is often compatible with *má huáng*, *gān cǎo*, etc. To treat asthma and cough with profuse yellow and thick phlegm due to internal heat and complex wind-cold, it is often used together with *má huáng*, *huáng qín*, *sāng bái pí*, etc. To treat deficiency-type panting due to deficiency of lung and kidney, it is often combined with *wǔ wèi zǐ*, *hú táo ròu* (Juglans regia L.), etc. To treat lung-heat dryness cough and asthma and cough without phlegm, it is often used together with *tiān dōng* (Asparagi Radix), *mài dōng*, *kuǎn dōng huā*, etc.

2. 带下，白浊，尿频，遗尿　本品苦涩收敛，具有收涩止带、固肾缩尿之功，兼能化湿浊。用治脾肾亏虚之带下清稀量多，常与山药、莲子、芡实等同用。用治湿热带下，色黄腥臭，常配伍芡实、黄柏、车前子等。用治小便白浊，可与萆薢、益智仁等同用。用治肾虚不固之遗精、尿频、遗尿，多与熟地黄、山茱萸、覆盆子等同用。

(2) **Leucorrhea, gonorrhea, frequent micturition and enuresis**　Bitter and astringent, *bái guǒ* has the functions of rescuing from astringency and arresting vaginal discharge, tonifying the kidney and reducing urination, and removing damp-turbidity concurrently. To treat clear and abundant vaginal discharge due to depletion of spleen and kidney, it is often used together with *shān yào* (Dioscoreae Rhizoma), *lián zǐ* (Nelumbinis Semen), *qiàn shí* (Euryales Semen), etc. To treat yellow and stinking damp-heat leucorrhea, it is often compatible with *qiàn shí*, *huáng bó* (Phellodendri Chinensis Cortex), *chē qián zǐ* (Plantaginis Semen), etc. To treat gonorrhea, it can be combined with *bì xiè* (Dioscoreae Hypoglaucae Rhizoma), *yì zhì rén* (Alpiniae Oxyphyllae Fructus), etc. To treat seminal emission, frequent micturition and enuresis due to kidney deficiency and insecurity, it is often used with *shú dì huáng*, *shān zhū yú* (Corni Fructus), *fù pén zǐ* (Rubi Fructus), etc.

【用法用量 / Usage and dosage】

煎服，5~10g。

Decoction, 5-10g.

【使用注意 / Precaution】

用量不宜过大，小儿尤当注意。

The dosage should not be too large. It should be used with caution especially for children.

【现代研究 / Modern research】

本品主要含山奈黄素、槲皮素、芦丁、白果素、银杏素、银杏内酯 A、银杏内酯 C、白果酸、银杏毒素、白果酚、白果醇等。具有平喘、祛痰、抑菌、降血压、降血脂、抗衰老、抗氧化等作用。

Bái guǒ mainly contains kaempferol, quercetin, rutin, bilobetin, ginkgetin, ginkgolide A, ginkgolide C, ginkgolic acid, ginkgotoxin, bilobol, ginnol and so on. It has the functions of relieving panting, dispelling phlegm, resisting bacteria, lowering blood pressure and blood lipid, resisting aging and oxidation, etc.

其他化痰止咳平喘药功用介绍见表18-1。

The efficacies of other phlegm-dissolving, cough and panting-relieving medicinals are shown in table 18-1.

表 18-1　其他化痰止咳平喘药功用介绍

分类	药物	药性	功效	应用	用法用量
温化寒痰药	白前	辛、苦,微温。归肺经	降气,祛痰,止咳	肺气壅实,咳嗽痰多,胸满喘急	煎服,3~10g
	皂荚	辛、咸,温;有小毒。归肺、大肠经	祛痰开窍,散结消肿	顽痰喘咳,咳痰不爽;中风,癫痫;痈疽肿毒	多入丸、散,1~1.5g。外用适量,研末吹鼻取嚏或研末调敷患处
清化热痰药	竹沥	甘,寒。归心、肺、肝经	清热豁痰,定惊利窍	痰热咳喘;中风痰迷,惊痫癫狂	冲服,30~50ml
	天竺黄	甘,寒。归心、肝经	清热豁痰,清心定惊	热病神昏,中风痰迷;小儿痰热惊痫,抽搐,夜啼	煎服,3~9g
	胖大海	甘,寒。归肺、大肠经	清热润肺,利咽开音,润肠通便	肺热声哑,咽喉干痛,干咳无痰;热结便秘,头痛目赤	2~3枚,沸水泡服或煎服
	海藻	苦、咸,寒。归肝、胃、肾经	消痰软坚散结,利水消肿	瘿瘤、瘰疬、睾丸肿痛;痰饮水肿	煎服,6~12g。不宜与甘草同用
	昆布	咸,寒。归肝、胃、肾经	消痰软坚散结,利水消肿	瘿瘤、瘰疬、睾丸肿痛;痰饮水肿	煎服,6~12g
	黄药子	苦,寒;有毒。归肺、肝、心经	化痰散结消瘿,清热凉血解毒	瘿瘤;疮疡肿毒,咽喉肿痛,毒蛇咬伤	煎服,5~15g;研末服,1~2g。外用适量。肝、肾功能损伤者慎用
清化热痰药	海蛤壳	苦、咸,寒。归肺、肾、胃经	清热化痰,软坚散结,制酸止痛;外用收湿敛疮	痰热咳喘;瘿瘤,瘰疬;胃痛吞酸;外治湿疮,烧烫伤	煎服,6~15g,先煎,蛤粉包煎。外用适量
	海浮石	咸,寒。归肺、肾经	清肺化痰,软坚散结,利尿通淋	痰热咳喘;瘰疬,瘿瘤;血淋、石淋	煎服,10~15g,打碎先煎
	瓦楞子	咸,平。归肺、胃、肝经	消痰化瘀,软坚散结,制酸止痛	顽痰胶结,瘿瘤,瘰疬;癥瘕痞块,胃痛泛酸	煎服,9~15g,先煎
	礞石	甘、咸,平。归肺、心、肝经	坠痰下气,平肝镇惊	气逆喘急,癫狂,惊痫	多入丸、散,3~6g;煎服,10~15g,布包先煎

续表

题库

分类	药物	药性	功效	应用	用法用量
止咳平喘药	枇杷叶	苦,微寒。归肺、胃经	清肺止咳,降逆止呕	肺热咳喘;胃热呕吐,烦热口渴	煎服,6~10g
	洋金花	辛,温;有毒。归肺、肝经	平喘止咳,解痉定痛	哮喘咳嗽,脘腹冷痛,风湿痹痛,小儿慢惊,癫痫,外科麻醉	0.3~0.6g,宜入丸、散。外用适量。孕妇、外感及痰热咳喘、青光眼、高血压及心动过速患者禁用

（张　艳）

第十九章　安　神　药
Chapter 19　Mind-calming medicinals

学习目标 ┊ Learning goals

1. **掌握**　安神药在性能、功效、主治、配伍及使用注意方面的共性；朱砂、龙骨、磁石、酸枣仁、柏子仁及远志的性能、功效、应用以及特殊的用法用量和特殊的使用注意。

2. **熟悉**　安神药的分类；琥珀、首乌藤的功效、主治以及特殊的用法用量和特殊的使用注意。

3. **了解**　安神药、重镇安神药及养心安神药功效术语的含义；珍珠、合欢皮的功效以及特殊的用法用量和特殊的使用注意。

1. Master the commonness of mind-calming medicinals in efficacy, indications, property, compatibility and cautions; as well as the property, efficacy, application, special usage and dosage and special precautions of *zhū shā, lóng gǔ, cí shí, suān zǎo rén, bǎi zǐ rén* and *yuǎn zhì*.

2. Familiar with the classification of mind-calming medicinals; and the efficacy, indications, special usage, dosage and special precautions of *hǔ pò* and *shǒu wū téng*.

3. Understand the definitions of mind-calming medicinals, heavy-sedative mind-calming medicinals, heart-nourishing and mind-calming medicinals; and the efficacy, special usage and dosage and special precautions of *zhēn zhū* and *hé huān pí*.

凡以安定神志为主要功效，常用于治疗心神不宁病证的药物，称为安神药。

Medicinals with the major efficacy of tranquilizing the (conscious) mind and commonly used for the treatment of restless heart disease are known as mind-calming medicinals.

安神药主入心、肝经，具有镇惊安神或养心安神之效。主治心悸、怔忡、失眠、多梦、健忘等心神不宁病证，亦可治疗惊风、癫痫、癫狂等心神失常。部分药物兼能平肝潜阳、纳气平喘、清热解毒、敛汗、活血、润肠、祛痰等，又可用治肝阳上亢、肾虚气喘、疮疡肿毒、自汗盗汗、瘀血阻滞、肠燥便秘、痰多咳喘等。

Acting on the liver and heart meridians, their major efficacies are to calm the mind with heavy sedatives or nourish the heart and calm the mind. They are mainly indicated to treat palpitations or severe palpitations, insomnia and profuse dreaming, convulsive epilepsy and mania. Some medicinals also have the efficacies of calming the liver and subduing yang, improving qi reception and relieving panting, treat ascendant hyperactivity of liver yang panting due to kidney deficiency and clearing heat and resolving toxins, invigorating blood, astringing sweating, moistening the intestines, and dispelling phlegm. Some can also treat hyperactivity of liver yang, asthma due to kidney deficiency, sores and ulcers with swelling and toxins, stagnation of blood stasis, spontaneous sweating and night sweating, constipation due to intestinal dryness, cough and panting with excessive phlegm.

根据安神药的药性及功效主治差异，可分为重镇安神药及养心安神药两类。

According to the different medicinal properties and efficacies, they are classified into two categories: heavy-sedative mind-calming medicinals and heart-nourishing and mind-calming medicinals.

应用安神药时，应根据病因、病机的不同，选用并配伍适宜的安神药。若因心火亢盛、肝郁化火、痰热内扰、肝阳上亢、痰扰心神，应选用重镇安神药，同时配伍清泻心火、清肝泻火、平肝潜阳、祛痰开窍药。若因心肝血虚阴亏、心脾两虚或心肾不交，应选用养心安神药，同时配伍补血养阴、补益心脾和滋阴降火、交通心肾之品。此外，对于癫狂、痫证、惊风等，则以化痰开窍或平肝息风药为主，本类药物多作辅助药。

Mind-calming medicinals should be appropriately selected to use according to different disease causes and pathogenesis, and correspondingly combined with other medicinals. For those with hyperactivity of heart fire, stagnation of liver qi, internal disturbance of phlegm heat, hyperactivity of liver yang, and disturbance of heart and mind by phlegm, the heavy-sedative mind-calming medicinals should be selected and combined with the medicinals of clearing heart and liver fire, calming liver yang, removing phlegm and opening up the orifices; for those with deficiency of heart and liver, blood and yin deficiency, deficiency of heart and spleen, or failure of intercourse between heart and kidney, heart-nourishing and mind-calming medicinals should be selected and combined with the ones of nourishing blood and yin, tonifying heart and spleen, nourishing yin to subdue fire, and intercoursing heart and kidney; as for epilepsy and convulsion, they are mainly treated with phlegm-dissolving and orifices-opening medicinals or liver-calming and wind extinguishing medicinals, and medicinals in this category are only the auxiliary ones.

使用本类药物特别是矿石类重镇安神药及有毒药物，入汤剂必须先煎，且只宜暂用，不可久服，应中病即止。矿石类安神药，如作丸、散剂服用，须配伍养胃健脾之品，以免伤胃耗气。

Mind-calming medicinals, especially minerals for heavy-sedative mind-calming and the toxic ones, should be decocted first and not suitable for long-term oral use. If mineral medicinals are made into pills or powder, they should be appropriately combined with stomach-nourishing and spleen-fortifying medicinals in order to avoid damage to the stomach and consuming qi.

第一节　重镇安神药

Section 1　Heavy-sedative mind-calming medicinals

PPT

本类药物多为矿石、化石和介类药物，具有质重沉降之性，重则能镇，重可去怯，以镇安心神、平惊定志、平肝潜阳等为主要功效。主治心火炽盛、阳气躁动、痰火扰心、肝郁化火及惊吓等引起的心悸、失眠、多梦等心神不宁之实证。惊风、癫狂、痫证以及肝阳上亢等亦可选用本类药物。

Most of heavy-sedative mind-calming medicinals are minerals, fossils and intermediates, which have the properties of heavy subsidence. Heavy weight can control and relieve timidity, with the main effects of calming the mind and the nerves and calming down the liver yang. It is mainly used to treat palpitation, insomnia and profuse dreaming caused by heartburn, yang agitation, phlegm and fire disturbing the heart, liver depression transforming into fire and fright. They can also be selected to treat convulsion, mania, epilepsy and hyperactivity of liver yang.

朱砂　*Zhū shā* (Cinnabaris)
《神农本草经》
Shen Nong's Classic of the Materia Medica (Shén Nóng Běn Cǎo Jīng)

【来源 / Origin】

为硫化物类矿物辰砂族辰砂，主含硫化汞（HgS）。主产于湖南、贵州、四川等地，传统以产于古之辰州（今湖南沅陵）者为道地药材。随时可采，除去杂石和泥沙，研细水飞，晾干或40℃以下干燥。本品气微，味淡。《中国药典》规定，含硫化汞不得少于96%，朱砂粉不得少于98.0%。

Zhū shā is the cinnabar of the sulfide minerals, pertaining to Cinnabaris. It mainly contains mercury sulfide (HgS) and mainly produced in Hunan, Guizhou, and Sichuan provinces in China. Traditionally, the genuine one is produced in ancient Chenzhou (now Yuanling, Hunan Province). It can be mined at any time and purified to remove the stones and sands. It is refined into powder with water, and then dried in the sun or dry under 40 ℃. It has slight odor and is bland in taste. According to *Chinese Pharmacopoeia*, the content of mercury sulfide should be no less than 96%, cinnabaris powder should not be less than 98.0%.

【性味归经 / Medicinal properties】

甘，微寒；有毒。归心经。

Sweet, slightly cold and toxic; act on the heart meridian.

【主要功效 / Medicinal efficacies】

清心镇惊，安神，明目，解毒。

Clear heart heat and suppress fright; calm the mind; improve vision and resolve toxin.

【临床应用 / Clinical application】

1. **心悸易惊，失眠多梦**　本品甘寒质重，专入心经，长于镇惊安神，可用治各种原因所致的心神不宁病证。因其性寒，又长于清泻心火以安神，故尤宜于心火亢盛，内扰神明之心神不宁、惊悸怔忡、烦躁不眠，常与黄连、甘草等同用。治心火亢盛，阴血不足之失眠多梦、心中烦热、心悸怔忡，常与当归、地黄等同用。本品安神效佳，随证配伍亦用治心血虚、心阴虚、心气虚等心神不宁之虚证。

(1) **Palpitations (due to fright), insomnia and profuse dreaming**　With the nature of cold and heavy and acting on the heart meridian, it is good at suppressing fright and calming the mind. It can be used to treat the restless disease caused by various reasons. Because of its cold nature, it is also good at clearing and purging heart fire to calm nerves. Therefore, it is particularly suitable for those with restlessness of heart-spirit, palpitations due to fright, severe palpitations, vexation and agitation, and insomnia due to hyperactivity of heart fire, and it is usually combined with *huáng lián* and *gān cǎo*; to treat insomnia and profuse dreaming, vexing heat in the heart, and palpitation due to hyperactivity of heart fire and yin deficiency, it is often combined with *dāng guī* and *dì huáng*. It has a good calming effect and can also be used to treat the deficiency of heart and blood, heart yin and heart qi deficiency in combination with other medicinals.

2. **惊风，癫痫**　本品性寒质重，具有清热镇惊止痉之功。用治温热病，热入心包或痰热内闭，高热烦躁，神昏谵语，惊厥抽搐，常与牛黄、麝香等同用。用治癫痫，卒昏抽搐，常与磁石同用。用治小儿高热惊风，常与牛黄、全蝎、钩藤等同用。

(2) Epilepsy and infantile convulsions With the nature of cold and heavy weight, it has the efficacy of clearing heat to suppress fright. To treat high fever, loss of consciousness, and convulsion in warm febrile disease due to heat entering the pericardium or phlegm-heat internal block, it is often combined with *niú huáng* (Calculus Bovis) and *shè xiāng* (Moschus); to treat epilepsy with sudden syncope and convulsion, it is often used with *cí shí*; to treat infantile convulsion due to high fever, it is used with *niú huáng*, *quán xiē* (Scorpio) and *gōu téng* (Uncariae Cum Uncis Ramulus).

3. 疮疡肿毒，咽痛口疮　本品性寒，不论内服、外用，均有清热解毒作用。用治疮疡肿毒，红肿热痛，常与雄黄、山慈菇、大戟等同用。用治咽喉肿痛，牙龈肿痛，口舌生疮，常与冰片、硼砂等同用。

(3) Aphtha, throat *bì* (pharyngitis), sore and ulcers with swelling and toxin With the nature of cold, it can be used internally and externally to clear heat and resolve toxin. To treat sore and ulcers with swelling and toxin, it is usually combined with *xióng huáng* (Realgar), *shān cí gū* (Cremastrae seu Pleiones Pseudobulbus) and *dà jǐ* (Euphorbiae Pekinensis Radix); to treat aphtha, throat *bì* (pharyngitis), swelling in the gum, it is often combined with *bīng piàn* and *péng shā* (Borax).

4. 视物昏花　本品微寒，可清心降火，明目。用治心肾不交之视物昏花，耳鸣耳聋，心悸失眠，常与磁石、神曲同用。

(4) Blurred vision With the nature of slightly cold, it can clear and purge heart fire to improve eyesight. To treat blurred vision, tinnitus and deafness, palpitation and insomnia due to failure of the heart and kidney to interact, it is often combined with *cí shí* and *shén qū* (Medicata Fermentata Massa).

【用法用量 / Usage and dosage】

内服，只宜入丸、散服，0.1~0.5g，不宜入煎剂。外用适量。

It is usually made into pills or powder for oral use, 0.1-0.5g, it should not be decocted. An appropriate amount is used externally.

【使用注意 / Precaution】

不宜大量服用，也不宜少量久服。孕妇及肝功能不全者禁用。

It should not be taken in a large dosage or small dosage for a long time. It should be contraindicated for patients with liver insufficiency and pregnant women.

【现代研究 / Modern research】

本品主要含硫化汞，尚含铅、钡、镁、铁、锌等多种微量元素及雄黄、磷灰石、沥青质、氧化铁等杂质。具有降低中枢神经兴奋性、镇静、催眠、抗惊厥、抗心律失常等作用。

It mainly contains mercury sulfide. In addition, it also contains lead, barium, magnesium, iron, zinc and other trace elements as well as realgar, apatite, asphaltene, iron oxide and other impurities. It has the functions of reducing central nervous excitability, sedation, hypnosis, anticonvulsion, antiarrhythmia, etc.

磁石　*Cí shí* (Magnetitum)

《神农本草经》

Shen Nong's Classic of the Materia Medica (Shén Nóng Běn Cǎo Jīng)

【来源 / Origin】

为氧化物类矿物尖晶石族磁铁矿，主含四氧化三铁（Fe_3O_4）。主产于河北、山东、辽宁等地。随时可采，砸碎，生用或煅用。本品具磁性，有土腥气，味淡。《中国药典》规定，含铁（Fe）

不得少于 50.0%，煅磁石不得少于 45%。

Cí shí is the magnetite of the oxide mineral, pertaining to the Spinel family. Mainly produced in Hebei, Shandong and Liaoning Province in China, it is mined and smashed, used in the raw form or calcined. It is magnetic, and is earthy and bland in taste. According to *Chinese Pharmacopoeia*, the iron content (Fe) should be no less than 50.0%, the iron content of calcined magnetite is not more than 48%.

【性味归经 / Medicinal properties】

咸，寒。归心、肝、肾经。

Salty and cold; act on the heart, liver and kidney meridians.

【主要功效 / Medicinal efficacies】

镇惊安神，平肝潜阳，聪耳明目，纳气平喘。

Suppress fright and calm the mind; calm the liver and subdue yang; improve hearing and vision; improve reception and relieve panting.

【临床应用 / Clinical application】

1. **心神不宁，惊悸失眠，癫痫** 本品质重沉降，性寒清热，入心、肝、肾经，既能清泻心肝之火，镇惊安神，又兼益肾滋阴。为护真阴、镇浮阳、安神志之佳品。主治肾虚肝旺，肝火上炎，扰动心神或惊恐气乱，神不守舍之心神不宁，惊悸失眠等，常与朱砂、神曲同用。若治痰浊蒙蔽心窍之癫狂，可与牛黄、远志等同用。

(1) **Restlessness of heart spirit, palpitation, insomnia and epilepsy** With the nature of heavy and cold, clearing heat and entering the heart, liver and kidney meridians, it can not only clear the fire of heart and liver, suppress fright and calm the mind but also benefit the kidney and yin. It is a good medicinal for protecting real yin, controlling floating yang and calming the mind. To treat kidney deficiency and liver hyperactivity, liver fire flaming upward and harassing the heart spirit, or fright with chaotic qi, and mental derangement manifested as restlessness of heart spirit, palpitation due to fright and insomnia, it is often combined with *zhū shā, shén qū* (Medicata Fermentata Massa); to treat epilepsy due to turbid phlegm blinds the mind, it is usually combined with *niú huáng* and *yuǎn zhì*.

2. **肝阳上亢，头晕目眩** 本品入肝、肾经，既能平肝阳，又能益肾阴。用治肝阳上亢之头晕目眩、急躁易怒等证，常与石决明、珍珠、牡蛎等同用。治阴虚甚者，可与生地黄、白芍、龟甲等同用；治热甚者，可与钩藤、菊花、夏枯草等同用。

(2) **Ascendant hyperactivity of liver yang with dizziness** It can not only calm the liver yang, but also benefit the kidney yin. To treat dizziness and irascibility due to ascendant hyperactivity of liver yang, it is often combined with *shí jué míng* (Haliotidis Concha), *zhēn zhū* (Margarita) and *mǔ lì* (Ostreae Concha); for those accompanied by more evident yin deficiency, it is often combined with *shēng dì huáng*, *bái sháo* and *guī jiǎ*; for those accompanied by more evident heat, it is usually combined with *gōu téng*, *jú huā* and *xià kū cǎo* (Prunellae Spica).

3. **耳鸣耳聋，视物昏花** 本品益肾阴，有聪耳明目之功。用治肾虚耳鸣、耳聋，多配伍熟地黄、山茱萸、山药等。用治肝肾不足、目暗不明、视物昏花，可配伍枸杞子、女贞子、菊花等。

(3) **Tinnitus and deafness, blurred vision** It can benefit kidney yin to improve hearing and vision. To treat tinnitus and deafness caused by kidney deficiency, it is often combined with *shú dì huáng*, *shān zhū yú* and *shān yào*; to treat blurred vision due to deficiency of liver and kidney, it is often combined with *gǒu qǐ zǐ*, *nǚ zhēn zǐ* (Ligustri Lucidi Fructus) and *jú huā*.

4. **肾虚气喘** 本品有益肾纳气平喘之功。用治肾气不足、摄纳无权之虚喘，常与五味子、胡桃肉、蛤蚧等同用。

(4) Panting due to kidney deficiency It can benefit kidney yin, improve reception and relieve panting. To treat deficiency-type panting due to kidney qi depletion and failure to receive sent down form the lung, it is usually combined with *wǔ wèi zǐ* (Schisandrae Chinensis Fructus), *hú táo ròu* and *gé jiè* (Gecko).

【用法用量 / Usage and dosage】

煎服，9~30g，先煎。入丸、散，每次 1~3g。

Decoction, 9-30g, it should be decocted first, or it is made into pills or powder for use, 1~3g each time.

【使用注意 / Precaution】

入丸、散不可多服。脾胃虚弱者慎用。

It can not be taken with overdosage when it is made into pills and powder.It should be used with caution for patients with weakness of the spleen and stomach.

【现代研究 / Modern research】

本品主要含四氧化三铁（Fe_3O_4），尚含钙、镁、钾、钠、铬、锰、镉、铜、锌、砷等微量元素。具有抑制中枢神经系统、镇静、催眠、抗惊厥、抗炎、镇痛等作用。

It mainly contains Fe_3O_4 and also contains calcium, magnesium, potassium, sodium, chromium, manganese, cadmium, copper, zinc, arsenic and other trace elements. It has the functions of inhibiting the central nervous system, sedation, hypnosis, anticonvulsion, anti-inflammatory and analgesic.

龙骨　*Lóng gǔ* (Draconis Os)
《神农本草经》
Shen Nong's Classic of the Materia Medica (Shén Nóng Běn Cǎo Jīng)

【来源 / Origin】

为古代大型哺乳动物象类、三趾马类、犀类、鹿类、牛类等骨骼的化石。主产于山西、内蒙古、河南等地。全年可采，生用或煅用。本品无臭，无味。

Lóng gǔ is the skeletal fossil of ancient large mammals, such as elephant, hippopotamus, rhinoceros, deer and oxen. Mainly produced in Shanxi Province, Inner Mongolia Autonomous Region and Henan Province in China, it can be collected all year round, used in the raw form or the calcined form. It has no odor and no flavor.

【性味归经 / Medicinal properties】

甘、涩，平。归心、肝、肾经。

Sweet, astringent and neutral; act on the heart, liver and kidney meridians.

【主要功效 / Medicinal efficacies】

镇惊安神，平肝潜阳，收敛固涩。

Suppress fright and calm the mind; calm the liver and subdue yang; astringe and consolidate essence.

【临床应用 / Clinical application】

1. 心神不宁，心悸失眠，惊痫癫狂　本品质重，入心、肝经，善镇心定惊安神，为治疗心神不宁的常用药。用治心神不宁，心悸失眠，健忘多梦等，可与朱砂、石菖蒲、酸枣仁等同用。用治痰热内盛，惊痫抽搐，癫狂发作等，多与牛黄、胆南星、钩藤等配伍。

(1) Restlessness, palpitations and insomnia, convulsive epilepsy and mania With the nature of heavy and acting on the heart and liver meridians, it is good at calming the heart and mind. It is a common medicine for the treatment of restlessness of heart spirit. To treat restlessness, palpitation, insomnia, forgetfulness, profuse dreaming, it is usually combined with *zhū shā*, *shí chāng pú* (Acori Tatarinowii Rhizoma) and *suān zǎo rén*; to treat convulsive epilepsy, tics and mania attack due to internal exuberance of phlegm-heat, it is often combined with *niú huáng* (Calculus Bovis), *dǎn nán xīng* (Arisaema cum Bile) and *gōu téng*.

2. 肝阳上亢，头晕目眩　本品入肝经，质重沉降，有较强的平肝潜阳作用。用治肝阴不足，肝阳上亢所致的头晕目眩、烦躁易怒等症，常与赭石、生牡蛎、生白芍等同用。

(2) **Ascendant hyperactivity of liver yang with dizziness**　Acting on the liver meridian and heavy, it has strong efficacy of calming the liver and subduing yang. To treat ascendant hyperactivity of liver yang with dizziness due to liver yin deficiency, fidgety and irritation, it is usually combined with *zhě shí* (Haematitum), *mǔ lì* (Ostreae Concha) and *bái sháo*.

3. 滑脱诸证　本品味涩能敛，有收敛固涩之功。凡遗精、滑精、尿频、遗尿、崩漏、带下、自汗、盗汗等多种正虚滑脱之证，皆可用之。若治肾虚遗精、滑精，常与芡实、沙苑子、牡蛎等配伍。若治心肾两虚，小便频数，常与桑螵蛸、龟甲、茯神等配伍。若治气虚不摄，冲任不固之崩漏，可与黄芪、海螵蛸、五倍子等同用。若治表虚自汗，阴虚盗汗，常与黄芪、牡蛎、五味子等配伍。若治大汗不止，脉微欲绝之亡阳证，可与牡蛎、人参、附子等同用。

(3) **Loss and desertion syndrome**　With the nature of astringent, it has the functions of astringing and consolidating essence. It can be used for many kinds of loss and desertion syndrome, such as seminal emission, spontaneous seminal emission, frequent urination, enuresis, metrorrhagia(*bēng lòu*), hypodermia, spontaneous sweating and night sweating, etc. To treat seminal emission and spontaneous seminal emission, it is often combined with *qiàn shí* (Euryales Semen), *shā yuàn zǐ* (Astragali Complanati Semen) and *mǔ lì*; to treat frequent micturition and enuresis due to deficiency of both the heart and kidney, it is often combined with *sāng piāo xiāo*, *guī jiǎ* and *fú líng* (Poria); to treat metrorrhagia and leucorrhea due to deficiency qi falling to control and insecurity of the Chong and Ren mai, it is often combined with *huáng qí*, *hǎi piāo xiāo* and *wǔ bèi zǐ*; to treat spontaneous sweating due to exterior deficiency and night sweating due to yin deficiency, it is usually combined with *huáng qí*, *mǔ lì* and *wǔ wèi zǐ*; to treat excessive sweating syndrome of losing yang, it is often combined with *mǔ lì*, *rén shēn* and *fù zǐ* (Aconiti Lateralis Radix Praeparata).

4. 湿疮痒疹，疮疡久溃不敛　本品性收涩，煅后外用有收湿、敛疮、生肌之效。用治湿疮流水、湿疹瘙痒，可配伍牡蛎研粉外敷。用治疮疡溃久不敛，与枯矾等分共研细末，擦敷患处。

(4) **Eczema, sores and ulcers with ulceration but no close**　With the nature of astringent, after calcination it has the effect of astringing dampness, closing sores and promoting muscle growth for externally use. To treat wet sores with fluid, eczema and pruritus, it is often combined with *mǔ lì* and ground into powder for external application; to treat sores and ulcers with chronic ulceration and no close, it is usually combined with *kū fán* (Dehydratum Alumen) and ground into powder for external application.

【用法用量 / Usage and dosage】

煎服，15~30g，先煎。外用适量。镇静安神，平肝潜阳多生用；收敛固涩宜煅用。

Decoction, 15-30g;it should be decocted first. An appropriate amount for external usage. For suppressing fright and calming the mind, calming the liver and subduing yang, it should be used in the raw form; for astringing and consolidating essence, it should be used in the calcined form.

【使用注意 / Precaution】

湿热积滞者不宜使用。

It is not suitable for those with damp heat accumulation.

【现代研究 / Modern research】

本品主要含碳酸钙、磷酸钙、氧化镁，尚含铁、钾、钠、氯、铜、锰、硫酸根等。具有镇静、催眠、抗惊厥、促进血液凝固、降低血管壁通透性、抑制骨骼肌兴奋、消除溃疡、促进伤口愈合等作用。

It mainly contains calcium carbonate, calcium phosphate and magnesium oxide. It also contains iron, potassium, sodium, chlorine, copper, manganese and sulfate, etc. It has the functions of sedation, hypnosis, anticonvulsion, promoting blood coagulation, reducing the permeability of blood vessel wall, inhibiting the excitation of skeletal muscle, eliminating ulcer and promoting wound healing.

第二节　养心安神药
Section 2　Heart-nourishing and mind-calming medicinals

PPT

本类药物多为植物类种子、种仁，具有甘润滋养之性，以滋养心肝、益阴补血为主要功效，主治阴血不足、心脾两虚、心肾不交等导致的心悸怔忡、虚烦不眠、健忘多梦等。

Most of the heart-nourishing and mind-calming medicinals are plant seeds, which are sweet and nourishing. They can nourish the heart and liver, benefit yin and replenish blood. They are mainly used to treat palpitation, insomnia and forgetfulness caused by deficiency of yin and blood, deficiency of heart and spleen, and heart and kidney and failure of intercourse between heart and kidney.

酸枣仁　*Suān zǎo rén* (Ziziphi Spinosae Semen)
《神农本草经》
Shen Nong's Classic of the Materia Medica (Shén Nóng Běn Cǎo Jīng)

【来源 / Origin】

为鼠李科植物酸枣 *Ziziphus jujuba* Mill. var. *spinosa*（Bunge）Hu ex H. F. Chou 的干燥成熟种子。主产于河北、陕西、辽宁等地。秋末冬初果实成熟时采收，晒干，生用或炒用。本品气微，味淡。《中国药典》规定，含酸枣仁皂苷 A（$C_{58}H_{94}O_{26}$）不得少于 0.030%，含斯皮诺素（$C_{28}H_{32}O_{15}$）不得少于 0.080%。

Suān zǎo rén is the dry and mature seed of *Ziziphus jujuba* Mill. var. *spinosa* (Bunge) Hu ex H. F. Chou, pertaining to Rhanaceae. Mainly produced in Hebei, Shaanxi and Liaoning Province in China, it is collected in late autumn and early winter when fruit is ripe, dried and used in the raw form or the stir-fried form. It has slight odor and tastes bland. According to *Chinese Pharmacopoeia*, the content of jujuboside A ($C_{58}H_{94}O_{26}$) in jujube kernel should be no less than 0.030%, the content of spironolacton should be no less than 0.080%.

【性味归经 / Medicinal properties】

甘、酸，平。归心、肝、胆经。

Sweet, sour and neutral; act on the heart, liver and gallbladder meridians.

【主要功效 / Medicinal efficacies】

养心补肝，宁心安神，敛汗，生津。

Nourish the heart and supplement the liver, tranquilized the heart and calm the mind, arrest sweat and promote fluid production.

【临床应用 / Clinical application】

1. **虚烦不眠，惊悸多梦**　本品味甘能补，入心、肝经，能滋养心肝阴血而宁心安神，为养心安神之要药。用治阴血不足，失眠多梦，心悸不安，常与麦冬、制何首乌、茯苓等同用。用治肝虚有热之虚烦不眠，常与知母、茯苓、川芎等配伍。若治心脾气血亏虚之心悸失眠，常与黄芪、当归、党参等同用。若治心肾不足，阴亏血少之心悸、失眠、健忘者，多与麦冬、地黄、远志等同用。

(1) Deficient restlessness and insomnia, palpitations due to fright and profuse dreaming　With the nature of sweet and acting on the heart and liver meridians, it can nourish yin blood of the heart and liver to tranquilize the mind. It's an essential medicine for nourishing the heart and tranquilizing the mind. To treat insomnia and profuse dreaming, palpitation and uneasiness due to yin and blood deficiency, it is often combined with *mài dōng* (Ophiopogonis Radix), *zhì hé shǒu wū* (Polygoni Multiflori Radix Praeparata cum Succo Glycines Sotae) and *fú líng* (Poria); to treat deficient restlessness and insomnia due to liver deficiency with heat, it is usually combined with *zhī mǔ* (Anemarrhenae Rhizoma), *fú líng* and *chuān xiōng* (Chuanxiong Rhizoma); to treat palpitations due to fright and profuse dreaming due to insufficiency of heart-spleen qi and blood, it can be combined with *huáng qí*, *dāng guī* and *dǎng shēn*; to treat palpitation, insomnia and forgetfulness due to heart-kidney insufficiency and yin-blood depletion, it is often combined with *mài dōng*, *dì huáng* and *yuǎn zhì* (Polygalae Radix).

2. **自汗，盗汗**　本品味酸能敛，有一定的收敛止汗功效。用治体虚自汗、盗汗，常与五味子、黄芪、山茱萸等同用。

(2) Spontaneous sweating and night sweating　with the nature of astringent, it has the function of arresting sweat. To treat spontaneous sweating and night sweating due to body weakness, it is usually combined with *wǔ wèi zǐ*, *huáng qí* and *shān zhū yú*.

3. **津伤口渴**　本品酸甘化阴，有生津止渴之功。可用治伤津口渴咽干，可与地黄、麦冬、天花粉等同用。

(3) Thirst due to fluid consumption　With the nature of sweet and sour, it can stanch thirst and promote fluid production. To treat thirst and dry throat due to fluid consumption, it is often combined with *dì huáng*, *mài dōng* and *tiān huā fěn* (Trichosanthis Radix).

【用法用量 / Usage and dosage】

煎服，10~15g。

Decoction, 10-15g.

【现代研究 / Modern research】

本品主要含酸枣仁皂苷 A 和 B、荷叶碱、欧鼠李叶碱、原荷叶碱、去甲异紫堇定碱、斯皮诺素等，尚含挥发油、糖类、蛋白质及有机酸等。具有镇静、催眠、中枢抑制、抗惊厥、镇痛、抗心律失常、降体温、降压、降血脂、抗缺氧、抑制血小板聚集、增强免疫功能等作用。

It mainly contains jujuboside A and B, lotus leaf alkali, rhamnophylline, protolotus leaf alkali, norisocorydine and spironolacton, and it also contains volatile oil, sugar, protein and organic acid, etc. It has the functions of sedation, hypnosis, central inhibition, anticonvulsion, analgesia, antiarrhythmia, hypothermia, hypotension, hypolipidemia, anti hypoxia, inhibition of platelet aggregation and enhancement of immune function, etc.

柏子仁 *Bǎi zǐ rén* (Platycladi Semen)
《神农本草经》
Shen Nong's Classic of the Materia Medica (Shén Nóng Běn Cǎo Jīng)

【来源 / Origin】

为柏科植物侧柏 *Platycladus orientalis*（L.）Franco 的干燥成熟种仁。主产于山东、河南、河北等地。秋、冬二季采收，晒干，生用或制霜用。本品气微香，味淡。

Bǎi zǐ rén is the seed of *Platycladus orientalis* (L.) Franco, pertaining to Cupressaceae. Mainly produced in Shandong, Henan and Hebei Province in China, it is collected in autumn and winter. It is dried in the sun and used for raw or wrapped with paper to be heated slightly and squeezed to remove the oil, thus *bǎi zǐ rén shuāng* is got. It has slight odor and is bland in taste.

【性味归经 / Medicinal properties】

甘，平。归心、肾、大肠经。

Sweet and neutral; act on the heart, kidney and large intestine meridians.

【主要功效 / Medicinal efficacies】

养心安神，润肠通便。

Nourish the heart and calm the mind, moisten the intestine and promote defecation.

【临床应用 / Clinical application】

1. **心悸失眠**　本品味甘质润，药性平和，具有滋养阴血、宁心安神之功，功似酸枣仁而药力稍逊。其主入心经，多用治心之阴血不足，心神失养，心悸怔忡，虚烦不眠，常与酸枣仁、麦冬、枸杞子等同用。若治心肾不交之心悸不宁、心烦少寐、健忘等，常与麦冬、熟地黄、石菖蒲等同用。

(1) Palpitation and insomnia　With the nature of sweet, moist and neutral, it has the functions of nourishing yin and blood, calming the heart and mind, which had similar efficacy to *suān zǎo rén* but with less power. To treat palpitation or severe palpitation, deficient restlessness and insomnia due to depletion of heart yin and heart-blood, it is often combined with *suān zǎo rén*, *mài dōng* and *gǒu qǐ zǐ*; to treat palpitation and restlessness, vexation and insomnia and forgetfulness due to failure of the heart and kidney to interact, it is often combined with *mài dōng*, *shú dì huáng* and *shí chāng pú*.

2. **肠燥便秘**　本品富含油脂，入大肠经，有润肠通便之功。用治阴虚血亏，老年、产后等肠燥便秘证，常与郁李仁、松子仁、杏仁等配伍。

(2) Constipation due to intestinal dryness　It is rich in grease, which can act on the large intestine meridian and has the functions of moistening the intestine and promoting defecation. To treat constipation of the elderly and postpartum due to dryness of intestines and yin deficiency and insufficiency of blood, it is usually combined with *yù lǐ rén* (Pruni Semen), *sōng zǐ rén* (Pini Koraiensis Semen) and *xìng rén* (Armeniacae Amarum Semen).

【用法用量 / Usage and dosage】

煎服，3~10g。

Decoction, 3-10g.

【使用注意 / Precaution】

便溏及多痰者慎用。

It should be used with caution for patients with thin and unformed stool and excessive phlegm.

【现代研究 / Modern research】

本品主要含脂肪油，并含少量挥发油、皂苷及植物甾醇、维生素 A、蛋白质等。具有延长睡眠时间、镇静、改善记忆、缓泻等作用。

It mainly contains fat oil and a small amount of volatile oil, saponin, phytosterol, vitamin A and protein, etc. It can prolong sleep, calm down the mind, improve memory and relieve diarrhea.

远志　*Yuǎn zhì* (Polygalae Radix)
《神农本草经》
Shen Nong's Classic of the Materia Medica (Shén Nóng Běn Cǎo Jīng)

【来源 / Origin】

为远志科植物远志 *Polygala tenuifolia* Willd. 或卵叶远志 *Polygala sibirica* L. 的干燥根。主产于山西、陕西、吉林等地。春、秋二季采挖，晒干，生用或炙用。本品气微，味苦、微辛，嚼之有刺喉感。《中国药典》规定，含细叶远志皂苷（$C_{36}H_{56}O_{12}$）不得少于 2.0%，饮片不得少于 2.0%；含远志𫫇酮Ⅲ（$C_{25}H_{28}O_{15}$）不得少于 0.15%，饮片不得少于 0.10%；含 3,6′–二芥子酰基蔗糖（$C_{36}H_{46}O_{17}$）不得少于 0.50%，饮片不得少于 0.30%。

Yuǎn zhì is the dry root of *Polygala tenuifolia* Wild. or *Polygala sibirica* L., pertaining to Polygalaceae, mainly produced in Shanxi, Shaanxi, and Jilin Province, collected in spring and autumn, dried, and used raw or processed. It has a slight odor, bitter and slightly acrid taste, and it has a tingling sensation when chewing. According to *Chinese Pharmacopoeia*, the content of the saponin ($C_{36}H_{56}O_{12}$) of *Polygala tenuifolia* should not be less than 2.0%, and not be less than 2.0% in decoction pieces; the content of polygalaxanthone Ⅲ ($C_{25}H_{28}O_{15}$) should not be less than 0.15%, and not be less than 0.10% in decoction pieces; the content of the 3,6′-dimustard sucrose ($C_{36}H_{46}O_{17}$) should not be less than 0.50%, and not be less than 0.30% in decoction pieces.

【性味归经 / Medicinal properties】

苦、辛，温。归心、肾、肺经。

Bitter, acrid and warm; act on heart, kidney and lung meridians.

【主要功效 / Medicinal efficacies】

安神益智，祛痰开窍，消散痈肿。

Calm mind and improve intelligence, dispel phlegm and open orifices, resolve abscess and swelling.

【临床应用 / Clinical application】

1. **失眠多梦，健忘惊悸**　本品苦辛性温，性善宣泄通达，既能开心气而宁心安神，又能通肾气而强志不忘，为交通心肾、安定心神、益肾强志之佳品。宜用治心肾不交之心神不宁、失眠、惊悸、健忘等，常与茯神、龙齿、朱砂等同用。治健忘症，常与人参、茯苓、石菖蒲等同用。

(1) **Insomnia, dream-disturbed sleep, poor memory and palpitation**　*Yuǎn zhì* is bitter, acrid and warm, good at diffusing and dredging with the functions of opening heart qi to calm heart and induce tranquilization, as well as dredging kidney qi to reinforce will and memory. It is the key medicinal for restoring normal coordination between heart and kidney, inducing tranquilization, improving intelligence and reinforcing will. For restlessness of heart-mind, insomnia, fright palpitations, and poor memory, it is combined with *fú shén*, *lóng chǐ* and *zhū shā*. For amnesia, it is combined with *rén shēn*, *fú líng* and *shí chāng pú*.

2. **癫痫惊狂**　本品味辛通利，能祛痰、开心窍。用治痰阻心窍所致之癫狂发作，神志恍惚等，可与石菖蒲、郁金、白矾等配伍。用治痫证抽搐，口吐白沫，神昏者，常与天麻、石菖蒲、天南星等同用。

(2) Epilepsy and mania *Yuǎn zhì* is acrid and dredging with the functions of dispelling phlegm and opening heart orifice. It treats epilepsy, mania and trance due to phlegm obstruction of heart in combination with *shí chāng pú*, *yù jīn* and *bái fán*. For epilepsy manifested as convulsion, foaming at the mouth and coma, it is combined with *tiān má*, *shí chāng pú* and *tiān nán xīng*.

3. 咳嗽痰多　本品苦温性燥，入肺经，能祛痰止咳。用治痰多黏稠、咳吐不爽者，可单用，或与桔梗、白前、贝母等同用。

(3) Cough with profuse phlegm *Yuǎn zhì* is bitter, warm and dry, acting on lung meridian with the functions of resolving phlegm and relieving cough. For cough with profuse phlegm, thick phlegm and difficulty to spit, it is used alone or with *jié gěng*, *bái qián* and *bèi mǔ*.

4. 痈疽疮毒，乳房肿痛　本品辛行苦泄，能疏通气血之壅滞而消散痈肿。用治痈疽疮毒，乳房肿痛，可单用，或配伍解毒消肿之品内服、外用。

(4) Abscess, carbuncle and sores, painful swollen breast *Yuǎn zhì* is acrid moving and bitter purging, and it can dissipate swollen abscess by smoothing obstruction of qi and blood. For abscess, carbuncle and sores, and painful swollen breast, it is used alone or in combination with medicinals of resolving toxins and dispersing swelling for internal and external use.

【用法用量 / Usage and dosage】

煎服，3~10g。外用适量。化痰止咳宜炙用。

Decoction, 3-10g. An appropriate amount is used for external application. It should be stir-fried with liquid adjuvant for resolving phlegm and relieving cough.

【使用注意 / Precaution】

实热或痰火内盛及胃溃疡或胃炎者慎用。

It should be used with caution for those with excess heat or phlegm fire, and gastric ulcer or gastritis.

【现代研究 / Modern research】

本品主要含皂苷，水解后可获得远志皂苷元 A 和远志皂苷元 B，尚含远志叫酮、生物碱、糖及糖苷、远志醇、细叶远志定碱、脂肪油、树脂等。具有镇静、催眠、抗惊厥、祛痰、镇咳、降血压、兴奋子宫等作用。

Yuǎn zhì mainly contains saponins, and can be divided into polygalagenin A and polygalagenin B after hydrolysis. It also contains polygala ketone, alkaloid, sugar and glycoside, polygala alcohol, polygala tenuifolia alkaloid, fat oil, resin, etc. It has the functions of sedation, hypnosis, anticonvulsion, dispelling phlegm, relieving cough, reducing blood pressure and stimulating uterus.

其他安神药功用介绍见表 19-1。

The efficacies of other mind-calming medicinals are shown in table 19-1.

表 19-1　其他安神药功用介绍

分类	药物	药性	功效	应用	用法用量
重镇安神药	琥珀	甘，平。归心、肝、膀胱经	镇惊安神，活血散瘀，利尿通淋	心神不宁，心悸失眠，惊风癫痫；血滞经闭痛经，心腹刺痛，癥瘕积聚；淋证，癃闭	研末冲服，或入丸、散，每次1.5~3g。外用适量
	珍珠	甘、咸，寒。归心、肝经	安神定惊，明目消翳，解毒生肌，润肤祛斑	惊悸失眠，惊风癫痫；目赤翳障，疮疡不敛，皮肤色斑	入丸、散，0.3~1g。外用适量

第十九章　安神药┊Chapter 19　Mind-calming medicinals

续表

分类	药物	药性	功效	应用	用法用量
养心安神药	首乌藤	甘，平。归心、肝经	养血安神，祛风通络	心神不宁，失眠多梦；血虚身痛，风湿痹痛；皮肤瘙痒	煎服，9~15g。外用适量
	合欢皮	甘，平。归心、肝经	解郁安神，活血消肿	心神不安，忿怒忧郁，失眠多梦，肺痈，疮肿，跌仆伤痛	煎服，6~12g。外用适量，研末调敷。孕妇慎用

题库

（杨青山）

第二十章 平肝息风药
Chapter 20 Liver-calming wind-extinguishing medicinals

 学习目标 | Learning goals

1. **掌握** 平肝息风药在性能、功效、主治、配伍及使用注意方面的共性；石决明、牡蛎、赭石、羚羊角、钩藤、天麻的性能、功效、应用以及特殊的用法用量和特殊的使用注意。

2. **熟悉** 平肝息风药的分类；全蝎、地龙、蜈蚣、僵蚕的功效、主治以及特殊的用法用量和特殊的使用注意。

3. **了解** 平抑肝阳药（平肝潜阳药）、息风止痉药及相关功效术语的含义；珍珠母、蒺藜、罗布麻叶的功效以及特殊的用法用量和特殊的使用注意。

1. Master the commonness of liver-calming wind-extinguishing medicinals in efficacy, indications, property, compatibility and cautions; as well as the property, efficacy, application, special usage and dosage and special precautions of *shí jué míng, mǔ lì, zhě shí, líng yáng jiǎo, gōu téng* and *tiān má*.

2. Familiar with classification of liver-calming wind-extinguishing medicinals; as well as the efficacy, indications, special usage, dosage and special precautions of *quán xiē, dì lóng, wú gōng* and *jiāng cán*.

3. Understand the definitions of medicinals for calming the liver yang (liver-calming yang-subduing medicinals) and wind-extinguishing convulsion-arresting medicinals, and related efficacy terms; and the efficacy, special usage and dosage and special precautions of *zhēn zhū mǔ, jí lí* and *luó bù má yè*.

凡以平肝潜阳、息风止痉为主要功效，常用以治疗肝阳上亢证或肝风内动证的药物，称为平肝息风药。

Medicinals with efficacies of calming the liver and subduing yang, extinguishing wind and arresting convulsion are known as liver-calming wind-extinguishing medicinals, which are often used in the treatment of the syndrome of ascendant hyperactivity of liver yang or internal stirring of liver wind.

平肝息风药主入肝经，药性多寒凉，少数性平或偏温，以平肝潜阳（或平抑肝阳）、息风止痉为主要功效，主治肝阳上亢之眩晕耳鸣、头目胀痛、面赤烦躁，或肝风内动之肢体抽搐、震颤等。

Most cold and cool and a few neutral or slightly warm, liver-calming wind-extinguishing medicinals mainly enter the liver meridian, with calming the liver and subduing yang (or restraining the liver yang), extinguishing wind and arresting convulsion as the main efficacies. They are mainly applied to treat syndromes of ascendant hyperactivity of liver yang such as dizziness and ringing in the ears, distending pain of head and eyes, vexation and agitation with flushed face, as well as syndromes of internal stirring of liver wind such as limb convulsion, vibration, etc.

根据平肝息风药的药性及功效主治差异，可分为平抑肝阳药及息风止痉药两类。

According to the differences in the properties, efficacies and indications, liver-calming wind-extinguishing medicinals can be classified into two groups: medicinals for calming the liver yang and wind-extinguishing convulsion-arresting medicinals.

应用平肝息风药时，须针对病因、病机以及兼证之不同，进行相应的配伍。若肝阳上亢，多配伍滋补肝肾之阴的药物。若肝阳化风致肝风内动，应将平肝潜阳药和息风止痉药同用；若热极生风致肝风内动，宜配伍清热泻火之药；若阴血亏虚致肝风内动，宜配伍滋阴养血之药。若兼窍闭神昏，当配伍开窍药；兼失眠多梦、心神不宁者，当配伍安神药；兼痰浊者，当配伍化痰药；对于血虚生风者，当配伍养血之药。

It is necessary to make corresponding compatibility according to the differences in etiology, disease mechanism and concurrent syndromes in the application of liver-calming wind-extinguishing medicinals. For the patients with internal stirring of liver wind due to liver yang transforming into wind, liver-calming yang-subduing medicinals and wind-extinguishing convulsion-arresting medicinals should be used together; in the case of internal stirring of liver wind due to extreme heat producing wind, it should be compatible with heat-clearing and fire-draining medicinals; for those with internal stirring of liver wind because of yin-blood depletion, it should be combined with yin-enriching and blood-nourishing medicinals. For those patients with concurrent orifice block and unconsciousness, it should go together with orifice-opening medicinals; for those with concurrent insomnia and profuse dreaming as well as uneasiness, it should be used together with mind-calming medicinals; for those with concurrent turbid phlegm, it should be compatible with phlegm-dissolving medicinals; for those with blood deficiency producing wind, it should be used together with blood-nourishing medicinal.

本类药物有药性寒凉与温燥之不同，故应区别使用，脾虚慢惊者勿用寒凉之品，阴血亏损者忌用温燥之品。介类或矿石类药物质地坚硬，入汤剂应打碎先煎。某些药物有毒，应注意用药安全，孕妇当慎用或忌服。

Such medicinals have different properties, to be specific, cold coolness and warm dryness, and thus should be used differently. While patients with weak spleen or chronic infantile convulsion should avoid cold cool medicinals, those with yin-blood depletion should avoid warm dry ones. Medicinals like mediators and minerals are hard, and thus should be crushed and decocted first. Some medicinals are toxic, so the safety of medication should be noted, and pregnant women should use them with caution or avoid taking them.

第一节 平抑肝阳药

Section 1 Medicinals for calming the liver yang

本类药物多为介类及矿物类，质重沉降，主入肝经，以平肝潜阳或平抑肝阳为主要功效，主治肝阳上亢证，症见眩晕耳鸣、头目胀痛、面红目赤、烦躁易怒、舌红苔黄、脉弦数等。部分药物兼能清肝明目、重镇安神等，可用治肝火上炎，目赤肿痛以及心神不宁、惊悸失眠等。

Mostly in the form of mediators and minerals, such medicinals, featuring their heaviness and subsidence, mainly enter the liver meridian, with calming the liver and subduing yang, restraining the liver yang as the major efficacies. They are mainly used to treat the syndromes of ascendant hyperactivity of liver yang, with the symptoms such as dizziness and ringing in the ears, distending pain of head and eyes, flushed face with red eyes, vexation and agitation with irascibility, red tongue with yellow coating, rapid wiry pulse, etc. Some medicinals also have concurrent actions of clearing liver to improve vision, calming the mind with heavy sedatives, etc. They also can be used to treat liver fire flaming upward, red swelling and pain eyes, uneasiness, palpitations due to fright and insomnia, etc.

石决明 *Shí jué míng* (Haliotidis Concha)
《名医别录》
Miscellaneous Records of Famous Physicians (Míng Yī Bié Lù)

【来源 / Origin】

为鲍科动物杂色鲍 *Haliotis diversicolor* Reeve、皱纹盘鲍 *Haliotis discus hannai* Ino、羊鲍 *Haliotis ovina* Gmelin、澳洲鲍 *Haliotis ruber*（Leach）、耳鲍 *Haliotis asinina* Linnacus 或白鲍 *Haliotis laevigata*（Donovan）的贝壳。主产于广东、福建、辽宁等沿海地区。夏、秋二季捕捉，干燥，生用或煅用，用时打碎。本品气微，味微咸。《中国药典》规定，含碳酸钙（$CaCO_3$）不得少于93%，煅石决明不得少于95%。

Shí jué míng is the shell of *Haliotis diversicolor* Reeve, *Haliotis discus hannai* Ino, *Haliotis ovina* Gmelin, *Haliotis ruber* (Leach), *Haliotis asinina* Linnacus, *Haliotis laevigata* (Donovan), pertaining to the Sisoridae. Mainly produced in Guangdong, Fujian, Liaoning and other coastal areas, it is captured in summer and autumn, dried and then used in raw or calcined form. It is bland in odor and slightly salty. According to *Chinese Pharmacopoeia*, the content of calcium carbonate ($CaCO_3$) should be no less than 93%, and as for calcined *shí jué míng*, no less than 95%.

【性味归经 / Medicinal properties】

咸，寒。归肝经。

Salty and cold; act on liver meridian.

【主要功效 / Medicinal efficacies】

平肝潜阳，清肝明目。

Calm the liver and subdue yang, clear liver to improve vision.

【临床应用 / Clinical application 】

1. 肝阳上亢证　本品咸寒清热，质重潜降，专入肝经，具有潜镇肝阳、清泻肝火之功，为平肝凉肝之要药。用治肝肾阴虚，肝阳上亢之眩晕、头痛等，常与白芍、牡蛎、生地黄等同用。用治肝阳上亢兼肝火亢盛之头晕头痛、烦躁易怒，常与夏枯草、钩藤、菊花等同用。

(1) Syndromes of ascendant hyperactivity of liver yang　Salty, cold and heat-clearing, *shí jué míng*, featuring its heaviness and subsidence, specially enters the liver meridian. Having the actions of subduing and restraining the liver yang as well as clearing and draining the liver fire, it is an important medicinal for calming and cooling the liver. To treat patients with liver-kidney yin deficiency, dizziness and headache due to ascendant hyperactivity of liver yang, it is often used together with *bái sháo* (Paeoniae Alba Radix), *mǔ lì*, *shēng dì huáng* (Rehmannia glutinosa Libosch), etc. To treat those with ascendant hyperactivity of liver yang with concurrent liver fire exuberance symptoms such as dizziness and headache as well as vexation and agitation with irascibility, it is often combined with *xià kū cǎo* (Prunellae Spica), *gōu téng*, *jú huā* (Chrysanthemi Flos).

2. 目赤翳障，视物昏花　本品性寒，具有清泻肝火、明目退翳之效，为治疗目疾之常用药。用治肝火上炎，目赤肿痛，常配伍决明子、夏枯草、菊花等。用治肝经风热，目赤羞明、翳膜遮睛，可与木贼、蝉蜕、菊花等同用。用治肝肾阴虚，视物模糊，常配伍熟地黄、枸杞子、谷精草等。

(2) Red eyes with nebula, dim-sightedness　Being cold, *shí jué míng*, with the efficacies of clearing and draining the liver fire as well as removing nebula to improve vision, is a common medicinal used to treat eye diseases. To treat patients with liver fire flaming upward and red swelling and pain eyes, it is often compatible with *jué míng zǐ* (Cassiae Semen), *xià kū cǎo*, *jú huā*, etc. To treat those with fire heat in the liver channel, red eyes with photophobia or nebula covering the eyes, it can be used together with *mù zéi* (Equiseti Hiemalis Herba), *chán tuì* (Cicadae Periostracum), *jú huā*, etc. To treat those with liver-kidney yin deficiency and dim-sightedness, it is often combined with *shú dì huáng* (Rehmanniae Radix Praeparata), *gǒu qǐ zǐ* (Lycii Fructus), *gǔ jīng cǎo* (Eriocauli Flos), etc.

【用法用量 / Usage and dosage 】

煎服，6~20g，宜打碎先煎。凉肝、镇肝宜生用；外用点眼宜煅用、水飞。

Decoction, 6-20g, suitable for being crushed and decocted first. For cooling and tranquilizing the liver, suitable for raw use and for exterior use, calcined form or grinding with water is more suitable.

【使用注意 / Precaution 】

脾胃虚寒、食少便溏者慎用。

It should be used with caution for those suffering deficiency-cold of the spleen and stomach, or small appetite and loose stool.

【现代研究 / Modern research 】

本品主要含碳酸钙，尚含少量有机质、镁、铁、硅酸盐、硫酸盐、氯化物和极微量的碘。具有镇静、解痉、解热、降血压、中和胃酸、抑菌、抗炎等作用。

Shí jué míng mainly contains calcium carbonate, and also contains a small amount of organic matter, magnesium, iron, silicate, sulfate, chloride and a very small amount of iodine. It has the functions of sedation, antispasmolysis, antipyresis, lowering blood pressure, neutralizing stomach acid, resisting bacteria and inflammation, etc.

牡蛎 *Mǔ lì* (Ostreae Concha)
《神农本草经》
Shen Nong's Classic of the Materia Medica (Shén Nóng Běn Cǎo Jīng)

【来源 / Origin】

为牡蛎科动物长牡蛎 *Ostrea gigas* Thunberg、大连湾牡蛎 *Ostrea talienwhanensis* Crosse 或近江牡蛎 *Ostrea rivularis* Gould 的贝壳。主产于广东、福建、浙江等沿海地区。全年均可捕捞。晒干，生用或煅用，用时打碎。本品气微，味微咸。《中国药典》规定，含碳酸钙（CaCO₃）不得少于94.0%。

Mǔ lì is the shell of *Ostrea gigas* Thunberg, *Ostrea talienwhanensis* Crosse, and *Ostrea rivularis* Gould, pertaining to the Ostreidae. It is mainly produced in Guangdong, Fujian, Zhejiang and other coastal areas, and can be captured all the year around. It is dried for raw or calcined use, and crushed in application. *Mǔ lì* is bland in odor and slightly salty. According to *Chinese Pharmacopoeia*, the content of calcium carbonate ($CaCO_3$) should be no less than 94.0%.

【性味归经 / Medicinal properties】

咸，微寒。归肝、胆、肾经。

Salty, slightly cold; act on liver, gallbladder and kidney meridians.

【主要功效 / Medicinal efficacies】

潜阳补阴，重镇安神，软坚散结，收敛固涩，制酸止痛。

Subdue yang and supplement yin, calm the mind with heavy sedatives, soften hardness and dissipate masses, astringe and consolidate essence, inhibit acidity to relieve pain.

【临床应用 / Clinical application】

1. 肝阳上亢证　本品咸寒质重，具有平肝潜阳、益阴清热作用。用治肝肾阴虚，肝阳上亢之眩晕耳鸣、头目胀痛、烦躁易怒等，常配伍赭石、龙骨、白芍等。

(1) Syndromes of ascendant hyperactivity of liver yang　*Mǔ lì*, salty, cold and heavy, has the functions of calming the liver and subduing yang, boosting yin and clearing heat. To treat patients with liver-kidney yin deficiency, symptoms caused by ascendant hyperactivity of liver yang, such as dizziness and tinnitus, distending pain of head and eyes, vexation and agitation with irascibility, etc., it is often compatible with *zhě shí*, *lóng gǔ* (Fossilia Ossis Mastodi), *bái sháo*, etc.

2. 心神不宁，惊悸失眠　本品有镇惊安神之功，功似龙骨而稍逊。用治心神不宁，惊悸怔忡，失眠多梦等，常与龙骨、酸枣仁等同用。

(2) Uneasiness, palpitations due to fright　Having similar actions as *lóng gǔ* but slightly inferior, *mǔ lì* has the fuction of suppressing fright and calming the mind. To treat patients with uneasiness, palpitations due to fright and severe palpitations, insomnia with profuse dreaming, it is often used together with *lóng gǔ*, *suān zǎo rén* (Ziziphi Spinosae Semen), etc.

3. 痰核瘰疬，瘿瘤癥瘕　本品咸寒，有清热软坚散结之效。用治痰火郁结之痰核、瘰疬、瘿瘤，多与浙贝母、玄参、夏枯草等同用。用治癥瘕痞块，常与鳖甲、莪术、丹参等同用。

(3) Phlegm node and scrofula, goiter, tumor, concretions and conglomerations　Salty and cold, *mǔ lì* has the efficacies of clearing heat, softening hardness and dissipating masses. To treat patients with symptoms due to binding constraint of phlegm fire, such as phlegm node, scrofula and concretions, it is often used together with *zhè bèi mǔ* (Fritillariae Thunbergii Bulbus), *xuán shēn* (Scrophulariae Radix), *xià kū cǎo*, etc. To treat those with conglomerations and *pǐ* clots, it is often combined with *biē jiǎ* (Trionycis

Carapax), *é zhú* (Curcumae Rhizoma), *dān shēn* (Salviae Miltiorrhizae Radix et Rhizoma), etc.

4. 正虚不固，滑脱诸证　本品煅用有固精、缩尿、止汗、止带、止血等收敛固涩功效。用治肾虚不固，滑泄、遗精，常与龙骨、芡实、沙苑子等同用。用治遗尿尿频，可与桑螵蛸、龙骨、金樱子等同用。用治自汗、盗汗，常与黄芪、麻黄根等同用。用治崩漏、带下，可与白芍、山茱萸、海螵蛸等配伍。

(4) Insecurity of vital qi deficiency, incontinence symptoms　For calcined use, *mŭ lì* has such astringing and consolidating efficacies as consolidating essence, reduinge urination, arresting sweating and vaginal discharge, stanching bleeding, etc. To treat patients with insecurity of kidney deficiency, efflux diarrhea and seminal emission, it is often combined with *lóng gŭ*, *qiàn shí* (Euryales Semen), *shā yuàn zĭ* (Astragali Complanati Semen), etc. To treat those with enuresis and frequent urination, it can be used together with *sāng piāo xiāo* (Mantidis Oötheca), *lóng gŭ*, *jīn yīng zĭ* (Rosae Laevigatae Fructus), etc. To treat those with spontaneous sweating and night sweat, it often goes with *huáng qí* (Astragali Radix), *má huáng gēn* (Ephedrae Radix et Rhizoma), etc. To treat those with flooding and spotting as well as abnormal vaginal discharge, it can be compatible with *bái sháo*, *shān zhū yú* (Corni Fructus), *hăi piāo xiāo* (Sepiae Endoconcha), etc.

5. 胃痛泛酸　本品煅用可制酸止痛。用治胃痛泛酸，常与乌贼骨、浙贝母共研细末服用。

(5) Stomachache with acid regurgitation　*Mŭ lì* can be used to inhibit acidity to relieve pain for calcined use. To treat patients with stomachache with acid regurgitation, it is often combined with *wū zéi gŭ* (Cleistocactus sepium) and *zhè bèi mŭ*, ground into powder and then taken.

【用法用量 / Usage and dosage】

煎服，9~30g，宜打碎先煎。收敛固涩、制酸止痛宜煅用，余皆生用。

Decoction, 9-30g, suitable for being crushed and decocted first. For astringing and consolidating essence, inhibiting acidity and relieving pain, it is advisable to be used in calcined form, and for other symptoms, raw use is recommended.

【现代研究 / Modern research】

本品主要含碳酸钙，尚含镁、铁、铝、硅等多种无机元素及多种氨基酸等。具有镇静、镇痛、抗惊厥、抗癫痫、抗胃溃疡、抗肿瘤、增强免疫等作用。

Mŭ lì mainly contains calcium carbonate, and also contains many inorganic elements such as magnesium, iron, aluminum, silicon and a variety of amino acids as well. It has the functions of sedation, analgesia, anti-convulsion, anti-epilepsy, anti-gastric ulcer, anti-tumor, immunity enhancement, etc.

赭石　*Zhě shí* (Haematitum)
《神农本草经》
Shen Nong's Classic of the Materia Medica (Shén Nóng Běn Căo Jīng)

【来源 / Origin】

为氧化物类矿物刚玉族赤铁矿，主含三氧化二铁（Fe_2O_3）。主产于山西、河北、河南等地。全年均可采集，打碎生用或醋淬研粉用。本品气微，味淡。《中国药典》规定，含铁（Fe）不得少于45.0%。

Zhě shí is corundum hematite, one oxide mineral. It mainly contains ferric oxide (Fe_2O_3), and is mainly produced in Shanxi, Hebei, Henan and other places. Mined all the year around, it can be crushed for raw use, or quenched in vinegar and then powdered. *Zhě shí* is mild and bland. According to *Chinese Pharmacopoeia*, the content of iron (Fe) should be no less than 45.0%.

【性味归经 / Medicinal properties】

苦，寒。归肝、心、肺、胃经。

Salty and cold; act on liver, heart, lung and stomach meridians.

【主要功效 / Medicinal efficacies】

平肝潜阳，重镇降逆，凉血止血。

Calm the liver and subdue yang, direct counterflow downward with heavy sedatives, cool the blood and stanch bleeding.

【临床应用 / Clinical application】

1. 肝阳上亢证　本品味苦性寒，质重坠降，主入肝经，善镇潜肝阳，清降火热，适宜于肝阳上亢兼有肝火旺者。用治肝阳上亢兼肝火上炎之头晕头痛、面红目赤、烦躁易怒等，多与石决明、夏枯草等同用。若治肝肾阴虚，肝阳上亢之眩晕耳鸣、头目胀痛等，常与牡蛎、龙骨、白芍等同用。

(1) Syndromes of ascendant hyperactivity of liver yang　Mainly entering the liver meridian, *zhě shí*, salty, cold and heavy, is good at tranquiliing and subduing liver yang as well as clearing and directing fire heat downward, and thus is especially suitable for those with ascendant hyperactivity of liver yang and concurrent vigorous liver fire. To treat patients with ascendant hyperactivity of liver yang and concurrent dizziness and headache caused by exuberance of liver fire, it is often used together with *shí jué míng*, *xià kū cǎo*, etc. To treat those with liver-kidney yin deficiency and symptoms brought by ascendant hyperactivity of liver yang, such as dizziness and ringing in the ears, distending pain of head and eyes, it is often combined with *mǔ lì*, *lóng gǔ*, *bái sháo*, etc.

2. 肺胃气逆证　本品质地沉重，有重镇降逆之功，入肺、胃经，既能降胃气上逆以止呕、止呃，又能降肺气上逆以平喘。用治胃气上逆之呕吐、呃逆、噫气不止等，常与旋覆花、半夏、生姜等配伍。若治肺气上逆之喘息痰鸣，可与苏子、苦杏仁、半夏等同用。若治肺肾不足，阴阳两虚之虚喘，常与人参、山茱萸、胡桃肉等同用。

(2) Qi counterflow of lung and stomach　*Zhě shí*, with a heavy quality, has the actions of directing counterflow downward with heavy sedatives. Entering the lung and stomach meridians, it can not only direct stomach qi ascending counterflow downward to arrest vomiting and relieve hiccup, but also direct lung qi ascending counterflow downward to relieve panting. To treat vomiting, hiccup and persistent belching brought by ascending counterflow of stomach qi, it is often compatible with *xuán fù huā* (Inulae Flos), *bàn xià* (Pinelliae Rhizoma), *shēng jiāng* (Zingiberis Recens Rhizoma), etc. To treat panting and gurgling with sputum, it is often used together with *sū zǐ* (Perillae Fructus), *kǔ xìng rén* (Armeniacae Amarum Semen), *bàn xià*, etc. To treat deficiency-type panting caused by insufficiency of lung and kidney and deficiency of both yin and yang, it is often combined with *rén shēn* (Ginseng Radix et Rhizoma), *shān zhū yú*, *hú táo ròu* (Juglandis Semen), etc.

3. 血热出血　本品苦寒，入肝心经，有凉血止血之效。用治血热妄行之吐血、衄血，可与竹茹、瓜蒌等配伍。若治血热崩漏下血，可与地榆、槐花等同用。

(3) Blood heat and bleeding　Bitter and cold, *zhě shí* invades the liver, heart and blood level, and has the efficacies of cooling the blood and stanching bleeding. To treat spitting of blood and nosebleed brought by frenetic transportation of blood heat, it is compatible with *zhú rú* (Bambusae Caulis in Taenia), *guā lóu*, etc. To treat blood heat flooding and spotting, it can be used together with *dì yú* (Sanguisorbae Radix), *huái huā* (Sophorae Flos), etc.

【用法用量 / Usage and dosage】

煎服，9~30g，宜打碎先煎。降逆平肝宜生用，止血宜煅用。

Decoction, 9-30g, suitable for being crushed and decocted first; direct counterflow downward and calm the liver in raw form, and stanch bleeding in calcined form.

【使用注意 / Precaution】

不宜长期服用。脾胃虚寒者及孕妇应慎用。

Not suitable for long-term use. Patients with deficiency-cold of the spleen and stomach and pregnant women should use it with caution.

【现代研究 / Modern research】

本品主要含氧化铁，尚含钙、锰、镁、锶等多种微量元素。具有镇静、抗惊厥、抗炎、促进肠蠕动、止血、促进红细胞和血红蛋白新生等作用。

Zhě shí mainly contains iron oxide, and also contains calcium, manganese, magnesium, strontium and many other trace elements. It has functions of sedation, anti-convulsion, anti-inflammation, intestinal peristalsis promotion, hemostasis, promotion of erythrocyte and hemoglobin regeneration, etc.

第二节 息风止痉药

Section 2 Wind-extinguishing convulsion-arresting medicinals

PPT

本类药物多为动物类，主入肝经，以平息肝风、制止痉挛抽搐为主要作用，主治热极生风、阳亢化风、血虚生风等所致的肝风内动证，症见眩晕欲仆，肢体痉挛、抽搐、震颤，或风中经络之口眼㖞斜、半身不遂等。部分药物兼有平肝潜阳、清泻肝火等功效，还可用治肝阳上亢之眩晕及肝火上炎之目赤肿痛等。

Mostly parts of animals, such medicinals mainly enter the liver meridian, with calming the liver and extinguishing wind as well as inhibiting spasm and convulsion as the major functions. They are mainly used to treat internal stirring of liver wind caused by extreme heat producing wind, yang hyperactivity transforming into wind, and blood deficiency producing wind, with the symptoms such as dizziness and likeliness to fall down, spasm, convulsion and vibration of limbs, or obliquity of mouth and eyes caused by wind striking the channels and collaterals, half-body paralysis, etc. Parts of the medicinals, with concurrent efficacies of calming the liver and subduing yang as well as clearing and draining liver fire, can also be used to treat dizziness brought by ascendant hyperactivity of liver yang, red swelling and pain eyes brought by liver fire flaming upward, etc.

微课

> 羚羊角 *Líng yáng jiǎo* (Saigae Tataricae Cornu)
> 《神农本草经》
> *Shen Nong's Classic of the Materia Medica (Shén Nóng Běn Cǎo Jīng)*

【来源 / Origin】

为牛科动物赛加羚羊 *Saiga tatarica* Linnaeus 的角。主产于新疆、青海、甘肃等地。全年均可捕捉。猎取后锯取其角，晒干，用时镑片或粉碎成细粉。本品气微，味淡。

Líng yáng jiǎo is the horn of *Saiga tatarica* Linnaeus, pertaining to the bovine. It is produced in Xinjiang Uygur Autonomous Region, Qinghai, Gansu and some other places. Captured all the year around, its horns are sawed, dried, and flaked in pieces or powdered for use. *Líng yáng jiǎo* is odorless and bland.

【 性味归经 / Medicinal properties 】

咸，寒。归肝、心经。

Salty and cold; act on liver and heart meridians.

【 主要功效 / Medicinal efficacies 】

平肝息风，清肝明目，清热解毒。

Calm the liver and extinguish wind, clear the liver and improve vision, clear heat stasis and resolve toxins.

【 临床应用 / Clinical application 】

1. 肝风内动证　本品性寒入肝经，具有良好的清泻肝火、息风止痉之功，为治疗肝风内动、惊痫抽搐的要药，尤宜于热极生风者。用治温热病火热炽盛，热极动风之高热神昏，痉厥抽搐，常与钩藤、菊花、白芍等同用。用治痰热痫证、惊风、中风等，可与天竺黄、牛黄、钩藤等同用。

(1) **Internal stirring of liver wind**　Cold in nature, *líng yáng jiǎo*, entering the liver meridian, has effective actions of clearing and draining the liver fire as well as extinguishing wind and arresting convulsion, and thus is an important medicinal for treating internal stirring of liver wind as well as fright epilepsy and convulsion, especially suitable for those with extreme heat producing wind. To treat warm febrile disease intense fire heat, hyperpyrexia and unconsciousness caused by extreme heat generating wind, and convulsive syncope and convulsion, it is often used with *gōu téng*, *jú huā*, *bái sháo*, etc. To treat phlegm-heat eclampsia, infantile convulsion, and wind-strike, it can be combined with *tiān zhú huáng* (Silicea Bambusae Concretio), *niú huáng* (Calculus Bovis), *gōu téng*, etc.

2. 肝阳上亢证　本品质重沉降，有显著的平肝潜阳作用。用治肝阳上亢之眩晕、头痛、头胀、耳鸣等，常配伍石决明、牡蛎、天麻等。

(2) **Syndromes of ascendant hyperactivity of liver yang**　Featuring its heaviness and subsidence, *líng yáng jiǎo* has obvious functions of calming the liver and subduing yang. To treat the dizziness, headache, head distention, and tinnitus caused by ascendant hyperactivity of liver yang, it is often compatible with *shí jué míng*, *mǔ lì*, *tiān má*, etc.

3. 肝火上炎，目赤翳障　本品善清泻肝火而明目，用治肝火上炎，目赤肿痛，羞明流泪，目生翳障等，常与决明子、龙胆草、黄芩等同用。

(3) **Liver fire flaming upward, red eyes with nebula**　*Líng yáng jiǎo* is good at clearing and draining the liver fire so as to improve the vision. To treat liver fire flaming upward, red swelling and pain eyes, photophobia and dacryorrhea, eye nebula, it is often used together with *jué míng zǐ*, *lóng dǎn cǎo* (Gentianae Radix et Rhizoma), *huáng qín* (Scutellariae Radix), etc.

4. 温热病，痈肿疮毒　本品入心、肝经，能清心凉肝，泻火解毒。用治温热病壮热神昏、谵语躁狂等，常与石膏、寒水石、麝香等同用。用治温毒发斑，可与生地黄、赤芍、水牛角等同用。用治痈肿疮毒，可与金银花、连翘等同用。

(4) **Warm febrile disease, abscess and sores**　*Líng yáng jiǎo* enters the heart and liver meridians, and can clear the heart and cool the liver, drain fire and resolve toxins. To treat warm febrile disease such

as high fever and dizziness, delirious speech, agitation and mania, it is often used together with *shí gāo* (Gypsum Fibrosum), *hán shuǐ shí* (Glauberitum), *shè xiāng* (Moschus), etc. To treat warm toxin with eruption, it can be combined with *shēng dì huáng*, *chì sháo* (Paeoniae Rubra Radix), *shuǐ niú jiǎo* (Bubali Cornu), etc. To treat abscess and sores, it can go with *jīn yín huā* (Lonicerae Japonicae Flos), *lián qiáo* (Forsythiae Fructus), etc.

此外，本品还能清肺止咳，用治肺热咳喘。

In addition, *líng yáng jiǎo* is also capable of clearing lung heat and relieving cough, and can be used to treat lung-heat cough and panting.

【用法用量 / Usage and dosage】

煎服，1~3g，宜单煎 2 小时以上。磨汁或研粉服，每次 0.3~0.6g。

Decoction, 1-3g, decocted alone for more than 2 hours; milled into juice or powdered before use, 0.3-0.6g per time.

【使用注意 / Precaution】

脾虚慢惊者忌用。

It is forbidden to patients with weak spleen or chronic infantile convulsion.

【现代研究 / Modern research】

本品主要含角蛋白、磷酸钙、不溶性无机盐、多种氨基酸等。具有抑制中枢神经系统、镇静、镇痛、抗惊厥、抗癫痫、解热、降压、镇咳、祛痰等作用。

Líng yáng jiǎo mainly contains keratin, calcium phosphate, insoluble inorganic salt, a variety of amino acids and so on. It has the functions of inhibiting central nervous system, sedation, analgesia, anti-convulsion, anti-epilepsy, antipyresis, resisting hypertension, relieving cough relieving, dispelling phlegm and so on.

钩藤　*Gōu téng* (Uncariae Ramulus Cum Uncis)
《名医别录》
Miscellaneous Records of Famous Physicians (Míng Yī Bié Lù)

【来源 / Origin】

为茜草科植物钩藤 *Uncaria rhynchophylla*（Miq.）Miq. ex Havil、大叶钩藤 *Uncaria macrophylla* Wall.、毛钩藤 *Uncaria hirsuta* Havil.、华钩藤 *Uncaria sinensis*（Oliv.）Havil. 或无柄果钩藤 *Uncaria sessilifructus* Roxb. 的干燥带钩茎枝。主产于浙江、福建、广东等地。秋、冬二季采收，晒干，生用。本品气微，味淡。

Gōu téng is the dry hooked stem or branch of *Uncaria rhynchophylla* (Miq.) Miq. ex Havil, *Uncaria macrophylla* Wall., *Uncaria hirsuta* Havil., *Uncaria sinensis* (Oliv.) Havil., or *Uncaria sessilifructus* Roxb., pertaining to the Rubiaceae. It is mainly produced in Zhejiang, Fujian, Guangdong and some other places. Harvested in autumn and winter, it is dried for raw use. *Gōu téng* is bland in odor.

【性味归经 / Medicinal properties】

甘，凉。归肝、心包经。

Sweet, cool; act on liver and pericardium meridians.

【主要功效 / Medicinal efficacies】

息风定惊，清热平肝。

Extinguish fire and relieve fright, clear heat and calm the liver.

【临床应用 / Clinical application】

1. **肝风内动证** 本品性凉，入肝经，具有与羚羊角类似的清肝热、息肝风作用，但其功力稍逊。亦为治疗肝风内动，惊痫抽搐的常用药，尤宜于热极生风者。若治温病热盛动风，痉挛抽搐，常与羚羊角、菊花、白芍等配伍。若治小儿急惊风，高热神昏，手足抽搐，常与全蝎、天麻等同用。

(1) Syndromes of internal stirring of liver wind Cold in nature, *gōu téng* enters the liver meridian, and has similar actions as *líng yáng jiǎo,* that is, clearing liver heat and extinguish liver wind, but doesn't have so good efficacies. It is also a common medicinal for treating internal stirring of liver wind as well as fright epilepsy and convulsion, also especially suitable for those with extreme heat producing wind. To treat warm disease such as excessive heat generating wind as well as spasm and convulsion, it is often compatible with *líng yáng jiǎo, jú huā, bái sháo*, etc. To treat acute infantile convulsion, unconsciousness caused by hyperpyrexia and and limb convulsion, it is often combined with *quán xiē, tiān má*, etc.

2. **肝阳上亢证** 本品既清肝热，又平肝阳。用治肝阳上亢，头痛眩晕，常与石决明、珍珠母、天麻等同用。若兼肝火上炎，多与夏枯草、栀子、黄芩等同用。

(2) Syndromes of ascendant hyperactivity of liver yang *Gōu téng* can not only clear liver heat but also calm liver yang. To treat ascendant hyperactivity of liver yang, headache and dizziness, it is often used together with *shí jué míng, zhēn zhū mǔ, tiān má*, etc. To treat those with concurrent liver fire flaming upward, it is often combined with *xià kū cǎo, zhī zǐ* (Gardeniae Fructus), *huáng qín*, etc.

此外，本品息风定惊之中兼能疏风透热，尚可用治感冒夹惊，风热头痛及小儿惊哭夜啼。

In addition, while extinguishing wind and relieving fright, *gōu téng* has concurrent action as pointing location according to proportional bone measurement, and also can be used to treat common cold with frightening or convulsion, wind-heat headache, and infantile frighting night crying.

【用法用量 / Usage and dosage】

煎服，3~12g，后下。

Decoction, 3-12g, added at the end.

【现代研究 / Modern research】

本品主要含钩藤碱、异钩藤碱、去氢钩藤碱、柯诺辛因碱、异柯诺辛因碱、柯楠因碱等多种吲哚类生物碱，尚含三萜类、黄酮类及东莨菪素、β-谷甾醇等。具有抗惊厥、镇静、催眠、镇痛、改善学习记忆、改善微循环、降血压、降血脂、抗心律失常、抗炎、抑制血小板聚集、抗血栓形成、增强免疫等作用。

Gōu téng mainly contains many kinds of indoles alkaloids such as rhynchophylline, isorhynchophylline, corynoxeine, isocorynoxein, and corynantheine, and also contains triterpenes, flavonoids, scopoletin, β-sitosterol, etc. It has the functions of anti-convulsion, sedation, hypnosis, analgesia, improving learning and memory, enhancing microcirculation, lowering blood pressure and fat, anti-arrhythmia, anti-inflammation, inhibiting platelet aggregation, anti-thrombosis and enhancing immunity.

天麻 *Tiān má* (Gastrodiae Rhizoma)
《神农本草经》
Shen Nong's Classic of the Materia Medica (Shén Nóng Běn Cǎo Jīng)

【来源 / Origin】

为兰科植物天麻 *Gastrodia elata* Blume. 的干燥块茎。主产于四川、云南、贵州等地。立冬后至次年清明前采挖，冬季茎枯时采挖者，为"冬麻"，质量优良；春季发芽时采挖者，为

"夏麻"，质量较差。干燥，切薄片，生用。本品气微，味甘。《中国药典》规定，含天麻素（$C_{13}H_{18}O_7$）和对羟基苯甲醇（$C_7H_8O_2$）的总量不得少于 0.25%。

Tiān má is the dry tuber of *Gastrodia elata* Blume., pertaining to the Orchid, and is mainly produced in Sichuan, Yunnan, Guizhou and some other places. It is collected from the beginning of winter to *Qingming* the next year. If dug in winter with withered stem, it is called *dōng má*, with a high quality. If dug in spring with buds, it is called *xià má*, with a comparatively worse quality. It is dried and cut into thin slices for raw use. *Tiān má* is mild and sweet. According to *Chinese Pharmacopoeia*, the content of gastrodin ($C_{13}H_{18}O_2$) P-hydroxybenzyl alcohol ($C_7H_8O_2$) should be no less than 0.25%.

【性味归经 / Medicinal properties】

甘，平。归肝经。

Sweet and neutral; act on liver meridian.

【主要功效 / Medicinal efficacies】

息风止痉，平抑肝阳，祛风通络。

Extinguish wind and arrest convulsion, restrain the liver yang, dispel wind and unblock the collaterals.

【临床应用 / Clinical application】

1. 肝风内动证 本品专入肝经，具有良好的息风止痉功效，且药性平和，可用治各种原因导致的肝风内动，惊痫抽搐。若治小儿急惊风，常与羚羊角、全蝎、钩藤等配伍。若治小儿脾虚慢惊，则与人参、白术、僵蚕等同用。若治破伤风之痉挛抽搐、角弓反张，常与白附子、天南星、防风等同用。

(1) Syndromes of internal stirring of liver wind Specially entering the liver meridian, *tiān má*, neutral, has a good efficacy of extinguishing wind and arresting convulsion, and can be used to treat internal stirring of liver wind as well as fright epilepsy and convulsion of various reasons. To treat acute infantile convulsion, it is often compatible with *líng yáng jiǎo*, *quán xiē*, *gōu téng*, etc. To treat infantile weak spleen or chronic convulsion, it can be used together with *rén shēn*, *bái zhú* (Atractylodis Macrocephalae Rhizoma), *jiāng cán*, etc. To treat spasm and convulsion and opisthotonus caused by tetanus, it is often combined with *bái fù zǐ* (Typhonii Rhizoma), *tiān nán xīng* (Arisaematis Rhizoma), *fáng fēng* (Saposhnikoviae Radix), etc.

2. 眩晕，头痛 本品既息肝风，又平肝阳，可用于多种原因所致的眩晕、头痛，尤宜于肝阳上亢者，常与牛膝、天麻、石决明等同用。若治风痰上扰，眩晕头痛，常与半夏、白术、茯苓等配伍。若治肝肾阴虚，头晕目眩，头痛耳鸣，可与熟地黄、何首乌等同用。若治血虚眩晕，可与当归、熟地黄、白芍等同用。

(2) Dizziness and headache Extinguishing liver wind and calming liver yang, *tiān má* can be used to treat dizziness and headache of various reasons, and is especially suitable for those with ascendant hyperactivity of liver yang, where it is often used together with *niú xī* (Achyranthis Bidentatae Radix), *tiān má*, *shí jué míng*, etc. To treat wind phlegm harassing the upper body, dizziness and headache, it is often compatible with *bàn xià*, *bái zhú*, *fú líng* (Poria), etc. To treat liver-kidney yin deficiency, light-headedness and dizziness, headache and tinnitus, it can be combined with *shú dì huáng*, *hé shǒu wū* (Polygoni Multiflori Radix), etc. To treat blood deficiency and dizziness, it can go together with *dāng guī* (Angelicae Sinensis Radix), *shú dì huáng*, *bái sháo*, etc.

3. 中风手足不遂，风湿痹痛 本品尚有祛风通络之效。用治中风手足不遂，肢体麻木，常与川芎、全蝎等同用。用治风湿痹痛，关节屈伸不利，多与羌活、秦艽、桑枝等配伍。

(3) Wind strike paralysis of the limbs, rheumatic arthralgia *Tiān má* has the effects of dispelling wind and unblocking the collaterals. To treat wind strike paralysis of the limbs and limb numbness, it is often used together with *chuān xiōng* (Chuanxiong Rhizoma), *quán xiē*, etc. To treat rheumatic arthralgia, disturbance of joint bending and stretching, it is often compatible with *qiāng huó* (Notopterygii Rhizoma et Radix), *qín jiāo* (Gentianae Macrophyllae Radix), *sāng zhī* (Mori Ramulus), etc.

【用法用量 / Usage and dosage】

煎服，3~10g。

Decoction, 3-10g.

【现代研究 / Modern research】

本品主要含天麻素、天麻苷元、天麻多糖、天麻醚苷、生物碱、氨基酸及微量元素等。具有镇静、催眠、抗惊厥、镇痛、抗缺氧、抗衰老、扩血管、降血压、降血脂、抗凝血、抗血栓、抗肿瘤、增强免疫等作用。

Tiān má mainly contains gastrodin, gastrodin aglycogen, gastrodia polysaccharide, gastrodia ether glycosides, alkaloids, amino acids and trace elements, etc. It has functions of sedation, hypnosis, anti-convulsion, analgesia, anti-hypoxia, anti-aging, vasodilation, blood pressure and lipid lowering, anti-coagulation, anti-thrombosis, anti-tumor, and immune enhancement, etc.

地龙 *Dì lóng* (Pheretima)
《神农本草经》
Shen Nong's Classic of the Materia Medica (Shén Nóng Běn Cǎo Jīng)

【来源 / Origin】

为钜蚓科动物参环毛蚓 *Pheretima aspergillum*（E. Perrier）、通俗环毛蚓 *Pheretima vulgaris* Chen、威廉环毛蚓 *Pheretima guillelmi*（Michaelsen）或栉盲环毛蚓 *Pheretima pectinifera* Michaelsen 的干燥体。前一种习称"广地龙"，主产于广东、广西、福建等地；后三种习称"沪地龙"，主产于上海一带。广地龙春季至秋季捕捉，沪地龙夏季捕捉。干燥，生用。本品气腥，味微咸。

Dì lóng is the dry bulk of *Pheretima aspergillum* (E. Perrier), *Pheretima vulgaris* Chen, *Pheretima guillelmi* (Michaelsen) or *Pheretima pectinifera* Michaelsen, pertaining to the Megascolecidae. Of the previous mentioned species, the first, commonly known as *guǎng dì lóng*, is mainly produced in Guangdong, Guangxi Zhuang Autonomous Region, Fujian and some other places, while the rest three, commonly known as *hù dì lóng*, are mainly produced around Shanghai. *Guǎng dì lóng* is harvested from spring to autumn, whereas *hù dì lóng* is captured in summer. They are dried for raw use. *Dì lóng* has a fishy flavor and tastes slightly salty.

【性味归经 / Medicinal properties】

咸，寒。归肝、脾、膀胱经。

Salty and cold; act on liver, spleen and bladder meridians.

【主要功效 / Medicinal efficacies】

清热定惊、通络、平喘、利尿。

Clear heat and relieve fright, unblock the collaterals, relieve panting, promote urination.

【临床应用 / Clinical application】

1. 肝风内动证 本品咸寒入肝经，有清热息风定惊之功。用治温病热极生风之神昏谵语、痉挛抽搐，多与钩藤、牛黄、僵蚕等同用。用治小儿急惊风，高热抽搐，可以本品研烂，与朱砂共为丸服。用治癫狂、痫证，可单用鲜品，加食盐搅拌化水后服用。

(1) Syndromes of internal stirring of liver wind　Being salty and cold and entering the liver meridian, *dì lóng* has the actions of clearing heat, extinguishing wind and relieving fright. To treat unconsciousness and delirious speech caused by warm disease extreme heat producing wind, it is often used together with *gōu téng, niú huáng, jiāng cán*, etc. To treat acute infantile convulsion and high fever convulsion, it can be smashed and taken together with *zhū shā* (Cinnabaris) in the form of pills. To treat mania and eclampsia, *dì lóng*, used alone in the fresh form, can be taken after salt is added and stirred in water.

2．中风偏瘫，痹证　本品性善走窜，善通经活络，可用于多种原因所致的经络痹阻，血脉不通病证。若治中风后气虚血滞，经络不通，半身不遂、口眼㖞斜等，常与黄芪、当归、赤芍等配伍。本品又善治痹证，因其性寒清热，故适宜于关节红肿疼痛、屈伸不利之热痹，常与秦艽、防己、桑枝等同用。若治风寒湿痹之关节麻木疼痛，可与川乌、没药、天南星等同用。

(2) Stroke hemiplegia, *bì* syndrome　Good at channeling, *dì lóng* is apt to unblock the channels and quicken the collaterals, and as a result can be used to treat channel obstruction caused by various reasons, and blockage of blood vessels. To treat qi deficiency and blood stagnation, blockage of channels and collaterals, half-body paralysis and obliquity of mouth and eyes, it can be compatible with *huáng qí, dāng guī, chì sháo*, etc. In addition, *dì lóng* is also good at treating *bì* syndrome. Since it is cold and can clear heat, it is suitable for heat *bì* caused by swollen and painful joints, and inhibited bending and stretching of joints as well. In such a case, it is often used together with *qín jiāo, fáng jǐ* (Stephaniae Tetrandrae Radix), *sāng zhī*, etc. To treat joint numbness and pain resulted from wind-cold dampness *bì*, it can be combined with *chuān wū* (Aconiti Radix), *mò yào* (Myrrha), *tiān nán xīng*, etc.

3．肺热喘咳　本品有清肺平喘之功。适用于肺热喘息，可与麻黄、杏仁、石膏等同用。用治痰热阻肺，咳嗽气喘，咳痰黄稠者，可与石膏、葶苈子、苦杏仁等配伍。

(3) Lung heat panting and cough　*Dì lóng* has the actions of clearing lung heat and relieving panting. To treat lung heat panting, it can be used together with *má huáng* (Ephedrae Herba), *xìng rén* (Armeniacae Amarum Semen), *shí gāo*, etc. For those with phlegm-heat obstructing the lung, cough and panting, thick and yellow sputum, it can be compatible with *shí gāo, tíng lì zǐ* (Lepidii Semen), *kǔ xìng rén*, etc.

4．水肿，小便不利　本品咸寒，入膀胱经，有清热利尿之效。用治湿热水肿，可配伍泽泻、木通等。用治热结膀胱之小便不利，甚至尿闭不通，可捣烂浸水，滤取浓汁服，或与木通、车前子、茯苓等同用。

(4) Edema, difficult urination　Salty and cold, *dì lóng*, entering the bladder channel, has the efficacies of clearing heat and promoting urination. To treat damp-heat edema, it can be compatible with *zé xiè* (Alismatis Rhizoma), *mù tōng* (Akebiae Caulis), etc. To treat difficult urination or even retention and blockage of urine caused by heat accumulation in the bladder, it can be crushed, soaked in water and filtered to extract thick juice, or it also can be used together with *mù tōng, chē qián zǐ* (Plantaginis Semen), *fú líng*, etc.

【用法用量 / Usage and dosage】

煎服，5~10g。

Decoction, 5-10g.

【使用注意 / Precaution】

脾胃虚寒者慎用。孕妇忌用。

It should be used with caution for those with deficiency-cold of the spleen and stomach, and forbidden for pregnant women.

【现代研究 / Modern research】

本品主要含蚯蚓解热碱、蚯蚓毒素、6-羟基嘌呤、黄嘌呤、腺嘌呤、鸟嘌呤、胆碱以及多种氨基酸、脂肪酸等。具有抗惊厥、解热、镇静、抗血栓、抗凝血、降压、镇痛、抗炎、平喘、抗肿瘤、利尿、抑菌、兴奋子宫、增强免疫等作用。

Dì lóng mainly contains lumbrofebin, terrestro-lumbrilysin, 6-hydroxypurine, xanthine, adenine, guanine, choline and a variety of amino acids, fatty acids, etc. It has such functions as anti-convulsion, antipyresis, sedation, antithrombosis, anticoagulation, antihypertension, analgesia, anti-inflammation, antiasthma, anti-tumor, diuresis, bacteriostasis, uterus stimulation and immunity enhancement.

全蝎 *Quán xiē* (Scorpio)
《蜀本草》
Materia Medica of Sichuan (Shǔ Běn Cǎo)

【来源 / Origin】

为钳蝎科动物东亚钳蝎 *Buthus martensii* Karsch 的干燥体。主产于河南、山东、湖北等地。春末至秋初捕捉。置沸水或沸盐水中，煮至全身僵硬，捞出，置通风处，阴干。本品气微腥，味咸。

Quán xiē is the dry bulk of *Buthus martensii* Karsch, pertaining to the Buthidae. It is mainly produced in Henan, Shandong, Hubei and some other places. Captured from later spring to early autumn, it is put into boiling water or boiling salty water, and fished out until the body becomes stiff. Then it will be put in a ventilate place and dried in shade. *Quán xiē* is slightly fishy and tastes salty.

【性味归经 / Medicinal properties】

辛，平；有毒。归肝经。

Acrid and neutral; toxic; act on liver meridian.

【主要功效 / Medicinal efficacies】

息风镇痉，攻毒散结，通络止痛。

Extinguish wind and suppress convulsion, attack toxins and dissipate masses, unblock the collaterals and relieve pain.

【临床应用 / Clinical application】

1. 痉挛抽搐　本品专入肝经，性善走窜，既平息肝风，又搜风定搐，为息风止痉之要药，适用于各种原因引起的痉挛抽搐，常与蜈蚣相须为用。如治小儿急惊风之高热、神昏、抽搐，常与羚羊角、钩藤、天麻等同用。如治小儿慢惊风之抽搐，常与人参、白术、天麻等同用。如治破伤风之痉挛抽搐，角弓反张，常与蜈蚣、蝉蜕、天南星等配伍。如治风中经络，口眼㖞斜，常与僵蚕、白附子配伍。如治癫痫抽搐，可与僵蚕、天麻、石菖蒲等配伍。

(1) Spasm and convulsion　Especially entering the liver meridian and being good at channeling, *quán xiē*, which can not only calm and extinguish liver wind but also remove wind and relieve convulsion, is an important medicinal to extinguish wind and arrest convulsion. To treat spasm and convulsion of various reasons, it is often used together with *wú gōng*. To treat high fever, unconsciousness and convulsion resulted from acute infantile convulsion, it is often combined with *líng yáng jiǎo*, *gōu téng*, *tiān má*, etc. To treat convulsion brought by chronic infantile convulsion, it often goes with *rén shēn*, *bái zhú*, *tiān má*, etc. To treat spasm and convulsion and opisthotonus caused by tetanus, it is often compatible with *wú gōng, chán tuì, tiān nán xīng*, etc. To treat obliquity of mouth and eyes caused by wind striking the channels and collaterals, it is often combined with *jiāng cán* and *bái fù zǐ*. To treat hieronosus and hyperspasmia, it can go with *jiāng cán, tiān má, shí chāng pú* (Acori Tatarinowii Rhizoma), etc.

2. 风湿顽痹，偏正头痛　本品味辛走窜，善于搜风通络止痛。用治风寒湿痹日久不愈，筋脉拘挛，甚至关节变形之顽痹，常与川乌、蕲蛇、没药等同用。若治顽固性偏正头痛，常与天麻、川芎、蜈蚣等配伍。

(2) Wind-damp obstinate impediment, hemilateral and over-all headache　Acrid and channelable, *quán xiē* does well in removing wind, unblocking the collaterals and relieving pain. To treat recurring wind-cold-dampness *bì* and such obstinate *bì* as hypertonicity of the sinews and even dysarthrose, it is often used together with *chuān wū* (Aconiti Radix), *qí shé, mò yào*, etc. To treat intractable hemilateral or over-all headache, it is often compatible with *tiān má, chuān xiōng* (Chuanxiong Rhizoma), *wú gōng*, etc.

3. 疮疡肿毒，瘰疬痰核　本品味辛而有毒，能以毒攻毒，散结消肿。用治疮疡肿毒、瘰疬痰核等，内服外用均可。如治诸疮肿毒，可与栀子、黄蜡制膏外用。如治瘰疬瘿瘤，可与马钱子、半夏、五灵脂等同用。

(3) Sores and pyogenic infections, scrofula and phlegm node　Acrid and toxic, *quán xiē*, can use poisons as antidotes, dissipate masses and diminish swelling. To treat sores and pyogenic infections, scrofula and phlegm node, it can be both of internal and external use. To treat all sores and pyogenic infections, it also can go together with *zhī zǐ* (Gardeniae Fructus) and *huáng là* (Cera Flava) to make paste for exterior use. To treat scrofula, goiter and tumor, it can be combined with *mǎ qián zǐ* (Strychni Semen), *bàn xià, wǔ líng zhī* (Trogopterori Faeces), etc.

【用法用量 / Usage and dosage】

煎服，3~6g。外用适量。

Decoction, 3-6g. Appropriate amount for external use.

【使用注意 / Precaution】

用量不宜过大。孕妇禁服。

The dosage should not be too large. Pregnant women should avoid using it.

【现代研究 / Modern research】

本品主要含蝎毒，尚含三甲胺、甜菜碱、牛磺酸、棕榈酸、油酸、胆甾醇、卵磷脂、铵盐、微量元素等。具有抗惊厥、抗癫痫、镇痛、抗凝、抗血栓、抗肿瘤、降压等作用。

Quán xiē mainly contains scorpion venom, and also contains trimethylamine, betaine, taurine, palmitic acid, oleic acid, cholesterol, lecithin, ammonium salt, trace elements, etc. It has the functions of anti-convulsion, anti-epilepsy, analgesia, anticoagulation, anti-thrombus, antitumor, antihypertensive, etc.

蜈蚣　***Wú gōng*** (Scolopendra)

《神农本草经》

Shen Nong's Classic of the Materia Medica (Shén Nóng Běn Cǎo Jīng)

【来源 / Origin】

为蜈蚣科动物少棘巨蜈蚣 *Scolopendra subspinipes mutilans* L. Koch 的干燥体。主产于湖北、浙江、江苏等地。春、夏二季捕捉，用竹片插入头尾，绷直，干燥，剪段用。本品气微腥，有特殊刺鼻的臭气，味辛、微咸。

Wú gōng is the dry bulk of *Scolopendra subspinipes mutilans* L. Koch, pertaining to the Scolopendridae. It is mainly produced in Hubei, Zhejiang, Jiangsu and some other places. Captured in spring and autumn, it will be inserted with a piece of bamboo on the head and tail, strained, dried and cut into pieces for use later. *Wú gōng*, with particularly pungent odor, is slightly fishy, acrid and a little salty.

【性味归经 / Medicinal properties 】

辛，温；有毒。归肝经。

Acrid and warm; toxic; act on liver meridian.

【主要功效 / Medicinal efficacies 】

息风镇痉，通络止痛，攻毒散结。

Extinguish wind and tranquilize convulsion, unblock the collaterals and relieve pain, attack toxins and dissipate masses.

【临床应用 / Clinical application 】

1. 痉挛抽搐　本品辛温，性善走窜，内通脏腑，外达经络，具有与全蝎相似的搜风定搐、息风镇痉功效，且作用和温燥毒烈之性更强。可用治多种原因引起的痉挛抽搐，常与全蝎相须为用。如治小儿急惊风，高热抽搐，常与天竺黄、全蝎等同用。如治破伤风之痉挛抽搐，可与天南星、防风等同用。如治风中经络，口眼㖞斜，可与全蝎、白附子等配伍。

(1) Spasm and convulsion　Being acrid and warm, and good at channeling, *wú gōng* goes interiorly to viscera and bowels, and exteriorly to channels and collaterals. It has similar functions of calming and extinguishing liver wind as well as removing wind and relieving convulsion as *quán xiē*, or even with a stronger effect as well as stronger warm dryness and toxicity. To treat spasm and convulsion of various reasons, it is often used together with *quán xiē*. To treat acute infantile convulsion and high fever convulsion, it is often combined with *tiān zhú huáng*, *quán xiē*, etc. To treat spasm and convulsion caused by tetanus, it can go with *tiān nán xīng*, *fáng fēng*, etc. To treat wind striking the channels and collaterals, obliquity of mouth and eyes, it can be compatible with *quán xiē*, *bái fù zǐ*, etc.

2. 风湿顽痹，偏正头痛　本品长于搜风，具有较好的祛风通络止痛作用，功似全蝎而药力更强。用治风湿顽痹，疼痛麻木，多与川乌、威灵仙、蕲蛇等同用。用治顽固性偏正头痛，可与天麻、川芎、地龙等同用。

(2) Wind-damp obstinate impediment, hemilateral and over-all headache　Being good at removing wind, *wú gōng* has a better efficacy of dispelling wind, unblocking the collaterals and relieving pain. It has similar actions as *quán xiē*, with even stronger effects. To treat wind-damp obstinate *bì* symdrome, pain and numbness, it is often used together with *chuān wū*, *wēi líng xiān* (Clematidis Radix et Rhizoma), *qí shé* (Agkistrodon), etc. To treat stubborn hemilateral and over-all headache, it can be combined with *tiān má*, *chuān xiōng*, *dì lóng*, etc.

3. 疮疡肿毒，瘰疬痰核，蛇虫咬伤　本品以毒攻毒，解毒散结，功似全蝎而力强。用治恶疮肿毒，可与雄黄、猪胆汁制膏外敷。用治瘰疬溃烂，可与玄参、浙贝母、金银花藤等同用。用治蛇虫咬伤，可与白芷、雄黄、樟脑等油调外搽患处。

(3) Sores and pyogenic infections, scrofula and phlegm node, snake bite and insect sting　Having similar actions as *quán xiē* and with even stronger effects, *wú gōng* can use poisons as antidotes, dissipate masses and diminish swelling. To treat malignant sores and pyogenic infections, it can be used together with *xióng huáng* (Realgar) and porcine bile to make paste for exterior use. To treat scrofula and fester, it can be combined with *xuán shēn*, *zhè bèi mǔ*, *jīn yín huā téng* (Lonicerae Japonicae Caulis), etc. To treat snake bite and insect sting, *wú gōng*, together with *bái zhǐ* (Angelicae Dahuricae Radix), *xióng huáng* and *zhāng nǎo* (Camphora), can be mixed with oil and then applied exteriorly to the afflicted part.

【用法用量 / Usage and dosage】

煎服，3~5g。外用适量。

Decoction, 3-5g. Appropriate amount for external use.

【使用注意 / Precaution】

本品有毒，用量不宜过大。孕妇禁服。

Wú gōng is toxic, so the dosage should not be too large; pregnant women should avoid using it.

【现代研究 / Modern research】

本品主要含组胺样物质和溶血性蛋白质两种类似蜂毒的成分，尚含酶类、脂肪油、胆甾醇、蚁酸、氨基酸、糖类、微量元素等。具有抗惊厥、镇痛、抗肿瘤、抑菌、抗炎、抗心肌缺血、抗衰老、改善微循环、抗凝血、降低血黏度等作用，并有溶血和组胺样作用。

Wú gōng mainly contains histamine substances and hemolytic proteins, two components similar to bee venom. It also contains enzymes, fat oils, cholesterols, formic acid, amino acids, sugars and trace elements, etc. It has the functions of anti-convulsion, analgesia, anti-tumor, bacteriostasis, anti-inflammation, anti-myocardial ischemia, anti-aging, microcirculation improvement, anti-coagulation, blood viscosity reduction and so on. It also has the actions of hemolysis and histamine.

僵蚕　*Jiāng cán* (Bombyx Batryticatus)
《神农本草经》
Shen Nong's Classic of the Materia Medica (Shén Nóng Běn Cǎo Jīng)

【来源 / Origin】

为蚕蛾科昆虫家蚕 *Bombyx mori* Linnaeus 4~5 龄的幼虫感染（或人工接种）白僵菌 *Beauveria bassiana*（Bals.）Vuillant 而致死的干燥体。主产于浙江、江苏、四川等地。多于春、秋二季生产，干燥，生用或炒用。本品气微腥，味微咸。

Jiāng cán is the dry bulk of *Bombyx mori* Linnaeus, which was infected with or artificially infected with *Beauveria bassiana* (Bals.) Vuillant to death at the age of 4-5. It pertains to the Saturniidae, and is mainly produced in Zhejiang, Jiangsu, Sichuan and some other places. Mainly produced in spring and autumn, it is dried, and then used in raw or dry-fried form. *Jiāng cán* smells a little fishy and tastes a little salty.

【性味归经 / Medicinal properties】

咸、辛，平。归肝、肺、胃经。

Salty, acrid and neutral; act on liver, lung and stomach meridians.

【主要功效 / Medicinal efficacies】

息风止痉、祛风止痛、化痰散结。

Extinguish wind and arrest convulsion, dispel wind and relieve pain, dissolve phlegm and dissipate masses.

【临床应用 / Clinical application】

1. 肝风内动证　本品既能息风止痉，又能化痰定惊，且性平偏凉，故宜于肝风内动夹有痰热者。若治小儿痰热急惊风，常与牛黄、全蝎、胆南星等配伍。若治小儿脾虚慢惊风，需与党参、白术、天麻等配伍。若治破伤风之痉挛抽搐、角弓反张，多与钩藤、全蝎、蜈蚣等同用。若治风中经络，口眼㖞斜，痉挛抽搐，常与全蝎、白附子等同用。

(1) Syndromes of internal stirring of liver wind　With the efficacies of extinguishing wind and arresting convulsion, as well as dissolving phlegm and arresting convulsion, *jiāng cán*, neutral and a little cool, is suitable for those with phlegm-heat internal stirring of liver wind. To treat acute infantile convulsion resulted from phlegm heat, it is often compatible with *niú huáng*, *quán xiē*, *dǎn nán xīng* (Arisaema cum Bile), etc. To treat chronic infantile convulsion causes by weak spleen, it is necessary to be combined with *dǎng shēn* (Codonopsis Radix), *bái zhú*, *tiān má*, etc. To treat spasm and convulsion and opisthotonus caused by tetanus, it often can go with *gōu téng*, *quán xiē*, *wú gōng*, etc. To treat wind striking the channels and collaterals, obliquity of mouth and eyes, spasm and convulsion, it is often combined with *quán xiē*, *bái fù zǐ*, etc.

2. 风热头痛，目赤咽痛，风疹瘙痒　本品味辛能散，具有疏风散热、止痛、利咽、止痒之效。用治肝经风热之头痛、目赤肿痛，可与荆芥、木贼、桑叶等同用。用治风热咽喉肿痛，可与桔梗、甘草、薄荷等同用。用治风疹瘙痒，可与蝉蜕、防风、地肤子等同用。

(2) Wind-heat headache, red eyes and sore throat, pruritus due to urticaria　Acrid and dispersing, *jiāng cán* has the efficacies of scattering wind and heat, relieving pain, sore throat and itching. To treat headache and red swelling and pain eyes caused by wind-heat in the liver channel, it can be used together with *jīng jiè* (Schizonepetae Herba), *mù zéi*, *sāng yè* (Mori Folium), etc. To treat wind-heat sore swollen throat, it can be combined with *jié gěng* (Platycodonis Radix), *gān cǎo* (Glycyrrhizae Radix et Rhizoma), *bò he* (Menthae Herba), etc. To treat pruritus due to urticaria, it can be compatible with *chán tuì*, *fáng fēng*, *dì fū zǐ* (Kochiae Fructus), etc.

3. 痰核瘰疬，发颐痄腮　本品咸能软坚散结，又兼化痰之效，用治痰火郁结之痰核瘰疬，可与浙贝母、夏枯草、牡蛎等同用。若治发颐、痄腮、疔疮，可与牛蒡子、连翘、板蓝根等同用。

(3) Phlegm node and scrofula, suppurative parotitis and mumps　Salty, *jiāng cán* has the actions of softening hardness and dissipating masses, and dissolving phlegm as well. To treat phlegm node and scrofula due to binding constraint of phlegm fire, it can be used together with *zhè bèi mǔ*, *xià kū cǎo*, *mǔ lì*, etc. To treat suppurative parotitis, mumps or boils, it can be combined with *niú bàng zǐ* (Arctii Fructus), *lián qiáo*, *bǎn lán gēn* (Isatidis Radix), etc.

【用法用量 / Usage and dosage】
煎服，5~10g。散风热多生用，其他多制用。

Decoction, 5-10g. Normally used in raw form to disperse wind heat and processed form for other uses.

【现代研究 / Modern research】
本品主要含蛋白质、脂肪、多种氨基酸以及多种微量元素等。具有镇静、催眠、抗惊厥、抗凝血、抑菌、降血糖、抗肿瘤等作用。

Jiāng cán mainly contains protein, fat, a variety of amino acids and trace elements. It has the functions of sedation, hypnosis, anti-convulsion, anti-coagulation, bacteriostasis, blood sugar reduction, anti-tumor, etc.

其他平肝息风药功用介绍见表20-1。
The efficacies of other liver-calming wind-extinguishing medicinals are shown in table 20-1.

表 20-1　其他平肝息风药功用介绍

分类	药物	药性	功效	应用	用法用量
平抑肝阳药	珍珠母	咸，寒。归肝、心经	平肝潜阳，安神定惊，明目退翳	肝阳上亢证，心神不宁证，目赤翳障，视物昏花	煎服，10~25g，先煎
	蒺藜	辛、苦，微温；有小毒。归肝经	平肝解郁，活血祛风，明目，止痒	肝阳上亢证，肝郁气滞证，目赤翳障，风疹瘙痒，白癜风	煎服，6~10g
	罗布麻叶	甘、苦，凉。归肝经	平肝安神，清热利水	肝阳上亢证，水肿	煎服，6~12g
息风止痉药	山羊角	咸，寒。归肝经	平肝，镇惊	肝阳上亢，头晕目眩；肝火上炎，目赤肿痛；惊风抽搐	煎服，10~15g

题库

（王科军）

第二十一章　开　窍　药

Chapter 21　Resuscitative medicinals

学习目标 | Learning goals

1. 掌握　开窍药在性能、功效、主治、配伍及使用注意方面的共性；麝香和石菖蒲的性能、功效、应用以及特殊的用法用量和特殊的使用注意。

2. 熟悉　冰片的功效、应用以及特殊的用法用量和特殊的使用注意。

3. 了解　开窍药以及有关功效术语的含义；苏合香、安息香的功效、应用特点以及特殊的用法用量和特殊的使用注意。

1. Master the commonness of resuscitative medicinals in efficacy, indications, property, compatibility and cautions; as well as the property, efficacy, application, special usage and dosage and special precautions of *shè xiāng*, *shí chāng pú*.

2. Familiar with the efficacy, indications, special usage, dosage and special precautions of *bīng piàn*.

3. Understand the definitions of resuscitative medicinals and related efficacy terms; the efficacy, special usage and dosage and special precautions of *sū hé xiāng* and *ān xī xiāng*.

凡具辛香走窜之性，以开窍醒神为主要功效，常用以治疗闭证神昏的药物，称为开窍药。

Medicinals with properties of acridness, aroma and wandering, which has main efficacies of opening the orifices and inducing resuscitation, are known as resuscitative medicinals. These medicinals are usually used to treat block syndrome with unconsciousness.

开窍药味辛，多具浓郁的芳香之气，性善走窜，主入心经，具有开通心窍、醒脑回苏之功。主治温病热陷心包、痰浊、瘀血等实邪蒙蔽清窍等所致的闭证神昏，以及惊风、癫痫、中风等卒然昏厥、痉挛抽搐等症。其中，闭证兼见面红、身热、苔黄、脉数者为热闭；闭证兼见面青、身凉、苔白、脉迟者为寒闭，均可应用本类药物。部分开窍药兼有活血、行气、止痛、解毒等功效，又可用治血瘀气滞，经闭癥瘕，心腹疼痛，目赤咽肿，痈疽疔疮等。

Resuscitative medicinals are usually acrid in flavor and aromatic in smell for wandering, and they mainly act on the heart meridian, which function to open heart orifice and resuscitate the mind. They are indicated to treat block with unconsciousness, sudden syncope, convulsion and spasm, such as infantile convulsion, epilepsy and stroke caused by excess pathogenic factors blocking orifices due to heat entering pericardium in warm disease, phlegm-turbidity as well as static blood. Block accompanied by flushed faces, fever, yellowish coating and rapid pulse is called heat block; while that accompanied by green-blue complexion, cold body, whitish coating and slow pulse is called cold block. The above-mentioned morbid condition can be treated with medicinals in this chapter. Some resuscitative medicinals also have actions

医药大学堂
WWW.YIYAODXT.COM

of invigorating blood, moving qi, relieving pain and resolving toxin, which can also be applied to treat amenorrhea, abdominal masses, pain in the heart and abdomen, red eyes, sore throat, carbuncle, abscess, sores and boils caused by blood stasis and qi stagnation.

应用开窍药须明辨热闭、寒闭，根据闭证的不同性质，选用适宜的药物，并做适当的配伍。若属热闭神昏者宜凉开，配伍清热泻火解毒药；若属寒闭神昏者宜温开，配伍温里祛寒药。若闭证神昏兼惊厥抽搐，宜配伍息风止痉药；若见烦躁不安，宜配伍安神药；若痰浊壅盛，应配伍化湿、祛痰药。

When using resuscitative medicinals, doctors should identify heat block and cold block first, and then select corresponding medicinals and make proper compatibility according to different natures of block. For heat block with unconsciousness, the therapeutic principle should be "resuscitating with cold medicinals", so resuscitative medicinals with pungent and cold nature should be applied, and they should be combined with medicinals that can clear heat, reduce fire as well as resolve toxin; for cold block with unconsciousness, the therapeutic principle should be "resuscitating with warm medicinals", so resuscitative medicinals with acrid and warm nature should be used, and they should be combined with medicinals that can warm the interior and dispel cold; for block with unconsciousness accompanied by syncope and convulsion, liver-calming, wind-extinguishing and convulsion-arresting medicinals should be combined. For the conditions manifested as vexation and agitation, mind-calming medicinals should be combined; for conditions with exuberance of phlegm-turbidity, damp-resolving and phlegm-eliminating medicinals should be combined.

开窍药辛香走窜，为救急、治标之品，宜耗伤正气，故只宜暂服，不可久用。因其芳香之气易于挥发，或受热有效成分易被破坏，或有效成分不易溶于水，故内服多宜入丸、散，不宜入煎剂。孕妇慎用或忌用。

Medicinals of this category are acrid, aromatic and wandering, so they are usually used for emergency and the branches of disease. But they tend to consume healthy qi, so they are only used temporally. They are usually taken orally in pills or powder instead of decoction, because its fragrance tends to volatilize, the effective ingredients are easily damaged after being heated, and the active ingredients should not dissolve in water. In addition, they should be used with caution or be contraindicated for pregnant women.

麝香　*Shè xiāng* (Moschus)
《神农本草经》
Shen Nong's Classic of the Materia Medica (Shén Nóng Běn Cǎo Jīng)

【来源 / Origin】

为鹿科动物林麝 *Moschus berezovskii* Flerov、马麝 *M. sifanicus* Przewalski 或原麝 *M. moschiferus* Linnaeus 成熟雄体香囊中的干燥分泌物。主产于四川、西藏、云南等地。野生麝多在冬季至次春猎取后，割取香囊，阴干，习称"毛壳麝香"，用时剖开香囊，除去囊壳，称"麝香仁"，其中呈颗粒状者称"当门子"；人工驯养麝直接从香囊中取出麝香仁，阴干。本品气香浓烈而特异，味微辣、微苦带咸。《中国药典》规定，含麝香酮（$C_{16}H_{30}O$）不得少于 2.0%。

Shè xiāng is the dried secretion from the mature male musk bag of *Moschus berezovskii* Flerov, *M. sifanicus* Przewalski or *M. moschiferus* Linnaeus, pertaining to Cervidae. It is mainly produced in Sichuan Province, Tibet Autonomous Region and Yunnan Province in China. The wild musk deer is hunted from winter to the next spring, and the musk bad is cut off and dried in the shade, which is called *máo ké shè*

xiāng. When in use, the musk bag is cut off and the shell is removed in order to take out the core, which is called *shè xiāng rén*, and the one appears like granule is called *dāng mén zǐ*. *Shè xiāng rén* is usually taken out directly from the musk bag of home musk deer and dried in the shade. It has strong and unique fragrance, and tastes slightly spicy, mildly bitter and salty. According to *Chinese Pharmacopoeia*, the content of muscone ($C_{16}H_{30}O$) should be no less than 2.0%.

【性味归经 / Medicinal properties】

辛，温。归心、脾经。

Acrid and warm; act on the heart and spleen meridians.

【主要功效 / Medicinal efficacies】

开窍醒神，活血通经，消肿止痛。

Open the orifices and induce resuscitation, invigorate blood to smooth meridians, remove swelling and relieve pain.

【临床应用 / Clinical application】

1. 闭证神昏　本品辛香走窜之性甚烈，具有较强的开窍通闭作用，为醒神回苏之要药。可用于各种原因所致的闭证神昏，无论热闭或寒闭，皆可应用。因其性温，为"温开"之品，故治寒闭神昏尤宜。若治温病热陷心包，痰热蒙蔽心窍，小儿惊风及中风痰厥等热闭神昏，常配伍牛黄、冰片、朱砂等。若治寒湿或痰浊闭阻心窍之寒闭神昏，常配伍苏合香、檀香、安息香等。

(1) Unconsciousness in block　*Shè xiāng* is aromatic with strong abilities of moving and wandering, which has strong effect of opening orifices and relieving block. It is an important medicinal for inducing resuscitation. It can be used to treat unconsciousness in block caused by various reasons, including both heat and cold block. It is warm in nature, thus, it is especially suitable to treat unconsciousness in cold block. To treat unconsciousness in cold block due to pathogenic heat entering pericardium, phlegm-heat blocking, infantile convulsion and phlegm syncope of wind-strike, it is often combined with *niú huáng* (Calculus Bovis), *bīng piàn* (Borneolum Syntheticum) and *zhū shā* (Cinnabaris). To treat unconsciousness in cold block caused by block and obstruction of cold-damp or phlegm-turbidity, it is often combined with *sū hé xiāng* (Styrax), *tán xiāng* (Santali Albi Lignum) and *ān xī xiāng* (Benzoinum).

2. 血瘀证　本品辛香，开通走窜，具有较好的活血通经、消癥、止痛、疗伤之效，可广泛用于瘀血阻滞病证。若治血瘀经闭，常与丹参、桃仁、红花等同用。若治癥瘕痞块等血瘀重证，可与水蛭、虻虫、三棱等配伍。若治心血瘀阻，胸痹疼痛不止或厥心痛，常配伍木香、桃仁等。若治偏正头痛，日久不愈，常与赤芍、川芎、桃仁等同用。若治跌仆肿痛、骨折扭挫，不论内服外用均有良效，常与乳香、没药、红花等配伍。若治风寒湿痹证顽固不愈者，可与独活、威灵仙、桑寄生等同用。

(2) Blood stasis　It is acrid and aromatic for moving and wandering, which is effective in invigorating blood to unblock meridians, resolving masses, relieving pain and curing injury. It can be widely used to treat disorders caused by blood stagnation. To treat amenorrhea due to blood stasis, it is often combined with *dān shēn* (Salviae Miltiorrhizae Radix et Rhizoma), *táo rén* (Persicae Semen) and *hóng huā* (Carthami Flos). To treat severe conditions caused by blood stagnation, such as concretions and conglomerations (lower abdominal masses), it is often combined with *shuǐ zhì* (Hirudo), *méng chóng* (Tabanus) and *sān léng* (Sparganii Rhizoma). To treat heart pain in chest impediment, precordial pain with cold limbs due to stagnation and obstruction of heart blood, it is often combined with *mù xiāng* (Aucklandiae Radix) and *táo rén* (Persicae Semen). To treat prolonged hemicrania, it is often combined with *chì sháo* (Paeoniae Rubra Radix), *chuān xiōng* (Chuanxiong Rhizoma) and *táo rén* (Persicae Semen). To treat injury due to fall, swelling and pain, fracture and contusion, it is effective either by oral taking or topical application, and is usually combined with *rǔ xiāng* (Olibanum), *mò yào* (Myrrha) and *hóng huā* (Carthami Flos). To treat stubborn wind-cold-damp *bì*, it is often combined with *dú huó* (Angelicae Pubescentis Radix), *wēi líng xiān* (Clematidis Radix et Rhizoma) and *sāng jì shēng* (Taxilli Herba).

3. 疮疡肿毒，咽喉肿痛　本品具有活血散结、消肿止痛作用，内服、外用均有良效。用治疮疡肿毒，常与雄黄、乳香、没药等同用。用治咽喉肿痛，可与牛黄、蟾酥、珍珠等配伍。

(3) Sores, ulcer, swelling and toxin, sore throat　It has efficacies of activating blood and dissolving masses, removing swelling to relieve pain, and is effective either by oral taking or topical application. To treat sores, ulcer, swelling and toxin, it is often used with *xióng huáng* (Realgar), *rǔ xiāng* (Olibanum) and *mò yào* (Myrrha). To treat sore throat with swelling and pain, it can be combined with *niú huáng* (Calculus Bovis), *chán sū* (Bufonis Venenum) and *zhēn zhū* (Margarita).

【用法用量 / Usage and dosage】

入丸、散，0.03~0.1g。不宜入煎剂。外用适量。

It is used in pills and powder, 0.03-0.1g. It should not be decocted. A proper amount is used for external application.

【使用注意 / Precaution】

孕妇禁用。

It should be contraindicated in pregnant women.

【现代研究 / Modern research】

本品主要含麝香大环化合物，如麝香酮、降麝香酮、麝香醇、麝香吡啶、麝香吡喃等，尚含睾丸酮、雌二醇、胆甾醇等甾类化合物以及蛋白质、多肽、氨基酸等。其对中枢神经系统（CNS）呈现双向影响，小剂量兴奋，大剂量则抑制，并有增强中枢神经系统耐缺氧能力、抗脑水肿、改善脑循环、强心、调节血压、抗炎、兴奋子宫、抗早孕、抗肿瘤等作用。

It mainly contains musk macro-cycles, such as muscone, normuscone, muscol, muscopyridine and mus-copyran. It also contains steroid, such as testosterone, estradiol and cholesterol, as well as proteins, polypeptide and amino acid. It may excite central nervous system (CNS) in a small dosage while inhibit CNS in a large dosage. In addition, it has other functions of strengthening CNS's resistance to anoxia, anti-cerebral edema, improving cerebral circulation, enhancing the heart, regulating blood pressure, antiinflammation, exciting the uterus, anti-early pregnancy and anti-tumor.

冰片　***Bīng piàn* (Borneolum Syntheticum)**

《新修本草》

Newly Revised Materia Medica (Xīn Xiū Běn Cǎo)

【来源 / Origin】

为龙脑香科植物龙脑香 *Dryobalanops aromatica* Gaertn. f. 树干蒸馏冷却所得的结晶，或菊科植物艾纳香（大艾）*Blumea balsamifera* DC. 的叶中提取的结晶。前者又称"龙脑冰片""梅片"，主产于东南亚地区，我国台湾有引种；后者又称"艾片"，主产于广东、广西、云南等地。现多用合成冰片，即用松节油、樟脑等经化学方法合成，又称"机制冰片""合成龙脑"。冰片成品须贮于阴凉处，密闭。研粉用。本品气清香，味辛、凉。《中国药典》规定，天然冰片含右旋龙脑（$C_{10}H_{18}O$）不得少于96.0%，合成冰片含龙脑（$C_{10}H_{18}O$）不得少于55%。

Bīng piàn is the crystals produced by distilling *Dryobalanops aromatica* Gaertn. f. tree trunk and cooling down, which is in the family of Dipterocarpaceae. Or it is produced by processing and chopping the leaves sublimate of *Blumea balsamifera* DC. in the family Compositae. The former is also named *lóng nǎo bīng piàn*, or *méi piàn*, which is mainly produced in the Southeast Asia, and it is also planted in Taiwan, China; the latter is also called *ài piàn*, which is mainly produced in Guangdong Province, Guangxi Zhuang Autonomous Region and Yunnan Province in China. Currently, it is synthesized with chemical methods mostly from the raw materials such as turpentine and camphor, which is called *jī zhì bīng piàn*, or *hé chéng lóng nǎo* The finished product of *bīng piàn* should be closed and stored in the shade. It is ground into powder for application. It has fragrance and tastes acrid and cool. According to *Chinese Pharmacopoeia*, the content of D-borneol ($C_{10}H_{18}O$) in natural *bīng piàn* should be no less than 96.0%, the content of borneol ($C_{10}H_{18}O$) in synthetic *bīng piàn* should be no less than 55%.

【性味归经 / Medicinal properties 】

辛、苦，微寒。归心、脾、肺经。

Acrid, bitter and slightly cold; act on the heart, spleen and lung meridians.

【主要功效 / Medicinal efficacies 】

开窍醒神，清热止痛。

Open the orifices and induce resuscitation, clear heat and relieve pain.

【临床应用 / Clinical application 】

1. 闭证神昏　本品辛凉清香，开窍醒神之功与麝香相似而药力稍逊。因其性偏寒凉，为"凉开"之品，故适宜于热闭神昏。用治热毒内陷心包、痰热内闭、暑热卒厥等热闭证，常与牛黄、麝香、黄连等同用。若治寒闭证，则配伍苏合香、安息香、丁香等温开之品。

(1) Unconsciousness in block　*Bīng piàn* is acrid, cool and aromatic. Its efficacies of opening the orifices and inducing resuscitation are not as strong as those of *shè xiāng* (Moschus). It is mildly cold in nature and is suitable to treat heat block with unconsciousness. To treat heat block caused by heat-toxin invading pericardium, phlegm-heat blocking internally, and sudden syncope due to summer-heat, it is often combined with *niú huáng* (Calculus Bovis), *shè xiāng* (Moschus) and *huáng lián* (Coptidis Rhizoma). To treat cold block, it is often combined with *sū hé xiāng* (Styrax), *ān xī xiāng* (Benzoinum) and *dīng xiāng* (Caryophylli Flos)

2. 胸痹心痛　本品辛香走窜，通窍止痛之力较佳。用治气滞血瘀所致的胸痹心痛，可与丹参、三七配伍。

(2) Heart pain in chest impediment　It is acrid and aromatic with effect of moving and wandering, which is powerful in inducing resuscitation to relieve pain. To treat heart pain in chest *bì* due to qi stagnation and blood stasis, it is often combined with *dān shēn* (Salviae Miltiorrhizae Radix et Rhizoma) and *sān qī* (Notoginseng Radix et Rhizoma).

3. 目赤肿痛，咽喉肿痛，耳道流脓　本品味苦微寒，具有良好的清热解毒、消肿止痛功效，为五官科及外科常用药。用治目赤肿痛，单用点眼即效，也可与炉甘石、硼砂等同用。用治咽喉肿痛、口舌生疮，常与硼砂、朱砂、玄明粉等配伍。治疗耳道流脓，可用本品搅溶于核桃油中滴耳。

(3) Red, swelling and painful eyes, sore throat, purulence in ear canal　It is bitter and slightly cold with effects of clearing heat and resolving toxin, as well as removing swelling and relieving pain. Which is a commonly used medicinal in Otorhinolaryngology and Department of Surgery. To treat red, swelling and painful eyes, it is effective when used singly for eye dropping, or it can be used with *lú gān*

shí (Calamina) and *péng shā* (Borax). To treat sore throat, mouth and tongue ulcer, it is often used with *péng shā* (Borax), *zhū shā* (Cinnabaris) and *xuán míng fěn* (Natrii Sulfas Exsiccatus). To treat ear canal purulence, it can be dissolved in walnut oil for ear dropping.

4. 疮疡肿痛，久溃不敛，水火烫伤　本品有清热解毒、防腐生肌的功效。用治疮疡溃后日久不敛，可配伍牛黄、珍珠、炉甘石等。若治水火烫伤，可与紫草、黄连等制成药膏外用。

(4) Unclosed ulcers and sores, burns and scald　It has functions of clearing heat and resolving toxin, as well as anti-septic and promoting growth of muscles. To treat chronic unclosed ulcers and sores, it is often combined with *niú huáng* (Calculus Bovis), *zhēn zhū* (Margarita) and *lú gān shí* (Calamina). To treat burns and scald, it is often made into paste with *zǐ cǎo* (Arnebiae Radix) and *huáng lián* (Coptidis Rhizoma) for external application.

【用法用量 / Usage and dosage】

入丸、散，0.15~0.3g。不宜入煎剂。外用适量，研粉点敷患处。

It is used in pills and powder, 0.15-0.3g. It should not be decocted. A proper amount is ground into powder and pasted at the affected areas.

【使用注意 / Precaution】

孕妇慎用。

It should be used with caution for pregnant women.

【现代研究 / Modern research】

龙脑冰片主要含右旋龙脑、葎草烯、β-榄香烯等倍半萜类成分，以及齐墩果酸、麦珠子酸、积雪草酸、龙脑香醇等三萜类成分。合成冰片主要含龙脑、异龙脑、樟脑等。对中枢神经系统有双向调节作用，并有抗炎、镇痛、镇静、催眠、抗脑损伤、抗心肌缺血、抗菌及防腐等作用。

Lóng nǎo bīng piàn mainly contains sesquiterpenes, such as D-borneol, caryophyllene, β-elemene, it also contains triterpenes, such as oleanic acid, alphitolic acid, asiatic acid and dipterocarpol. *Hé chéng bīng piàn* mainly contains camphol, isoborneol and camphor. It has two-way regulation to central nervous system. It also has functions of antiinflammation, relieving pain, sedation, hypnotizing, anti-brain damage, anti-myocardial ischemia, anti-bacteria and antiseptic.

苏合香　*Sū hé xiāng* (Styrax)
《名医别录》
Miscellaneous Records of Famous Physicians (*Míng Yī Bié Lù*)

【来源 / Origin】

为金缕梅科植物苏合香树 *Liquidambar orientalis* Mill. 的树干渗出的香树脂经加工精制而成。主产于非洲、印度及土耳其等地，我国广西、云南有引种栽培。初夏采集。本品气芳香。《中国药典》规定，含肉桂酸（$C_9H_8O_2$）不得少于 5.0%。

Sū hé xiāng is processed and refined from resin secreted from the tree trunk of *Liquidambar orientalis* Mill., pertaining to Hamamelidales. It is mainly produced in Africa, India and Turkey, and is also planted in Guangxi Zhuang Autonomous Region and Yunnan Province in China. It is collected in early summer. *Sū hé xiāng* has fragrance. According to *Chinese Pharmacopoeia*, the content of cinnamic acid ($C_9H_8O_2$) should be no less than 5.0%.

【性味归经 / Medicinal properties】

辛，温。归心、脾经。

Acrid and warm; act on the heart and spleen meridians.

【主要功效 / Medicinal efficacies】

开窍，辟秽，止痛。

Open the orifices, repel foulness, relieve pain.

【临床应用 / Clinical application】

1. 寒闭神昏　本品味辛香而性温，有开窍醒神之效，但作用稍逊于麝香，其长于温通辟秽，为"温开"之品。故宜用治中风、惊痫等属于寒邪、痰浊闭阻心窍所致的寒闭神昏，常与麝香、安息香、檀香等同用。

(1) **Cold block with unconsciousness**　It is acrid, aromatic and warm in nature with effect of opening orifices and inducing resuscitation. But it is milder than *shè xiāng* (Moschus), and is good at warming and repelling foulness. To treat cold block with unconsciousness, manifested as wind-strike, fright epilepsy due to pathogenic cold or phlegm-turbidity blocking internally, it is combined with *shè xiāng* (Moschus), *ān xī xiāng* (Benzoinum) and *tán xiāng* (Santali Albi Lignum).

2. 胸痹心痛，脘腹冷痛　本品辛能行散，性温祛寒，功善温里散寒，并有良好的止痛作用。用治寒凝气滞，心脉瘀阻的胸痹心痛，可与乳香、冰片、檀香等配伍。用治寒凝痰浊之胸脘痞满冷痛，常与冰片同用。

(2) **Heart pain in chest impediment**　It is acrid for moving and dispersing, warm in nature for eliminating cold, which is effective in warming the interior and eliminating cold to relieving pain. To treat stagnation of heart vessel caused by qi stagnation due to cold coagulation, manifested as heart pain in chest impediment, it can be combined with *rŭ xiāng* (Olibanum), *bīng piàn* (Borneolum Syntheticum) and *tán xiāng* (Santali Albi Lignum). To treat stuffiness and fullness in the chest and stomach cavity with cold pain due to phlegm-turbidity and congealing cold, it is often combined with *bīng piàn* (Borneolum Syntheticum).

【用法用量 / Usage and dosage】

入丸剂，0.3~1g。不入煎剂。外用适量。

It is used in pills, 0.3-1g. It should not be decocted. A proper amount for external application.

【现代研究 / Modern research】

本品主要含萜类和挥发油，如肉桂酸、α-蒎烯、β-蒎烯、月桂烯、柠檬烯、桂皮醛等。具有兴奋中枢、抗脑损伤、抗缺氧、抗心肌缺血、抗心律失常、抑制血小板聚集、抗血栓形成、祛痰、抗菌等作用。

It mainly contains terpene, volatile oil, such as cinnamic acid, α-pinene, β-pinene, myrcene, limonene and cinnamaldehyde. It has the functions of exciting central nervous system, anti-brain damage, anti-myocardial ischemia, anti-arrhythmia, inhibiting platelet aggregation, antithrombus, eliminating phlegm and inhibiting bacteria.

石菖蒲　*Shí chāng pú* (Acori Tatarinowii Rhizoma)

《神农本草经》

Shen Nong's Classic of the Materia Medica (Shén Nóng Běn Cǎo Jīng)

【来源 / Origin】

为天南星科植物石菖蒲 *Acorus tatarinowii* Schott 的干燥根茎。我国长江流域以南各省均有分布，主产于四川、浙江、江苏等地。秋、冬二季采挖，晒干，生用。本品气芳香，味苦、微辛。《中国药典》规定，含挥发油不得少于 1.0%（ml/g），饮片不得少于 0.7%（ml/g）。

Shí chāng pú is the dried rhizome of *Acorus tatarinowii* Schott, pertaining to Araceae. It is produced in the southern provinces of the Yangtze River valley, and mainly includes Sichuan, Zhejiang and Jiangsu Province. It is collected in the fall and winter, dried in the sun and used in the raw. *Shí chāng pú* is fragrant and tastes bitter, slightly acrid. According to *Chinese Pharmacopoeia*, the content of volatile oil should be no less than 1.0% (ml/g), while that in prepared herbal pieces should be no less than 0.7% (ml/g).

【性味归经 / Medicinal properties】

辛、苦，温。归心、胃经。

Acrid, bitter and warm; act on the heart and stomach meridians.

【主要功效 / Medicinal efficacies】

开窍豁痰，醒神益智，化湿开胃。

Open the orifices and eliminate phlegm, induce resuscitation and benefit intelligence, resolve dampness and prompt appetite.

【临床应用 / Clinical application】

1. **闭证神昏**　本品辛香走窜，入心经，开窍醒神作用比较和缓，但其苦温性燥，长于化湿、豁痰、辟秽，适宜于痰湿秽浊蒙蔽清窍之神昏。若治中风痰迷心窍，神志昏乱，常与半夏、天南星等同用。若治痰热蒙蔽，高热、神昏谵语，常与郁金、半夏、竹沥等配伍。若治痰热癫痫抽搐，可与枳实、竹茹、黄连等同用。

(1) Unconsciousness in block　It is acrid and aromatic for moving and wandering. It acts on the heart meridian with mild effect of opening the orifices and inducing resuscitation. But it is bitter, warm and dry in nature, which is good at resolving dampness, eliminating phlegm and repelling foulness. It is suitable to treat unconsciousness due to phlegm-damp, turbid and foul pathogens blocking the clear orifices. To treat unconsciousness in wind-strike due to phlegm blocking the heart orifices, it is combined with *bàn xià* (Pinelliae Rhizoma) and *tiān nán xīng* (Arisaematis Rhizoma). To treat high fever, unconsciousness and delirium speech due to phlegm-heat blocking the clear orifices, it is often combined with *yù jīn* (Curcumae Radix), *bàn xià* (Pinelliae Rhizoma) and *zhú lì* (Bambusae Succus). To treat convulsion, mania and epilepsy due to phlegm-heat, it can be combined with *zhǐ shí* (Aurantii Immaturus Fructus), *zhú rú* (Bambusae Caulis in Taenia) and *huáng lián* (Coptidis Rhizoma).

2. **健忘失眠，耳鸣耳聋**　本品有宁心安神益智、聪耳明目之功。用治健忘，常与人参、茯苓、石菖蒲等配伍。用治劳心过度、心神失养之失眠、多梦、心悸，常与远志、茯苓、朱砂等同用。用治心血不足、虚火内扰之心悸失眠、头晕耳鸣，可与丹参、五味子、首乌藤等同用。用治湿浊蒙蔽所致的头晕、嗜睡、健忘、耳鸣、耳聋，常与茯苓、远志、龙骨等配伍。

(2) Poor memory, insomnia, tinnitus and deafness　It has efficacies of calming heart, tranquilizing the mind, benefiting intelligence, improving hearing and vision. To treat poor memory, it is often combined with *rén shēn* (Ginseng Radix et Rhizoma), *fú líng* (Poria) and *shí chāng pú* (Acori Tatarinowii Rhizoma). To treat malnutrition of heart mind due to spiritual exhaustion, manifested as insomnia, dreaminess and palpitation, it is often combined with *yuǎn zhì* (Polygalae Radix), *fú líng* (Poria) and *zhū shā* (Cinnabaris). To treat internal disturbance of deficiency-fire due to shortage of heart blood, manifested as palpitation, insomnia, dizziness and tinnitus, it is often combined with *dān shēn* (Salviae Miltiorrhizae Radix et Rhizoma), *wǔ wèi zǐ* (Schisandrae Chinensis Fructus) and *shǒu wū téng* (Polygoni Multiflori Caulis). To treat dizziness, somnolence, tinnitus, deafness due to damp-turbidity blocking the clear orifices, it is often used with *fú líng* (Poria), *yuǎn zhì* (Polygalae Radix) and *lóng gǔ* (Fossilia Ossis Mastodi).

3. **湿阻中焦证** 本品辛香苦燥，善化湿醒脾，开胃进食。用治湿阻中焦，运化失常之脘腹痞满、食欲不振、苔腻，常与广藿香、苍术、厚朴等同用。若治湿浊、热毒蕴结肠中所致的水谷不纳、里急后重，可与黄连、茯苓、石莲子等同用。

(3) Damp obstruction in the middle energizer It is acrid, aromatic, bitter and dry with effects of resolving damp and awakening spleen, as well as stimulating appetite. To treat dysfunction of spleen in transporting and transforming due to damp obstructing middle energizer, manifested as stuffiness and fullness in the gastric cavity and abdomen, poor appetite and greasy coating, it is often combined with *guǎng huò xiāng* (Pogostemonis Herba), *cāng zhú* (Atractylodis Rhizoma) and *hòu pò* (Magnoliae Officinalis Cortex). To treat rejecting to water and food, as well as tenesmus due to damp-turbidity or heat-toxin accumulating in the intestine, it is often combined with *huáng lián* (Coptidis Rhizoma), *fú líng* (Poria) and *shí lián zǐ* (Nelumbo nucifera Gaerth).

【用法用量 / Usage and dosage】

煎服，3~10g。鲜品加倍。

Decoction, 3-10g. The fresh one is applied in double dosage.

【现代研究 / Modern research】

本品含挥发油如细辛醚、石竹烯、α-葎草烯、石菖醚、细辛醛、百里香酚等，尚含氨基酸、有机酸和糖类。具有镇静、抗惊厥、抗抑郁、抗脑损伤、改善学习记忆、促进消化液分泌、调节胃肠运动、抗心律失常、抗心肌缺血、平喘、祛痰、镇咳等作用。

It mainly contains volatile oil, which includes asarone, caryophyllene, α-humulene, sekishone, asarylaldehyde and thymol. It also contains amino acid, organic acid and saccharides. It has the functions of sedation, anti-convulsion, anti-depression, anti-brain damage, improve memory, promoting secretion of digestive juice, regulating gastric and intestinal movement, anti-myocardial ischemia, anti-arrhythmia, relieve asthma, eliminating sputum and relieving cough.

其他开窍药功用介绍见表21-1。

The efficacies of other resuscitative medicinals are shown in table 21-1.

表21-1　其他开窍药功用介绍

分类	药物	药性	功效	应用	用法用量
开窍药	安息香	辛、苦，平。归心、脾经	开窍醒神，行气活血，止痛	闭证神昏，心腹疼痛，风湿痹痛	入丸、散剂，0.6~1.5g

（杨青山）

第二十二章 补 虚 药
Chapter 22 Supplementing medicinals

 学习目标 ┊ **Learning goals**

    1. 掌握 补虚药在性能、功效、主治、配伍及使用注意方面的共性；人参、党参、黄芪、白术、甘草、鹿茸、淫羊藿、杜仲、补骨脂、菟丝子、当归、熟地黄、白芍、阿胶、北沙参、麦冬、枸杞子、龟甲、鳖甲的性能、功效、应用以及特殊的用法用量和特殊的使用注意。

    2. 熟悉 补虚药的分类；西洋参、大枣、山药、紫河车、巴戟天、续断、肉苁蓉、蛤蚧、冬虫夏草、何首乌、天冬、百合、石斛的功效、主治以及特殊的用法用量和特殊的使用注意。

    3. 了解 补虚药及相关功效术语的含义；太子参、刺五加、白扁豆、绞股蓝、红景天、沙棘、饴糖、蜂蜜、鹿角、鹿角胶、鹿角霜、仙茅、锁阳、益智仁、沙苑子、核桃仁、韭菜子、阳起石、海狗肾、海马、龙眼肉、南沙参、玉竹、黄精、墨旱莲、女贞子、桑椹、黑芝麻、楮实子、蛤蟆油的功效以及特殊的用法用量和特殊的使用注意。

    1. Master the commonness of supplementing medicinals in efficacy, indications, property, compatibility and cautions; as well as the property, efficacy, application, special usage and dosage and special precautions of *rén shēn, dǎng shēn, huáng qí, bái zhú, gān cǎo, lù róng, yín yáng huò, dù zhòng, bǔ gǔ zhī, tù sī zǐ, dāng guī, shú dì huáng, bái sháo, ē jiāo, běi shā shēn, mài dōng, gǒu qǐ zǐ, guī jiǎ* and *biē jiǎ*.

    2. Familiar with the classifications of supplementing medicinals; the efficacy, indications, special usage, dosage and special precautions of *xī yáng shēn, dà zǎo, shān yào, zǐ hé chē, bā jǐ tiān, xù duàn, ròu cōng róng, gé jiè, dōng chóng xià cǎo, hé shǒu wū, tiān dōng, bǎi hé* and *shí hú*.

    3. Understand the definitions of supplementing medicinals and related efficacy terms; and the efficacy, special usage and dosage and special precautions of *tài zǐ shēn, cì wǔ jiā, bái biǎn dòu, jiāo gǔ lán, hóng jǐng tiān, shā jí, yí táng, fēng mì, lù jiǎo, lù jiǎo jiāo, lù jiǎo shuāng, xiān máo, suǒ yáng, yì zhì rén, shā yuàn zǐ, hé táo rén, jiǔ cài zǐ, yáng qǐ shí, hǎi gǒu shèn, hǎi mǎ, lóng yǎn ròu, nán shā shēn, yù zhú, huáng jīng, mò hàn lián, nǚ zhēn zǐ, sāng shèn, hēi zhī ma, chǔ shí zǐ* and *há ma yóu*.

    凡以补虚扶弱，纠正人体气血阴阳不足为主要功效，常用以治疗虚证的药物，称为补虚药，又称补益药或补养药。

Medicinals with the major efficacies of supplementing the deficiency, reinforcing weakness, supplementing qi, blood, yin and yang are known as supplementing medicinals, or reinforcing medicinals, or supplementing-nourishing medicinals. This kind of medicinals are usually used to treat deficiency syndrome.

补虚药多具有甘味，性质有温、寒之分，补气药多归脾、肺经；补阳药多归肾经；补血药多归心、肝经；补阴药多归肺、胃、肝、肾经。本类药物具有补益虚损之功，具体又有补气、补阳、补血、补阴之别，主要用于治疗虚证。虚证的临床表现比较复杂，但其证型概括起来不外气虚证、阳虚证、血虚证、阴虚证。

Supplementing medicinals are mostly sweet with warm or cold nature. Qi-supplementing medicinals mostly act on spleen and lung meridians; yang-supplementing medicinals mainly act on the kidney meridian; blood-supplementing medicinals mainly act on the heart and liver meridians; yin-supplementing medicinals mostly act on the lung, stomach, liver and kidney meridians. They have the efficacies of supplementing deficiency and reinforcing weakness. Specifically speaking, they function to supplementing qi, yang, blood and yin, which are mainly used to treat deficiency syndrome. Clinical manifestations of deficiency syndrome are quite complicated, but it can be generalized into qi deficiency syndrome, yang deficiency syndrome, blood deficiency syndrome and yin deficiency syndrome.

应用补虚药时，首先必须针对气虚、阳虚、血虚、阴虚的证候不同，选用相应的补虚药。其次，应充分考虑人体气血阴阳相互依存、相互影响的关系，有选择地将两类或两类以上的补虚药配伍使用。如治气虚证常配伍补血药，使气有所归；治血虚证常配伍补气药，使气旺生血；治阳虚证常配伍补阴药，阴中求阳，使阳得阴助而生化无穷；治阴虚证常配伍补阳药，阳中求阴，使阴得阳升而泉源不竭。再如，气阴两虚者，则补气药与补阴药同用；血虚与阴亏并呈之证，则补血药与补阴药同用。

When using supplementing medicinals, doctors should firstly differentiate qi deficiency, yang deficiency, blood deficiency and yin deficiency, and then select corresponding medicinals. In addition, when in use, supplementing medicinals are required to be combined with each other based on the interdependent and mutually affect relations among qi, blood, yin and yang. For instance, blood-supplementing medicinals are often combined to treat qi deficiency, because blood is the carrier of qi; qi-supplementing medicinals are often combined to treat blood deficiency, because sufficient qi can generate blood; yin-supplementing medicinals are usually combined to treat yang deficiency, so that yang generates endlessly from origination of yin; yang-supplementing medicinals are often used to treat yin deficiency, so that yin grows with generation of yang. Moreover, qi-supplementing and blood-supplementing medicinals are applied together to treat dual deficiency of qi and yin; for co-existence of blood deficiency and yin deficiency, blood-supplementing and yin-supplementing medicinals should be used together.

补虚药是为虚证而设，若邪实而正不虚，应以祛邪为要，误用补虚药有"误补益疾"之弊。若正气虚弱、余邪未尽或邪盛正衰，应当攻补兼施，使祛邪不伤正，补虚不留邪。部分补虚药滋腻碍胃，不易消化，应顾护脾胃，适当配伍健脾消食药，对于湿阻中焦，脾胃气滞，脘腹满闷者，应当慎用。虚证一般病程较长，故补虚药宜采用丸剂、膏剂、片剂等便于服用的剂型，若入汤剂宜文火久煎，使药味尽出。

Supplementing medicinals are intended to treat deficiency syndrome. For the condition of combined pathogen excess and vigorous healthy qi, doctors should take elimination of pathogenic factors as priority. Improper usage of supplementing medicinals may lead to "wrong supplement and retained pathogen". For healthy qi deficiency with lingered pathogen, or pathogen excess with healthy qi deficiency, the pathogen should be dispelled without damaging healthy qi, and the deficiency should be supplemented without inducing pathogen retention. Some supplementing medicinals are greasy and over-nourishing, which tend to block the stomach and influence digestion. Thus spleen-invigorating and digestion-promoting medicinals should be combined to strengthen spleen and stomach. They should be used with caution for those with fullness and stuffiness in the gastric cavity and abdomen due to qi stagnation of spleen and stomach caused by damp obstructing middle energizer. The course of deficiency syndrome is usually long, so supplementing medicinals are often applied in the forms of pills, pastes and tablets, which are convenient for application. When used for decoction, they are required to be decocted in slow fire for a long time in order to release the active ingredients completely.

第一节　补气药

Section 1　Qi-supplementing medicinals

PPT

　　本类药物多味甘，性温或平，主归脾、肺经，以补脾气和补肺气为主要功效，部分补气药又归心、肾经，还能补心气、补肾气和补元气。相应的主治为：脾气虚证，症见食欲不振，脘腹胀满，食后胀甚，大便溏稀，体倦神疲，面色萎黄，消瘦或一身虚浮，甚或脱肛、脏器下垂等。肺气虚证，症见气短而喘，动则尤甚，咳嗽无力，声低懒言，自汗等；心气虚证，症见心悸怔忡、胸闷气短，活动后加剧等；肾气虚证，症见腰膝酸软，尿频或尿后余沥不尽，或遗尿，或男子早泄遗精，女子带下清稀等；元气虚极欲脱，可见气息短促，脉微欲绝等。某些药物还兼有养阴、生津、养血等功效，还可用治气阴（津）两伤或气血俱虚之证。

　　Qi-supplementing medicinals are mostly sweet and warm or neutral in flavor and property. They mainly act on the spleen and lung meridians with major efficacies of tonifying spleen and lung qi. Some act on the heart and kidney meridians to supplement heart qi, kidney qi and primordial qi. They are respectively used to treat spleen qi deficiency, manifested as poor appetite, distension and fullness in the gastric cavity and abdomen, worsened after meals, loose stool, fatigue and spiritual lassitude, sallow complexion, emaciation or general edema, or even proctoptosis and prolapse of internal organs; lung qi deficiency with symptoms of panting due to shortage of breath, aggravated with movement, cough, flaccidity, low voice, less speech and spontaneous sweating; heart qi deficiency, manifested as palpitation, severe palpitation, chest oppression, dyspnea, worsened with movement; kidney qi deficiency, manifested as soreness and weakness of waist and knees, frequency urination or dribble of urine, or enuresis, or male premature ejaculation, seminal emission, female thin leukorrhea; original qi depletion with symptoms of shortness of breath, fatigue and faint pulse verging on expiry. Some medicinals also has functions of nourishing yin, generating fluid and nourishing blood, which can be applied to treat dual damage of qi and yin(fluid), as well as deficiency of both qi and blood.

　　补气药多味甘壅中，碍气助湿，湿盛中满者应慎用，必要时辅以理气除湿之品。

　　Qi-supplementing medicinals are mostly sweet and tend to obstruct middle energizer and stagnate qi movement, leading to production of damp, so they should be used with caution for those with fullness of middle energizer due to exuberant damp. They are usually used with qi-rectifying and damp-removing medicinals under necessary conditions.

人参　*Rén shēn* (Ginseng Radix et Rhizoma)
《神农本草经》
Shen Nong's Classic of the Materia Medica (*Shén Nóng Běn Cǎo Jīng*)

【来源 / Origin】

为五加科植物人参 *Panax ginseng* C.A. Mey. 的干燥根和根茎。主产于吉林、辽宁、黑龙江。栽培者俗称"园参"；播种在山林野生状态下自然生长者称"林下山参"，习称"籽海"。多于秋季采挖。鲜参洗净后干燥者称"生晒参"；蒸制后干燥者称"红参"。切薄片或粉碎用。本品香气特异，味微苦、甘。《中国药典》规定，含人参皂苷 Rg$_1$（C$_{42}$H$_{72}$O$_{14}$）和人参皂苷 Re（C$_{48}$H$_{82}$O$_{18}$）的总量不得少于 0.30%，人参皂苷 Rb$_1$（C$_{54}$H$_{92}$O$_{23}$）不得少于 0.20%。

Rén shēn is the root and rhizome of *Panax ginseng* C.A. Mey., pertaining to Araliaceae. It is mainly produced in Jilin, Liaoning and Heilongjiang Province in China. Those cultivated artificially are called *yuán shēn* (garden ginseng); those which are sowed in mountains and woods and grow naturally in the wild are called *lín xià shān shēn* (ginseng under forest), and they are habitually named as *zǐ hǎi* (sea of the seed). *Rén shēn* is usually collected in autumn. The fresh ones which are dried after being washed clean are called *shēng shài shēn* (sun-dried ginseng); those which are dried after being steam-processed are called *hóng shēn* (red ginseng). It is sliced or ground into powder for application. It has a unique fragrance and tastes slightly bitter and sweet. According to *Chinese Pharmacopoeia*, the total content of ginsenoside Rg$_1$ (C$_{42}$H$_{72}$O$_{14}$) and ginsenoside Re (C$_{48}$H$_{82}$O$_{18}$) should be no less than 0.30%, and the content of ginsenoside Rb$_1$ (C$_{54}$H$_{92}$O$_{23}$) should be no less than 0.20%.

【性味归经 / Medicinal properties】

甘、微苦，微温。归脾、肺、心、肾经。

Sweet, slightly bitter and mildly warm; act on the spleen, lung, heart and kidney meridians.

【主要功效 / Medicinal efficacies】

大补元气，复脉固脱，补脾益肺，生津养血，安神益智。

Supplement original qi powerfully, restore pulse to rescue from desertion, supplement spleen and boost the lung, promote fluid production and nourish blood, calm the mind and benefit intelligence.

【临床应用 / Clinical application】

1. 元气虚脱证　本品甘温补虚，能大补元气，复脉固脱，为拯危救脱之要药。对于元气虚极欲脱，气息微弱，汗出不止，脉微欲绝的急危重证，可单用人参浓煎服。若气虚欲脱兼见汗出、四肢逆冷等亡阳征象者，应与附子同用。若气虚欲脱兼见汗出身暖、渴喜冷饮、舌红干燥等亡阴征象者，常与麦冬、五味子配伍。

(1) Original qi desertion　*Rén shēn* is sweet and warm for supplementing deficiency. It has functions of supplementing original qi powerfully, restoring pulse and stopping collapse, which is an essential medicinal to rescue desertion. It can be used alone in large dosage for oral taking to treat severe pattern of extreme deficient original qi, manifested as feeble breath, profuse sweating and faint pulse verging on expiry. For the condition accompanied with yang collapse manifestations, such as sweating and counterflow cold of four limbs, it can be used with *fù zǐ* (Aconiti Lateralis Radix Praeparata). For the condition accompanied with yin collapse manifestations, such as profuse sweating with warm body, thirst and preference for cold drink, red and dry tongue, it is often combined with *mài dōng* (Ophiopogonis Radix) and *wǔ wèi zǐ* (Schisandrae Chinensis Fructus).

2. 脾肺气虚证　本品归脾、肺经，为补脾肺气之要药。用治脾气虚弱，倦怠乏力，食少便溏者，常与白术、茯苓、甘草配伍。用治脾气虚弱，不能统血而致失血者，常与黄芪、白术、当归等同用。用治脾气虚衰，气虚不能生血，以致气血两虚者，多与白术、当归、熟地黄等配伍。用治脾气虚衰，中气下陷，短气不足以息，脏器脱垂者，常与黄芪、白术、升麻等同用。用治肺气虚弱，咳嗽无力，气短喘促，声低懒言者，常与黄芪、五味子、紫菀等同用。用治肺肾两虚，肾不纳气之短气虚喘，常与蛤蚧、胡桃仁等同用。

(2) Qi deficiency of spleen and lung　It acts on the spleen and lung meridians, which serves as an essential medicinal to supplementing spleen and lung qi. to treat fatigue, lassitude, poor appetite and loose stool due to weakness of spleen, it is often combined with *bái zhú* (Atractylodis Macrocephalae Rhizoma), *fú líng* (Poria) *and gān cǎo* (Glycyrrhizae Radix et Rhizoma). To treat failure of spleen to controlling blood due to spleen qi deficiency, manifested as various hemorrhages, it is often combined with *huáng qí* (Astragali Radix), *bái zhú* (Atractylodis Macrocephalae Rhizoma) and *dāng guī* (Angelicae Sinensis Radix). To treat failure of qi to generate blood due to spleen qi deficiency, manifested as dual deficiency of qi and blood, it is often combined with *bái zhú* (Atractylodis Macrocephalae Rhizoma), *dāng guī* (Angelicae Sinensis Radix) and *shú dì huáng* (Rehmanniae Radix Praeparata). To treat sinking of middle qi due to spleen qi deficiency, with symptoms of short breath, panting and prolapse of internal viscera, it is often used with *huáng qí* (Astragali Radix), *bái zhú* (Atractylodis Macrocephalae Rhizoma) and *shēng má* (Cimicifugae Rhizoma). To treat cough, flaccidity, short breath, panting, low voice and less speech caused by lung qi deficiency, it is often combined with *huáng qí* (Astragali Radix), *wǔ wèi zǐ* (Schisandrae Chinensis Fructus) and *zǐ wǎn* (Asteris Radix et Rhizoma). To treat short breath and deficient panting due to failure of kidney to receive qi and dual deficiency of lung and kidney, it is often combined with *gé jiè* (Gecko) and *hú táo rén* (Juglans Regia).

3. 气虚津伤口渴及消渴　本品有益气生津止渴之功。用治热病气津两伤之口渴、多汗、脉大无力者，常与知母、石膏等同用。用治气阴两虚之消渴，症见口渴喜饮、倦怠乏力、五心烦热等，常与天花粉、五味子、麦冬等同用。

(3) Qi deficiency, fluid consumption and thirst, consumptive thirst　It has effects of tonifying qi, producing fluid and relieving thirst. To treat consumption of qi and fluid in febrile disease, manifested as thirst, profuse sweating, large and weak pulse, it is often used together with *zhī mǔ* (Anemarrhenae Rhizoma) and *shí gāo* (Gypsum Fibrosum). To treat *xiāo kě* resulting from dual deficiency of qi and yin, with symptoms of thirst with desire to drink, fatigue, lassitude, feverish sensation over palms and soles, it is often combined with *tiān huā fěn* (Trichosanthis Radix), *wǔ wèi zǐ* (Schisandrae Chinensis Fructus) and *mài dōng* (Ophiopogonis Radix).

4. 心气不足，心悸失眠　本品归心经，能补益心气，安神益智。用治心气虚弱，心悸怔忡，失眠多梦，健忘等，常与茯苓、远志、石菖蒲等同用。用治心脾两虚，心悸失眠，体倦食少等，常配伍黄芪、当归、龙眼肉等。用治心肾不足，虚烦不眠，心悸健忘，多配伍生地黄、当归、酸枣仁等。

(4) Insufficiency of heart qi, palpitation and insomnia　It acts on the heart meridian with effects of reinforcing heart qi, tranquilizing the mind and benefiting intelligence. To treat palpitation, severe palpitation, insomnia, dreaminess and amnesia due to heart qi deficiency, it is often combined with *fú líng* (Poria), *yuǎn zhì* (Polygalae Radix) and *shí chāng pú* (Acori Tatarinowii Rhizoma). To treat palpitation, insomnia, fatigue and poor appetite due to deficiency of heart and spleen, it is often combined with *huáng qí* (Astragali Radix), *dāng guī* (Angelicae Sinensis Radix) and *lóng yǎn ròu* (Longan Arillus). To treat deficient vexation, insomnia, palpitation and amnesia due to deficiency of heart and kidney, it is often combined with *dì huáng* (Rehmanniae Radix), *dāng guī* (Angelicae Sinensis Radix) and *suān zǎo rén* (Ziziphi Spinosae Semen).

5. 阳痿，宫冷 本品入肾经，能益肾气、助肾阳。用治肾阳虚衰，肾精亏虚之阳痿、宫冷，多与鹿茸、肉苁蓉等同用。

(5) Impotence, cold uterus It acts on kidney meridian with effects of reinforcing kidney qi and strengthening kidney yang. To treat impotence, cold uterus caused by kidney yang deficiency and shortage of kidney essence, it is often combined with *lù róng* (Cervi Cornu Pantotrichum) and *ròu cōng róng* (Cistanches Herba).

【用法用量 / Usage and dosage】

煎服 3~9g，挽救虚脱可用 15~30g，文火另煎兑服。研末吞服，一次 2g，一日 2 次。

Decoction, 3-9g; to rescue desertion, 15-30g. It should be decocted singly with moderate fire and taken orally in divided doses mixed with decoction. Or it can be ground into powder for swallow, 2g each time, twice a day.

【使用注意 / Precaution】

实证、热证而正气不虚者忌用。不宜与藜芦、五灵脂同用。

It should be contraindicated in those with excess syndrome, heat syndrome and insufficient healthy qi. It is not proper to be used with *lí lú* and *wǔ líng zhī*.

【现代研究 / Modern research】

本品主要含人参皂苷 R_0、人参皂苷 Ra_1、人参皂苷 Rb_1、人参皂苷 Rc、人参皂苷 Re、人参皂苷 Rg_1 等，尚含多糖、氨基酸、挥发油、有机酸、黄酮类、维生素、微量元素等。具有增强免疫、抗休克、抗心肌缺血、抗心律失常、调节血压、促进食欲和蛋白质合成、性激素样作用、促进造血、降血糖、提高记忆力、延缓衰老、抗骨质疏松及抗肿瘤等作用。

It mainly contains ginsenoside R_0, Ra_1, Rb_1, Rc, Re, Rg_1. It also contains polysaccharide, amino acid, volatile oil, organic acid, flavonoids, vitamin and micro-elements. It has the efficacies of strengthening immunity, anti-shock, anti-myocardial ischemia, anti-arrhythmia, regulating blood pressure, promoting appetite and protein synthesis. It also has hormone-like actions. In addition, it also has the functions of promoting hematopoiesis, lowering blood glucose, improving memory, delaying aging, anti-osteoporosis and anti-tumor.

西洋参　*Xī yáng shēn* (Panacis Quinquefolii Radix)
《增订本草备要》
Revised and Expanded Essentials of Materia Medica (Zēng Dìng Běn Cǎo Bèi Yào)

【来源 / Origin】

为五加科植物西洋参 *Panax quinquefolium* L. 的干燥根。主产于美国、加拿大，我国亦有栽培。秋季采挖，干燥，切薄片或用时捣碎，生用。本品气微而特异，味微苦、甘。《中国药典》规定，含人参皂苷 Rg_1（$C_{42}H_{72}O_{14}$）、人参皂苷 Re（$C_{48}H_{82}O_{18}$）和人参皂苷 Rb_1（$C_{54}H_{92}O_{23}$）的总量不得少于 2.0%。

Xī yáng shēn is the root of *Panax quinquefolium* L., pertaining to Araliaceae. It is mainly produced in America and Canada, and it is also cultivated in China. It is collected in autumn and dried in the sun, used raw and sliced or pounded into pieces for application. It has mild and unique smell and tastes slightly bitter and sweet. According to *Chinese Pharmacopoeia*, the total content of ginsenoside Rg_1 ($C_{42}H_{72}O_{14}$), ginsenoside Re ($C_{48}H_{82}O_{18}$) and ginsenoside Rb_1 ($C_{54}H_{92}O_{23}$) should be no less than 2.0%.

【性味归经 / Medicinal properties】

甘、微苦，凉。归心、肺、肾经。

Sweet, slightly bitter and cool; act on the heart, lung and kidney meridians.

【主要功效 / Medicinal efficacies】

补气养阴，清热生津。

Supplement qi and nourish yin, clear heat and produce fluid.

【临床应用 / Clinical application】

1. 气阴两脱证　本品味甘能补，补气之力较强，具有与人参类似的益气救脱之功而药力稍逊，因其性偏凉，兼能清热养阴生津，故适用于气阴两脱证，症见神疲乏力、气短息促、汗出不止、心烦口渴、脉细数无力，常与麦冬、五味子等同用。

(1) Desertion of both qi and yin　It is sweet for supplementing with strong effect of tonifying qi. Its efficacy of strengthening qi to rescue collapse is similar to that of *rén shēn* (Ginseng Radix et Rhizoma), but it is milder. It is cool in nature with actions of clearing heat, nourishing yin and producing fluid, which is suitable to treat depletion of both qi and yin. To treat depletion of both qi and yin, manifested as spiritual lassitude, fatigue, short and quick breath, profuse sweating, vexation, thirst, thin, rapid and weak pulse, it is often combined with *mài dōng* (Ophiopogonis Radix) and *wǔ wèi zǐ* (Schisandrae Chinensis Fructus).

2. 气阴两虚证　本品味甘补气、养阴生津，性凉清热，为补气药中"清补"之品。归肺经，长于补肺气，兼能养肺阴、清肺热，用治火热耗伤肺脏气阴所致的短气喘促、咳嗽痰少，或痰中带血者，常与玉竹、麦冬、川贝母等同用。归心经，亦能补心气、养心阴，用治心之气阴两虚所致的心悸心痛、失眠多梦，常与甘草、麦冬、生地黄等同用。归肾经，又能补肾气、益肾阴，用治肾之气阴两虚所致的腰膝酸软、遗精滑精，常与山茱萸、枸杞子、沙苑子等同用。

(2) Deficiency of both qi and yin　It is sweet for reinforcing qi, nourishing yin and producing blood, cool in nature for clearing heat, which is "moistening tonification" in qi-supplementing medicinals. It acts on the lung meridian and is effective in reinforcing lung qi, nourishing lung yin and clearing lung heat. To treat short breath, panting, cough with less sputum, or blood-stained sputum caused by fire-heat consuming qi and yin of lung, it is often combined with *yù zhú* (Polygonati Odorati Rhizoma), *mài dōng* (Ophiopogonis Radix) and *chuān bèi mǔ* (Fritillariae Cirrhosae Bulbus). It acts on heart meridian to supplementing heart qi and nourish heart yin. To treat palpitation, heart pain, insomnia and dreaminess caused by deficiency of heart qi and yin, it is often combined with *gān cǎo* (Glycyrrhizae Radix et Rhizoma), *mài dōng* (Ophiopogonis Radix) and *dì huáng* (Rehmanniae Radix). It acts on the kidney meridian to supplement kidney qi and nourish kidney yin. To treat soreness and weakness of waist and knees, seminal emission and spermatorrhea due to deficiency of kidney qi and yin, it is often combined with *shān zhū yú* (Corni Fructus), *gǒu qǐ zǐ* (Lycii Fructus) and *shā yuàn zǐ* (Astragali Complanati Semen).

3. 热病气虚津伤口渴及消渴　本品既能补气、养阴生津，又能清热，用治热伤气津所致身热汗多、口渴心烦、体倦少气、脉虚数，常与西瓜翠衣、竹叶、麦冬等同用。若治消渴气阴两伤，常与黄芪、山药、天花粉等同用。

(3) Qi deficiency, fluid consumption and thirst in febrile disease, consumptive thirst　It has efficacies of reinforcing qi, nourishing yin and producing fluid, as well as clearing heat. To treat fever, profuse sweating, thirst, vexation, fatigue, shortage of qi, deficient and rapid pulse due to heat impairing qi and fluid, it is often combined with *xī guā cuì yī* (Citrulli Exocarpium), *zhú yè* (Phyllostachydis

Henonis Folium) and *mài dōng* (Ophiopogonis Radix). To treat *xiāo kě* with consumption of qi and yin, it is often combined with *huáng qí* (Astragali Radix), *shān yào* (Dioscoreae Rhizoma) and *tiān huā fěn* (Trichosanthis Radix).

【用法用量 / Usage and dosage】

另煎兑服，3~6g。

Decoction, 3-6g. It is decocted alone, and mixed with the decoction for oral administration.

【使用注意 / Precaution】

不宜与藜芦同用。

It is not proper to be used with *lí lú*.

【现代研究 / Modern research】

本品主要含人参皂苷、拟人参皂苷，尚含挥发油、多糖、黄酮类、蛋白质、氨基酸、甾醇类、脂肪酸、有机酸等成分。具有增强免疫、抗疲劳、降血糖、降血脂、升高白细胞等作用。

It mainly contains ginsenoside and pseuoginsenoside. It also contains amino acid, volatile oil, polysaccharide, organic acid, flavonoids, proteins, sterols and fatty acids. It has the functions of strengthening immunity, anti-fatigue, lowering blood glucose, lowering blood fat and elevating white cells.

党参　*Dǎng shēn* (Codonopsis Radix)
《增订本草备要》
Revised and Expanded Essentials of Materia Medica (Zēng Dìng Běn Cǎo Bèi Yào)

【来源 / Origin】

为桔梗科植物党参 *Codonopsis pilosula*（Franch.）Nannf.、素花党参 *Codonopsis pilosula* Nannf. var. *modesta*（Nannf.）L. T. Shen 或川党参 *Codonopsis tangshen* Oliv. 的干燥根。主产于甘肃、四川、山西等地。秋季采收，切厚片，生用或米炒用。本品有特殊香气，味微甜。

Dǎng shēn is the root of *Codonopsis pilosula* (Franch.) Nannf., *Codonopsis pilosula* Nannf. var. *modesta* (Nannf.) L. T. Shen or *Codonopsis tangshen* Oliv., pertaining to Campanulaceae. It is mainly produced in Gansu, Sichuan and Shanxi Province in China, collected in autumn cut into thick slices, used raw or stir-fried with rice. *Dǎng shēn* has a unique fragrance and tastes slightly sweet.

【性味归经 / Medicinal properties】

甘，平。归脾、肺经。

Sweet and neutral; act on the spleen and lung meridians.

【主要功效 / Medicinal efficacies】

补脾益肺，养血生津。

Supplement spleen and boost lung, nourish blood and produce fluid.

【临床应用 / Clinical application】

1. 脾肺气虚证　本品甘平，归脾、肺经，补脾肺气之功与人参相似而药力较弱。因其药性平和，凡脾肺气虚之轻证需用人参者，皆可用党参代替。若治脾气虚弱、倦怠乏力、食少便溏等，常与白术、茯苓等同用。若治肺气亏虚，咳嗽气短、语声低弱等，常与黄芪、蛤蚧等同用。

(1) **Qi deficiency of spleen and lung**　*Dǎng shēn* is sweet, neutral and acts on the spleen and lung meridians. Its efficacy of supplementing spleen and lung qi is similar to *rén shēn* (Ginseng Radix et Rhizoma), but it is milder than *rén shēn* (Ginseng Radix et Rhizoma). For its neutral nature, it can substitute *rén shēn* (Ginseng Radix et Rhizoma) to treat patients with light deficiency of spleen and

stomach qi. To treat lassitude, fatigue, poor appetite and loose stool due to spleen qi deficiency, it is often used with *bái zhú* (Atractylodis Macrocephalae Rhizoma) and *fú líng* (Poria). To treat cough, short breath and low voice due to lung qi deficiency, it is often combined with *huáng qí* (Astragali Radix) and *gé jiè* (Gecko).

2. 气血两虚证　本品有补气养血之功。用治气血不足，面色苍白或萎黄、体倦乏力、头晕心悸等，常与黄芪、当归、熟地黄等同用。

(2) **Deficiency of both qi and blood**　It functions to reinforce qi and nourish blood. To treat pale or sallow complexion, fatigue and weakness, dizziness and palpitation due to shortage of qi and blood, it is often combined with *huáng qí* (Astragali Radix), *dāng guī* (Angelicae Sinensis Radix) and *shú dì huáng* (Rehmanniae Radix Praeparata).

3. 气津两伤证　本品有补气生津的作用。用治气津两伤之气短口渴及内热消渴，可与麦冬、五味子等同用。

(3) **Consumption of both qi and fluid**　It has functions of reinforcing qi and producing blood. To treat short breath, thirst due to consumption of qi and fluid, it is often combined with *mài dōng* (Ophiopogonis Radix) and *wǔ wèi zǐ* (Schisandrae Chinensis Fructus).

【用法用量 / Usage and dosage】
煎服，9~30g。
Decoction, 9-30g.

【使用注意 / Precaution】
不宜与藜芦同用。
It is not proper to be used with *lí lú*.

【现代研究 / Modern research】
本品主要含党参苷、党参多糖、党参内酯、植物甾醇、黄酮类、香豆素类、氨基酸、微量元素等。具有增强免疫、提高记忆能力、抗肺损伤、改善胃肠功能、抗缺氧、抗衰老、降血糖、调节血脂等作用。

It mainly contains tangshenoside, codonopisis pilosula polysaccharide, codonolactone, phytosterin, flavonoids, coumarins, amino acid and micro-element. It has the functions of strengthening immunity, improving memory, anti-lung injury, improving gastrointestinal functions, anti-hypoxia, anti-aging, lowering blood glucose and regulating blood fat.

黄芪　*Huáng qí* (Astragali Radix)
《神农本草经》
Shen Nong's Classic of the Materia Medica (Shén Nóng Běn Cǎo Jīng)

【来源 / Origin】
为豆科植物蒙古黄芪 *Astragalus membranaceus*（Fisch.）Bge. var. *mongholicus*（Bge.）Hsiao 或膜荚黄芪 *Astragalus membranaceus*（Fisch.）Bge. 的干燥根。主产于内蒙古、山西、黑龙江等地。春、秋二季采挖，切厚片，生用或蜜炙用。本品气微，味微甜。《中国药典》规定，含黄芪甲苷（$C_{41}H_{68}O_{14}$）不得少于 0.080%，炙黄芪不得少于 0.060%；含毛蕊异黄酮葡萄糖苷（$C_{22}H_{22}O_{10}$）不得少于 0.020%，炙黄芪不得少于 0.020%。

Huáng qí is the root of *Astragalus membranaceus* (Fisch.) Bge. var. *mongholicus* (Bge.) Hsiao or *Astragalus membranaceus* (Fisch.) Bge., pertaining to Leguminosae. It is mainly produced in Inner Mongolia Autonomous Region, Shanxi and Heilongjiang Province in China, collected in spring and autumn, cut into thick slices, and used raw or honey-fried. It has slight flavor and tastes slightly sweet. According to *Chinese Pharmacopoeia*, the content of astragaloside A ($C_{41}H_{68}O_{14}$) should be no less than 0.080%, and that in honey-fried *huáng qí* should be no less than 0.060%. The content of calycosin-7-glucoside ($C_{22}H_{22}O_{10}$) should be no less than 0.020%, and that in honey-fried *huáng qí* should be no less than 0.020%.

【性味归经 / Medicinal properties】

甘，微温。归肺、脾经。

Sweet and slightly warm; act on the lung and spleen meridians.

【主要功效 / Medicinal efficacies】

补气升阳，固表止汗，利水消肿，生津养血，行滞通痹，托毒排脓，敛疮生肌。

Supplement qi and raise yang, consolidate the exterior and arrest sweat, promote urination to relieve edema, produce fluid and nourish blood, move stagnation and relieve impediment, express toxin and expel pus, promote granulation.

【临床应用 / Clinical application】

1. **脾虚气陷证**　本品甘温，入脾经，善于补益脾气，升举中阳，故长于治疗脾虚中气下陷所致的久泻脱肛、内脏下垂，常与人参、升麻、柴胡等同用。若治脾气虚弱，倦怠乏力，食少便溏，可单用熬膏服，或与人参、白术等同用。本品还可补气以摄血，若治脾虚不能统血之失血证，多与人参、白术等同用。

(1) Qi sinking due to spleen deficiency　It is sweet and warm, and acts on the spleen meridian. It is effective in tonifying spleen qi and elevating spleen yang. To treat middle qi sinking due to spleen deficiency, with symptoms of prolonged diarrhea, rectal prolapse and prolapse of internal viscera, it is often combined with *rén shēn* (Ginseng Radix et Rhizoma), *shēng má* (Cimicifugae Rhizoma) and *chái hú* (Bupleuri Radix). To treat lassitude, fatigue, poor appetite and loose stool due to spleen qi deficiency, it can be used alone and decocted into cream for oral taking, or combined with *rén shēn* (Ginseng Radix et Rhizoma) and *bái zhú* (Atractylodis Macrocephalae Rhizoma). It can also reinforce qi to control blood. To treat loss of blood due to spleen deficiency failing to control blood, it is often used with *rén shēn* (Ginseng Radix et Rhizoma) and *bái zhú* (Atractylodis Macrocephalae Rhizoma).

2. **肺气虚证，表虚自汗**　本品入肺经，能补肺气，益卫气，固表止汗。用治肺气虚弱，咳喘气短、声低懒言，常与人参、紫菀、五味子等同用。若治脾肺气虚，卫气不固，表虚自汗，常与牡蛎、麻黄根等同用。若治卫气不固，表虚自汗而易感风邪，常与白术、防风同用。

(2) Lung qi deficiency, spontaneous sweating due to exterior deficiency　It acts on the lung with effects of reinforcing lung qi, strengthening defensive qi, and consolidating the exterior to stanch sweating. To treat cough, panting, short breath, low voice and less speech due to lung qi deficiency, it is often combined with *rén shēn* (Ginseng Radix et Rhizoma), *zǐ wǎn* (Asteris Radix et Rhizoma) and *wǔ wèi zǐ* (Schisandrae Chinensis Fructus). To treat failure of defensive qi to protect body surface and spontaneous sweating due to deficiency of spleen and lung qi, it is often combined with *mǔ lì* (Ostreae Concha) and *má huáng gēn* (Ephedrae Radix et Rhizoma). To treat spontaneous sweating due to exterior deficiency and susceptibility to pathogenic wind, it is often combined with *bái zhú* (Atractylodis Macrocephalae Rhizoma) and *fáng fēng* (Saposhnikoviae Radix).

3. **气虚水肿**　本品既能补气，又能利水消肿，故为治气虚水肿之要药。用治脾虚水湿失运，浮肿尿少，常与白术、茯苓、防己等同用。

(3) Edema due to qi deficiency　It has efficacies of tonifying qi, promoting urination to relieve edema, which is an essential medicinal to treat edema due to qi deficiency. To treat edema and scanty urine due to spleen deficiency and water-damp, it is often combined with *bái zhú* (Atractylodis Macrocephalae Rhizoma), *fú líng* (Poria) and *fáng jǐ* (Stephaniae Tetrandrae Radix).

4. 血虚萎黄，气血两虚证　本品有补气养血之功，用治血虚或气血两虚所致的面色萎黄、神疲体倦、脉虚等，常与当归、白芍等同用。

(4) **Sallow complexion due to blood deficiency, deficiency of both qi and blood**　It has effect of tonifying qi and nourishing blood. To treat sallow complexion, spiritual lassitude, fatigue and deficient pulse due to blood deficiency or insufficiency of both qi and blood, it is used with *dāng guī* (Angelicae Sinensis Radix) and *bái sháo* (Paeoniae Alba Radix).

5. 消渴　本品有益气生津的作用，用治气虚津亏之消渴，口渴引饮，常与天花粉、葛根等同用。

(5) **consumptive thirst**　It functions to supplement qi and produce fluid. To treat consumptive thirst, thirst with desire for drinking due to qi deficiency and fluid consumption, it is often combined with *tiān huā fěn* (Trichosanthis Radix) and *gé gēn* (Puerariae Lobatae Radix).

6. 半身不遂，痹痛麻木　本品有补气行滞通痹之效。对于气虚血滞之半身不遂、风湿痹痛或肌肤麻木者，常用本品治疗。若治中风后遗症，常与当归、川芎、地龙等同用。若治风湿痹痛、肌肤麻木，常与羌活、当归、姜黄等同用。若治气虚血滞之胸痹心痛，常与红花、丹参、三七等同用。

(6) **Hemiplegia, pain and numbness of impediment**　It has actions of reinforcing qi, moving stagnation and relieving impediment, which is often used to treat hemiplegia, pain and numbness of wind-damp impediment or skin numbness. To treat sequelae of wind-strike, it is often combined with *dāng guī* (Angelicae Sinensis Radix), *chuān xiōng* (Chuanxiong Rhizoma) and *dì lóng* (Pheretima). To treat pain and numbness of wind-damp *bì* or skin numbness, it is often used with *qiāng huó* (Notopterygii Rhizoma et Radix), *dāng guī* (Angelicae Sinensis Radix) and *jiāng huáng* (Curcumae Longae Rhizoma). To treat chest impediment and heart pain due to qi deficiency and blood stasis, it is often combined with *hóng huā* (Carthami Flos), *dān shēn* (Salviae Miltiorrhizae Radix et Rhizoma) and *sān qī* (Notoginseng Radix et Rhizoma)

7. 痈疽难溃或久溃不敛　本品补气养血，使正气旺盛，可收托毒排脓、生肌敛疮之效。用治疮疡中期，正虚毒盛不能托毒外达，疮形平塌，根盘散漫，难溃难腐者，常与人参、当归、升麻等同用。若治溃疡后期，脓水清稀，疮口难敛者，常与人参、当归、肉桂等同用。

(7) **Unerupted sores and carbuncles, or unclosed sores and carbuncles after eruption**　It has functions of reinforcing qi and nourishing blood to strengthen healthy qi, which helps to reach effects of expelling pus and expressing toxin, as well as astringing sores and promoting granulation. To treat sores with flat, collapsed shape and diffuse root in the middle stage of sores and ulcers, which is chronic and hard to erupt induced by healthy qi deficiency failing to expel toxin to the external, it is often combined with *rén shēn* (Ginseng Radix et Rhizoma), *dāng guī* (Angelicae Sinensis Radix) and *shēng má* (Cimicifugae Rhizoma). For late stage of sores and ulcers, manifested as unclosed sores with clear and thin pus, it is often combined with *rén shēn* (Ginseng Radix et Rhizoma), *dāng guī* (Angelicae Sinensis Radix) and *ròu guì* (Cinnamomi Cortex).

【用法用量 / Usage and dosage 】

煎服，9~30g。补中益气宜蜜炙用，其余多生用。

Decoction, 9-30g. It is mostly used raw except that the honey-fried form can strengthen the efficacy of supplementing the center and boosting qi.

【现代研究 / Modern research】

本品主要含黄芪皂苷Ⅰ~Ⅳ（黄芪甲苷）、荚膜黄芪苷Ⅰ和Ⅱ、大豆皂苷、芒柄花素、毛蕊异黄酮葡萄糖苷，尚含多糖及氨基酸等。具有增强免疫、促进胃肠运动、利尿与抗肾损伤、促进造血、抗心肌缺血、抗衰老、保肝、降血糖、降血脂、降血压等作用。

It mainly contains astragaloside Ⅰ-Ⅳ (astragaloside A), astramembrannin Ⅰ and Ⅱ, pureonebio, formononetin and calycosin-7-glucoside. It also contains polysaccharide and amino acid. It has the functions of strengthening immunity, promoting gastrointestinal movement, promoting diuresis, anti-kidney injury, promoting hematopoiesis, anti-myocardial ischemia, anti-aging, protecting the liver, and lowering blood glucose, blood fat and blood pressure.

白术　*Bái zhú* (Atractylodis Macrocephalae Rhizoma)
《神农本草经》
Shen Nong's Classic of the Materia Medica (Shén Nóng Běn Cǎo Jīng)

【来源 / Origin】

为菊科植物白术 *Atractylodes macrocephala* Koidz. 的干燥根茎。主产于浙江、安徽。冬季采挖，切厚片，生用或麸炒用。本品气清香，味甘、微辛。

Bái zhú is the rhizome of *Atractylodes macrocephala* Koidz., pertaining to Compositae. It is mainly produced in Zhejiang and Anhui Province in China, collected in winter, cut into thick slices, and used raw or stir-fried with bran. This medicinal has clear fragrance and tastes sweet, slightly acrid.

【性味归经 / Medicinal properties】

甘、苦，温。归脾、胃经。

Sweet, bitter and warm; act on the spleen and stomach meridians.

【主要功效 / Medicinal efficacies】

健脾益气，燥湿利水，止汗，安胎。

Invigorate spleen and supplement qi, dry dampness and promote urination, arrest sweating, calm fetus.

【临床应用 / Clinical application】

1. **脾气虚证**　本品甘温补虚，主入脾、胃经，功善补气健脾，被前人誉为"补气健脾第一要药"。用治脾气虚弱，运化无力，食少体倦，便溏或泄泻等，常与人参、茯苓、炙甘草同用。若治脾胃虚寒，腹满泄泻，多与人参、干姜、炙甘草同用。

(1) **Spleen qi deficiency**　It is sweet and warm for reinforcing the deficiency, and acts on the spleen and stomach meridians with effects of tonifying qi and invigorating spleen, which was considered to be "the first medicinal to tonify qi and invigorate spleen" by predecessors. To treat dysfunction of spleen in transportation and transformation due to spleen qi deficiency, manifested as poor appetite, fatigue, loose stool or diarrhea, it is often combined with *rén shēn* (Ginseng Radix et Rhizoma), *fú líng* (Poria) and *zhì gān cǎo* (Glycyrrhizae Radix et Rhizoma Praeparata cum Melle). To treat abdominal fullness and diarrhea due to deficiency cold of spleen and stomach, it is often used with *rén shēn* (Ginseng Radix et Rhizoma), *gān jiāng* (Zingiberis Rhizoma) and *zhì gān cǎo* (Glycyrrhizae Radix et Rhizoma Praeparata cum Melle).

2. **痰饮、水肿**　本品甘温补虚，苦温燥湿，既能补气健脾，又能燥湿利水，对于脾虚水湿失运所导致的痰饮、水肿有标本兼顾之效。若治脾虚中阳不振，痰饮内停，常与桂枝、茯苓、甘草同用。若治脾虚水肿，常与茯苓、泽泻等同用。若治脾虚湿浊下注，带下量多清稀，常与山药、苍术、车前子等同用。

(2) Phlegm-fluid retention and edema　It is sweet and warm for reinforcing the deficiency, bitter and warm for drying damp. It has efficacies of tonifying qi and invigorating spleen, as well as drying dampness and promoting urination. For phlegm-fluid retention and edema caused by water-damp resulting from spleen deficiency, it can treat both the root and the branch. To treat internal retention of phlegm rheum due to inactivation and deficiency of spleen yang, it is often combined with *guì zhī* (Cinnamomi Ramulus), *fú líng* (Poria) and *gān cǎo* (Glycyrrhizae Radix et Rhizoma). To treat edema caused by spleen deficiency, it is often combined with *fú líng* (Poria) and *zé xiè* (Alismatis Rhizoma). To treat profuse and thin leukorrhea due to damp-heat draining downward resulting from spleen deficiency, it is often used with *shān yào* (Dioscoreae Rhizoma), *cāng zhú* (Atractylodis Rhizoma) and *chē qián zǐ* (Plantaginis Semen).

3. **气虚自汗**　本品能益气健脾，固表止汗，作用与黄芪相似而力稍弱。用治脾肺气虚，卫气不固，表虚自汗，常与黄芪、防风等同用。

(3) Spontaneous sweating due to qi deficiency　It has functions of tonifying qi and invigorating spleen, as well as consolidating the exterior and arresting sweating. Its effect is milder than that of *huáng qí* (Astragali Radix). To treat deficiency of spleen and lung qi, manifested as dysfunction of defensive qi in consolidating, spontaneous sweating due to superficies deficiency, it is often used with *huáng qí* (Astragali Radix) and *fáng fēng* (Saposhnikoviae Radix).

4. **胎动不安**　本品益气健脾，使脾健气旺，则胎儿得养而自安，故有安胎之功。可用于多种原因所致的胎动不安，尤宜于脾虚胎动不安，常与人参、甘草、丁香等同用。若兼内热，常与黄芩同用；兼气滞胸腹胀满者，常与紫苏梗、砂仁等同用；兼肾虚者，常与杜仲、川断、阿胶等同用。

(4) Threatened miscarriage due to spleen deficiency　It has effects of tonifying qi and invigorating spleen. Sufficient spleen qi promotes fetal nourishment, so *bái zhú* also has functions of calming the fetus, which can be used to treat various threatened miscarriages. It is especially effective to treat threatened miscarriage caused by spleen deficiency in combination with *rén shēn* (Ginseng Radix et Rhizoma), *gān cǎo* (Glycyrrhizae Radix et Rhizoma) and *dīng xiāng* (Caryophylli Flos). If accompanied by internal heat, it is often combined with *huáng qín* (Scutellariae Radix); if accompanied by distension and fullness in the chest and abdomen due to qi stagnation, it is often used with *zǐ sū gěng* (Perillae Caulis) and *shā rén* (Amomi Fructus); if accompanied by kidney deficiency, it is often used with *dù zhòng* (Eucommiae Cortex), *xù duàn* (Dipsaci Radix) and *ē jiāo* (Corii Asini Colla).

【用法用量 / Usage and dosage】

煎服，6~12g。燥湿利水宜生用，补气健脾宜炒用，健脾止泻宜炒焦用。

Decoction, 6-12g. The raw form should be used for drying damp and promoting urination, the fried form should be used for tonifying qi and invigorating spleen, and the charcoaled form should be used for strengthening spleen to arresting diarrhea.

【现代研究 / Modern research】

本品主要含苍术酮、苍术醇、苍术内酯、白术内酯，尚含东莨菪素、甘露醇糖、氨基酸等。具有促进胃肠运动、增强免疫、抑制子宫平滑肌收缩、利尿、抗衰老、抗肿瘤等作用。

It mainly contains atractylon, atractylol, and atractylenolide. It also contains pureonebio, mannitol and amino acid. It has the functions of strengthening immunity, promoting gastrointestinal movement, inhibiting contraction of uterus smooth muscle, promoting diuresis, anti-aging and anti-tumor.

山药 *Shān yào* (Dioscoreae Rhizoma)
《神农本草经》
Shen Nong's Classic of the Materia Medica (Shén Nóng Běn Cǎo Jīng)

【来源 / Origin 】

为薯蓣科植物薯蓣 *Dioscorea opposite* Thunb. 的干燥根茎。主产于河南。冬季茎叶枯萎后采挖，切厚片，干燥，生用或麸炒用。本品味淡、微酸。

Shān yào is the dry rhizome of *Dioscorea opposite* Thunb., pertaining to Dioscoreaceae, mainly produced in Henan Province. It is collected after stems and leaves wither in winter, cut into thick slices, dried, used raw or stir-fried with bran. It is light and slightly sour.

【性味归经 / Medicinal properties 】

甘，平。归脾、肺、肾经。

Sweet and neutral; act on spleen, lung and kidney meridians.

【主要功效 / Medicinal efficacies 】

补脾养胃，生津益肺，补肾涩精。

Tonify spleen and nourish stomach, promote fluid production and replenish lung, and tonify kidney to astringe essence.

【临床应用 / Clinical application 】

1. 脾虚证　本品甘平，入脾经，补脾气、益脾阴，兼能收涩止泻，适用于脾胃气阴两虚者。若治脾虚食少、便溏、泄泻，常与人参、白术、茯苓等同用。若治脾阴亏虚，口干唇燥，乏力食少，常与白扁豆、莲子等同用。对慢性久病或病后虚弱羸瘦者，可作为营养调补品长期服用。

(1) Spleen deficiency　*Shān yào* is sweet and neutral, enters spleen meridian, with the functions of supplementing spleen qi and replenishing spleen yin, as well as checking diarrhea by astringing therapy, which is suitable for those with spleen-stomach qi and yin deficiency. To treat spleen deficiency manifested as poor appetite, loose stool, and diarrhea, it is usually used with *rén shēn*, *bái zhú*, and *fú líng*. To treat spleen yin deficiency manifested as dry mouth and tips, fatigue and poor appetite, it is used with *bái biǎn dòu* (Lablab Album Semen) and *lián zǐ* (Nelumbinis Semen). For those who are chronically ill or weak and emaciated, it can be taken for long as a nutritional tonic.

2. 肺虚证　本品入肺经，能补肺气、滋肺阴。用治肺虚久咳或虚喘，可与太子参、南沙参等同用。

(2) Lung deficiency　*Shān yào* enters lung meridian, and can supplement lung qi as well as nourish lung yin. To treat lung deficiency manifested as chronic cough or deficiency-type panting, it is usually combined with *tài zǐ shēn* (Pseudostellariae Radix) and *nán shā shēn* (Adenophorae Radix).

3. 肾虚证　本品入肾经，能补肾气，兼滋肾阴，并可固精止带。用治肾虚不固，夜尿频多或遗尿，常与乌药、益智仁同用。若治肾虚不固，带下清稀，多与熟地黄、山茱萸、五味子等同用。若治肾阴亏虚，形体消瘦，腰膝酸软，遗精等，常配伍熟地黄、山茱萸、茯苓等。

(3) Kidney deficiency　*Shān yào* enters spleen meridian, and can supplement spleen qi as well as nourish kidney yin, secure essence and leukorrhagia. To treat kidney qi deficiency manifested as frequent urination or enuresis, it is usually combined with *wū yào* (Linderae Radix) and *yì zhì rén* (Alpiniae Oxyphyllae Fructus). To treat kidney qi deficiency manifested as clear vaginal discharge, it is used with

398

shú dì huáng (Rehmanniae Radix Praeparata), *shān zhū yú* (Corni Fructus) and *wǔ wèi zǐ* (Schisandrae Chinensis Fructus). To treat kidney yin deficiency manifested as emaciation, weak waist and knees and spermatorrhea, it is often combined with *shú dì huáng* (Rehmanniae Radix Praeparata), *shān zhū yú* (Corni Fructus) and *fú líng*.

4. 消渴　本品既补脾肺肾之气，又补脾肺肾之阴，用治消渴属于气阴两虚者，常与黄芪、天花粉、知母等同用。

(4) Consumptive thirst　*Shān yào* supplements both qi and yin of spleen, lung and kidney, and treats consumptive thirst due to qi-yin deficiency in combination with *huáng qí* (Astragali Radix), *tiān huā fěn* (Trichosanthis Radix) and *zhī mǔ* (Anemarrhenae Rhizoma).

【用法用量 / Usage and dosage】

煎服，15~30g。麸炒山药可增强补脾止泻作用。

Decoction, 15-30g. Stir-frying with bran can strengthen the effects of supplementing spleen and arresting diarrhea.

【现代研究 / Modern research】

本品主要含氨基酸、甾醇、多糖、薯蓣皂苷元、多巴胺、山药碱、尿囊素、粗纤维、微量元素等。具有调节胃肠功能、降血糖、增强免疫、抗衰老、保肝等作用。

It mainly contains amino acid, sterol, polysaccharide, diosgenin, dopamine, dioscorea alkaloid, allantoin, crude fiber, trace elements, etc. It has the functions of regulating gastrointestinal function, reducing blood sugar, enhancing immunity, resisting aging and protecting liver.

甘草　*Gān cǎo* (Glycyrrhizae Radix et Rhizoma)
《神农本草经》
Shen Nong's Classic of the Materia Medica (Shén Nóng Běn Cǎo Jīng)

【来源 / Origin】

为豆科植物甘草 *Glycyrrhiza uralensis* Fisch.、胀果甘草 *Glycyrrhiza inflata* Bat. 或光果甘草 *Glycyrrhiza glabra* L. 的干燥根和根茎。主产于内蒙古、甘肃、新疆。春、秋二季采挖，切厚片，生用或蜜炙用。本品气微，味甜而特殊。《中国药典》规定，含甘草苷（$C_{21}H_{22}O_9$）不得少于 0.50%，饮片不得少于 0.45%，炙甘草不得少于 0.50%；含甘草酸（$C_{42}H_{62}O_{16}$）不得少于 2.0%，饮片不得少于 1.8%，炙甘草不得少于 1.0%。

Gān cǎo is the dry root and rhizome of *Glycyrrhiza uralensis* Fisch., *Glycyrrhiza inflata* Bat., or *Glycyrrhiza glabra* L., pertaining to Leguminosae, mainly produced in Inner Mongolia Autonomous Region, Gansu Province, and Xinjiang Uygur Autonomous Region, collected in spring and autumn, sliced into thick pieces, and used raw or burned with honey. It is slight in odor, sweet and special in taste. According to *Chinese Pharmacopoeia*, the content of glycyrrhizin ($C_{21}H_{22}O_9$) should not be less than 0.50%, 0.45% in decoction pieces, and no less than 0.50% in *zhì gān cǎo* (Glycyrrhizae Radix et Rhizoma Praeparata cum Melle); the content of glycyrrhizic acid ($C_{42}H_{62}O_{16}$) should not be less than 2.0%, no less than 1.8% in decoction pieces, and on less than 1.0% in *zhì gān cǎo*.

【性味归经 / Medicinal properties】

甘，平。归心、肺、脾、胃经。

Sweet and neutral; act on heart, lung, spleen and stomach meridians.

【主要功效 / Medicinal efficacies】

补脾益气，清热解毒，祛痰止咳，缓急止痛，调和诸药。

Supplement spleen and replenish qi, clear heat and resolve toxins, dispel phlegm and relieve cough, relax spasms and relieve pain, and harmonize all medicinals.

【临床应用 / Clinical application】

1. 脾气虚证　本品味甘能补，入脾胃经，能补脾胃、益中气，但其作用和缓，故多作辅助药用。用治脾胃虚弱，体倦乏力、食欲不振、腹胀便溏等，常与人参、白术、茯苓同用。

(1) Spleen qi deficiency　*Gān cǎo* can supplement with sweet, enters spleen and stomach meridians with the functions of supplementing spleen-stomach and replenishing middle qi. It is often used as a supplementary medicinal because of its moderate efficacy. To treat spleen-stomach deficiency manifested as fatigue, poor appetite, abdominal distention and loose stools, it is used with *rén shēn, bái zhú,* and *fú líng*.

2. 心气不足，心动悸，脉结代　本品入心经，能补益心气，益气复脉。用治心气不足所致的脉结代，心动悸，常与人参、阿胶、生地黄等同用。

(2) Heart qi deficiency, palpitations, irregularly and regularly intermittent pulse　*Gān cǎo* enters heart meridian, with the functions of tonifying and heart qi, replenishing qi and restore pulse. To treat irregular and regular intermittent pulse, palpitations due to heart qi insufficiency, it is usually used with *rén shēn, ē jiāo* and *shēng dì huáng*.

3. 咳喘痰多　本品性平，入肺经，能祛痰止咳。凡是咳喘，不论寒热虚实、有痰无痰均可配伍使用。如治风寒咳嗽，常与麻黄、苦杏仁同用；治肺热咳喘，常与石膏、麻黄、苦杏仁同用；治寒痰咳嗽，常与干姜、细辛等同用；治湿痰咳嗽，常与半夏、陈皮、茯苓同用；治肺虚咳嗽，常与黄芪、太子参等同用。

(3) Cough and panting with profuse sputum　*Gān cǎo* is neutral in nature, enters lung meridian with the functions of dispelling phlegm and relieving cough. It treats all cough and panting of cold, heat, deficiency or excess pattern, with phlegm or without in combination. To treat cough and panting of wind-cold pattern, it is used with *má huáng* and *kǔ xìng rén*; to treat cough and panting due to lung heat, it is used with *shí gāo, má huáng* and *kǔ xìng rén*; to treat cough with cold phlegm, it is used with *gān jiāng* and *xì xīn*; to treat cough with damp phlegm, it is used with *bàn xià, chén pí* and *fú líng*; to treat cough due to lung deficiency, it is used with *huáng qí* and *tài zǐ shēn*.

4. 脘腹、四肢挛急疼痛　本品味甘，善于缓急止痛，适用于脘腹及四肢挛急作痛，常与白芍同用。临床常以芍药甘草汤为基础，随证配伍，可用于血虚、血瘀、寒凝等多种原因所致的脘腹、四肢挛急作痛。

(4) Spasms and pain of stomach, abdomen and four limbs　*Gān cǎo* is sweet, good at relaxing spasms and relieving pain, and suitable for spasms and pain of stomach, abdomen and four limbs usually in combination with *bái sháo*. Based on *Sháo Yào Gān Cǎo Tāng* (Peony and Licorice Decoction), it can be used in combination with syndrome for spasms and pain of stomach, abdomen and four limbs caused by blood deficiency, blood stasis and cold congeal.

5. 痈肿疮毒，咽喉肿痛　本品生用药性偏凉，能清解热毒，可用于多种热毒证。用治热毒疮疡，多与金银花、连翘等同用。用治热毒咽喉肿痛，可单用本品煎服，或与桔梗同用；若病情较重，多与山豆根、牛蒡子等同用。

(5) Sores, abscess, swellings and toxins, sore and swelling throat　*Gān cǎo* is cool in nature with the functions of clearing heat and removing toxins, and it is suitable for many kinds of heat toxin syndromes. To treat sore due to heat toxin, it is used with *jīn yín huā* and *lián qiáo*. To treat sore and swelling throat due to heat toxin, it is used alone or in combination with *jié gěng*; for severe cases, it is used with *shān dòu gēn* and *niú bàng zǐ*.

6. **缓解药物毒性、烈性**　本品甘平，药性和缓，与寒热补泻各类药物同用，能缓和烈性或减轻毒性和副作用，有调和百药之功，故有"国老"之称。如与石膏、知母等寒药同用，可防寒凉伤胃；与附子、干姜等热药同用，可防温燥伤阴，并能降低附子的毒性；与大黄、芒硝等泻下药同用，可缓其峻下之势，使泻不伤正，并能缓解大黄、芒硝刺激胃肠引起的腹痛；与人参、黄芪、熟地黄等补药同用，以调和脾胃，使补虚药效缓慢持久；与黄芩、黄连、干姜、半夏等寒药、热药同用，能调其寒热、升降之偏，以得其平。此外，本品对药物或食物所致中毒，有一定的解毒作用。

(6) Resolving toxins and drastic properties of medicinals　*Gān cǎo* is sweet and neutral with mild efficacies. It can resolve toxins and drastic properties if used with cold, heat, tonic or purgative medicinals, and it has the function of harmonizing hundreds of medicines, so it is called *guǒ lǎo* (illustrious elders of a country). It is combined with cold medicinals like *shí gāo* and *zhī mǔ* to protect stomach from cold; with heat medicinals like *fù zǐ* and *gān jiāng* to avoid damaging yin by warm-dryness and reduce the toxicity of *fù zǐ*; with purgative medicinals like *dà huáng* and *máng xiāo* to relieve the drastic purgation, avoid damaging healthy qi, and relieve the abdominal pain caused by *dà huáng* and *máng xiāo* stimulating the gastrointestinal tract; with tonics like *rén shēn*, *huáng qí* and *shú dì huáng* to harmonize spleen and stomach, making tonic effect slow and lasting; with cold and heat medicinal simultaneously like *huáng qín*, *huáng lián*, *gān jiāng* and *bàn xià* to adjust its cold and heat, ascending and descending to get its balance. In addition, it has certain effect of medicinal poisoning or food poisoning.

【 用法用量 / Usage and dosage 】

煎服，2~10g。清热解毒宜生用；补中缓急、益气复脉宜蜜炙用。

Decoction, 2-10g. It should be used raw for clearing heat and resolving toxins, and should be honeyed for supplementing the middle, relaxing spasms, replenishing qi and restoring pulse.

【 使用注意 / Precaution 】

不宜与海藻、京大戟、红大戟、甘遂、芫花同用。湿盛胀满、水肿者不宜用。不宜大剂量、长期服用。

Gān cǎo is not proper to be used together with *hǎi zǎo* (Sargassum), *jīng dà jǐ* (Euphorbiae Pekinensis Radix), *hóng dà jǐ* (Knoxiae Radix), *gān suí* (Kansui Radix) and *yuán huā* (Genkwa Flos). It is not suitable for distension, fullness and edema due to dampness exuberance. Long-term application in large dose should be avoided.

【 现代研究 / Modern research 】

本品主要含甘草酸、甘草苷、异甘草苷、甘草甜素、甘草黄酮，尚含香豆素类、生物碱、多糖等。具有抗消化道溃疡、调节胃肠运动、保肝、调节免疫、抗衰老、抗病毒、抗菌、解毒、抗肺损伤、抑制子宫平滑肌收缩和皮质激素样等作用。

It mainly contains glycyrrhizic acid, glycyrrhizin, isoliquiritigenin, liquorice flavonoids, coumarins, alkaloids, polysaccharides, etc. It has the functions of anti peptic ulcer, regulating gastrointestinal movement, protecting liver, regulating immunity, anti-aging, anti-virus, antibacterial, detoxification, anti lung injury, inhibiting contraction of uterine smooth muscle and corticosteroid like.

PPT

第二节 补阳药
Section 2 Yang-supplementing medicinals

本类药物味多甘、辛、咸，性多温热，主入肾经，以温补肾阳为主要功效，主要用于肾阳虚证，症见畏寒肢冷，腰膝酸软，性欲淡漠，阳痿早泄，遗精滑精，尿频遗尿，精寒不育或宫冷不孕等，以及肾阳虚衰，脾失温运之腹中冷痛，五更泄泻；肾阳虚不能纳气之虚喘；阳虚水泛之水肿；肾阳虚而精髓亦亏之眩晕耳鸣，须发早白，筋骨痿软或小儿发育不良，囟门不合，齿迟行迟；肾阳不足，下元虚冷，冲任不固之崩漏不止、带下清稀等。某些药物还兼有祛风湿、强筋骨、温脾阳、补肺气、养肝等功效，还可用治风湿痹证、脾肾阳虚证、肺肾两虚证及肝肾亏虚证。补阳药性多燥烈，易助火伤阴，故阴虚火旺者忌用。

Yang-supplementing medicinals are mostly sweet, acrid and salty in flavor, warm and hot in property, and they mainly act on kidney meridian with the main functions of warming and tonifying kidney yang. They are mainly used to treat syndromes of kidney yang deficiency, manifested as aversion to cold, chilly limbs, soreness and weakness of waist and knees, apathy of sexual desire, impotence and premature ejaculation, spermatorrhea, frequent urination, infertility due to spermatic cold or sterility due to uterine cold, as well as cold pain in the abdomen, diarrhea before dawn due to deficiency of kidney yang, and dysfunction of spleen in warming and transporting; deficiency-type dyspnea due to deficiency of kidney yang failing to receive qi; edema due to yang deficiency and water diffusion; vertigo and tinnitus, premature graying of hairs, flaccid sinew and bones or infantile dysplasia, non-closure of fontanels, retardation of tooth eruption and walking due to deficiency of kidney yang and essence; metrorrhagia and mentrostaxis, clear and thin vaginal discharge due to kidney yang deficiency, deficiency-cold of lower jiao, and insecurity of thoroughfare and conception vessels. Some medicinals can also be used not only to eliminate wind-dampness, strengthen sinews and bones, warm spleen yang, invigorate lung qi, and nourish liver, but also to treat wind-dampness *bì* (impediment) syndrome, spleen-stomach yang deficiency syndrome, lung-spleen deficiency syndrome and liver-kidney depletion. Yang-supplementing medicinals are mostly dry and drastic in property, and tend to assist fire to damage yin, so it is contraindicated in patients with vigorous fire due to yin deficiency.

鹿茸 *Lù róng* (Cervi Cornu Pantotrichum)
《神农本草经》
Shen Nong's Classic of the Materia Medica (Shén Nóng Běn Cǎo Jīng)

【来源 / Origin】
为鹿科动物梅花鹿 *Cervus nippon* Temminck 或马鹿 *Cervus elaphus* Linnaeus 的雄鹿未骨化密生茸毛的幼角。前者习称"花鹿茸"，后者习称"马鹿茸"。主产于吉林、辽宁、黑龙江等地。夏、秋二季锯取鹿茸，切薄片或研成细粉用。花鹿茸气微腥，味微咸；马鹿茸气腥臭，味咸。

Lù róng is the young horn of *Cervus nippon* Temminck or *Cervus elaphus* Linnaeus, pertaining to Cervidae, mainly produced in Jilin, Liaoning, and Heilongjiang Province. The former is known as *huā lù*

róng, while the latter *mǎ lù róng*. The pilose antler is sawed in summer and autumn, sliced or ground into fine powder. *Huā lù róng* is slightly fishy and salty; *mǎ lù róng* is fishy and salty.

【性味归经 / Medicinal properties】

甘、咸，温。归肾、肝经。

Sweet, salty, and warm; act on kidney and liver meridians.

【主要功效 / Medicinal efficacies】

壮肾阳，益精血，强筋骨，调冲任，托疮毒。

Supplement kidney yang, replenish essence and blood, strengthen the sinews and bones, regulate thoroughfare and conception vessels, and promoting pus discharge of sores.

【临床应用 / Clinical application】

1. 肾阳虚证　本品甘温能补，味咸入肾，能峻补肾阳，益精血，适宜于肾阳亏虚，精血不足之阳痿遗精、宫冷不孕、腰膝酸软、畏寒肢冷、眩晕耳鸣、尿频遗尿等，可单用，或与山药浸酒服，或与山茱萸、枸杞子、熟地黄等同用。

(1) Kidney yang deficiency　*Lù róng* can tonify with sweet and warm, salty property entering kidney, and can drastically tonify kidney yang, replenishing essence and blood. It treats impotence and spermatorrhea, infertility due to uterine cold, soreness and weakness waist and knees, aversion to cold and chilly limbs, dizziness and tinnitus, frequent urination and enuresis due to kidney yang deficiency and insufficiency of essence and blood, used alone or soaked in wine with *shān yào*, or in combination with *shān zhū yú*, *gǒu qǐ zǐ* and *shú dì huáng*.

2. 肝肾亏虚，筋骨不健　本品入肝、肾经，能补肾阳，益精血，强筋健骨。用治肝肾不足，精血亏虚之筋骨痿软，或小儿发育不良，行迟齿迟，囟门不合等，常与五加皮、熟地黄、怀牛膝等同用。若治骨折后期，愈合不良，多与骨碎补、续断、自然铜等同用。

(2) Liver-kidney deficiency, flaccid sinews and bones　*Lù róng* enters liver and kidney meridians with the functions of tonifying kidney yang, replenishing essence and blood, and strengthening sinews and bones. It treats flaccid sinew and bones or infantile dysplasia, retardation of tooth eruption and walking and non-closure of fontanels due to deficiency of kidney yang and essence in combination with *wǔ jiā pí*, *shú dì huáng* and *huái niú xī*. To treat undesirable healing in the later stage of bone fracture, it is used with *gǔ suì bǔ*, *xù duàn* and *zì rán tóng*.

3. 冲任虚寒，崩漏带下　本品补肝肾，固冲任，止崩带。用治肝肾亏虚，冲任虚寒之崩漏不止、带下过多，前者常与当归、阿胶、蒲黄等同用；后者可与桑螵蛸、菟丝子、沙苑子等同用。

(3) Deficiency-cold of thoroughfare and conception vessels, metrorrhagia, metrostaxis and abnormal vaginal discharge　*Lù róng* can tonify liver and kidney, secure thoroughfare and conception vessels, and relieve metrorrhagia, metrostaxis and abnormal vaginal discharge. To treat liver-kidney deficiency, deficiency cold thoroughfare and conception vessels, continuous metrorrhagia and metrostaxis, and excessive abnormal vaginal discharge, the former is used with *dāng guī*, *ē jiāo* and *pú huáng*, while the latter with *sāng piāo xiāo*, *tù sī zǐ* and *shā yuàn zǐ*.

4. 疮疡内陷不起或久溃不敛　本品补阳气、益精血而有托毒生肌之效，用治阳气不足，精血亏虚之阴疽疮肿内陷不起或疮疡久溃不敛，常与熟地黄、肉桂、白芥子等同用。

(4) Deteriorated or chronic ulcer without healing　*Lù róng* can tonify yang qi, replenishing essence and blood, promoting pus discharge and tissue regeneration. It treats deteriorated or chronic ulcer caused by deficiency of yang qi, essence and blood in combination with *shú dì huáng*, *ròu guì* and *bái jiè zǐ*.

【用量用法 / Usage and dosage】

研末冲服，1~2g。

Powdered and mixed with water, 1-2g.

【使用注意 / Precaution】

服用本品宜从小剂量开始，缓慢增加，不可骤用大剂量，以免阳升风动，头晕目赤，或伤阴动血。凡热证均当忌服。

The dosage should be increased gradually from small one. Large dosage is not allowed to be applied suddenly in order to avoid raising yang and stirring of wind, vertigo and red eyes, or damaging yin and inducing bleeding. It should be contraindicated in all heat syndromes.

【现代研究 / Modern research】

本品主要含雌二醇、胆固醇、雌酮、磷脂、磷脂酰胆碱、核糖核酸、脱氧核糖核酸、前列腺素、蛋白质、多糖、氨基酸、脂肪酸及无机元素等。具有性激素样作用，能抗骨质疏松、促进子宫发育、增强性功能、增强免疫、延缓衰老、抗疲劳、促进红细胞和血红蛋白新生、促进核酸和蛋白质合成、促进伤口和骨折愈合、抗心肌缺血、抗炎、保肝、抗辐射等。

Lù róng mainly contains estradiol, cholesterol, estrone, phospholipid, phosphatidylcholine, ribonucleic acid, deoxyribonucleic acid, prostaglandin, protein, polysaccharide, amino acid, fatty acid and inorganic elements. It has the function of sex hormone, and can resist osteoporosis, promote the development of uterus, improve sexual function, enhance immunity, delay aging, resist fatigue, promote the regeneration of red blood cell and hemoglobin, promote the synthesis of nucleic acid and protein, promote the healing of wound and fracture, resist myocardial ischemia, resist inflammation, protect liver, and resist radiation.

淫羊藿 *Yín yáng huò* (Epimedii Folium)
《神农本草经》
Shen Nong's Classic of the Materia Medica (Shén Nóng Běn Cǎo Jīng)

【来源 / Origin】

为小檗科植物淫羊藿 *Epimedium brevicornu* Maxim.、箭叶淫羊藿 *Epimedium sagittatum*（Sieb. et Zucc.）Maxim.、柔毛淫羊藿 *Epimedium Pubescens* Maxim. 或朝鲜淫羊藿 *Epimedium koreanum* Nakai. 的干燥叶。主产于山西、四川、湖北等地。夏、秋二季茎叶茂盛时采收，生用或以羊脂油炙用。本品气微，味微苦。《中国药典》规定，含总黄酮以淫羊藿苷（$C_{33}H_{40}O_{15}$）计不得少于 0.50%，饮片不得少于 0.40%；炙淫羊藿含羊藿苷（$C_{33}H_{40}O_{15}$）和宝羊藿苷 I（$C_{27}H_{30}O_{10}$）的总量不得少于 0.60%。

Yín yáng huò is the dried leaves of *Epimedium brevicornu* Maxim., *Epimedium sagittatum* (Sieb. Et Zucc.) Maxim., *Epimedium pubescens* Maxim., or *Epimedium koreanum* Nakai., pertaining to Berberidaceae, mainly produced in Shanxi, Sichuan, Hubei and other places, collected in summer and autumn when the stems and leaves are luxuriant, and used raw or roasted with Lanolin oil. It has a slight odor and bitter taste. According to *Chinese Pharmacopoeia*, the content of total flavonoids in Herba Epimedii glycosides ($C_{33}H_{40}O_{15}$) shall not be less than 0.50%, and not less than 0.40% in decoction pieces. The total content of icariin ($C_{33}H_{40}O_{15}$) and pogostemin I ($C_{27}H_{30}O_{10}$) in processed *yín yáng huò* should not be less than 0.60%.

【性味归经 / Medicinal properties】

辛、甘，温。归肝、肾经。

Acrid, sweet and warm; act on liver and kidney meridians.

【主要功效 / Medicinal efficacies】

补肾阳，强筋骨，祛风湿。

Tonify kidney yang, strengthen the sinews and bones, and dispel wind-dampness.

【临床应用 / Clinical application】

1. 肾阳虚证　本品味辛甘，性温燥烈，主入肾经，长于补肾壮阳起痿，宜用于肾阳虚衰之男子阳痿不育，可单用浸酒服，或与巴戟天、枸杞子等同用。若治肾虚阳痿遗精，腰酸腿软，精神倦怠，多与肉苁蓉、巴戟天、杜仲等同用。

(1) **Kidney yang deficiency**　*Yín yáng huò* is acrid and sweet in flavor, warm, dry and drastic in property, entering in kidney meridian and good at tonifying kidney and strengthening yang, which can be used alone in wine or in combination with *bā jǐ tiān* and *gǒu qǐ zǐ* in treating impotence and infertility in men due to kidney yang deficiency. To treat impotence, spermatorrhea, lumbago, leg weakness, mental fatigue due to kidney deficiency, it is used with *ròu cōng róng*, *bā jǐ tiān* and *dù zhòng*.

2. 风寒湿痹，筋骨痿软　本品甘温，入肝肾经，能强健筋骨，辛温发散而祛风散寒除湿，用治风寒湿痹，日久不愈，累及肝肾，筋骨不健，或肝肾不足，筋骨不健，常与威灵仙、杜仲、桑寄生等同用。

(2) **Wind-cold-dampness impediment, weakness of sinews and bones**　*Yín yáng huò* is sweet and warm, entering liver and kidney meridians with the functions of strengthening the sinews and bones, expelling wind, dispersing cold and removing dampness with acrid warm. It treats weak sinews and bones due to persisting wind-cold-dampness impediment, involving liver and kidney, or weak sinews and bones due to liver-kidney insufficiency in combination with *wēi líng xiān*, *dù zhòng* and *sāng jì shēng*.

【用量用法 / Usage and dosage】

煎服，6~10g。

Decoction, 6-10g.

【使用注意 / Precaution】

阴虚火旺者忌服。

It is contraindicated in patients with vigorous fire due to yin deficiency.

【现代研究 / Modern research】

本品主要含淫羊藿苷、宝羊藿苷、淫羊藿次苷、大花淫羊藿苷、箭藿苷、金丝桃苷等，尚含多糖、生物碱、脂肪酸、挥发油等。具有性激素样作用，能抗骨质疏松、增强免疫、抗肝肾损伤、抗甲状腺损伤、抗心肌缺血、抗阿尔茨海默病、抗血栓、抗衰老及促进造血等作用。

Yín yáng huò mainly contains icariin, pogoside, hypericin, as well as polysaccharides, alkaloids, fatty acids, volatile oil, etc. It has the function of sex hormone, which can resist osteoporosis, enhance immunity, resist liver and kidney injury, resist thyroid injury, resist myocardial ischemia, resist Alzheimer's disease, resist thrombosis, resist aging and promote hematopoiesis.

巴戟天　*Bā jǐ tiān* (Morindae Officinalis Radix)
《神农本草经》
Shen Nong's Classic of the Materia Medica (*Shén Nóng Běn Cǎo Jīng*)

【来源 / Origin】

为茜草科植物巴戟天 *Morinda officinalis* How 的干燥根。主产于广东、广西及福建。全年均可采挖。晒干，生用或抽取木心，分别加工炮制成巴戟肉、盐巴戟天、制巴戟天用。本品气微，味甘而微涩。《中国药典》规定，含耐斯糖（$C_{24}H_{42}O_{21}$）不得少于 2.0%。

Bā jǐ tiān is the dry root of *Morinda officinalis* How, pertaining to Rubiaceae, mainly produced in Guangdong, Guangxi Zhuang Autonomous Region and Fujian, collected all year round, dried, and used raw or extracted woody heart, prepared and processed into *bā jǐ ròu*, *yán bā jǐ tiān* and *zhì bā jǐ tiān* respectively. It has a slight odor, sweet and astringent taste. According to *Chinese Pharmacopoeia*, the content of nexose ($C_{24}H_{42}O_{21}$) should not be less than 2.0%.

【性味归经 / Medicinal properties】

甘、辛，微温。归肾、肝经。

Sweet, acrid and slightly warm; act on kidney and liver meridians.

【主要功效 / Medicinal efficacies】

补肾阳，强筋骨，祛风湿。

Tonify kidney yang, strengthen the sinews and bones, and dispel wind-dampness.

【临床应用 / Clinical application】

1. 肾阳虚证　本品甘温，入下焦，能补肾壮阳益精。用治肾阳不足，命门火衰之阳痿、不育，常与淫羊藿、仙茅、枸杞子等同用。用治肾阳亏虚，宫冷不孕，月经不调，少腹冷痛，常与肉桂、吴茱萸、高良姜等同用。

(1) Kidney yang deficiency　*Bā jǐ tiān* is sweet and warm, entering lower energizer with the functions of tonifying kidney, strengthening yang and replenishing essence. It treats impotence and infertility due to kidney yang insufficiency, and declining of the fire of life gate in combination with *yín yáng huò*, *xiān máo* and *gǒu qǐ zǐ*. To treat kidney yang deficiency manifested as infertility due to cold uterus, irregular menstruation and cold and pain in lower abdomen, it is used with *ròu guì*, *wú zhū yú* and *gāo liáng jiāng*.

2. 风湿痹痛，筋骨痿软　本品辛温能散，甘温助阳，具有补肾阳、强筋骨、祛风湿之效，用治肾阳不足，兼有风湿痹痛，筋骨痿软，肢体拘挛等，常与肉苁蓉、杜仲、菟丝子等同用。用治风冷腰胯疼痛、行步不利，常与羌活、杜仲、五加皮等同用。

(2) Pain of wind-dampness impediment, weakness of sinews and bones　*Bā jǐ tiān* can dispersing with acrid warm, and assist yang with sweet warm, and has the efficacies of tonify kidney yang, strengthen the sinews and bones, and dispel wind-dampness. It treats kidney yang insufficiency with pains of wind-dampness impediment manifested as weakness of sinews and bones, and hypertonicity of the limbs in combination with *ròu cōng róng*, *dù zhòng* and *tù sī zǐ*. To treat pain in waist and crotch due to cold wind, and difficult walking, it is used with *qiāng huó*, *dù zhòng* and *wǔ jiā pí*.

【用量用法 / Usage and dosage】

煎服，3~10g。

Decoction, 3-10g.

【使用注意 / Precaution】

阴虚火旺及有热者不宜服。

It is contraindicated in patients with heat or with vigorous fire due to yin deficiency.

【现代研究 / Modern research】

本品主要含甲基异茜草素、大黄素甲醚、水晶兰苷、四乙酰车叶草苷、耐斯糖等，尚含甾醇、有机酸、维生素 C 等。具有雄激素样作用，能增强免疫、抗缺氧、抗疲劳、抗衰老、抗肿瘤等。

Bā jǐ tiān mainly contains methyl isorubicin, emodin methyl ether, crystal orchid glycoside, tetraacetyl plantain, nexose, as well as sterol, organic acid, vitamin C, etc. It has androgen-like effect, and can enhance immunity, resist hypoxia, fatigue, aging and tumor.

杜仲 *Dù zhòng* (Eucommiae Cortex)
《神农本草经》
Shen Nong's Classic of the Materia Medica (Shén Nóng Běn Cǎo Jīng)

【来源 / Origin】

为杜仲科植物杜仲 *Eucommia ulmoides* Oliv. 的干燥树皮。主产于陕西、四川、云南等地。4~6月剥取，晒干，生用或盐水炒用。本品气微，味稍苦。《中国药典》规定，含松脂醇二葡萄糖苷（$C_{32}H_{42}O_{16}$）不得少于 0.10%。

Dù zhòng is the dry bark of *Eucommia ulmoides* Oliv., pertaining to Eucommiaceae, mainly produced in Shaanxi, Sichuan, and Yunnan Province. It is peeled in April to June, dried in the sun, and used raw or stir-fried with salted water. It has a slight odor and a slightly bitter taste. According to *Chinese Pharmacopoeia*, the content of rosin diglucoside ($C_{32}H_{42}O_{16}$) shall not be less than 0.10%.

【性味归经 / Medicinal properties】

甘，温。归肝、肾经。

Sweet and warm; act on liver and kidney meridians.

【主要功效 / Medicinal efficacies】

补肝肾，强筋骨，安胎。

Tonify liver and kidney, strengthen sinews and bones, and prevent miscarriage.

【临床应用 / Clinical application】

1. 肾阳虚证 本品甘温，入肾经，能温补肾阳。用治肾阳不足之阳痿、尿频，常与山茱萸、菟丝子、覆盆子等同用。

(1) **Kidney yang deficiency** *Dù zhòng* sweet and warm, entering kidney meridian with the functions of warming and tonifying kidney yang. It treats impotence and frequent urination due to kidney yang insufficiency in combination with *shān zhū yú*, *tù sī zǐ* and *fù pén zǐ*.

2. 肝肾不足，腰膝酸痛，筋骨无力 本品甘温，入肝肾经，以补肝肾、强筋骨见长，用治肝肾不足之腰膝酸痛，筋骨痿软，可单用浸酒服，或与胡桃肉、补骨脂等同用。用治风寒湿痹日久，腰膝冷痛，常与独活、桑寄生、细辛等同用。用治外伤腰痛，常与川芎、丹参、红花等同用。用治妇女经期腰痛，常与当归、川芎等同用。用治肝肾不足，头晕目眩，常与牛膝、枸杞子、菟丝子等同用。

(2) **Liver-kidney insufficiency, soreness and pain of loins and knees, weakness of sinews and bones** *Dù zhòng* is sweet and warm, entering liver and kidney meridian with the functions of tonifying liver-kidney, strengthen sinews and bones. It treats soreness and pain of loins and knees, weakness of sinews and bones due to liver-kidney insufficiency alone in wine or in combination with *hú táo ròu* and *bǔ gǔ zhī*. To treat cold and pain waist and knees due to persistent wind-cold-dampness impediment, it is used with *dú huó*, *sāng jì shēng* and *xì xīn*. To treat traumatic lumbago, it is used with *chuān xiōng*, *dān shēn* and *hóng huā*. To treat women's low back pain during menstruation, it is used with *dāng guī* and *chuān xiōng*. To treat dizziness due to insufficiency of liver and kidney, it is used with *niú xī*, *gǒu qǐ zǐ* and *tù sī zǐ*.

3. 胎漏，胎动不安 本品甘温，能补肝肾、固冲任而安胎。用治肝肾不足，冲任不固，胎漏下血，胎动不安或滑胎，常与续断、桑寄生、白术等同用。

(3) Vaginal bleeding during pregnancy, threatened abortion *Dù zhòng* is sweet and warm, and can prevent miscarriage by tonifying liver-kidney and secure thoroughfare and conception vessels. It is often combines with *xù duàn*, *sāng jì shēng* and *bái zhú* in treating vaginal bleeding during pregnancy, threatened abortion or habitual abortion due to liver-kidney insufficiency and insecurity of thoroughfare and conception vessels.

【用量用法 / Usage and dosage】

煎服，6~10g。

Decoction, 6-10g.

【使用注意 / Precaution】

阴虚火旺者慎用。

It should be used with caution in patients with vigorous fire due to yin deficiency.

【现代研究 / Modern research】

本品主要含松脂醇二葡萄糖苷、杜仲胶、杜仲苷、杜仲树脂醇双吡喃葡萄糖苷、京尼平、京尼平苷、桃叶珊瑚苷、鞣质、黄酮等。具有促进骨折愈合、降血压、抗疲劳、镇静、镇痛、增强免疫、延缓衰老及抗肿瘤等作用。

Dù zhòng mainly contains rosin diglucoside, eucommia gum, eucommia glycoside, eucommia resin alcohol dipyran glucoside, genipin, geniposide, aucubin, tannin, flavonoids, etc. It has the functions of promoting fracture healing, lowering blood pressure, resist fatigue, sedation, analgesia, enhancing immunity, delaying aging and anti-tumor.

续断　*Xù duàn* (Dipsaci Radix)
《神农本草经》
Shen Nong's Classic of the Materia Medica (Shén Nóng Běn Cǎo Jīng)

【来源 / Origin】

为川续断科植物川续断 *Dipsacus asper* Wall. ex Henry 的干燥根。主产于湖北、四川、湖南等地。秋季采挖，干燥，切厚片，生用或酒炙、盐炙用。本品气微香，味苦、微甜而后涩。《中国药典》规定，含川续断皂苷Ⅵ（$C_{47}H_{76}O_{18}$）不得少于 2.0%，饮片不得少于 1.5%。

Xù duàn is the dry root of *Dipsacus asper* wall. ex Henry, pertaining to Dipsacaceae, mainly produced in Hubei, Sichuan, and Hunan, collected in autumn, dried, sliced into thick pieces, and used raw or processed with wine or salt. It is slightly fragrant, bitter, sweet and astringent. According to *Chinese Pharmacopoeia*, the content of dipsacus saponin Ⅵ ($C_{47}H_{76}O_{18}$) shall not be less than 2.0%, and that in pieces shall not be less than 1.5%.

【性味归经 / Medicinal properties】

苦、辛，微温。归肝、肾经。

Bitter, acrid and slightly warm; act on liver and kidney meridians.

【主要功效 / Medicinal efficacies】

补肝肾，强筋骨，续折伤，止崩漏。

Tonify liver and kidney, strengthen sinews and bones, heal bone fracture and trauma, and relieve metrorrhagia and metrostaxis.

【临床应用 / Clinical application】

1. **肝肾不足，腰膝酸软，风湿痹痛**　本品补而能行，既能补肝肾，强筋骨，又能通利血脉，用治肝肾亏虚，腰膝酸痛，足膝痿软，常与杜仲、牛膝、五加皮等同用。用治肝肾不足兼寒湿痹痛，常与防风、牛膝、萆薢等同用。

(1) Liver-kidney insufficiency, soreness and pain of loins and knees, wind-dampness pain of impediment *Xù duàn* tonifies and moves, not only tonifying liver and kidney, strengthen sinews and bones, but also dredging blood vessels. It treats soreness and pain in the back and knees, impotence in the feet and knees due to liver-kidney deficiency in combination with *dù zhòng*, *niú xī* and *wǔ jiā pí*. To treat liver-kidney insufficiency with wind-dampness pain of impediment, it is used with *fáng fēng*, *niú xī* and *bì xiè*.

2. 跌仆损伤，筋伤骨折 本品辛散温通，能活血祛瘀，续筋疗伤，为伤科常用药。用治跌打损伤，瘀血肿痛，筋伤骨折，常与骨碎补、自然铜等配伍。用治足膝折损愈后失补，筋缩疼痛，可与当归、木瓜、黄芪等同用。

(2) Injury from falls, tendon injury and bone fracture *Xù duàn* is dispersing with acrid and dredging with warm with the functions of activating blood, dissolving blood stasis, reinforcing tendons and healing wounds and is a commonly used medicinal in traumatology. It treats injury from fall, bruise, swelling and pain, tendon injury and bone fracture in combination with *gǔ suì bǔ* and *zì rán tóng*. To treat pain of muscle contraction due to the loss of tonic after the recovery of knee fracture, it is used with *dāng guī*, *mù guā* and *huáng qí*.

3. 胎漏，胎动不安 本品补益肝肾，调理冲任，固经安胎。用治肝肾不足，冲任不固所致的胎漏下血，胎动不安或滑胎，常与桑寄生、阿胶、菟丝子等同用。若治肝肾亏虚所致的崩漏、月经过多，可与黄芪、地榆、艾叶等配伍。

(3) Vaginal bleeding during pregnancy, threatened abortion *Xù duàn* tonifies and replenishes liver and kidney, regulates thoroughfare and conception vessels and astringes menses to prevent miscarriage. It is often combines with *sāng jì shēng*, *ē jiāo* and *tù sī zǐ* in treating vaginal bleeding during pregnancy, threatened abortion or habitual abortion due to liver-kidney insufficiency and insecurity of thoroughfare and conception vessels. To treat metrorrhagia and menorrhagia, it is used with *huáng qí*, *dì yú* and *ài yè*.

【用法用量 / Usage and dosage】

煎服，9~15g。

Decoction, 9-15g.

【现代研究 / Modern research】

本品主要含川续断皂苷、常春藤苷、喜树次碱、川续断碱、熊果酸、番木鳖苷以及黄酮类、甾醇及多糖等。具有促进骨折愈合、抗骨质疏松、抑制子宫收缩、抗炎、镇痛、抗氧化、抗维生素 E 缺乏等作用。

Xù duàn mainly contains dipsacus saponin, ivy glycoside, camptothecin, dipsacus aspectus alkaloid, ursolic acid, chitin, flavonoids, sterols and polysaccharides. It has the functions of promoting fracture healing, anti osteoporosis, inhibiting uterine contraction, anti inflammation, analgesia, anti-oxidation, anti vitamin E deficiency and so on.

肉苁蓉 *Ròu cōng róng* (Cistanches Herba)
《神农本草经》
Shen Nong's Classic of the Materia Medica (Shén Nóng Běn Cǎo Jīng)

【来源 / Origin】

为列当科植物肉苁蓉 *Cistanche deserticola* Y. C. Ma 或管花肉苁蓉 *Cistanche tubulosa*（Schenk）

Wight 的干燥带鳞叶的肉质茎。主产于内蒙古、新疆及甘肃。春季苗刚出土时或秋季冻土之前采收。生用或酒制用。本品气微，味甜、微苦。《中国药典》规定，肉苁蓉含松果菊苷（$C_{35}H_{46}O_{20}$）和毛蕊花糖苷（$C_{29}H_{36}O_{15}$）的总量不得少于 0.30%，管花肉苁蓉含松果菊苷和毛蕊花糖苷的总量不得少于 1.5%。

Ròu cōng róng is the dried scaly fleshy stem of *Cistanche deserticola* Y. C. Ma or *Cistanche tubulosa* (Schenk) Wight, pertaining to Orobanchaceae, mainly produced in Inner Mongolia Autonomous Region, Xinjiang Uygur Autonomous Region and Gansu Province, collected in spring when it has not or just come out of the ground, or before the soil frozen in autumn. Used raw or processed with wine, it is slight in odor, sweet and slightly bitter in taste. According to *Chinese Pharmacopoeia*, the total content of echinacoside ($C_{35}H_{46}O_{20}$) and mulleioside ($C_{29}H_{36}O_{15}$) in *Cistanche deserticola* Y. C. Ma should not be less than 0.30%, and not be less than 1.5% in *Cistanche tubulosa* (Schrenk) Wight.

【性味归经 / Medicinal properties】

甘、咸，温。归肾、大肠经。

Sweet, salty and warm; act on kidney and large intestine meridians.

【主要功效 / Medicinal efficacies】

补肾阳，益精血，润肠通便。

Supplement kidney yang, replenish essence and blood, and moisten the intestines to promote defecation.

【临床应用 / Clinical application】

1. 肾阳不足，精血亏虚证　本品甘温助阳，质润滋养，咸以入肾，能补肾阳，益精血，且温而不燥，补而不腻，作用从容和缓。用治肾阳不足，精血亏虚所致的阳痿不育、宫冷不孕、腰膝酸软、筋骨无力，畏寒怕冷，常与鹿角胶、淫羊藿、熟地黄等同用。

(1) **Insufficiency of kidney yang, essence and blood depletion**　*Ròu cōng róng* assists yang with sweet warm, moistening and nourishing in nature, entering kidney with its salty property, and it can tonify kidney yang and replenish essence and blood, warm but not dry, tonifying but not slimy with slow and mild efficacies. To treat impotence and infertility, uterine cold and sterility, weak waist and knees, inability of the extremities, and aversion to cold due to kidney yang insufficiency, essence and blood depletion, it is usually used with *lù jiǎo jiāo*, *yín yáng huò* and *shú dì huáng*.

2. 肠燥便秘　本品甘咸质润，入大肠经，能润肠通便。适用于老人或病后肠燥便秘属于肾阳不足，精血亏虚者，常与当归、牛膝、枳壳等同用。

(2) **Constipation due to intestinal dryness**　*Ròu cōng róng* is sweet, salty and moistening, entering large intestine and can moistening intestines to promote defecation. It is suitable for the elderly or those with constipation caused by dryness of intestines after illness due to kidney yang insufficiency and essence and blood depletion in combination with *dāng guī*, *niú xī* and *zhǐ qiào*.

【用量用法 / Usage and dosage】

煎服，6~10g。

Decoction, 6-10g.

【使用注意 / Precaution】

阴虚火旺、热结便秘、大便溏泄者忌服。

It should be contraindicated in patients with fire exuberance due to yin deficiency, constipation due to heat accumulation, or loose stool.

【现代研究 / Modern research】

本品主要含松果菊苷、毛蕊花糖苷、肉苁蓉苷 A、肉苁蓉苷 B、肉苁蓉苷 C、肉苁蓉苷 H、洋丁香酚苷、海胆苷、鹅掌楸苷、甜菜碱、氨基酸及多糖等。具有激活肾上腺、释放皮质激素作用及增强记忆、延缓衰老、通便、增强免疫、促进代谢、抗阿尔茨海默病、抗肝损伤等作用。

Ròu cōng róng mainly contains echinacoside, mulleioside, cistanche glycoside A, B, C, H, eugenol glycoside, sea urchin, liriodendrin, betaine, amino acids and polysaccharides, etc. It has the functions of activating adrenal glands, releasing corticosteroids, enhancing memory, delaying senility, defecating, enhancing immunity, promoting metabolism, resisting Alzheimer's diease and resisting liver injury.

锁阳　*Suǒ yáng* (Cynomorii Herba)
《本草衍义补遗》
Supplement to the Extension of the Materia Medica (Běn Cǎo Yǎn Yì Bǔ Yí)

【来源 / Origin】

为锁阳科植物锁阳 *Cynomorium songaricum* Rupr. 的干燥肉质茎。主产于内蒙古、甘肃及新疆。春季采挖，切薄片，生用。本品气微，味甘而涩。

Suǒ Yáng is the dried fleshy stem of *Cynomorium songaricum* Rupr., pertaining to Cynomoriaceae. It is mainly produced in Inner Mongolia Autonomous Region, Gansu Province and Xinjiang Uygur Autonomous Region, collected in spring, sliced and used raw. It has a slight odor, and is sweet and astringent in taste.

【性味归经 / Medicinal properties】

甘，温。归肝、肾、大肠经。

Sweet and warm; act on the liver, kidney and large intestine meridians.

【主要功效 / Medicinal efficacies】

补肾阳，益精血，润肠通便。

Tonify kidney yang, benefit essence and blood, moisten intestines and relieve constipation.

【临床应用 / Clinical application】

1. 肾阳不足，精血亏虚证　本品甘温入肾经，能补肾阳、益精血，功用与肉苁蓉相似而偏于补阳。用治肾阳虚阳痿滑精、不孕，常与巴戟天、补骨脂、菟丝子等同用。用治肾阳不足，腰膝酸软，头晕耳鸣、遗精早泄，常与巴戟天、补骨脂、菟丝子等同用。

(1) **Deficiency syndromes of blood and essence due to deficiency of kidney yang** *Suǒ yáng* can nourish kidney yang and blood essence by warming the kidney meridian. Its function is similar to *ròu cōng róng* (Cistanches Herba), but it is partial to tonifying yang. To treat impotence, involuntary emission and asthenia due to kidney defficiency, it is often combined with *bā jǐ tiān*, *bǔ gǔ zhī* (Psoraleae Fructus) and *tù sī zǐ* (Cuscutae Semen); to treat deficiency of kidney yang, weakness of waist and knees, dizziness, tinnitus and premature ejaculation, it is also combine with *bā jǐ tiān*, *bǔ gǔ zhī* (Psoraleae Fructus) and *tù sī zǐ* (Cuscutae Semen).

2. 肠燥便秘　本品甘温质润，能益精养血，润肠通便。用治肾阳不足，精血亏虚之肠燥便秘，常与肉苁蓉、火麻仁、当归等同用。

(2) **Constipation due to dryness of intestine** With the nature of sweet, warm and moist, it can benefit essence, nourish blood, moisten intestines and relieve constipation. To treat constipation due to deficiency of kidney yang and essence, it is often combined with *ròu cōng róng*, *huǒ má rén* (Cannabis

Fructus) and *dāng guī*.

【用量用法 / Usage and dosage】

煎服，5~10g。

Decoction, 5-10g.

【使用注意 / Precaution】

阴虚阳亢、脾虚泄泻、实热便秘者不宜使用。

It is not suitable for the patients with yin deficiency and yang hyperactivity, diarrhea due to spleen deficiency, and constipation due to excess heat.

【现代研究 / Modern research】

本品主要含锁阳苷、熊果酸及挥发油、黄酮、氨基酸等。具有增强免疫、延缓衰老、抗缺氧、抗疲劳、促进性成熟、降血压等作用。

It mainly contains cynomolgin, ursolic acid, volatile oil, flavonoids, and amino acids, etc. It has the functions of enhancing immunity, delaying aging, anti hypoxia, anti fatigue, promoting sexual maturity, and lowering blood pressure, etc.

补骨脂 *Bǔ gǔ zhī* (Psoraleae Fructus)
《药性论》
Treatise on Medicinal Properties (*Yào Xìng Lùn*)

【来源 / Origin】

为豆科植物补骨脂 *Psoralea corylifolia* L. 的干燥成熟果实。主产于河南、四川、安徽等地。秋季果实成熟时采收，晒干，生用，炒或盐水炒用。本品气香，味辛、微苦。《中国药典》规定，含补骨脂素（$C_{11}H_6O_3$）和异补骨脂素（$C_{11}H_6O_3$）的总量不得少于 0.70%。

Bǔ gǔ zhī is the mature dry fruit of *Psoralea corylifolia* L., pertaining to Leguminosae. It is mainly produced in Henan, Sichuan, Anhui and other places in China, collected in autumn, when the fruit is ripe, dried and used raw, or stir-fried with saline water. It is fragrant, and tastes acrid and slightly bitter. According to *Chinese Pharmacopoeia*, the total content of psoralen ($C_{11}H_6O_3$) and isopsoralen ($C_{11}H_6O_3$) should be no less than 0.70%.

【性味归经 / Medicinal properties】

辛、苦，温。归肾、脾经。

Acrid, bitter and warm; act on kidney and spleen meridians.

【主要功效 / Medicinal efficacies】

温肾助阳，纳气平喘，温脾止泻；外用消风祛斑。

Warm the kidney and assist yang, improve qi reception and relieve asthma, warm the spleen and arrest diarrhea; disperse wind and remove patches in topical application.

1. 肾阳虚证　本品性温入肾经，有温补命门、补肾强腰、壮阳固精之效。用治肾虚阳痿，遗精滑精，常与菟丝子、胡桃肉、沉香等同用。用治肾阳不足，腰膝冷痛，常与杜仲、胡桃肉等同用。用治肾阳不足，遗尿尿频，可与小茴香配伍。

(1) Kidney yang depletion syndrome　With warm nature and acting on the kidney meridian, it has the effects of warming the life-gate, tonifying the kidney and strengthening the waist, strengthening yang and the essence. To treat impotence due to kidney deficiency and seminal emission, it is often combined with *tù sī zǐ*, *hú táo ròu* and *chén xiāng* (Aquilariae Resinatum Lignum); to treat cold pain of the loins and knees due to kidney yang depletion, it is usually applied with *dù zhòng* (Eucommiae Cortex) and *hú táo*

ròu; to treat frequent urination due to deficiency-cold of kidney qi, it is often used in combination with *xiǎo huí xiāng* (Foeniculi Fructus).

2. **肾虚作喘**　本品能补肾助阳，纳气平喘，用治肾阳亏虚，肾不纳气之虚喘，常与附子、肉桂、沉香等同用。

(2) Panting and asthma due to kidney-deficiency　With the efficacy of warming kidney and assisting yang, improving qi reception and relieving asthma, it can treat panting and asthma in combination with *fù zǐ* (Aconiti Lateralis Radix Praeparata), *ròu guì* (Cinnamomi Cortex) and *chén xiāng*.

3. **五更泄泻**　本品入脾肾二经，补中兼涩，能温肾阳、补脾阳、涩肠止泻，用治脾肾阳虚之五更泄泻，常与吴茱萸、五味子、肉豆蔻等同用。

(3) Diarrhea before dawn　With the nature of astringent, tonifying the middle and acting on the spleen and kidney meridians, it can warm kidney yang, invigorate spleen yang, astringent intestines and relieve diarrhea and often combined with *wú zhū yú*, *wǔ wèi zǐ* and *ròu dòu kòu*.

此外，本品外用能消风祛斑，还可用治白癜风、斑秃等。

In addition, it is able to disperse wind and remove patches in topical application, so it can treat vitiligo and alopecia.

【用量用法 / Usage and dosage】

煎服，6~10g。外用 20%~30% 酊剂涂患处。

Decocting, 6-10g. Apply 20%-30% tincture to the affected area.

【使用注意 / Precaution】

阴虚火旺及大便秘结者忌服。

It is contraindicated in those with vigorous fire due to yin deficiency and constipation.

【现代研究 / Modern research】

本品主要含补骨脂素、异补骨脂素、补骨脂定、异补骨脂定、补骨脂异黄酮、紫云英苷、补骨脂苯并呋喃酚、异补骨脂苯并呋喃酚、脂肪酸、多糖及氨基酸等。具有性激素样作用，能抗骨质疏松、平喘、延缓衰老、抗心肌缺血、调节免疫、抗前列腺增生等。

It mainly contains psoralen, isopsoralen, isopsoralen, psoralen isoflavone, astragaloside, psoralen benzofuranol, isopsoralen benzofuranol, fatty acid, polysaccharide and amino acid, etc. It has sex hormone-like effect and can resist osteoporosis, antiasthmatic, delay aging, resist myocardial ischemia, regulate immunity, and resist prostatic hyperplasia, etc.

菟丝子　*Tù sī zǐ* (Cuscutae Semen)

《神农本草经》

Shen Nong's Classic of the Materia Medica (Shén Nóng Běn Cǎo Jīng)

【来源 / Origin】

为旋花科植物南方菟丝子 *Cuscuta australis* R.Br. 或菟丝子 *Cuscuta chinensis* Lam. 的干燥成熟种子。全国大部分地区均产。秋季果实成熟时采收，生用或盐水炙用。本品气微，味淡。《中国药典》规定，含金丝桃苷（$C_{21}H_{20}O_{12}$）不得少于 0.10%。

Tù sī zǐ is the dry and mature seed of Cuscuta australis R.Br., or Cuscuta chinensis Lam, pertaining to Convolvulaceae. It is produced in most areas of China, collected in autumn when the fruit is ripe, and used in raw or stir-fried with saline water. It has a slight odor and tastes bland. According to *Chinese Pharmacopoeia*, the content of hyperoside ($C_{21}H_{20}O_{12}$) should not be less than 0.10%.

【性味归经 / Medicinal properties】

辛、甘，平。归肝、肾、脾经。

Acrid, sweet and neutral; act on the liver, kidney and spleen meridians.

【主要功效 / Medicinal efficacies】

补肝益肾，固精缩尿，安胎，明目，止泻；外用消风祛斑。

Supplement the liver and kidney, consolidate essence and reduce urination, stabilize the fetus, improve vision and stop diarrhea;disperse wind and remove patches in topical application.

【临床应用 / Clinical application】

1. 肾阳虚证，肾气不固证　本品味甘性平，既补肾阳，又益肾精，为平补阴阳之品，兼能固精、缩尿、止带。用治肾虚精亏所致的阳痿遗精，常与枸杞子、覆盆子、车前子等同用。用治小便过多或失禁，常与桑螵蛸、肉苁蓉、鹿茸等同用。用治肾虚腰痛，常与杜仲、山药等同用。用治肾虚不固之遗精、带下、白浊、尿有余沥，常与茯苓、石莲子等同用。

(1) Kidney yang depletion and insufficiency of the kidney qi the nature of sweet and neutral　It can not only boost essence but also assist yang of kidney, so it is an important medicinal for neutrally supplementing yin and yang. In addition, it can secure essence, reduce urination and arrest leukorrhagia. To treat impotence and seminal emission caused by deficiency of kidney essence, it is often combined with *gǒu qǐ zǐ*, *fù pén zǐ* (Rubi Fructus) and *chē qián zǐ* (Plantaginis Semen); to treat polyuria or urine incontinence, it is often combined with *sāng piāo xiāo*, *ròu cōng róng* and *lù róng* (Cervi Cornu Pantotrichum); to treat seminal emission, morbid leukorrhea, gonorrhea and dysuria, it is often combined with *fú líng* and *shí lián zǐ*.

2. 胎漏，胎动不安　本品能补肝肾，益精血而安胎，用治肝肾不足，冲任不固之胎动不安、滑胎，常与续断、桑寄生、阿胶等同用。

(2) Threatened abortion and habitual miscarriage　It can nourish the liver and kidney, benefit the essence and blood to stabilize the fetus. To treat threatened abortion and habitual miscarriage due to insufficiency of liver and kidney, debility of chong and ren channels, it is usually combined with *xù duàn*, *sāng jì shēng* (Taxilli Herba) and *ē jiāo* (Corii Asini Colla)

3. 肝肾不足，目暗耳鸣　本品能补肝肾而明目，用治肝肾不足，耳目失养之目暗耳鸣，眼干涩、视物模糊，常与熟地黄、枸杞子、黄精等同用。

(3) Blurred vision and tinnitus due to insufficiency of the liver and kidney　It can nourish the liver and kidney to improve eyesight. To treat blurred, tinnitus and dry eyes cause by deficiency of liver and kidney, it is usually combined with *shú dì huáng*, *gǒu qǐ zǐ* and *huáng jīng* (Polygonati Rhizoma).

4. 脾肾虚泻　本品能补肾益脾止泻，用治脾肾两虚之便溏泄泻，常与补骨脂、白术、肉豆蔻等同用。

(4) Diarrhea due to deficiency of spleen and kidney　It can arrest diarrhea by supplementing the kidney and fortifying spleen, so it is usually combined with *bǔ gǔ zhī*, *bái zhú* and *ròu dòu kòu* to treat thin and unformed stool or diarrhea due to deficiency of spleen and kidney.

此外，本品外用能消风祛斑，用治白癜风，可单用酒浸外涂。

In addition, it is used to disperse wind and remove patches by topical application. To treat vitiligo, it is soaked in wine to be pasted on the affected area.

【用量用法 / Usage and dosage】

煎服，6~12g。外用适量。

Decoction, 6-12g. Proper amount for external use.

【使用注意 / Precaution】

阴虚火旺，大便燥结，小便短赤者不宜服。

It is not proper for those with vigorous fire due to yin deficiency, dry stool or constipation, scanty and dark yellow urine.

【现代研究 / Modern research】

本品主要含金丝桃苷、菟丝子苷、绿原酸及微量元素、氨基酸等。具有性激素样作用，能延缓衰老、抗骨质疏松、促进造血功能、增强免疫、抗心脑缺血、降血脂、降血压等。

It mainly contains hyperoside, dodder glycoside, chlorogenic acid, trace elements and amino acids, etc. It has sex hormone like effects and can delay aging, anti osteoporosis, promote hematopoiesis, enhance immunity, anti cardio cerebral ischemia, reduce blood lipid and blood pressure.

沙苑子 *Shā yuàn zǐ* (Astragali Complanati Semen)
《本草衍义》
Extension of the Materia Medica (Běn Cǎo Yǎn Yì)

【来源 / Origin】

为豆科植物扁茎黄芪 *Astragalus complanatus* R.Br. 的干燥成熟种子。主产于陕西、河北。秋末冬初果实成熟尚未开裂时采收，生用或盐水炙用。本品气微，味淡，嚼之有豆腥味。《中国药典》规定，含沙苑子苷（$C_{28}H_{32}O_{16}$）不得少于 0.060%，饮片不得少于 0.050%。

Shā yuàn zǐ is the dried and mature seed of *Astragalus complanatus* R.Br., pertaining to Leguminosae. It is mainly produced in Shaanxi and Hebei Province. It is collected at the end of autumn and the beginning of winter when the fruit is mature but not yet cracked, used in raw or stir-fired with saline water. It has a slight odor and tastes bland with a beany smell. According to *Chinese Pharmacopoeia*, the content of astragaloside ($C_{28}H_{32}O_{16}$) should be no less than 0.060%, and that in pieces should be no less than 0.050%.

【性味归经 / Medicinal properties】

甘，温。归肝、肾经。

Sweet and warm; act on the liver and kidney meridians.

【主要功效 / Medicinal efficacies】

补肾助阳，固精缩尿，养肝明目。

Supplement the kidney and assist yang, secure essence and relieve polyuria, supplement the liver to improve vision.

【临床应用 / Clinical application】

1. 肾虚腰痛，遗精早泄，遗尿尿频，白浊带下　本品甘温补益，兼具涩性，功效与菟丝子相似，但其补益之力不如菟丝子，而收涩之力强于菟丝子。用治肾虚不固之遗精早泄，白带过多，常与龙骨、牡蛎、莲子等同用。用治肾虚腰痛，常与杜仲、续断、桑寄生等同用。用治肾虚精亏之阳痿，可与淫羊藿、巴戟天等配伍。

(1) Low back pain due to kidney deficiency, seminal emission, premature ejaculation, enuresis and frequent urination, white turbid and abnormal vaginal discharge　With the nature of sweet, warm and astringent, it has the similar efficacy with *tù sī zǐ*. Its tonic power is not as good as *tù sī zǐ* but its astringent power is stronger. To treat excessive leucorrhea and spermatorrhea caused by deficiency of kidney, it is often used in combination with *lóng gǔ*, *mǔ lì* and *lián zǐ*; to treat low back pain due to kidney deficiency, often combined with *dù zhòng, xù duàn* and *sāng jì shēng*; to treat impotence due to deficiency of kidney and essence, it is often combined with *yín yáng huò* and *bā jǐ tiān*.

2. **肝肾不足，头晕目眩，目暗昏花** 本品入肝、肾经，能温肾养肝明目，用治肝肾不足，目失所养，目暗不明，头晕目眩，常与枸杞子、菟丝子、菊花等同用。

(2) Dizziness and lured vision due to deficiency of liver and kidney With the nature of acting on the liver and kidney meridians, it has the functions of warming the kidney and supplement the liver to improve vision. To treat dizziness and lured vision due to deficiency of liver and kidney, it is often combined with *gǒu qǐ zǐ, tù sī zǐ* and *jú huā* (Chrysanthemi Flos).

【用量用法 / Usage and dosage】

煎服，9~15g。

Decoction, 9-15g.

【使用注意 / Precaution】

阴虚火旺及小便不利者不宜服用。

It is not proper for those with vigorous fire and dysuria due to yin deficiency.

【现代研究 / Modern research】

本品主要含沙苑子苷、沙苑子杨梅苷及脂肪酸类、酚类、鞣质、蛋白质、多糖等。具有抗肝损伤、降血脂、降血压、增强免疫、抗肿瘤、镇静、镇痛、抗炎等作用。

It mainly contains astragaloside, myricomplanoside, fatty acids, phenols, tannins, proteins, and polysaccharides, etc. It has the functions of anti liver injury, reducing blood fat, blood pressure, enhancing immunity, anti-tumor, sedation, analgesia, anti-inflammatory, etc.

蛤蚧　*Gé Jiè* (Gecko)
《雷公炮炙论》
Master Lei's Discourse on Medicinal Processing (Léi Gōng Páo Zhì Lùn)

【来源 / Origin】

为壁虎科动物蛤蚧 *Gekko gecko* Linnaeus 的干燥体。主产于我国广东、广西，进口蛤蚧主产于越南。全年均可捕捉，生用或酒制用。本品气腥，味微咸。

Gé jiè is the dried body of *Gekko gecko* Linnaeus, pertaining to Gekkonidae. It is mainly produced in Guangdong Province and Guangxi Zhuang Autonomous Region of China. Imported gecko is mainly produced in Vietnam. It can be collected all year round, used raw or prepared with liquor. It smells fishy and tastes slightly salty.

【性味归经 / Medicinal properties】

咸，平。归肺、肾经。

Salty and neutral; act on the lung and kidney meridians.

【主要功效 / Medicinal efficacies】

补肺益肾，纳气定喘，助阳益精。

Supplement the lung and boost the kidney, receive qi and relieve panting, assist yang and enrich essence.

【临床应用 / Clinical application】

1. **肺肾两虚之喘咳** 本品咸平，入肺、肾经，长于补益肺肾，纳气定喘，为治虚劳喘咳之佳品。用治虚劳咳嗽，常与川贝母、紫菀、苦杏仁等同用。用治肺肾虚喘咯血，常与人参、川贝母、苦杏仁等同用。用治气阴两虚之久咳气喘，常与黄芪、麦冬、麻黄等同用。

(1) Panting and cough due to deficiency of both lung and kidney　With the nature of salty and neutral and act on the lung and kidney meridians, it is good at supplement the lung and boost the kidney, receive qi and relieve panting. To treat cough due to deficiency and fatigue, it is often combined with *chuān bèi mǔ* (Fritillariae Cirrhosae Bulbus), *zǐ wǎn* (Asteris Radix et Rhizoma) and *kǔ xìng rén*; to treat asthma and hemoptysis caused by lung and kidney deficiency, it is often combined with *rén shēn, chuān bèi mǔ* and *kǔ xìng rén*; to treat chronic cough and asthma due to deficiency of qi and yin, it is usually combined with *huáng qí, mài dōng* and *má huáng* (Ephedrae Herba).

2. **肾虚阳痿，遗精**　本品补肾助阳，兼能益精养血。用治肾阳不足，精血亏虚之阳痿遗精，可单用浸酒服，或与淫羊藿、山茱萸等同用。

(2) Impotence and seminal emission due to kidney deficiency　It can nourish the kidney and assist yang as well as benefit the essence and blood. To treat impotence and seminal emission caused by deficiency of kidney yang and blood essence, it is soaked singly in liquor for oral administration or in combination with *yín yáng huò* (Epimedii Herba) and *shān zhū yú* (Corni Fructus).

【用量用法 / Usage and dosage】

多入丸、散或酒剂，3~6g。

It is often used in pills, powder or prepared with liquor, 3-6g.

【使用注意 / Precaution】

咳喘实证不宜使用。

It is not suitable for those with excess syndrome of panting and cough.

【现代研究 / Modern research】

本品主要含磷脂类、脂肪酸类、蛋白质、氨基酸及微量元素等。具有性激素样作用，能延缓衰老、解痉平喘、增强免疫、耐缺氧、抗炎等。

It mainly contains phospholipids, fatty acids, proteins, amino acids and trace elements. It has sex hormone-like effect, and can delay aging, relieve spasm and asthma, enhance immunity, bear hypoxia and anti inflammation, etc.

冬虫夏草　*Dōng chóng xià cǎo* (Cordyceps)
《本草从新》
Thoroughly Revised Materia Medica (Běn Cǎo Cóng Xīn)

【来源 / Origin】

为麦角菌科真菌冬虫夏草菌 *Cordyceps sinensis*（Berk.）Sacc. 寄生在蝙蝠蛾科昆虫幼虫上的子座和幼虫尸体的干燥复合体。主产于四川、西藏、青海。夏初子座出土、孢子未发散时挖取，生用。本品气微腥，味微苦。《中国药典》规定，含腺苷（$C_{10}H_{13}N_5O_4$）不得少于 0.010%。

Dōng chóng xià cǎo is the dry compound of the stroma of *Cordyceps sinensis* (Berk.) Sacc., of the family Calvicipitaceae parasitized on the insect larva of Hepialus armoricanus and the dead body of the parasitized insect larva. It is mainly produced in Sichuan, Tibet Autonomous Region and Qinghai, collected in early summer when the stroma comes up but the spores haven't spread. It is used raw and with slightly fishy smell and bitter taste. According to *Chinese Pharmacopoeia*, the content of adenosine ($C_{10}H_{13}N_5O_4$) should be no less than 0.010%.

【性味归经 / Medicinal properties】

甘，平。归肺、肾经。

Sweet and neutral; act on the lung and kidney meridians.

【主要功效 / Medicinal efficacies】

补肾益肺，止血化痰。

Supplement the lung and boost the kidney, stanch bleeding and dissolve phlegm.

【临床应用 / Clinical application】

1. 肾阳不足，精血亏虚证　本品味甘能补，性平偏温，有补肾益精、助阳起痿之功。用治肾阳不足，精血亏虚之阳痿遗精、腰膝酸痛、宫冷不孕等，可单用，或与人参、鹿角胶、补骨脂等同用。

(1) **Syndrome due to insufficiency of kidney yang, blood deficiency and essence depletion**　With the nature of sweet, warm and neutral, it has the functions of tonifying the kidney and benefiting the essence to assist the yang and treat impotence. It can be used alone to treat impotence, seminal emission, lumbago and knee pain and infertility due to uterine cold, or in combination with *rén shēn*, *lù jiǎo jiāo* (Cervi Cornus Colla) and *bǔ gǔ zhī*.

2. 肺肾两虚之喘咳　本品甘平，入肺、肾经，能补肾益肺、止血化痰、平喘止咳，为平补肺肾之品。用治肺虚或肺肾两虚之久咳虚喘，可单用，或与人参、黄芪、蛤蚧等同用。用治劳嗽痰血，常与北沙参、川贝母、阿胶等同用。

(2) **Cough and panting due to deficiency of both lung and kidney**　With the nature of sweet and neutral and act on the lung and kidney meridians, it can tonify the lung and kidney to stop hemorrhage and reduce phlegm, relieve asthma and cough. To treat chronic cough and deficiency-type panting, it can be used singly or combined with *rén shēn*, *huáng qí* and *gé jiè*; to treat consumptive cough with sputum and blood, it is often combined with *běi shā shēn* (Glehniae Radix), *chuān bèi mǔ* (Fritillariae Cirrhosae Bulbus) and *ē jiāo* (Corii Asini Colla).

此外，对于病后体虚不复，自汗畏寒，头晕乏力等，可与鸭、鸡、猪肉等同炖服，具有补虚扶弱，促进机体功能恢复的作用。

In addition, *dōng chóng xià cǎo* can be used to treat body deficiency after disease or spontaneous sweating and fear of cold, dizziness and fatigue, and it is stewed with chicken, duck and pork for oral-taking.

【用量用法 / Usage and dosage】

煎汤或炖服，3~9g。

Decoction or stewing, 3-9g.

【使用注意 / Precaution】

有表邪者不宜用。

It is not advised for the conditions with exterior pathogen.

【现代研究 / Modern research】

本品主要含腺苷、腺嘌呤核苷、肌苷（次黄嘌呤核苷）、麦角甾醇、蛋白质、脂肪酸、氨基酸、维生素及多糖等。具有调节免疫、抗衰老、祛痰、平喘、抗炎、抗心肌缺血、抗肝损伤、抗肾损伤、抗肺损伤、降血糖、降血脂等作用。

It mainly contains adenosine, adenine nucleoside, hypoxanthine nucleoside, ergosterol, protein, fatty acid, amino acid, vitamin and polysaccharide, etc. It has the functions of regulating immunity, anti-aging, eliminating phlegm, relieving asthma, anti-inflammatory, anti myocardial ischemia, anti liver and kidney injury, anti lung injury, lowering blood sugar and blood lipid.

第三节 补血药
Section 3 Blood-supplementing medicinals

本类药物多味甘，性温或平，质地滋润，主入心肝血分，以补血为主要功效，主要用于血虚证，症见面色淡白或萎黄，眼睑、口唇、爪甲色淡，头晕目眩，心悸失眠，肢体麻木，妇女月经量少色淡、愆期甚至经闭，舌淡苔白，脉细无力等。某些药物兼能滋养肝肾、润肺等，还可用治肝肾阴虚证、阴虚肺燥证。补血药多滋腻黏滞，故脾虚湿阻，气滞食少者慎用。

Blood-supplementing medicinals are sweet in taste, warm and moistening. They mainly act on the heart and liver meridian and have the main efficacy of supplementing blood. So they are used for heart-liver blood deficiency manifested as pale or sallow yellow complexion, pale mouth lips and nails, dizziness, palpitation and insomnia, numbness of limbs, menstruation irregularities, scanty and light menses, amenorrhea, pale tongue and thready pulse, etc. Some of them can nourish the liver and kidney; moisten the lung and so on. They can also be used to treat syndrome caused by yin deficiency of liver and kidney, yin deficiency and lung dryness. Blood-supplementing medicinals are mostly greasy and sticky, so they should be used with caution for those with spleen deficiency and dampness obstruction, qi stagnation and poor appetite.

当归 *Dāng guī* (Angelicae Sinensis Radix)
《神农本草经》
Shen Nong's Classic of the Materia Medica (Shén Nóng Běn Cǎo Jīng)

微课

【来源 / Origin】
为伞形科植物当归 *Angellica sinensis*（Oliv.）Diels 的干燥根。主产于甘肃。秋末采收，干燥，切薄片，生用或酒炒用。本品有浓郁的香气，味甘、辛、微苦。《中国药典》规定，含阿魏酸（$C_{10}H_{10}O_4$）不得少于 0.050%，含挥发性不得少于 0.4%（ml/g）。

Dāng guī is the root of *Angellica sinensis* (Oliv.) Diels, pertaining to Umberlliferae. It is mainly produced in Gansu Province and collected in late autumn, used raw or stir-fried with liquor after being dried and sliced. It is hugely aromatic, sweet, acrid and slightly bitter in flavor. According to *Chinese Pharmacopoeia*, the content of ferulic acid ($C_{10}H_{10}O_4$) should be no less than 0.050%, the content of volatile oil should not be less than 0.4% (ml/g).

【性味归经 / Medicinal properties】
甘、辛，温。归肝、心、脾经。

Sweet acrid and warm; act on the live heart and spleen meridians.

【主要功效 / Medicinal efficacies】
补血调经，活血止痛，润肠通便。

Supplement blood to regulate menstruation, invigorate blood to relieve pain, moisten the intestines to promote defecation.

【临床应用 / Clinical application】
1. **血虚证** 本品甘温质润，功善补血养血，为补血要药。用治心肝血虚之面色萎黄、头晕心悸、失眠多梦等，常与熟地黄、白芍、酸枣仁等同用。若治血虚兼见气虚，常与黄芪配伍。

(1) Syndrome due to blood deficiency With the nature of sweet, warm and moist, it's good at nourishing and supplementing blood. It's an important medicine for nourishing blood. To treat heart-liver blood deficiency manifested as pale or sallow yellow complexion, dizziness, palpitation and insomnia, it is often combined with *shú dì huáng*, *bái sháo* (Paeoniae Alba Radix) and *suān zǎo rén* (Ziziphi Spinosae Semen); to treat syndrome due to deficiency of both qi and blood, it is usually in combination with *huáng qí*.

2. 月经不调，经闭痛经 本品入肝心血分，甘温补血，辛温活血，并能调经止痛，为妇科要药。凡妇女月经不调、经闭痛经等，不论寒热虚实，皆可选用，尤以血虚、血瘀所致者最为适宜。若治血虚所致者，常与熟地黄、当归、白芍配伍；血瘀所致者，常与桃仁、红花、川芎等同用；冲任虚寒，瘀血阻滞所致者，可与白芍、桂枝、吴茱萸等同用；肝郁气滞所致者，可与柴胡、白芍等同用；肝郁化火，迫血妄行所致者，可与柴胡、牡丹皮、栀子等同用；气血亏虚所致者，可与人参、熟地黄、白术等同用。

(2) Menstruation irregularities, amenorrhea and dysmenorrhea With the nature of sweet, warm and acting on the liver and heart meridians, it has the function of invigorating blood regulating menstruation and relieving pain so it is an essential medicine for gynecology. It can be selected to treat irregular menstruation, amenorrhea and dysmenorrhea regardless of deficiency or excess, cold or heat, especially the one caused by blood deficiency and stagnation. To treat that due to blood deficiency, it is often combined with *shú dì huáng*, *dāng guī* and *bái sháo*; for that due to blood stagnation, it is often combined with *táo rén*, *hóng huā* and *chuān xiōng*; for that caused by cold-deficiency of thoroughfare and conception vessels and blood stasis, it is usually in combination with *bái sháo*, *guì zhī* (Cinnamomi Ramulus) and *wú zhū yú*; for that due to liver depression and qi stagnation, often combined with *chái hú* (Bupleuri Radix) and *bái sháo*; that due to liver depression transform into fire and force blood to flourish, it is combined with *chái hú*, *mǔ dān pí* (Moutan Cortex) and *zhī zǐ* (Gardeniae Fructus); that due to deficiency of both qi and blood, it is usually in combination with *rén shēn*, *shú dì huáng* and *bái zhú*.

3. 虚寒腹痛，风湿痹痛，跌仆损伤，痈疽疮疡 本品辛散温通，又为活血化瘀的良药，兼能止痛，可用治血瘀诸证。若治血虚寒凝血瘀之腹痛，多与桂枝、生姜、芍药等同用。若治风寒痹痛，常与羌活、防风、秦艽等同用。若治跌打损伤，瘀血作痛，常与乳香、没药、桃仁等同用。若治疮疡初起，肿胀疼痛，可与金银花、赤芍、天花粉等同用。若治痈疽溃后不敛，可与黄芪、人参、肉桂等同用。若治寒凝血瘀之头痛，常与川芎、白芷等同用。若治气血瘀滞之胸痛、胁痛，常与郁金、香附等同用。

(3) Abdominal pain due to deficiency-cold, wind-dampness *bì*, injury of falling and swelling, carbuncle and sore With the nature of warm and astringent, it is a good medicinal for promoting blood circulation and removing blood stasis, and it can also relieve pain. It is often used to treat various syndromes of blood stasis. To treat abdominal pain due to blood deficiency, blood stasis and cold congealing, it is often combined with *guì zhī* (Cinnamomi Ramulus), *shēng jiāng* (Zingiberis Recens Rhizoma) and *sháo yào* (Paeoniae Radix); to treat wind-cold *bì*, it is often combined with *qiāng huó* (Notopterygii Rhizoma et Radix), *fáng fēng* (Saposhnikoviae Radix) and *qín jiāo* (Gentianae Macrophyllae Radix); to treat injuries from falling, swelling and pain due to blood stasis, it is combined with *rǔ xiāng*, *mò yào* and *táo rén*; to treat sores and ulcers in the early stage, with scorching sensation and pain, it is used with *jīn yín huā*, *chì sháo* and *tiān huā fen* (Trichosanthis Radix); to treat disunion of sores and ulcer, it is often combined with *huáng qí*, *rén shēn* and *ròu guì*; to treat headache of cold coagulation and blood stasis, it is often combined with *chuān xiōng* and *bái zhǐ*; to treat chest pain and hypochondriac pain with stagnation of qi and blood, it is usually used in combination with *yù jīn* and *xiāng fù*.

4. 肠燥便秘　本品能养血润肠通便。用治血虚津亏之肠燥便秘，常与肉苁蓉、火麻仁、熟地黄等同用。

(4) Constipation due to blood deficiency and intestine dryness　It can nourish blood, moisten intestines and relieve constipation. To treat constipation due to dryness of intestines with deficiency of blood and body fluid, it is usually used with *ròu cōng róng* (Cistanches Herba), *huǒ má rén* (Cannabis Fructus) and *shú dì huáng*.

【用量用法 / Usage and dosage】

煎服，6~12g。酒炒可增加活血通经之力。

Decoction, 6-12g. Stir-frying with liquor can increase the power of promoting blood circulation and dredging channels.

【使用注意 / Precaution】

湿盛中满、大便溏泄者忌服。

It is contraindicated in patients with the center fullness due to dampness exuberance with thin and unformed stool or diarrhea.

【现代研究 / Modern research】

本品主要含藁本内酯、正丁烯呋内酯、当归酮、香荆芥酚、阿魏酸、当归多糖、多种氨基酸、维生素及微量元素等。具有促进骨髓造血、改善冠脉循环、抗血栓、增强免疫、降血脂、抑制子宫平滑肌收缩、抗肝损伤、抗炎、镇痛等作用。

It mainly contains ligustilide, N-butenolactone, angelione, kaempferol, ferulic acid, angelica polysaccharide, a variety of amino acids, vitamins and trace elements. It has the functions of promoting bone marrow hematopoiesis, improving coronary circulation, antithrombotic, enhancing immunity, reducing blood fat, inhibiting contraction of uterine smooth muscle, anti liver injury, anti-inflammatory and analgesic.

熟地黄　*Shú dì huáng* (Rehmanniae Radix Praeparata)
《本草拾遗》
Supplement to the Materia Medica (Běn Cǎo Shí Yí)

【来源 / Origin】

为玄参科植物地黄 *Rehmannia glutinosa* Libosch. 的干燥块根经加工炮制而成。切厚片或块。本品气微，味甜。《中国药典》规定，含地黄苷 D（$C_{27}H_{42}O_{20}$）不得少于 0.050%。

Shú dì huáng is the tuberous root of *Rehmannia glutinosa* Libosch., pertaining to Scrophulariaceae, which is produced by processing *shēng dì huáng*. Cut into thick piece or block, it has slight odor and taste sweet. According to *Chinese Pharmacopoeia*, the content of rehmannoside D ($C_{27}H_{42}O_{20}$) should be no less than 0.050%.

【性味归经 / Medicinal properties】

甘，微温。归肝、肾经。

Sweet and mildly warm; act on the live and kidney meridians.

【主要功效 / Medicinal efficacies】

补血滋阴，益精填髓。

Supplement blood and enrich yin, boost essence and replenish marrow.

【临床应用 / Clinical application】

1. 血虚证　本品甘温质润，为补血要药。用治血虚面色萎黄、眩晕、心悸失眠、月经不调、崩漏等，常与当归、川芎、白芍同用。

(1) **Blood deficiency**　With the nature of sweet, warm and moist, it is an important medicinal to supplement blood. To treat sallow yellow complexion, vertigo, palpitation, insomnia, menstruation irregularities and flooding and spotting (*bēng lòu*), it is usually combined with *dāng guī*, *chuān xiōng* and *bái sháo*.

2. 肝肾阴虚证　本品入肝、肾经，长于滋肾阴、益肾精、养肝阴，为滋阴主药。用治肝肾阴虚之腰膝酸软、头目眩晕、视物昏花、耳鸣耳聋、骨蒸潮热、盗汗、遗精、消渴等，常与山茱萸、山药、牡丹皮等同用。若治肝肾精血亏虚之须发早白，常与何首乌、枸杞子、菟丝子等同用。若治肝肾不足，精血亏虚所致的五迟、五软，可与龟甲、狗脊等同用。

(2) **Yin deficiency of the liver and kidney**　It acts on the liver and kidney meridians and good at nourishing kidney yin, tonifying kidney essence and liver yin, so it is also the main medicinal for nourishing yin. To treat yin deficiency of liver and kidney manifested as soreness and weakness of the loins and knees, dizziness, tinnitus and deafness, bone steaming and hot flashes, night sweating, seminal emission and consumptive thirst, it is often combined with *shān zhū yú*, *shān yào* and *mǔ dān pí*; to treat early graying hair due to essence and blood depletion, it is often used in combination with *hé shǒu wū*, *gǒu qǐ zǐ* and *tù sī zǐ*; to treat developmental delay due to deficiency of liver and kidney, insufficiency of blood essence, it is often combined with *guī jiǎ* (Testudinis Carapax et Plastrum) and *gǒu jǐ* (Cibotii Rhizoma).

【用法用量 / Usage and dosage】

煎服，9~15g。

Decoction, 9-15g.

【使用注意 / Precaution】

气滞痰多、湿盛中满、食少便溏者忌服。

It is contraindicated in the patients with qi stagnation, profuse sputum, the center fullness due to dampness exuberance, eating less and with thin and unformed stool or diarrhea.

【现代研究 / Modern research】

本品主要含梓醇、毛蕊花糖苷、环烯醚萜苷、地黄苷、地黄素、糖类、氨基酸等。具有促进骨髓造血、增强学习记忆能力、增强免疫、抗焦虑、抗肿瘤、抗衰老、降血糖等作用。

It mainly contains catalpol, mullein glycoside, iridoid glycoside, digitalis glycoside, digitalis, sugars and amino acids, etc. It has the functions of promoting the hematopoiesis of bone marrow, enhancing the ability of learning and memory, enhancing immunity, anti anxiety, anti-tumor, anti-aging, and reducing blood sugar.

白芍　*Bái sháo* (Paeoniae Radix Alba)

《神农本草经》

Shen Nong's Classic of the Materia Medica (Shén Nóng Běn Cǎo Jīng)

【来源 / Origin】

本品为毛茛科植物芍药 *Paeonia lactiflora* Pall. 的干燥根。主产于浙江、安徽、四川等地。夏、秋二季采收，晒干，切薄片，生用或炒用、酒炙用。本品气微，味微苦、酸。《中国药典》规定，含芍药苷（$C_{23}H_{28}O_{11}$）不得少于 1.2%。

Bái sháo is the dried root of *Paeonia lactiflora* Pall., pertaining to Ranunculaceae. It is mainly produced in Zhejiang, Anhui and Sichuan Province in China, collected in summer and autumn, dried in the sun, sliced and used raw, dry-fried or stir fried with liquor. It has a mild odor and tastes slightly bitter and sour. According to *Chinese Pharmacopoeia*, paeoniflorin ($C_{23}H_{28}O_{11}$) should be no less than 1.2%.

【性味归经 / Medicinal properties 】

苦、酸，微寒。归肝、脾经。

Bitter, sour and slightly cold; act on the liver and spleen meridians.

【主要功效 / Medicinal efficacies 】

养血调经，敛阴止汗，柔肝止痛，平抑肝阳。

Nourish blood and regulate menstruation; astringe yin and arrest sweating; soften the liver and relieve pain; calm and subdue liver yang.

【临床应用 / Clinical application 】

1. 血虚证　本品味酸入肝经，长于养血调经，用治血虚面色萎黄、眩晕心悸、月经不调或崩漏等，常与当归、熟地黄等同用。若治血虚而月经不调，常与当归、丹参等同用。

(1) **Blood deficiency**　With the nature of sour and acting on the liver meridian, it is good at nourishing blood and regulating menstruation. To treat sallow yellow complexion, vertigo, palpitation, menstruation irregularities and flooding and spotting (*bēng lòu*), it is often combined with *dāng guī* and *shú dì huáng*; to treat menstrual irregularities and dysmenorrhea due to blood deficiency, it is usually in combination with *dāng guī* and *dān shēn*.

2. 肝阳上亢证　本品有养血敛阴、平抑肝阳之功。用治肝阳上亢之眩晕、头痛，常与生地黄、牛膝、赭石等同用。

(2) **Syndrome caused by hyperactivity of liver yang**　It has the efficacy of nourishing blood and astringing yin, calming and subduing liver yang. To treat headache and vertigo due to ascendant hyperactivity of liver yang, it is usually in combination with *shēng dì huáng, niú xī* and *zhě shí*.

3. 胁腹、四肢挛急疼痛　本品能养血柔肝、缓急止痛。用治血虚肝郁，胁肋疼痛，常与柴胡、当归等同用。用治脾虚肝旺，腹痛泄泻，可与白术、白芍、陈皮同用。用治痢疾腹痛，可与木香、黄连等同用。用治阴血亏虚，筋脉失养之手足挛急作痛，常与甘草同用。

(3) **Rib-side and abdominal pain, spastic pain in four limbs**　It has the functions of nourishing blood, softening liver and relieving pain. To treat rib-side pain due to blood deficiency and liver depression, it is often combined with *chái hú* and *dāng guī*; to treat abdominal pain and diarrhea due to spleen deficiency and liver hyperactivity, it is usually in combination with *bái zhú, bái sháo* and *chén pí*; to treat dysentery and abdominal pain, it is often used with *mù xiāng* and *huáng lián*; to treat acute pain of hand and foot due to blood deficiency and malnutrition of tendon and vessel, it is often combined with *gān cǎo*.

4. 盗汗、自汗　本品有敛阴止汗之功效。用治阴虚盗汗，常与牡蛎、浮小麦等同用。用治气虚自汗，常与黄芪、白术等同用。用治外感风寒，营卫不和之汗出恶风，常与桂枝配伍。

(4) **Night sweating and spontaneous sweating**　It has the efficacy of astringing yin and arresting sweating. To treat night sweating due to yin deficiency, it is usually in combination with *mǔ lì* and *fú xiǎo mài*; to treat spontaneous sweating due to qi deficiency, it is often combined with *huáng qí* and *bái zhú*; to treat sweating and aversion to wind due to externally contracted wind-cold and disharmony between nutrient and defensive qi, it is often combined with *guì zhī*.

【用法用量 / Usage and dosage】

煎服，6~15g。

Decoction, 6-15g.

【使用注意 / Precaution】

不宜与藜芦同用。

It should not be combined with *lí lú* (Veratri Nigri Radix et Rhizoma).

【现代研究 / Modern research】

本品主要含芍药苷、氧化芍药苷、苯甲酰芍药苷、白芍苷、芍药苷元酮等，尚含甾醇、鞣质、多糖、挥发油等。具有保肝、解痉、镇痛、抗炎、调节免疫、抗抑郁、镇静、调节胃肠功能等作用。

It mainly contains paeoniflorin, oxidized paeoniflorin, benzoyl paeoniflorin, paeoniflorin and paeoniflorin ketone, etc., and it also contains sterol, tannin, polysaccharide and volatile oil, etc. It has the functions of liver protection, spasmolysis, analgesia, anti inflammation, immunity regulation, anti depression, sedation and gastrointestinal function regulation, etc.

阿胶　*Ē jiāo* (Asini Corii Colla)
《神农本草经》
Shen Nong's Classic of the Materia Medica (Shén Nóng Běn Cǎo Jīng)

【来源 / Origin】

本品为马科动物驴 *Equus asinus* L. 的干燥皮或鲜皮经煎煮、浓缩制成的固体胶。主产于山东。捣成碎块用，或采用烫法用蛤粉或蒲黄烫成阿胶珠用。本品气微，味微甘。《中国药典》规定，含 L- 羟脯氨酸不得少于 8.0%，甘氨酸不得少于 18.0%，丙氨酸不得少于 7.0%，L- 脯氨酸不得少于 10.0%；含特征多肽以驴源多肽 A$_1$（C$_{41}$H$_{68}$N$_{12}$O$_{13}$）和驴源多肽 A$_2$（C$_{51}$H$_{82}$N$_{18}$O$_{15}$）的总量计不得少于 0.15%。

Ē jiāo is a solid glue decocted from the dry or fresh skin by soaking of donkey *Equus asinus* L., pertaining to Equidae. It is mainly produced in Shandong Province. It is used by being mashed into pieces, or in the form of *ē jiāo zhū* (Asini Corii Colla Pilula) which is the product of *ē jiāo* fried with calm shell powder or *pú huáng* (Typhae Pollen). It has a mild odor and tastes slightly sweet. According to *Chinese Pharmacopoeia*, the content of L-hydroxyproline, glycine, alanine and L-proline should be no less than 8.0%, 18.0%, 7.0% and 10.0% respectively. The total content of characteristic polypeptide such as donkey peptide A$_1$ (C$_{41}$H$_{68}$N$_{12}$O$_{13}$) and donkey peptide A$_2$ (C$_{51}$H$_{82}$N$_{18}$O$_{15}$) should be no less than 0.15%.

【性味归经 / Medicinal properties】

甘，平。归肺、肝、肾经。

Sweet and neutral; act on the lung, liver and kidney meridians.

【主要功效 / Medicinal efficacies】

补血滋阴，润燥，止血。

Supplement blood and enrich yin, moisten dryness and stanch bleeding.

【临床应用 / Clinical application】

1. 血虚证　本品味甘质润，为补血要药，广泛用于血虚诸证。用治血虚心失所养之心悸怔忡、心烦、失眠、健忘等，常与当归、酸枣仁等同用。用治血虚肝失所养之眩晕、筋脉拘挛、月经不调、闭经等，常与当归、熟地黄、枸杞子等同用。

(1) **Blood deficiency**　With the nature of sweet and moist, it is an effective medicinal for

supplementing blood. To treat depletion of both qi and blood manifested as palpitation, knotted pulse or intermittent pulse, upset, insomnia and bad memory, it is often combined with *dāng guī* and *suān zǎo rén*; to treat vertigo, muscle contracture, irregular menstruation and amenorrhea caused by blood deficiency and malnutrition of liver, it is usually in combination with *dāng guī*, *shú dì huáng* and *gǒu qǐ zǐ*.

2. 阴虚证　本品能滋养肺、心、肾阴，尤以滋阴润肺见长。用治阴虚肺燥，燥咳痰少，咽喉干燥，痰中带血，常与麦冬、川贝母、百部等同用。用治心阴不足，心火偏亢，心烦不眠，多与黄连、白芍等同用。用治肝肾阴虚，虚风内动，手足瘛疭，常与白芍、龟甲、牡蛎等同用。

(2) Yin deficiency　It can nourish lung, heart and kidney yin, especially nourish yin and moisten the lung. To treat dry cough with less phlegm, dry throat and blood in phlegm due to yin deficiency and lung dryness, it is often combined with *mài dōng*, *chuān bèi mǔ* and *bǎi bù* (Stemonae Radix); to treat deficiency of wind and internal movement, special movements of hand and foot caused by deficiency of liver and kidney yin, it is often combined with *bái sháo*, *guī jiǎ* and *mǔ lì*.

3. 出血　本品有止血之功，可用于多种出血。因其长于补血、滋阴，故对于出血兼有血虚、阴虚者尤为适宜，常与当归、熟地黄等同用。

(3) Bleeding　It is an effective medicinal for stanching bleeding. Because it is good at tonifying blood and nourishing yin, it is especially suitable for those with blood deficiency and yin deficiency and often combined with *dāng guī* and *shú dì huáng*.

【用法用量 / Usage and dosage】

烊化兑服，3~9g。

It should be melted singly and mixed in decoction for oral administration, 3-9g.

【使用注意 / Precaution】

脾胃虚弱，食少便溏者慎用。

It should be used with caution for those with deficiency of the spleen and stomach, eating less and with thin and unformed stool or diarrhea.

【现代研究 / Modern research】

本品主要含蛋白及肽类成分，水解可产生多种氨基酸，如甘氨酸、L-脯氨酸、L-羟脯氨酸、谷氨酸、精氨酸等。具有补血、增强免疫、抗疲劳、抗辐射、提高耐缺氧和耐寒能力等作用。

It mainly contains protein and peptide components. It can produce many kinds of amino acids by hydrolysis, such as glycine, L-proline, L-hydroxyproline, glutamic acid, and arginine, etc. It has the functions of replenishing blood, enhancing immunity, anti fatigue, anti radiation, improving hypoxia tolerance and cold tolerance.

何首乌　*Hé shǒu wū* (Polygoni Multiflori Radix)
《开宝本草》
Materia Medica of the Kaibao Era (Kāi Bǎo Běn Cǎo)

【来源 / Origin】

本品为蓼科植物何首乌 *Polygonum multiflorum* Thunb. 的干燥块根。主产于湖北、贵州、四川等地。秋季茎叶枯萎时采挖，个大的切成块，干燥，称"生何首乌"；清蒸或用黑豆汁拌匀后蒸，蒸至内外均呈黑褐色，晒至半干，切片，干燥，称"制何首乌"。生何首乌气微、味微苦而甘涩；制何首乌气微，味微甘而苦涩。《中国药典》规定，含结合蒽醌以大黄素（$C_{15}H_{10}O_5$）和大黄素甲醚（$C_{16}H_{12}O_5$）的总量计不得少于 0.10%；饮片不得少于 0.05%。

Hé shǒu wū is the dried tuberous root of *Polygonum multiflorum* Thunb., pertaining to Polygonaceae.

It is mainly produced in Hubei, Guizhou and Sichuan Province in China, collected in autumn when the stems and leaves are withered. Cut the large ones into pieces and dry them. Thus *shēng* (raw) *hé shǒu wū* is obtained, which has a slight odor and tastes slightly bitter and astringent. If *hé shǒu wū* is steamed or mixed with black bean juice, it becomes black and sliced and dried, thus *zhì* (processed) *hé shǒu wū* is obtained, which has a slight odor and tastes slightly sweet, bitter and astringent. According to *Chinese Pharmacopoeia*, the content of combined anthraquinone based on the total amount of emodin ($C_{15}H_{10}O_5$) and emodin methyl ether ($C_{16}H_{12}O_5$) in dried medicinal materials should be no less than 0.10%, and that in the *zhì hé shǒu wū* should be no less than 0.05%.

【性味归经 / Medicinal properties】

苦、甘、涩，微温。归肝、心、肾经。

Bitter, sweet, astringent, and mildly warm; act on the liver, heart and kidney meridians.

【主要功效 / Medicinal efficacies】

制何首乌：补肝肾，益精血，乌须发，强筋骨，化浊降脂；生何首乌：解毒消痈，截疟，润肠通便。

The processed one can supplement the liver and kidney, boost essence and blood, blacked beard and hair, strengthen the sinews and bones, transform turbidity and reduce blood fat. The raw one can resolve toxin, relieve carbuncle, prevent attack of malaria, and moisten the intestines to promote defecation.

【临床应用 / Clinical application】

1. 血虚证　制何首乌味甘微温，入肝、心经，具有补血作用。用治血虚面色萎黄，心悸怔忡，失眠健忘，常与熟地黄、当归、酸枣仁等同用。用治肝血不足之两目干涩，视力减退，常与熟地黄、枸杞子、女贞子等同用。

(1) Blood deficiency　With the nature of sweet and warm and acting on the liver and heart meridians, *zhì hé shǒu wū* has the effect of nourishing blood. To treat yellow complexion due to blood deficiency, palpitation, insomnia and poor memory, it is often combined with *shú dì huáng, dāng guī and suān zǎo rén*; to treat dry eyes and poor vision due to liver blood deficiency, it is usually in combination with *shú dì huáng, gǒu qǐ zǐ and nǚ zhēn zǐ*.

2. 肝肾阴虚证　制何首乌甘涩而温，补中兼收，能补血养肝，益精固肾，乌须发，强筋骨，且性质温和，不燥不腻，为滋补良药。治肝肾不足，精亏血虚之腰膝酸软，肢体麻木，头晕目眩，须发早白及肾虚无子，常与菟丝子、枸杞子、当归等同用。若治肝肾不足，气血亏虚之须发早白、斑秃等，常与地黄、女贞子、桑椹等同用。

(2) Liver kidney-yin deficiency syndrome　It can nourish blood and liver, boost essence, blacked beard and hair, strengthen the sinews and bones, and it is mild, not so dry or greasy. To treat soreness and weakness of loins and knees, numbness of limbs and dizziness, early white hair ans azoospermia due to deficiency of essence and blood, it is often combined with *tù sī zǐ, gǒu qǐ zǐ and dāng guī*; to treat early white hair and bald due to deficiency of liver and kidney, deficiency of qi and blood, it is usually in combination with *dì huáng* (Rehmanniae Radix), *nǚ zhēn zǐ and sāng shèn* (Mori Fructus).

3. 高脂血症　制何首乌能化浊降脂，用治高脂血症，单用或与山楂、泽泻、决明子等同用。

(3) Hyperlipidemia　*Zhì hé shǒu wū* can transform turbidity and reduce blood fat. To treat hyperlipidemia, it can be used alone or combined with *shān zhā* (Crataegi Fructus), *zé xiè* and *jué míng zǐ* (Cassiae Semen).

4. 疮痈，瘰疬，风疹瘙痒　生何首乌有解毒消痈散结之功。用治痈肿疮毒，可与金银花、连翘、苦参等同用。用治瘰疬痰核，可与夏枯草、贝母、玄参等同用。用治风疹瘙痒，多与荆芥、防风、苦参等同用。

(4) Carbuncles, deep-rooted abscesses and scrofula, rubella and pruritus *Shēng hé shǒu wū* has the functions of resolving toxin, relieving carbuncle and preventing attack of malaria. To treat carbuncles and ulcers, it is often combined with *jīn yín huā*, *lián qiáo* and *kǔ shēn* (Sophorae Flavescentis Radix); to treat deep-rooted abscesses and scrofula, it is usually used in combination with *xià kū cǎo* (Prunellae Spica), *bèi mǔ* (Fritillaria Bulbus) and *xuán shēn* (Scrophulariae Radix); to treat rubella and pruritus, it is often combined with *jīng jiè* (Schizonepetae Herba), *fáng fēng* and *kǔ shēn*.

5. 久疟体虚 生何首乌具有截疟作用，用治久疟气血不足，常与人参、当归等同用。

(5) Body deficiency with chronic malaria *Shēng hé shǒu wū* has the function of preventing attack of malaria. To treat depletion of qi and blood due to chronic malaria, it is usually combined with *rén shēn* and *dāng guī*.

6. 肠燥便秘 生首乌具有润肠通便之效，用治血虚津亏，肠燥便秘，可单用或与当归、火麻仁、肉苁蓉等同用。

(6) Constipation due to intestinal dryness *Shēng hé shǒu wū* has the function of moistening the intestines to promote defecation. To treat constipation due to depletion of essence and blood with intestinal dryness, it can be used alone or combined with *dāng guī*, *huǒ má rén* and *ròu cōng róng*.

【用法用量 / Usage and dosage】

煎服，制何首乌 6~12g，生何首乌 3~6g。

Decoction, *zhì hé shǒu wū* 6-12g; *shēng hé shǒu wū* 3-6g.

【使用注意 / Precaution】

大便溏泄及湿痰壅盛者忌用。不宜长期、大剂量服用。

It is not proper for those with thin and unformed stool, diarrhea and severe damp-phlegm retention, and should not be taken in large quantities for a long time.

【现代研究 / Modern research】

本品主要含大黄素、大黄酚、大黄素甲醚、大黄酸、大黄酚蒽酮、2,3,5,4′- 四羟基二苯乙烯 –2-*O*-*β*-D- 葡萄糖苷，尚含卵磷脂、粗脂肪等。制何首乌具有增强免疫、促进骨髓造血、抗衰老、抗骨质疏松、降血脂、抗动脉粥样硬化等作用；生何首乌具有泻下、抗菌、抗炎、抗病毒等作用。

It mainly contains emodin, chrysophanol, emodin methyl ether, rhein acid, chrysophanol anthrone, 2,3,5,4′-tetrahydroxystilbene-2-*O*-*β*-D-glucoside, lecithin and crude fat, etc. *Zhì hé shǒu wū* has the functions of enhancing immunity, promoting bone marrow hematopoiesis, anti-aging, anti osteoporosis, reducing blood fat, anti atherosclerosis and so on. *Shēng hé shǒu wū* has the functions of purgative, antibacterial, anti-inflammatory and antiviral.

第四节 补阴药

Section 4 Yin-supplementing medicinals

PPT

本类药物多味甘，药性寒凉，质润多汁，主入肺、胃、肝、肾经，以补阴滋液、生津润燥为主要作用，主要用于阴虚证。补阴具体包括补肺阴、补胃阴、补肝阴、补肾阴等，分别主治肺、胃、肝、肾等阴虚证。临床主要表现为皮肤、咽喉、口鼻、眼干燥等阴液不足，以及午后潮热、盗汗、五心烦热、两颧发红等阴虚内热两类症状。不同脏腑的阴虚证又具有各自的临床特征性表现，如肺阴不足者，多见干咳少痰，或痰中带血、咯血、潮热等；胃阴不足者，多见口渴、咽干，或胃中嘈杂、干呕，或大便燥结、舌绛苔剥等；肝肾阴虚者，多见眼干涩昏花、眩晕、腰膝酸软、手足心热、遗精、盗汗等。某些药物兼能养心阴，又可用于心阴虚证。

Yin-supplementing medicinals are mostly sweet in flavor and cold in property and act on the lung, stomach and kidney meridians. They have the major efficacies of enriching yin, promoting fluid production and moistening dryness. Yin-supplementing medicinals are different in their efficacies, including supplementing lung yin, stomach yin, liver yin and kidney yin, which are respectively used to treat lung yin deficiency syndrome, stomach yin deficiency, liver yin deficiency and kidney yin deficiency. The major clinical manifestations of yin deficiency are as followings: first, dry skin and throat, dry nose and mouth, dry eyes, etc., caused by lacking of nourishing and moistening in organs due to yin deficiency; second, internal heat induced by yin deficiency, manifested as tidal fever in in the afternoon, night sweating, vexing heat in the five centers (chest, palms and soles) and flashes of cheeks. The yin deficiency syndrome of different *zang-fu* organs has its own clinical characteristics: in the case of lung yin deficiency, common syndromes are dry cough and less phlegm, phlegm with blood, hemoptysis and tidal fever; in the case of stomach yin deficiency, thirst, dry throat, blenching and epigastric upset, retch, dry stool and purplish tongue are common to see; for those with yin deficiency of liver and kidney, dry eyes, dizziness, soreness and weakness of loins and knees, hotness in palms and feet, seminal emission and night sweating are major syndromes. Some of them can also nourish heart yin and can be used for heart yin deficiency.

北沙参　*Běi shā shēn* (Glehniae Radix)
《本草汇言》
Treasury of Words on the Materia Medica (Běn Cǎo Huì Yán)

【来源 / Origin】

本品为伞形科植物珊瑚菜 *Glehnia littoralis* Fr. Schmidt ex Miq. 的干燥根。主产于山东、河北、辽宁等地。夏、秋二季采收，干燥，切段，生用。本品气特异，味微甘。

Běi shā shēn is the dried root of *Glehnia littoralis* Fr. Schmidt ex Miq., pertaining to Umbelliferae. It is mainly produced in Shandong, Hebei and Liaoning Province in China, collected in summer and autumn, dried, cut into sections and used raw. It has a unique odor and tastes slightly sweet.

【性味归经 / Medicinal properties】

甘、微苦，微寒。归肺、胃经。

Sweet, slightly bitter and cold; act on the lung and stomach meridians.

【主要功效 / Medicinal efficacies】

养阴清肺，益胃生津。

Enrich yin and clear lung heat; boost stomach and promote fluid production.

【临床应用 / Clinical application】

1. **肺阴虚证**　本品甘润苦寒，归肺经，能养肺阴、润肺燥，兼清肺热。用治阴虚肺燥之干咳少痰，或劳嗽久咳，咽干音哑等，常与麦冬、玉竹、冬桑叶等同用。用治阴虚劳热，咳嗽咯血，常与知母、川贝母等同用。

(1) Lung yin deficiency　With the nature of bitter and cold and acting on the lung meridian, it has the functions of nourishing lung yin, moistening lung dryness and clearing lung heat. To treat dry cough with less phlegm, or chronic cough and hoarseness of throat, it is usually combined with *mài dōng*, *yù zhú* and *sāng yè*; to treat yin deficiency manifested as consumptive fever, cough and hemoptysis, it is often combined with *zhī mǔ* and *chuān bèi mǔ*.

2. 胃阴虚证　本品归胃经，能养胃阴，生津止渴，兼清胃热。用治胃阴虚有热之口干多饮、饥不欲食、大便干结、舌苔光剥或舌红少津，以及胃脘隐痛、胃脘嘈杂、干呕等，常与麦冬、玉竹、石斛等同用。

(2) Stomach yin deficiency　Acting on the stomach meridian, it can nourish stomach yin, promote body fluid, quench thirst and clear stomach heat. To treat stomach yin deficiency, with heat manifested as dry mouth, polydipsia, hunger with no desire to eat, dry and hard stool, red tongue with less coating, or gastric cavity dull pain, blenching and epigastric upset, it is often combined with *mài dōng*, *yù zhú* and *shí hú*.

【用法用量 / Usage and dosage 】

煎服，5~12g。

Decoction, 5-12g.

【使用注意 / Precaution 】

不宜与藜芦同用。

It is not proper to be used with *lí lú*.

【现代研究 / Modern research 】

本品主要含法卡林二醇、补骨脂素、欧前胡素、异欧前胡素、花椒毒素、佛手柑内酯、挥发油、有机酸、三萜酸、豆甾醇、多糖及氨基酸等。具有镇咳、祛痰、平喘、解热、镇痛、免疫调节、抗肿瘤、抗胃溃疡、抑菌、抗氧化等作用。

It mainly contains fakalin diol, psoralen, imperatorin, isoimperatorin, zanthoxylin, bergamot lactone, volatile oil, organic acid, triterpenoid acid, stigmasterol, polysaccharide and amino acid, etc. It has the functions of relieving cough, eliminating sputum, relieving asthma, and antipyretic, analgesic, immunomodulatory, antitumor, anti gastric ulcer, bacteriostatic, and antioxidant.

麦冬　*Mài dōng* (Ophiopogonis Radix)

《神农本草经》

Shen Nong's Classic of the Materia Medica (*Shén Nóng Běn Cǎo Jīng*)

微课

【来源 / Origin 】

本品为百合科植物麦冬 *Ophiopogon japonicus*（L.f）Ker-Gawl. 的干燥块根。主产于浙江、四川等地。夏季采收，干燥，生用。本品气微香，味甘、微苦。《中国药典》规定，含麦冬总皂苷以鲁斯可皂苷元（$C_{27}H_{42}O_4$）计，不得少于 0.12%。

Mài dōng is the tuberous root of *Ophiopogon japonicus* (L.f) Ker-Gawl., pertaining to Liliaceae. It is mainly produced in Zhejiang and Sichuan Province in China, collected in summer, dried, and used raw. It has a slight odor and tastes sweet and slightly bitter. According to the *Chinese Pharmacopoeia*, the total saponins of ophiopogon japonicus based on ruscosapogenin ($C_{27}H_{42}O_4$) contained in dried medicinal materials should be no less than 0.12%.

【性味归经 / Medicinal properties 】

甘、微苦，微寒。归心、肺、胃经。

Sweet, slightly bitter and cold; act on the heart, lung and stomach meridians.

【主要功效 / Medicinal efficacies】

养阴生津，润肺清心。

Enrich yin and promote fluid production; moisten the lung and clear heart heat.

【临床应用 / Clinical application】

1. 肺阴虚证　本品甘寒入肺，能养肺阴、润肺燥；苦寒入肺，兼清肺热。用治肺阴不足、内有燥热之燥咳痰黏、咽干鼻燥，常与桑叶、阿胶、杏仁等同用。用治肺肾阴虚之劳嗽咯血，常与天冬同用。用治阴虚火旺，虚火上浮之口鼻干燥、咽喉肿痛，常与玄参、桔梗、甘草等同用。

(1) **Lung yin deficiency**　With the nature of sweet and cold and acting on the lung meridian, it can nourish lung yin, moisten lung dryness and clear lung heat. To treat warm-dry damaging lung yin manifested as dry cough with less sputum, dry throat and nose, it is often combined with *sāng yè* (Mori Folium), *ē jiāo* and *xìng rén* (Armeniacae Amarum Semen); to treat cough, hemoptysis and sore throat, it is often combined with *tiān dōng*; to treat dry mouth and nose, swelling and sore throat due to fire excess from yin deficiency and deficiency fire floating up, it is usually used in combination with *xuán shēn*, *jié gēng* and *gān cǎo*.

2. 胃阴虚证　本品入胃经，能养胃阴、生津止渴，兼清胃热，为治疗胃阴虚证之佳品。用治胃阴不足，胃脘隐隐灼痛、口干舌燥、纳呆干呕等，常与北沙参、石斛、玉竹等同用。用治津伤口渴，或内热消渴，常与天花粉、乌梅、太子参等同用。用治热病伤津之肠燥便秘，常与玄参、生地黄等同用。用治胃阴不足之气逆呕吐、口渴咽干、纳少，常与人参、半夏等同用。

(2) **Stomach yin deficiency**　Acting on the stomach meridian, it can enrich the stomach yin and promote fluid production to relieve thirst, and can clear stomach heat, so it is a good medicinal for treating stomach yin deficiency syndrome. To treat dull burning pain in the stomach, dry mouth and dry tongue, nauseous and retching caused deficiency of stomach yin, it is often combined with *běi shā shēn*, *shí hú* and *yù zhú*; to treat thirst due to fluid damaging, internal heat and heat due to consumptive thirst, it is combined with *tiān huā fen*, *wū méi* (Mume Fructus) and *tài zǐ shēn*; to treat constipation due to pathogenic heat damage fluid, it is used with *xuán shēn* and *shēng dì huáng*; to treat qi counterflow vomiting, thirst and dry throat, it is usually used in combination with *rén shēn* and *bàn xià* (Pinelliae Rhizoma).

3. 心阴虚证　本品入心经，具有养阴清心除烦之功。用治阴虚内热之心烦不眠，常与生地黄、酸枣仁等同用。用治热入心营，身热烦躁，舌绛而干等，常与生地黄、玄参、金银花等同用。

(3) **Heart yin deficiency**　Acting on the heart meridian, it has the function of enriching yin and clearing heart heat. To treat heart yin deficiency with heat manifested as vexation and insomnia, it is often combined with *shēng dì huáng* and *suān zǎo rén*; to treat body heat and fidgety, tongue crimson and dry, it is usually used in combination with *shēng dì huáng*, *xuán shēn* and *jīn yín huā*.

【用法用量 / Usage and dosage】

煎服，6~12g。

Decoction, 6-12g.

【现代研究 / Modern research】

本品主要含麦冬皂苷 B 和 D 以及高异黄酮成分、多糖、生物碱、谷甾醇、氨基酸等。具有增强免疫、降血糖、抗疲劳、镇静、催眠、抗心律失常、抗心肌缺血、抗肿瘤等作用。

It mainly contains ophiopogon japonicus saponin B and D, high isoflavones, polysaccharides, alkaloids, sitosterol, and amino acids etc. It has the functions of enhancing immunity, reducing blood sugar, anti fatigue, sedation, hypnosis, anti arrhythmia, anti myocardial ischemia, and anti-tumor, etc.

百合 *Bǎi hé* (Lilii Bulbus)
《神农本草经》
Shen Nong's Classic of the Materia Medica (Shén Nóng Běn Cǎo Jīng)

【来源 / Origin 】

为百合科植物卷丹 *Lilium lancifolium* Thunb.、百合 *Lilium brownii* F.E.Brown var.*viridulum* Baker 或细叶百合 *Lilium pumilum* DC. 的干燥肉质鳞叶。全国各地均产。秋季采挖，干燥，生用或蜜炙用。本品气微，味微苦。

Bǎi hé is the fleshly scale leaf of *Lilium lancifolium* Thunb., *Lilium brownii* F.E. Brown var. *viridulum* or *Lilium pumilum* DC. It's produced all over China, collected in autumn, dried, and used raw or honey-fried. It has a slight odor and tastes slightly bitter.

【性味归经 / Medicinal properties 】

甘，寒。归心、肺经。

Sweet and cold; act on the heart and lung meridians.

【主要功效 / Medicinal efficacies 】

养阴润肺，清心安神。

Enrich yin and moisten lung, clear heart heat and calm the mind.

【临床应用 / Clinical application 】

1. 肺阴虚证　本品甘寒入肺经，功能养阴润肺，兼止咳祛痰。用治肺阴虚之燥热咳嗽，痰中带血，常与款冬花同用。用治肺虚久咳，劳嗽咯血，常与生地黄、麦冬、川贝母等同用。

(1) **Lung yin deficiency**　With the nature of sweet and cold and acting on the lung meridian, it has the functions of enriching and moistening the lung, arresting cough and eliminating phlegm. To treat hot and dry cough and blood in sputum due to yin deficiency of the lung, it is usually combined with *kuǎn dōng huā* (Farfarae Flos); to treat chronic cough due to lung deficiency, cough and hemoptysis due to fatigue, it is often combined with *shēng dì huáng*, *mài dōng* and *chuān bèi mǔ*.

2. 心阴虚证　本品入心经，能清心安神。用治心阴亏虚，虚热上扰之失眠、心悸，可与麦冬、酸枣仁、生地黄等同用。用治心肺阴虚内热之百合病，症见神志恍惚，情绪不能自主，口苦，小便赤，脉微数，常与生地黄、知母等同用。

(2) **Heart yin deficiency**　Acting on the heart meridian, it has the function of clearing heart heat and calming the mind. To treat insomnia and palpitation caused by deficiency of heart yin and disturbance of deficiency heat, it is often combined with *mài dōng*, *suān zǎo rén* and *shēng dì huáng*; to treat lily disease due to deficiency of heart yin and lung yin and malnutrition of the heart spirit, which is manifested as blurred mind, uncontrolled emotions, bitter taste in mouth, dark urine, faint and rapid pulse, it is usually in combination with processed *shēng dì huáng* and *zhī mǔ*.

【用法用量 / Usage and dosage 】

煎服，6~12g。

Decoction, 6-12g.

【现代研究 / Modern research 】

本品主要含岷江百合苷 A 和 D、百合皂苷、去乙酰百合皂苷、百合多糖，以及甾醇、生物碱、蛋白质、氨基酸、维生素等。具有镇咳、祛痰、耐缺氧、抗疲劳、镇静、免疫调节、抗肿瘤、抗炎、降血糖等作用。

It mainly contains lilioside A and D, lilioside, deacetylated lilioside, lilium polysaccharide, sterol, alkaloid, protein, amino acid and vitamin, etc. It has the functions of arresting cough, relieving sputum, anti hypoxia, anti fatigue, sedative, immunomodulatory, anti-tumor, anti-inflammatory and reducing blood glucose.

天冬 *Tiān dōng* (Asparagi Radix)
《神农本草经》
Shen Nong's Classic of the Materia Medica (Shén Nóng Běn Cǎo Jīng)

【来源 / Origin】
为百合科植物天冬 *Asparagus cochinchinensis*（Lour.）Merr. 的干燥块根。主产于贵州、四川、广西等地。秋、冬二季采挖，干燥，切薄片，生用。本品气微，味甜、微苦。

Tiān dōng is the dry root tuber of *Asparagus cochinchinensis* (Lour.) Merr., mainly produced in Guizhou, Sichuan Province, and Guangxi Zhuang Autonomous Region, collected in autumn and winter, dried, sliced, and used raw. It is slight in odor, sweet and slightly bitter in flavor.

【性味归经 / Medicinal properties】
甘、苦，寒。归肺、肾经。
Sweet, bitter and cold; act on lung and kidney meridians.

【主要功效 / Medicinal efficacies】
养阴润燥，清肺生津。
Nourish yin and moisten dryness, clear lung and promote fluid production.

【临床应用 / Clinical application】
1. 肺阴虚证 本品入肺经，甘寒养阴润肺，苦寒清肺降火，清润之力强于麦冬。用治燥邪伤肺，干咳无痰，或痰少而黏，或痰中带血，可单用或与麦冬同用。用治阴虚劳嗽，痰中带血，常与麦冬、生地黄、阿胶等同用。

(1) Lung-yin deficiency *Tiān dōng* enters lung meridian, nourishing yin and moistening lung with sweet cold, clearing lung and reducing fire with bitter cold, with more powerful efficacy of clearing and moistening than *mài dōng*. It treats dry pathogen damaging lung manifested as dry cough with no sputum, or less but glutinous sputum, or sputum with blood, singly or in combination with *mài dōng*. For yin deficiency manifested as consumptive cough, sputum with blood, it is often used with *mài dōng*, *shēng dì huáng* and *ē jiāo*.

2. 肾阴虚证 本品入肾经，具有滋肾阴、清降虚火、生津润燥之效。用治肾阴亏虚，腰膝酸痛，眩晕耳鸣，常与熟地黄、枸杞子、牛膝等同用。用治阴虚火旺，骨蒸潮热、遗精等，常与生地黄、知母、黄柏等同用。

(2) Kidney-yin deficiency *Tiān dōng* enters kidney meridian and has the functions of nourishing kidney yin, clear and reducing deficiency fire, promoting fluid production and moistening dryness. It treats kidney yin deficiency manifested as soreness and pain of loins and knees, dizziness and tinnitus in combination with *shú dì huáng*, *gǒu qǐ zǐ* and *niú xī*. For yin deficiency with effulgent fire manifested as steaming bone fever, tidal fever, and spermatorrhea, it is often used with *shēng dì huáng*, *zhī mǔ* and *huáng bó* (Phellodendri Chinensis Cortex).

3. 胃阴虚证 本品还可养胃阴、清胃热、生津、润肠。用治热病伤津口渴或内热消渴，可与人参、生地黄等同用。用治津伤肠燥便秘，可与麦冬、玄参、火麻仁等同用。

(3) Stomach-yin deficiency　*Tiān dōng* can tonify stomach yin, clear stomach heat, promote fluid production and moisten intestines. It treats febrile disease damaging fluid manifested as thirst or consumptive thirst due to internal heat, in combination with *rén shēn* and *shēng dì huáng*. For constipation due to fluid depletion and intestinal dryness, it is often used with *mài dōng*, *xuán shēn* and *huǒ má rén*.

【用法用量 / Usage and dosage】

煎服，6~12g。

Decoction, 6-12g.

【使用注意 / Precaution】

脾胃虚寒，食少便溏及外感风寒咳嗽者忌服。

It is contraindicated in those with spleen-stomach deficiency cold, poor appetite and loose stool, and cough due to external-contraction wind cold.

【现代研究 / Modern research】

本品主要含甲基原薯蓣皂苷、伪原薯蓣皂苷、寡糖、天冬多糖、氨基酸、蛋白质等。具有镇咳、祛痰、抗肿瘤、抗炎、抗菌、抗衰老、降血糖等作用。

Tiān dōng mainly contains methyl protodioscin, pseudoprotodioscin, oligosaccharide, aspartic polysaccharide, amino acid, protein, etc. It has the functions of antitussive, expectorant, anti-tumor, anti-inflammatory, antibacterial, anti-aging, and decreasing blood glucose.

石斛　*Shí hú* (Dendrobii Caulis)

《神农本草经》

Shen Nong's Classic of the Materia Medica (Shén Nóng Běn Cǎo Jīng)

【来源 / Origin】

为兰科植物金钗石斛 *Dendrobium nobile* Lindl.、霍山石斛 *Dendrobium huoshanense* C.Z. Tang et S.J. Cheng、鼓槌石斛 *Dendrobium chrysotoxum* Lindl. 或流苏石斛 *Dendrobium fimbriatum* Hook. 的栽培品及其同属植物近似种的新鲜或干燥茎。主产四川、云南、贵州等地。全年均可采收，生用。本品味淡或微苦，嚼之有黏性。《中国药典》规定，金钗石斛含石斛碱（$C_{16}H_{25}NO_2$）不得少于 0.40%，霍山石斛含多糖以无水葡萄糖（$C_6H_{12}O_6$）计，不得少于 17.0%，鼓槌石斛含毛兰素（$C_{18}H_{22}O_5$）不得少于 0.030%。

Shí hú is the cultivated product of *Dendrobium nobile* Lindl., *Dendrobium huoshanense* C.Z. Tang et S.J. Cheng, *Dendrobium chrysotoxum* Lindl. or *Dendrobium fimbriatum* Hook., or the fresh or dry stem of similar species of the same genus, mainly produced in Sichuan, Yunnan, and Guizhou Province, collected all year round and used raw. It tastes light or slightly bitter, and sticky when chewed. According to *Chinese Pharmacopoeia*, *Dendrobium nobile* Lindl. contains dendrobine ($C_{16}H_{25}NO_2$) no less than 0.40%, *Dendrobium huoshanense* contains polysaccharide such as anhydrous glucose ($C_6H_{12}O_6$) no less than 17.0%, and *Dendrobium chrysotoxum* Lindl. contains maolanin ($C_{18}H_{22}O_5$) no less than 0.030%.

【性味归经 / Medicinal properties】

甘，微寒。归胃、肾经。

Sweet and slightly cold; act on stomach and kidney meridians.

【主要功效 / Medicinal efficacies】

益胃生津，滋阴清热。

Boost stomach and promote fluid production, nourish yin and clear heat.

【临床应用 / Clinical application 】

1. **胃阴虚证** 本品甘寒，入胃经，善养胃阴、生津止渴。用治胃阴不足之胃脘隐隐灼痛、口干舌燥、纳呆干呕等，常与北沙参、玉竹、麦冬等同用。用治热病伤津之低热烦渴、舌干苔黑，常与天花粉、麦冬、生地黄等同用。

(1) Stomach-yin deficiency *Shí hú* is sweet and cold, entering stomach meridian, and good at tonifying stomach yin, and promoting fluid production to quench thirst. It treats stomach yin insufficiency manifested as dull burning pain in stomach, dry mouth, anorexia and retch in combination with *běi shā shēn*, *yù zhú* and *mài dōng*. For febrile disease damaging fluid manifested as mild fever, excessive thirst, and dry tongue with black coating, it is often used with *tiān huā fěn*, *mài dōng* and *shēng dì huáng*.

2. **肾阴虚证** 本品入肾经，既能滋养肾阴，又能清退虚热。用治阴虚火旺，骨蒸劳热，可与知母、黄柏、生地黄等同用。用治肾阴亏虚，筋骨痿软，常与熟地黄、杜仲、山茱萸等同用。用治肝肾阴虚，目暗不明，视物昏花等，常与菊花、枸杞子、决明子等同用。

(2) Kidney-yin deficiency *Shí hú* enters kidney meridian with the functions of nourishing kidney yin as well as clear deficiency heat. It treats yin deficiency with fire hyperactivity manifested as steaming bone fever and consumptive fever, in combination with *zhī mǔ*, *huáng bó* and *shēng dì huáng*. For flaccid sinews and bones due to kidney yin deficiency, it is often used with *shú dì huáng*, *dù zhòng* and *shān zhū yú* (Corni Fructus). For blurred vision due to liver-kidney yin deficiency, it is often used with *jú huā*, *gǒu qǐ zǐ* and *jué míng zǐ*.

【用法用量 / Usage and dosage 】

煎服，干品 6~12g，鲜品 15~30g。

Decoction, 6-12g in dry form and 15-30g in fresh form.

【现代研究 / Modern research 】

本品主要含石斛碱、石斛酮碱、鼓槌菲、毛兰菲、毛兰素，以及多糖、生物碱、氨基酸、鞣质、淀粉、黏液质等。具有促进胃液分泌、改善肠胃功能、增强免疫、降血糖、抗肿瘤、抗氧化、抗炎、镇痛、解热等作用。

Shí hú mainly contains dendrobine, nobilonine, chrysotoxene, confusarin, erianin, as well as polysaccharides, alkaloids, amino acids, tannins, starch, mucus, etc. It has the functions of promoting the secretion of gastric juice, improving gastrointestinal function, enhancing immunity, reducing blood sugar, resisting tumor, oxidation, and inflammation, relieving pain and resolving fever.

枸杞子 *Gǒu qǐ zǐ* (Lycii Fructus)

《神农本草经》
Shen Nong's Classic of the Materia Medica (Shén Nóng Běn Cǎo Jīng)

【来源 / Origin 】

为茄科植物宁夏枸杞 *Lycium barbarum* L. 的干燥成熟果实。主产于宁夏、内蒙古、甘肃等地。夏、秋二季采收，干燥，生用。本品气微，味甜。《中国药典》规定，含甜菜碱（$C_5H_{11}NO_2$）不得少于 0.50%。

Gǒu qǐ zǐ is the dried and mature fruit of *Lycium barbarum* L. of Ningxia, a solanaceous plant, mainly produced in Ningxia Hui Autonomous Region, Inner Mongolia Autonomous Region, and Gansu Province, collected in summer and autumn, dried and used raw. It is mild in odor and sweet in taste. According to *Chinese Pharmacopoeia*, the content of betaine ($C_5H_{11}NO_2$) should be no less than 0.50%.

【性味归经 / Medicinal properties】

甘，平。归肝、肾经。

Sweet and neutral; act on liver and kidney meridians.

【主要功效 / Medicinal efficacies】

滋补肝肾，益精明目。

Nourish liver and kidney, boost essence and improve vision.

【临床应用 / Clinical application】

肝肾阴虚证　本品甘润滋养，药性平和，入肝肾经，长于补肝肾、益精血，并有较好的明目功效，为滋补肝肾的佳品。用治肝肾不足，精血亏虚之腰膝酸软，耳鸣耳聋，须发早白，发脱齿松，不育不孕，健忘呆钝或生长发育迟缓等，常与熟地黄、龟甲胶、山茱萸等同用。用治肝肾阴虚之两目昏花，视物模糊或眼干涩等，常与菊花、熟地黄、山茱萸等同用。用治肾虚腰痛，阳痿不育，遗精早泄，尿后余沥等，可与菟丝子、覆盆子、五味子等同用。用治血虚之面色萎黄，失眠多梦，头昏耳鸣等，常与龙眼肉同用。

Liver-kidney yin deficiency　*Gǒu qǐ zǐ* is sweet, nourishing and tonifying, and mild in temperament. It enters liver-kidney meridians, and is good at nourishing liver and kidney, boosting essence and blood, and improving vision, and is a good tonic for liver and kidney. For liver-kidney insufficiency, essence and blood deficiency manifested as soreness and weakness of loins and knees, tinnitus, deafness, early white hair, hair loss, loose teeth, infertility, forgetfulness or growth retardation, it is often combined with *shú dì huáng*, *guī jiǎ jiāo* (Testudinis Carapax et Plastrum Colla) and *shān zhū yú*. For liver-kidney yin deficiency manifested as blurred or dry eyes, it is used with *jú huā*, *shú dì huáng* and *shān zhū yú*. For kidney-deficiency-induced backache, impotence, infertility, spermatorrhea, premature ejaculation, and residual urine, it is used with *tù sī zǐ*, *fù pén zǐ* and *wǔ wèi zǐ*. For blood deficiency manifested as pale complexion, insomnia, dreaminess, dizziness and tinnitus, it is used with *lóng yǎn ròu*.

【用法用量 / Usage and dosage】

煎服，6~12g。

Decoction, 6-12g.

【现代研究 / Modern research】

本品主要含甜菜碱、莨菪亭、枸杞多糖、玉蜀黍黄素、枸杞素A和B、胡萝卜素、维生素C、氨基酸、微量元素等。具有免疫调节、抗衰老、促进造血、提高视力、抗肿瘤、保肝、降血脂、降血糖、降血压、抗脂肪肝等作用。

Gǒu qǐ zǐ mainly contains betaine, hyoscyamine, lycium polysaccharide, zeaxanthin, lycium A and B, carotene, vitamin C, amino acid, trace elements, etc. It has the functions of immune regulation, anti-aging, promoting hematopoiesis, improving vision, anti-tumor, protecting liver, reducing blood fat, blood sugar and blood pressure, and anti fatty liver.

龟甲　*Guī jiǎ* (Testudinis Carapax et Plastrum)
《神农本草经》
Shen Nong's Classic of the Materia Medica (Shén Nóng Běn Cǎo Jīng)

【来源 / Origin】

为龟科动物乌龟 *Chinemys reevesii*（Gray）的背甲及腹甲。主产浙江、湖北、湖南等地。全年均可捕捉，以秋、冬二季为多，晒干，生用或砂烫后醋淬用，用时捣碎。本品气微腥，味微咸。

Guī jiǎ is the carapace and plastron of tortoise *Chinemys reevesii* (Gray), mainly produced in Zhejiang, Hubei, and Hunan Province, caught all year round, mostly in autumn and winter, dried in the sun, used raw, or quenched with vinegar after being fried with sands and mashed when used. It is slightly fishy and salty.

【性味归经 / Medicinal properties】

咸、甘，微寒。归肝、肾、心经。

Salty, sweet and slightly cold; act on liver, kidney and heart meridians.

【主要功效 / Medicinal efficacies】

滋阴潜阳，益肾强骨，养血补心，固经止崩。

Nourish yin and subdue yang, boost kidney and strengthen bones, nourish blood and supplement heart, secure menses and stanch profuse uterine bleeding.

【临床应用 / Clinical application】

1. 肝肾阴虚证　本品甘寒质重，入肝肾经，既能滋补肝肾之阴而清虚热，又可潜降肝阳而息内风，适宜于肝肾阴虚诸证。用治阴虚阳亢之头晕目眩，常与白芍、天冬、牡蛎等同用。用治阴虚内热，骨蒸潮热，盗汗遗精，常与熟地黄、知母、黄柏等同用。用治阴虚风动之手足瘛疭，常与阿胶、生地黄、鳖甲等同用。

(1) **Liver-kidney yin deficiency**　*Guī jiǎ* is sweet, cold and heavy, enters liver and kidney meridians. It has the functions of nourishing liver-kidney yin and clearing deficiency heat as well as subduing liver yang and extinguishing internal wind, and is suitable for syndromes of liver-kidney yin deficiency. For dizziness due to yin deficiency with yang hyperactivity, it is often used with *bái sháo*, *tiān dōng* and *mǔ lì*. For internal heat due to yin deficiency, steaming bone fever and tidal fever, night sweat and spermatorrhea, it is often used with *shú dì huáng, zhī mǔ* and *huáng bó*. For stirring wind due to yin deficiency and convulsions of the extremities, it is used with *ē jiāo, shēng dì huáng* and *biē jiǎ*.

2. 肾虚筋骨痿弱　本品有滋肾养肝、强健筋骨之功。用治肝肾不足之腰膝酸软、下肢痿弱、步履艰难等，常与熟地黄、牛膝、豹骨等同用。用治小儿先天不足，精血亏损之行迟、齿迟、囟门难合、发育迟缓等，常与黄芪、龙骨、牡蛎等同用。用治小儿脾肾不足，阴血亏虚，发育不良，出现鸡胸、龟背等，常与鹿茸、紫河车、山药等同用。

(2) **Flaccid sinews and bones due to kidney deficiency**　*Guī jiǎ* has the functions of nourishing kidney and liver, strengthening sinews and bones. It treats liver-kidney-insufficiency-induced weak waist and knees, flaccid lower limbs, difficult walking in combination with *shú dì huáng, niú xī* and *bào gǔ* (Pardi Os). For walking retardation, teeth retardation, delayed fontanelle closure and delayed development due to infantile congenital deficiency and deficiency of blood and essence, it is often used with *huáng qí, lóng gǔ* and *mǔ lì*. For infantile spleen-kidney insufficiency, yin-blood deficiency and poor development manifested as pigeon breast and tortoise back, it is used with *lù róng, zǐ hé chē* and *shān yào*.

3. 心神不宁，惊悸失眠　本品入心经，能养血补心而安定神志。用治阴血亏虚，心神失养之惊悸、失眠、健忘等，常与石菖蒲、远志、龙骨等同用。

(3) **Restlessness, palpitation and insomnia**　*Guī jiǎ* enters heart meridian and can nourish blood and tonify heart to tranquilize spirit and stabilize mind. It treats yin-blood deficiency and failure of nourishment of heart manifested as palpitation, insomnia and forgetfulness in combination with *shí chāng*

pú, yuǎn zhì and *lóng gǔ*.

4. 崩漏，月经过多 本品具有滋肾降火、固冲止血之效。用治阴虚血热，冲脉不固之崩漏、月经过多，常与白芍、黄芩、椿皮等配伍。

(4) Metrorrhagia, menorrhagia *Guī jiǎ* has the efficacy of nourishing kidney and reducing fire, securing thoroughfare and stopping bleeding. It treats metrorrhagia and menorrhagia due to yin deficiency and blood heat, and insecurity of thoroughfare vessel, in combination with *bái sháo*, *huáng qín* and *chūn pí* (Ailanthi Cortex).

【用法用量 / Usage and dosage】

煎服，9~24g，打碎先煎。

Decoction, 9-24g. It should be broken and decocted firstly.

【使用注意 / Precaution】

孕妇及脾胃虚寒者忌服。

It is contraindicated in pregnant women and those with deficiency-cold of spleen and stomach.

【现代研究 / Modern research】

本品主要含动物胶、角蛋白、骨胶原蛋白、氨基酸、胆甾醇、脂肪、维生素、甾体类、微量元素等。具有增强免疫、兴奋子宫、延缓衰老、抗骨质疏松、抗凝血、增加冠脉血流量、补血、镇静等作用。

Guī jiǎ mainly contains animal glue, keratin, bone collagen, amino acids, cholesterol, fat, vitamins, steroids, trace elements, etc. It can enhance immunity, excite uterus, delay aging, resist osteoporosis, resist coagulation, increase blood flow of coronary artery, replenish blood, calm mind and so on.

鳖甲　*Biē jiǎ* (Trionycis Carapax)
《神农本草经》
Shen Nong's Classic of the Materia Medica (Shén Nóng Běn Cǎo Jīng)

【来源 / Origin】

为鳖科动物鳖 *Trionyx sinensis* Wiegmann 的背甲。主产湖北、江苏、河南等地。全年可捕捉，晒干，生用或砂烫后醋淬用，用时捣碎。本品气微腥，味淡。

Biē jiǎ is the dorsal shell of *Trionyx sinensis* Wiegmann, mainly produced in Hubei, Jiangsu, and Henan Province, caught all year round, dried in the sun, and used raw or scalded with sand and then quenched with vinegar and mashed when used. It is slightly fishy and tastes bland.

【性味归经 / Medicinal properties】

咸，微寒。归肝、肾经。

Salty and slightly cold; act on liver and kidney meridians.

【主要功效 / Medicinal efficacies】

滋阴潜阳，退热除蒸，软坚散结。

Nourish yin and subdue yang, relieve steaming hone fever, soften hardness and dissipate masses.

【临床应用 / Clinical application】

1. 肝肾阴虚证 本品入肝、肾经，咸寒质重，具有滋阴潜阳和清退虚热功效，适用于肝肾阴虚诸证。其功用与龟甲相似，常相须为用，但其滋补之力不如龟甲。其善清虚热、除骨蒸，故为治阴虚发热之要药。用治肝肾阴虚，虚火内扰之骨蒸潮热、盗汗，或低热日久不退，常与秦艽、知母、胡黄连等同用。用治温病后期，阴液耗伤，邪伏阴分，夜热早凉，热退无汗，常与青蒿、生地黄、牡丹皮等同用。用治阴虚阳亢，头晕目眩，常与生地黄、牡蛎、菊花等同用。用治阴虚风动，手指瘈疭，常与牡蛎、生地黄、阿胶等同用。用治肝肾阴虚，筋骨不健，腰膝酸软，步履乏力及小儿鸡胸、龟背、囟门不合等，多与熟地黄、知母等同用。

(1) Liver-kidney yin deficiency *Biē jiǎ* enters liver and kidney meridians, salty, cold and heavy, with the functions of nourishing yin, subduing yang and relieving deficiency heat and is suitable for syndromes of liver-kidney yin deficiency. It is often combined with *guī jiǎ* since they have the similar function but its nourishing efficacy is not as good as that of *guī jiǎ*, so it is especially good at clearing deficiency heat and eliminating steaming bone fever. Therefore, it is an essential medicine for the treatment of yin deficiency fever. It treats liver-kidney yin deficiency and internal disturbing of deficiency fire manifested as steaming bone fever and tidal fever, night sweating, or persistent low fever in combination with *qín jiāo*, *zhī mǔ* and *hú huáng lián* (Picrorhizae Rhizoma). For yin fluid consumption, pathogenic heat damaging yin in the later stage of warm disease manifested as night fever abating at dawn, and no sweating during fever relief, it is usually combined with *qīng hāo* (Artemisiae Annuae Herba), *shēng dì huáng* (Rehmanniae Radix) and *mǔ dān pí*. For yin deficiency with yang hyperactivity and dizziness, it is usually combined with *shēng dì huáng*, *mǔ lì* and *jú huā*. For stirring wind due to yin deficiency and convulsions of the fingers, it is used with *mǔ lì*, *shēng dì huáng* and *ē jiāo*. For liver-kidney yin deficiency manifested as weak sinews and bones, soreness and weakness of waist and knees, weak walking and pigeon breast, tortoise back and failure of closure of fontanel in children, it is often used with *shú dì huáng* (Rehmanniae Radix Praeparata) and *zhī mǔ*.

2. 癥瘕积聚　本品味咸，有软坚散结之功。用治癥瘕积聚，或疟疾日久不愈，胁下痞硬成块等，常与桃仁、土鳖虫、大黄等同用。

(2) Accumulation of abdominal masses *Biē jiǎ* is slightly salty and has the function of softening hardness and dissipating masses. It treats accumulation of abdominal masses or prolonged malaria, concretions and conglomerations of lower abdominal masses, in combination with *táo rén*, *tǔ biē chóng* (Eupolyphaga seu Steleophaga) and *dà huáng*.

【 用法用量 / Usage and dosage 】

煎服，9~24g，打碎先煎。

Decoction, 9-24g. It should be broken and decocted firstly.

【 使用注意 / Precaution 】

孕妇及脾胃虚寒者忌服。

It is contraindicated in pregnant women and those with deficiency-cold of spleen and stomach.

【 现代研究 / Modern research 】

本品主要含骨胶原、碳酸钙、磷酸钙、氨基酸、微量元素、多糖、多肽、维生素等。具有增强免疫、促进造血功能、提高血红蛋白含量、抗肝纤维化、抑制结缔组织增生、抗肿瘤、抗疲劳、抗突变、增加骨密度、镇静等作用。

Biē jiǎ mainly contains bone collagen, calcium carbonate, calcium phosphate, amino acids, trace elements, polysaccharides, polypeptides, vitamins, etc. It has the functions of enhancing immunity, promoting hematopoiesis, increasing hemoglobin content, resisting liver fibrosis, inhibiting hyperplasia of connective tissue, anti-tumor, anti fatigue, anti mutation, increasing bone density, and tranquilization.

其他补虚药功用介绍见表 22-1。

The efficacies of other supplementing medicinals are shown in table 22-1.

表 22-1 其他补虚药功用介绍

分类	药物	药性	功效	应用	用法用量
补气药	太子参	甘、微苦，平。归脾、肺经	益气健脾，生津润肺	脾虚体倦，食欲不振，病后虚弱，气阴不足，自汗口渴；肺燥干咳	煎服，9~30g
	大枣	甘，温。归脾、胃、心经	补中益气，养血安神	脾虚食少，乏力便溏，妇人脏躁	劈破煎服，6~15g
	刺五加	辛、微苦，温。归脾、肾、心经	益气健脾，补肾安神	脾肺气虚，体虚乏力，食欲不振，肺肾两虚，久咳虚喘，肾虚腰膝酸痛，心脾不足，失眠多梦	煎服，9~27g
	白扁豆	甘，微温。归脾、胃经	健脾化湿，和中消暑	脾胃虚弱，食欲不振，大便溏泄，白带过多，暑湿吐泻，胸闷腹胀	煎服，9~15g
	绞股蓝	甘、苦，寒。归脾、肺经	益气健脾，化痰止咳，清热解毒	脾虚证，肺虚咳嗽	煎服，10~20g
	红景天	甘、苦，平。归肺、心经	益气活血，通脉平喘	气虚血瘀，胸痹心痛，中风偏瘫，倦怠气喘	煎服，3~6g
	沙棘	酸、涩，温。归脾、胃、肺、心经	健脾消食，止咳祛痰，活血散瘀	脾虚食少，食积腹痛，咳嗽痰多，胸痹心痛，瘀血经闭，跌仆瘀肿	煎服，3~10g
	饴糖	甘，温。归脾、胃、肺经	补中益气，缓急止痛，润肺止咳	脾胃虚寒，脘腹疼痛，肺虚燥咳	入汤剂须烊化服，15~20g
	蜂蜜	甘，平。归肺、脾、大肠经	补中，润燥，止痛，解毒；外用生肌敛疮	脘腹虚痛，肺燥干咳，肠燥便秘，解乌头类药毒；外治疮疡不敛，水火烫伤	冲服，15~30g。外用适量
补阳药	仙茅	辛，热；有毒。归肾、肝、脾经	补肾阳，强筋骨，祛寒湿	阳痿精冷，筋骨痿软，腰膝冷痛，阳虚冷泻	煎服，3~10g
	益智仁	辛，温。归脾、肾经	暖身固精缩尿，温脾止泻摄唾	肾虚遗尿，小便频数，遗精白浊；脾寒泄泻，腹中冷痛，口多涎唾	煎服，3~10g
	狗脊	苦、甘，温。归肝、肾经	祛风湿，补肝肾，强腰膝	风湿痹痛，腰膝酸软，下肢无力	煎服，6~12g
	核桃仁	甘，温。归肾、肺、大肠经	补肾，温肺，润肠	肾阳不足，腰膝酸软，阳痿遗精，虚寒喘嗽，肠燥便秘	煎服，6~9g
	韭菜子	辛、甘，温。归肝、肾经	温补肝肾，壮阳固精	肝肾亏虚，腰膝酸痛，阳痿遗精，遗尿尿频，白浊带下	煎服，3~9g
	阳起石	咸，温。归肾经	温肾壮阳	肾阳亏虚，阳痿不举，宫冷不孕	煎服，3~6g
	海狗肾	咸，热。归肾经	暖肾壮阳，益精补髓	肾阳亏虚，阳痿精冷，精少不孕，心腹冷痛	研末服，每次1~3g，每日2~3次
	紫河车	甘、咸，温。归肺、肝、肾经	温肾补精，益气养血	肾阳不足，精血亏虚证，肺肾两虚之咳喘，气血两虚证	研末吞服，2~3g
	海马	甘、咸，温。归肝、肾经	温肾壮阳，散结消肿	阳痿，遗尿，肾虚作喘，癥瘕积聚，跌仆损伤；外治痈肿疔疮	煎服，3~9g

续表

分类	药物	药性	功效	应用	用法用量
补阳药	鹿角	咸、温。归肝、肾经	温肾阳，强筋骨，行血消肿	肾阳不足，阳痿遗精，腰脊冷痛，阴疽疮疡，乳痈初起，瘀血肿痛	煎服，6~15g
	鹿角胶	甘、咸，温。归肾、肝经	温补肝肾，益精养血	肝肾不足所致的腰膝酸冷，阳痿遗精，虚劳羸瘦，崩漏下血，便血尿血，阴疽肿痛	烊化兑服，3~6g
	鹿角霜	咸、涩，温。归肝、肾经	温肾助阳，收敛止血	脾肾阳虚，白带过多，遗尿尿频，崩漏下血，疮疡不敛	先煎，9~15g
补血药	龙眼肉	甘，温。归心、脾经	补益心脾，养血安神	气血不足，心悸怔忡，健忘失眠，血虚萎黄	煎服，9~15g
补阴药	南沙参	甘，微寒。归肺、胃经	养阴清肺，益胃生津，化痰，益气	肺热燥咳，阴虚劳嗽，干咳痰黏，胃阴不足，食少呕吐，气阴不足，烦热口干	煎服，9~15g
	玉竹	甘，微寒。归肺、胃经	养阴润燥，生津止渴	肺胃阴伤，燥热咳嗽，咽干口渴，内热消渴	煎服，6~12g
	黄精	甘，平。归脾、肺、肾经	补气养阴，健脾，润肺，益肾	脾胃气虚，体倦乏力，胃阴不足，口干食少，肺虚燥咳，劳嗽咯血，精血不足，腰膝酸软，须发早白，内热消渴	煎服，9~15g
	墨旱莲	甘、酸，寒。归肾、肝经	滋补肝肾，凉血止血	肝肾阴虚，牙齿松动，须发早白，眩晕耳鸣，腰膝酸软，阴虚血热吐血、衄血、尿血，血痢，崩漏下血，外伤出血	煎服，6~12g
	女贞子	甘、苦，凉。归肝、肾经	滋补肝肾，明目乌发	肝肾阴虚，眩晕耳鸣，腰膝酸软，须发早白，目暗不明，内热消渴，骨蒸潮热	煎服，6~12g
	桑椹	甘、酸，寒。归心、肝、肾经	滋阴补血，生津润燥	肝肾阴虚，眩晕耳鸣，心悸失眠，须发早白，津伤口渴，内热消渴，肠燥便秘	煎服，9~15g
	黑芝麻	甘，平。归肝、肾、大肠经	补肝肾，益精血，润肠燥	精血亏虚，头晕目眩，耳鸣耳聋，须发早白，病后脱发，肠燥便秘	煎服，9~15g
	楮实子	甘，寒。归肝、肾经	补肾清肝，明目，利尿	肝肾不足，腰膝酸软，虚劳骨蒸，头晕目昏，目生翳膜，水肿胀满	煎服，6~12g
	蛤蟆油	甘、咸，平。归肺、肾经	补肾益精，养阴润肺	病后体弱，神疲乏力，心悸失眠，盗汗，劳嗽咯血	煎服，5~15g

（王英豪　郝二伟）

题库

第二十三章 收 涩 药
Chapter 23　Astringent medicinals

学习目标︱Learning goals

　　1. 掌握　收涩药在性能、功效、主治、配伍及使用注意方面的共性；麻黄根、五味子、乌梅、山茱萸、肉豆蔻的性能、功效、应用以及特殊的用法用量和特殊的使用注意。

　　2. 熟悉　收涩药的分类；浮小麦、莲子、诃子、赤石脂、桑螵蛸、椿皮、海螵蛸的功效、应用以及特殊的用法用量和特殊的使用注意。

　　3. 了解　固表止汗药、敛肺涩肠药、固精缩尿止带药以及相关功效术语的含义；糯稻根、罂粟壳、石榴皮、五倍子、覆盆子、芡实、金樱子的功效以及特殊的用法用量和特殊的使用注意。

　　1. Master the commonness of astringent medicinals in efficacy, indications, property, compatibility and precautions; as well as the property, efficacy, application, special usage and dosage and precautions of *má huáng gēn, wǔ wèi zǐ, wū méi, shān zhū yú* and *ròu dòu kòu*.

　　2. Familiar with the classification of astringent medicinals and the efficacy, indications, special usage, dosage and precautions of *fú xiǎo mài, lián zǐ, hē zǐ, chì shí zhī, sāng piāo xiāo , chūn pí* and *hǎi piāo xiāo*.

　　3. Understand the classification and related efficacy of exterior-consolidating and sweat-arresting medicinals, lung-intestine astringing medicinals, and essence-securing, urination-reducing and leukorrhagia-arresting medicinals; and the efficacy, special usage and precaution of *nuò dào gēn, yīng sù qiào, shí liú pí, wǔ bèi zǐ, fù pén zǐ, qiàn shí* and *jīn yīng zǐ*.

　　凡以收敛固涩为主要功效，常用以治疗各种滑脱病证的药物，称为收涩药，又称固涩药。收涩药味多酸、涩，性温或平，主入肺、脾、肾、大肠经，能够收敛耗散，固涩滑脱，主要具有固表止汗、敛肺止咳、涩肠止泻、固精缩尿、收敛止血、收涩止带等作用。主治久病体虚、正气不固、脏腑功能衰退所致的自汗、盗汗、久咳虚喘、久泻久痢、遗精滑精、遗尿尿频、崩带不止等滑脱不禁的病证。

　　Medicinals with the main efficacies of astringing and consolidating are known as astringent medicinals, or consolidating medicinals. So they are usually used to treat various disorders due to insecurity and desertion. Astringent medicinals are usually sour and astringent in flavor, warm or neutral in property and they can astringe consumption and dispersing, consolidate insecurity and rescue from desertion. They have the main efficacies of consolidating the exterior and arresting sweating, astringing the lung and relieving cough, astringing the intestines and arresting diarrhea, consolidating essence and reducing urination, stanching profuse uterine bleeding and arresting vaginal discharge. So they are usually used to treat various disorders due to insecurity and desertion manifested as spontaneous sweating, night sweating, chronic cough, panting of deficiency pattern, chronic diarrhea, chronic dysentery, seminal emission, spontaneous seminal emission, enuresis, frequent urination, profuse uterine bleeding and vaginal discharge, which are induced by chronic diseases and weak constitution, insecurity of healthy qi and declined *zang-fu* organs.

根据收涩药的药性及功效主治差异，可分为固表止汗药、敛肺涩肠药、固精缩尿止带药三类。

According to the difference of efficacies, properties and clinical applications, astringent medicinals can be classified into three categories: exterior-consolidating and sweat-arresting medicinals, lung-intestine astringing medicinals, and essence-securing, urination-reducing and leukorrhagia-arresting medicinals.

收涩药多为治标之品，但导致滑脱病证的根本原因是正气虚弱，故在使用时须与相应的补虚药配伍，以标本兼顾。如气虚自汗、阴虚盗汗者，分别配伍补气药、补阴药；脾肾阳虚，久泻久痢者，应配伍温补脾肾药；肾虚遗精滑精，遗尿尿频者，当配伍补肾药；冲任不固，崩漏不止者，应配伍补肝肾、固冲任药；肺肾虚损，久咳虚喘者，宜配伍补肺益肾纳气药等。

The root of insecurity and desertion is healthy qi deficiency, so application of astringent medicinals for insecurity and desertion is just to treat the branch of disease. In clinical practice, astringent medicinals should be combined with corresponding supplementing medicinals to treat both the root and branch.For instance, to treat spontaneous sweating due to qi deficiency and night sweating due to yin deficiency, qi-supplementing medicinals and yin-supplementing medicinals should be combinedrespectively. To treat chronic diarrhea and chronic dysentery due to yang deficiency of the spleen and kidney, medicinals for warm-supplementing the spleen and kidney should be combined. To treat seminal emission, spontaneous seminal emission, enuresis and frequent urination, kidney-supplementing medicinals should be combined. To treat flooding and spotting due to insecurity of thoroughfare and conception vessels, medicinals for supplementing the liver and kidney and medicinals for securing the thoroughfare and conception vessels. To treat chronic cough and panting of deficiency type due to depletion of the lung and kidney, medicinals for supplementing the lung, boosting the kidney and receiving qi should be combined.

收涩药性涩敛邪，故凡表邪未解，湿热内蕴之泻痢、带下、血热出血以及郁热未清者，均不宜用，以防"闭门留寇"。但某些收涩药除收涩作用之外，兼有清湿热、解毒等功效，则当区别对待。

Astringent medicinals are astringent in property and they can astringe pathogens, so they are not proper for the conditions with unreleased exterior, internal damp stagnation and uncleared heat stagnation. In case they are misused, they will close the gate for dispelling pathogens so that pathogens will be retained. However, in addition to the astringent effect, some astringent medicinals have the functions of clearing damp heat and detoxification, so they should be treated separately.

第一节 固表止汗药

Section 1 Exterior-consolidating and sweat-arresting medicinals

PPT

本类药物多味甘涩而性平，主入肺、心经，以固表止汗为主要功效，主要用于气虚自汗、阴虚盗汗病证。

Exterior-consolidating and sweat-arresting medicinals are usually sour and astringent in flavor, neutral in property and act on the lung and heart meridians. They are commonly used to treat spontaneous sweating due to qi deficiency and night sweating due to yin deficiency.

麻黄根 *Má huáng gēn* (Ephedrae Radix et Rhizoma)
《本草经集注》
Collective Commentaries on the Classic of Materia Medica (Běn Cǎo Jīng Jí Zhù)

【来源 / Origin】

为麻黄科植物草麻黄 *Ephedra sinica* stapf 或中麻黄 *Ephedra intermedia* Schrenk et C.A.Mey. 的干燥根及根茎。主产于河北、山西、内蒙古等地。秋末采挖，干燥，切厚片，生用。本品气微，味微苦。

Má huáng gēn is the dry root and rhizome of *Ephedra sinica* stapf or *Ephedra intermedia* Schrenk et C. A. Mey., pertaining to Ephedraceae. It is mainly produced in Hebei Province, Shanxi Province and Inner Mongolia Autonomous Region in China, collected in late autumn, dried, cut into thick sections and used raw. It has a slight odor and tastes slightly bitter.

【性味归经 / Medicinal properties】

甘、涩，平。归心、肺经。

Sweet, astringent and neutral; act on the heart and lung meridians.

【主要功效 / Medicinal efficacies】

固表止汗。

Consolidate the exterior and arrest sweating.

【临床应用 / Clinical application】

自汗、盗汗 本品味涩收敛，主入肺经，功专敛肺固表止汗。用治气虚自汗，常与黄芪、牡蛎等同用。用治阴虚盗汗，常与生地黄、五味子、当归等同用。用治产后虚汗不止，多与当归、黄芪等配伍。

Spontaneous sweating and night sweating With the nature of astringent and acting on the lung meridian, *má huáng gēn* has the functions of exterior-consolidating and sweat-arresting. To treat spontaneous sweating due to qi deficiency, it is usually combined with *huáng qí* (Astragali Radix) and *mǔ lì* (Ostreae Concha); to treat night sweating due to yin deficiency, it is usually used with *shēng dì huáng*, *wǔ wèi zǐ* (Schisandrae Chinensis Fructus) and *dāng guī*; to treat postpartum incessant sweating of deficiency, it is often combined with *dāng guī* and *huáng qí*.

此外，本品配伍牡蛎共研细末，撒扑于身上，可治各种虚汗证。

In addition, to treat sweating of deficiency pattern, it can be ground into powder with *mǔ lì* and

医药大学堂
WWW.YIYAODXT.COM

dusted on the body for topical application.

【用法用量 / Usage and dosage】

煎服，3~9g。外用适量，研粉撒扑。

Decoction, 3-9g. Appropriate amount for external application, and it should be ground into powder and dusted on the body.

【使用注意 / Precaution】

有表邪者忌用。

It should be contraindicated in patients with exterior pathogen.

【现代研究 / Modern research】

本品主要含麻黄根碱 A、麻黄根碱 B、麻黄根碱 C、麻黄根碱 D、阿魏酰组胺等生物碱类，尚含麻黄宁 A、麻黄宁 B、麻黄宁 C、麻黄宁 D 和麻黄酚等双黄酮类。具有止汗、降血压、兴奋呼吸、扩张血管等作用。

It mainly contains various alkaloids, such as ephedrine A, B, C, D and feruloylhistamine, and also contains biflavonoids, such as epinine A, B, C, D and ephedrol. It has the functions of arresting sweating, descending blood pressure, exciting breath and vasodilation.

第二节　敛肺涩肠药

Section 2　Lung-intestine astringing medicinals

本类药物味多酸涩，主入肺、大肠经，以敛肺止咳喘或涩肠止泻痢为主要作用。主要用于肺虚喘咳，久治不愈或肺肾两虚之虚喘；脾肾阳虚或大肠虚寒，不能固摄之久泻、久痢。

This kind of medicinals have a sour and astringent taste and mainly act on the lung and large intestine meridians Its main functions are astringing lung to stop coughing and asthma and astringing intestine to stop diarrhea. It is mainly used for asthma and cough due to deficiency of lung and kidney, and for diarrhea due to deficiency of spleen and kidney yang or deficiency of large intestine.

五味子　*Wǔ wèi zǐ* (Schisandrae Fructus)
《神农本草经》
Shen Nong's Classic of the Materia Medica (Shén Nóng Běn Cǎo Jīng)

【来源 / Origin】

为木兰科植物五味子 *Schisandra chinesis*（Turcz.）Baill. 或华中五味子 *Schisandra sphenanthera* Rehd. et Wils. 的成熟果实。前者习称 "北五味子"，主产于东北；后者习称 "南五味子"，主产于西南及长江流域以南各省。秋季果实成熟时采摘，晒干，生用或醋、蜜拌蒸晒干用。本品果肉气微，味酸；种子破碎后有香气，味辛、微苦。《中国药典》规定，五味子含五味子醇甲（$C_{24}H_{32}O_7$）不得少于 0.40%；南五味子含五味子酯甲（$C_{30}H_{32}O_9$）不得少于 0.20%。

Wǔ wèi zǐ is the mature fruit of *Schisandra chinesis* (Turcz.) Baill. or *Schisandra sphenanthra* Rehd. et Wils., pertaining to Magnoliaceae. The former is habitually called North *wǔ wèi zǐ* and it is mainly produced in northeast of China. The latter is habitually called South *wǔ wèi zǐ* and it is mainly produced in the provinces in southwest China and the south of the Yangtze River basin. The fruit is harvested in autumn when it is ripe, used raw, or steamed after being mixed with vinegar and honey. It has a mild odor and tastes sour. After the seed is crashed, the seed smells fragrant, and tastes acrid and mildly bitter. According to *Chinese Pharmacopoeia*, the content of schisandrin alcohol ($C_{24}H_{32}O_7$) in *Schisandra chinesis* (Turcz) Baill. should be no less than 0.40%; the content of schisandrin A ($C_{30}H_{32}O_9$) in *Schisandra sphenanthera* Rehd. et Wils. should be no less than 0.20%.

【 性味归经 / Medicinal properties 】

酸、甘，温。归肺、心、肾经。

Sour, sweet and warm; act on the lung, heart and kidney meridians.

【 主要功效 / Medicinal efficacies 】

收敛固涩，益气生津，补肾宁心。

Astringe and consolidate; boost qi and promote fluid production, supplement the kidney and calm the heart.

【 临床应用 / Clinical application 】

1. 久咳虚喘　本品酸能收敛，甘能补虚，性温而润，既能敛肺止咳喘，又能益肺气、滋肾阴，为治疗久咳虚喘之要药。用治肺虚久咳，可与罂粟壳同用。用治肺肾两虚喘咳，常与山茱萸、熟地黄、山药同用。用治寒饮咳喘，常配伍麻黄、细辛、干姜等。

(1) Chronic cough and deficiency-type panting *Wǔ wèi zǐ* is astringe, sweet to tonify deficiency, and warm to moisten. It can astringe lung qi to relieve cough and dyspnea, replenish lung qi and enrich kidney yin, so it is an important medicinal to treat chronic cough and deficiency-type panting. To treat chronic cough due to lung deficiency, it is combined with *yīng sù qiào* (Papaveris Pericarpium); to treat panting and cough due to deficiency of both lung and kidney, it is usually combined with *shān zhū yú, shú dì huáng* and *shān yào*; to treat cough and panting due to cold fluid, it is used with *má huáng, xì xīn* (Asari Radix et Rhizoma) and *gān jiāng* (Zingiberis Rhizoma).

2. 自汗，盗汗　本品能益气固表止汗，亦为治疗虚汗证的常用药。用治自汗、盗汗，可与麻黄根、牡蛎等同用。

(2) Spontaneous sweating and night sweating *Wǔ wèi zǐ* can arrest sweating not only by boosting qi to consolidate the exterior and astringe the lung, but also by enriching yin to promote fluid production and astringe sweating. To treat spontaneous sweating and night sweating, it is usually combined with *má huáng gēn* (Ephedrae Radix et Rhizoma) and *mǔ lì*.

3. 遗精，滑精　本品酸甘而温，入肾经，能补肾涩精止遗，适用于肾虚精关不固之遗精、滑精，可与桑螵蛸、附子、龙骨等同用。

(3) Seminal emission, spontaneous seminal emission With the nature of sour, sweet and warm and acting on the spleen meridian, *wǔ wèi zǐ* can supplement the kidney and consolidate essence to arrest enuresis and emission, so it is a common medicinal for seminal emission and spontaneous seminal emission due to kidney deficiency, often combined with *sāng piāo xiāo* (Mantidis Oötheca), *fù zǐ* (Aconiti Lateralis Radix Praeparata) and *lóng gǔ* (Draconis Os).

4. 久泻不止　本品能涩肠止泻。用治脾肾虚寒，久泻不止，常与补骨脂、肉豆蔻、吴茱萸等同用。

(4) Chronic diarrhea It can astringe intestines and stop diarrhea and be used to treat chronic diarrhea due to deficiency-cold of the spleen and kidney combined with *bǔ gǔ zhī, ròu dòu kòu* (Myristicae Semen) and *wú zhū yú* (Evodiae Fructus).

5. **津伤口渴，消渴** 本品酸甘，有益气生津止渴之功。用治热伤气阴，汗多口渴，常与人参、麦冬等同用。用治阴虚内热，口渴多饮之消渴，多与山药、知母、天花粉等同用。

(5) Thirst due to fluid consumption With the nature of sour and sweet, it has the functions of invigorating qi, promoting body fluid and relieving thirst. To treat profuse sweating and thirst due to heat damaging qi-yin, it is often combined with *rén shēn* and *mài dōng*; to treat consumptive thirst manifested as thirst and polydipsia, induced by yin deficiency with internal heat, it is usually combined with *shān yào* (Dioscoreae Rhizoma), *zhī mǔ* (Anemarrhenae Rhizoma) and *tiān huā fěn* (Trichosanthis Radix).

6. **心悸，失眠，多梦** 本品既能补益心肾，又能宁心安神。用治阴血亏损，心神失养，或心肾不交之虚烦心悸、失眠多梦，常与麦冬、当归、酸枣仁等同用。

(6) Palpitation, insomnia and profuse dreaming With the functions of not only nourishing the heart and kidney, but also calming the heart and mind, it can be used to treat palpitation, insomnia and profuse dreaming due to yin-blood depletion, or non-interaction between the heart and kidney, it is usually combined with *mài dōng*, *dāng guī* and *suān zǎo rén*.

【用法用量 / Usage and dosage】

煎服，2~6g。

Decoction, 2-6g.

【使用注意 / Precaution】

凡表邪未解，内有实热，咳嗽初起，麻疹初期者均不宜用。

It is not suitable for those suffering unreleased exterior pathogen, internal excess heat, early stage of cough and measles.

【现代研究 / Modern research】

本品主要含五味子甲素和乙素、五味子醇甲和醇乙等，尚含挥发油、有机酸、鞣质、维生素、多糖等。具有保肝、镇静、催眠、抗衰老、增强免疫、镇咳、祛痰、抑菌、抗氧化等作用。

It mainly contains schisandrin A, B, schisandrin alcohol A, B, etc., and also contains volatile oil, organic acid, tannin, vitamins, polysaccharides, etc. It has the functions of liver protection, sedation, hypnosis, anti-aging, strengthening immunity, antitussive, expectorant, bacteriostatic, antioxidant, etc.

乌梅 *Wū méi* (Mume Fructus)

《神农本草经》

Shen Nong's Classic of the Materia Medica (Shén Nóng Běn Cǎo Jīng)

【来源 / Origin】

为蔷薇科植物梅 *Prunus mume*（Sieb.）Sieb.et Zucc. 的干燥近成熟果实。主产于浙江、福建、云南等地。夏季果实近成熟时采收，低温烘干，生用或炒炭用。本品气微，味极酸。《中国药典》规定，含枸橼酸（$C_6H_8O_7$）不得少于 12.0%。

Wū méi is the nearly matured fruit of *Prunus mume* (Sieb.) Sieb.et Zucc., pertaining to Rosaceae. It is mainly produced in Zhejiang, Fujian and Yunnan and other places in China. The fruit is collected when it is nearly ripe in summer, dried at low temperature and used raw or stir-fried to scorch. It has a slight odor and an extremely sour taste. According to *Chinese Pharmacopoeia*, the content of citric acid ($C_6H_8O_7$) should be no less than 12.0%.

【性味归经 / Medicinal properties】

酸、涩，平。归肝、脾、肺、大肠经。

Sour, astringent and neutral; act on the live, spleen, lung and large intestine meridians.

【主要功效 / Medicinal efficacies】

敛肺止咳，涩肠止泻，安蛔止痛，生津止渴。

Astringe the lung to stop cough and astringe the intestine to arrest diarrhea; calm roundworms to relieve pain; promote fluid production to stop thirst.

【临床应用 / Clinical application】

1. 肺虚久咳　本品酸涩收敛，入肺经，能敛肺止咳。用治肺虚久咳少痰或干咳无痰，可与罂粟壳、杏仁等同用。

(1) **Chronic cough due to lung deficiency**　It is astringent and sour and acting on the lung meridian, so it can restrain the lung qi to stop coughing. To treat chronic cough with little phlegm or dry cough without phlegm, it is often combined with *yīng sù qiào* and *kǔ xìng rén*.

2. 久泻，久痢　本品入大肠经，又有良好的涩肠止泻作用。用治久泻久痢，多与罂粟壳、诃子等同用。用治湿热泻痢，可与黄连、黄柏等同用。

(2) **Chronic diarrhea or chronic dysentery**　It can act on the large intestine meridian and has a good effect of astringent bowel to stop diarrhea. To treat chronic diarrhea or chronic dysentery, it is often combined with *yīng sù qiào* and *hē zǐ*; to treat diarrhea due to damp-heat, it is often combined with *huáng bó* (Phellodendri Chinensis Cortex) and *huáng lián* (Coptidis Rhizoma).

3. 蛔厥腹痛，呕吐　蛔虫得酸则静，本品味极酸，具有安蛔止痛、和胃止呕的功效。用治蛔虫引起的腹痛、呕吐、四肢厥冷之蛔厥病证，常与细辛、川椒、黄连等同用。

(3) **Vomiting, abdominal pain and syncope due to roundworms**　Roundworms become static when it gets acid. *Wū méi* tastes extremely sour, so it is good at calming roundworms with the effect of relieving pain and stomach nausea. To treat abdominal pain, vomiting and cold limbs caused by roundworms, it is often combined with *xì xīn* (Asari Radix et Rhizoma), *chuān jiāo* and *huáng lián*.

4. 虚热消渴　本品味酸性平，善生津液，止烦渴。用治虚热消渴，可单用煎服，或与天花粉、麦冬、人参等同用。

(4) **Deficiency-heat and consumptive thirst**　With the nature of sour and neutral, it is good at promoting the production of body fluids and quenching vexing thirst. To treat thirst due to deficiency-heat, it is decocted alone for oral administration, or combined with *tiān huā fěn*, *mài dōng* and *rén shēn*.

此外，本品炒炭后能收敛止血，可用于崩漏不止、便血等；外敷能消疮毒，可治胬肉外突、头疮等。

In addition, *wū méi* can astringe and stop bleeding, so it is used to treat metrorrhagia, metrostaxis and bloody stool. It can resolve sore toxin in topical application, so it is used to treat pterygium and head sores.

【用法用量 / Usage and dosage】

煎服，6~12g，大剂量可用至30g。外用适量，捣烂或炒炭研末外敷。止泻、止血宜炒炭用。

Decocting, 6-12g; the maximum dosage can reach 30g. Appropriate amount for external use, mashed, stir-fried to scorch or ground into powder. To stop diarrhea and bleeding, it should be stir-fried to scorch.

【使用注意 / Precaution】

外有表邪或内有实热积滞者均不宜服。

It is not suitable for those suffering exterior pathogen or internal excess heat accumulation and stagnation.

【现代研究 / Modern research】

本品主要含苹果酸、枸橼酸、琥珀酸、酒石酸、齐墩果酸、谷甾醇、熊果酸、油菜甾醇、豆甾醇及胆甾醇等。具有镇咳、止血、止泻、驱虫、抑菌、抗肿瘤、抗过敏等作用。

Wū méi mainly contains malic acid, citric acid, succinic acid, tartaric acid, oleanolic acid, sitosterol, ursolic acid, brassinol, stigmasterol and cholesterol, etc. It has the functions of antitussive, hemostasis, antidiarrheal, insect repellent, bacteriostatic, antitumor and antiallergic.

肉豆蔻 *Ròu dòu kòu* (Myristicae Semen)
《药性论》
Treatise on Medicinal Properties (Yào Xìng Lùn)

【来源 / Origin】

为肉豆蔻科植物肉豆蔻 *Myristica fragrans* Houtt 的干燥种仁。主产于马来西亚、印度尼西亚，我国广东、广西、云南亦有栽培。冬、春二季果实成熟时采收，干燥，煨制去油用。本品气香浓烈，味辛。《中国药典》规定，含挥发油不得少于 6.0%（ml/g）；含去氢二异丁香酚（$C_{20}H_{22}O_4$）不得少于 0.10%。

Ròu dòu kòu is the mature seed of *Myristica fragrans* Houtt, pertaining to Houtt. It is mainly produced in Malaysia and Indonesia, and also cultivated in Guangdong, Guangxi Zhuang Autonomous Region and Yunnan in China. The fruits are collected in winter and spring when they are ripe. It has strong fragrance and pungent taste. The seed is dried after the shell is removed, and used after being roasted and deoiled. According to *Chinese Pharmacopoeia*, the content of volatile oil should be no less than 6.0% (ml/g); the content of dehydroisobutanol ($C_{20}H_{22}O_4$) should be no less than 0.10%.

【性味归经 / Medicinal properties】

辛，温。归脾、胃、大肠经。

Acrid and warm; act on the spleen, stomach and large intestine meridians.

【主要功效 / Medicinal efficacies】

涩肠止泻，温中行气。

Astringe intestines and arrest diarrhea; warm the middle energizer and move qi.

【临床应用 / Clinical application】

1. 久泻久痢　本品辛温而涩，既能涩肠止泻，又能温暖脾胃，为治疗虚寒性泻痢之要药。用治脾胃虚寒之久泻、久痢，常与党参、白术、干姜等同用。用治脾肾阳虚，五更泄泻，常与补骨脂、五味子、吴茱萸等同用。

(1) Chronic diarrhea or chronic dysentery　With the nature of acrid and warm, it has a good effect of astringent bowel to stop diarrhea and warm the spleen and stomach, so it is an important medicinal to treat diarrhea and dysentery due to cold-deficiency. To treat chronic diarrhea or chronic dysentery, it is often combined with *dǎng shēn* (Codonopsis Radix), *bái zhú* (Atractylodis Macrocephalae Rhizoma) and *gān jiāng* (Zingiberis Rhizoma). To treat diarrhea before dawn due to spleen and kidney yang deficiency, it is often used with *bǔ gǔ zhǐ*, *wǔ wèi zǐ* and *wú zhū yú*.

2. 胃寒胀痛，食少呕吐　本品辛香温燥，能温中散寒，行气止痛，开胃进食。用治胃寒气滞、脘腹胀痛、食少呕吐等，常与木香、干姜、半夏等同用。

(2) Distending pain due to stomach cold, eating less and vomiting　With the nature of spicy, warm and dry, it can warm middle energizer and disperse cold, promote qi to relieve pain and stimulate appetite. To treat stomach cold and qi stagnation, abdominal distention and pain, less food and vomiting, it is often used with *mù xiāng* (Aucklandiae Radix), *gān jiāng* and *bàn xià* (Pinelliae Rhizoma).

【用法用量 / Usage and dosage】

煎服，3~10g。内服须煨熟去油用。

Decoction, 3-10g; it should be roasted and deoiled for oral administration.

【使用注意 / Precaution】

湿热泻痢者忌用。

It is not suitable for those suffering from diarrhea due to damp heat.

【现代研究 / Modern research】

本品主要含去氢二异丁香酚、香桧烯、α−蒎烯、β−蒎烯、γ−松油烯、肉豆蔻醚等挥发油，尚含脂肪油、蛋白质、色素、脂肪酶及三萜皂苷等。具有止泻、镇痛、抗炎、减慢心率、抗肿瘤、抗氧化、保肝等作用。

It mainly contains dehydroisobutanol, sabinene, α-pinene, β-pinene, γ-terpinene, nutmeg ether and other volatile oils, also fat oil, protein, pigment, lipase and triterpenoid saponins. It has the functions of anti diarrhea, analgesia, anti-inflammatory, slowing down heart rate, anti-tumor, anti-oxidation and liver protection, etc.

诃子　*Hē zǐ* (Chebulae Fructus)
《药性论》
Treatise on Medicinal Properties (Yào Xìng Lùn)

【来源 / Origin】

为使君子科植物诃子 *Terminalia chebula* Retz. 或绒毛诃子 *Terminalia chebula* Retz.var. *tomentella* Kurt. 的干燥成熟果实。主产于云南、广东、广西等地。秋、冬二季果实成熟时采收，晒干，生用或煨用。若用果肉，则去核。本品气微，味酸涩后甜。

Hē zǐ is the dried and mature fruit of *Terminalia chebula* Retz. or *Terminalia chebula* Retz. var. *tomentella* Kurt., pertaining to the Combreaceae. It is mainly produced in Yunnan, Guangdong, Guangxi Zhang Autonomous Region and other places in China. The fruits are collected when they are ripe in autumn and winter, dried in the sun and used raw or roasted. The pulp is used by removing the core. It has a slight odor and sour and sweet taste.

【性味归经 / Medicinal properties】

苦、酸、涩，平。归肺、大肠经。

Bitter, sour, astringent and neutral; act on the lung and large intestine meridians.

【主要功效 / Medicinal efficacies】

涩肠止泻，敛肺止咳，降火利咽。

Astringe intestines to arrest diarrhea, astringing the lung to stop cough; purge fire to open voice.

【临床应用 / Clinical application】

1. 久泻久痢　本品酸涩收敛，入大肠经，善涩肠止泻，为治疗久泻、久痢之常用药。若治久泻、久痢属虚寒者，常与干姜、罂粟壳、陈皮配伍。若治泻痢日久，中气下陷之脱肛，可与人参、黄芪、升麻等同用。若治肠风下血，可配伍防风、秦艽、白芷等。

(1) Chronic diarrhea or chronic dysentery　With the nature of sour and astringent and acting on the large intestine meridian, it has a good effect of astringent bowel to stop diarrhea, so it is an important medicinal to treat diarrhea and dysentery. To treat chronic diarrhea or chronic dysentery due to deficiency-cold, it is often combined with *gān jiāng* (Zingiberis Rhizoma), *yīng sù qiào* and *chén pí* (Citri Reticulatae

Pericarpium); to treat prolapse of the anus due to sinking of middle qi, it is often combined with *rén shēn*, *huáng qí* and *shēng má* (Cimicifugae Rhizoma); to treat bleeding due to intestine-wind, it is often combined with *fáng fēng* (Saposhnikoviae Radix), *qín jiāo* (Gentianae Macrophyllae Radix) and *bái zhǐ*.

2. 久咳，失音　本品生用偏凉，既能敛肺下气止咳，又能清肺利咽开音，为治失音之要药。用治肺虚久咳、失音，可与人参、五味子等同用。用治痰热郁肺，久咳失音，多与桔梗、甘草等同用。用治久咳失音，咽喉肿痛，常与硼酸、青黛、冰片等配伍。

(2) Chronic cough and aphonia　With the nature of cool for raw, it can not only astringe lung and descend qi to stop cough, but also clear the lung and relieve sore-throat to restore voice. It is an essential medicine for the treatment of aphonia. To treatment chronic cough and aphasia due to deficiency of lung, it is often combined with *rén shēn* and *wǔ wèi zǐ*; to treat chronic cough and aphasia due to phlegm-heat and lung stagnation, it is often combined with *jié gěng* (Platycodonis Radix) and *gān cǎo* (Glycyrrhizae Radix et Rhizoma); to treat chronic cough, aphonia and sore throat, it is often combined with *péng shā* (Borax), *qīng dài* (Indigo Naturalis) and *bīng piàn* (Borneolum Syntheticum).

【用法用量 / Usage and dosage】

煎服，3~10g。涩肠止泻宜煨用，敛肺清热、利咽开音宜生用。

Decoction, 3-10g; it is suitable to use the roasted form for astringing bowel to stop diarrhea; and the raw form for astringing lung and clearing heat to relieve sore-throat and restore voice.

【使用注意 / Precaution】

外有表邪、内有湿热积滞者忌用。

It can not be used for those suffering from exterior pathogen and interior dampness and heat stagnation.

【现代研究 / Modern research】

本品主要含大量鞣质（可达 20%~40%），其主要成分为诃子酸、诃黎勒酸、原诃子酸等，尚含诃子素、鞣酸酶、番泻苷 A 等。具有收敛、止泻、抑制气管平滑肌收缩、抑菌、强心、抗氧化、抗肿瘤等作用。

It mainly contains a large amount of tannins (up to 20%-40%), and the main components are chebulic acid, terminalia acid, protochebulic acid, etc., and also contains chebulin, tannase, and sennoside A, etc. It has the functions of astringent, antidiarrheal, inhibiting contraction of tracheal smooth muscle, bacteriostatic, cardiotonic, antioxidant and antitumor, etc.

第三节　固精缩尿止带药

Section 3　Essence-securing, urination-reducing and leukorrhagia-arresting medicinals

本类药物味多酸涩，主入肾、膀胱经，以固精、缩尿、止带为主要作用，某些甘温之品兼有补肾之功，主要用于肾虚不固所致的遗精滑精、遗尿尿频以及带下清稀等。

This kind of medicinals have a sour and astringent taste and mainly act on the kidney and gallbladder meridians. Its main functions are essence-securing, urination-reducing and leukorrhagia-arresting. Some sweet and warm ones have the function of invigorating the kidney. It is mainly used for seminal emission, spontaneous seminal emission, enuresis, frequent urination and morbid leukorrhea caused by deficiency of kidney.

山茱萸　*Shān zhū yú* (Corni Fructus)
《神农本草经》
Shen Nong's Classic of the Materia Medica (*Shén Nóng Běn Cǎo Jīng*)

【来源 / Origin】

为山茱萸科植物山茱萸 *Cornus officinalis* Sieb.et Zucc. 的成熟果肉。主产于浙江、河南、安徽等地。秋末冬初果实变红时采收，干燥，生用或酒制用。本品气微，味酸、涩、微苦。《中国药典》规定，含莫诺苷（$C_{17}H_{26}O_{11}$）和马钱苷（$C_{17}H_{26}O_{10}$）的总量不得少于 1.2%；酒萸肉不得少于 0.70%。

Shān zhū yú is the mature pulp of *Cornus officinalis* Sieb.et Zucc., pertaining to Cornaceae.It is mainly produced in Zhejiang, Henan and Anhui Province in China, collected when the fruit turns red at the end of autumn and the beginning of winter. The fruit is dried and used raw or prepared with wine. It has a slight odor and tastes sour, astringent and bitter. According to *Chinese Pharmacopoeia*, the total content of monetin ($C_{17}H_{26}O_{11}$) and loganin ($C_{17}H_{26}O_{10}$) should be no less than 1.2%, while no less than 0.70% in the wine processed evodia rutae carpa.

【性味归经 / Medicinal properties】

酸、涩，微温。归肝、肾经。

Sour, astringent and slightly warm; act on the liver and kidney meridians.

【主要功效 / Medicinal efficacies】

补益肝肾，收敛固涩。

Tonify the liver and kidney, rescue from desertion with astringency.

【临床应用 / Clinical application】

1. 肝肾亏虚证　本品酸温质润，温而不燥，补而不峻，既能补肾益精，又可温肾助阳，为平补肝肾阴阳之要药。用治肝肾阴虚，头晕目眩、腰酸耳鸣，常与熟地黄、山药等配伍。用治肾阳不足，腰膝冷痛，小便不利或频数，常与肉桂、附子等同用。用治肾虚阳痿，多与鹿茸、补骨脂、淫羊藿等配伍。

(1) Deficiency of liver and kidney syndrome　*Shān zhū yú* is sour and astringent in flavor slightly warm in property and moistening in texture. It is warm but not dry, and it is supplementing but not drastic. It is good at supplementing and boosting the liver and the kidney, and it not only boosts essence, but also assists yang, so it is an important medicinal for neutrally supplementing yin and yang. To treat yin deficiency of the liver and the kidney manifested as vertigo, blurred vision, lumbar soreness and tinnitus, it is usually used with *shú dì huáng* and *shān yào*; to treat declined cold pain in the loins and the knees and disturbance of urination due to deficiency of kidney yang, it is often combined with *ròu guì* and *fù zǐ*; to treat impotence due to kidney deficiency, it is usually combined with *lù róng*, *bǔ gǔ zhī* and *yín yáng huò* (Epimedii Herba).

2. 遗精滑精，遗尿尿频　本品既能补肾益精，又能固精缩尿，为益肾固精止遗之要药。用治肾虚精关不固，遗精滑精，常与熟地黄、山药等同用。用治肾虚膀胱失约，遗尿尿频，多与覆盆子、金樱子、沙苑子等同用。

(2) Seminal emission, spontaneous seminal emission, enuresis and frequent urination　*Shān zhū yú* can not only tonify the kidney and essence, but also secure essence and reduce urination. To treat kidney deficiency failing to consolidate essence gate manifested as seminal emission and spontaneous seminal emission, it is usually combined with *shú dì huáng* and *shān yào*. To treat urinary bladder failing to ensure retention due to kidney deficiency manifested as enuresis and frequent urination, it is usually combined with *fù pén zǐ* (Rubi Fructus), *jīn yīng zǐ* (Rosae Laevigatae Fructus) and *shā yuàn zǐ* (Astragali Complanati Semen).

3．崩漏带下，月经过多　本品入下焦，能补肝肾、固冲任以止血止带。用治肝肾亏损，冲任不固之崩漏及月经过多，常与熟地黄、白芍、当归等同用。用治脾气虚弱，冲任不固而漏下不止，常与龙骨、黄芪、五味子等同用。用治带下不止，可与芡实、煅龙骨等配伍。

(3) Metrorrhagia and metrostaxis, abnormal vaginal discharge and profuse menstruation　It enters the lower energizer and can nourish the liver and kidney, secure thoroughfare and conception vessels to stop bleeding. To treat deficiency of the liver and the kidney manifested as metrorrhagia and metrostaxis and profuse menstruation, it is usually combined with *shú dì huáng*, *dāng guī* and *bái sháo* (Paeoniae Alba Radix); to treat metrostaxis due to spleen qi deficiency and insecurity of thoroughfare and conception vessels, it is often combined with *lóng gǔ*, *huáng qí* and *wǔ wèi zǐ*; to treat abnormal vaginal discharge, it can be combined with *qiàn shí* (Euryales Semen) and *duàn lóng gǔ*.

4．大汗不止，体虚欲脱　本品能收敛止汗，补虚固脱。用治大汗欲脱或久病虚脱，常与人参、附子、龙骨等同用。

(4) Desertion due to profuse sweating　It is astringent and can stop perspiration and tonify deficiency and rescue from desertion for the emergency. To treat prostration due to profuse sweating or chronic disease collapse, it is often combined with *rén shēn*, *fù zǐ* and *lóng gǔ*.

此外，本品亦治肝肾阴虚，内热消渴，多与生地黄、天花粉等同用。

In addition, it also can be used to treat deficiency of liver and kidney yin, internal heat and consumptive thirst in combination with *shēng dì huáng* and *tiān huā fěn*.

【用法用量 / Usage and dosage】

煎服，6~12g，救急固脱 20~30g。

Decoction, 6-12g; to rescue from desertion for the emergency, 20-30g.

【使用注意 / Precaution】

素有湿热而致小便淋涩者不宜服用。

It is not proper for difficult or continuous dribbling urination due to retained damp-heat.

【现代研究 / Modern research】

本品主要含山茱萸苷、乌索酸、莫罗忍冬苷、7-O-甲基莫罗忍冬苷、獐牙菜苷、番木鳖苷等，尚含没食子酸、苹果酸、酒石酸、原维生素 A 以及皂苷、鞣质等。具有免疫调节、强心、升压、降血糖、抗心律失常、抑菌、抗肿瘤、改善认知能力、防治骨质疏松等作用。

It mainly contains cornoside, ursolic acid, molobioside, 7-O-methyl molobioside, swertide, muscarinic turtle glycoside, etc., and gallic acid, malic acid, tartaric acid, protovitamin A, saponin and tannin, etc. It has the functions of immunoregulation, cardiotonic, pressor, hypoglycemic, antiarrhythmic, bacteriostatic, antitumor, cognitive improvement, prevention and treatment of osteoporosis.

桑螵蛸　*Sāng piāo xiāo* (Mantidis Oötheca)

《神农本草经》

Shen Nong's Classic of the Materia Medica (Shén Nóng Běn Cǎo Jīng)

【来源 / Origin】

为螳螂科昆虫大刀螂 *Tenodera sinensis* Saussure、小刀螂 *Statilia maculata*（Thunberg）或巨

斧螳螂 *Hierodula patellifera*（Serville）的干燥卵鞘。分别习称"团螵蛸""长螵蛸"及"黑螵蛸"。全国大部分地区均产。深秋至次春采集，蒸至虫卵死后，干燥。本品气微腥，味淡或微咸。

Sāng piāo xiāo is the ootheca of *Tenodera sinensis* Saussure, *Statilia maculata* (Thunberg) or *Hierodula patellifera* (Serville), pertaining to Mantidae, which are habitually called *tuán piāo xiāo, cháng piāo xiāo* and *hēi piāo xiāo* respectively. It is produced in most areas of China, and collected from late autumn to next spring. For application, it is boiled to kill the eggs, or it is steamed and dried in the sun. It smells slightly fishy, and tastes bland or slightly salty.

【性味归经 / Medicinal properties】

甘、咸，平。归肝、肾经。

Sweet, salty and neutral; act on the liver and kidney meridians.

【主要功效 / Medicinal efficacies】

固精缩尿，补肾助阳。

Consolidate essence and reduce urination; supplement the kidney and assist yang.

【临床应用 / Clinical application】

1. **遗精滑精，遗尿尿频，白浊**　本品甘咸入肾，性收敛，既能固精缩尿，又兼补肾阳，尤以缩尿止遗见长，常用治肾虚遗尿尿频、遗精滑精等。用治小儿遗尿，可单用为末，米汤送服。用治肾虚遗精、滑精，常与龙骨、五味子、制附子等同用。用治心神恍惚，小便频数，遗尿，白浊，可与远志、龙骨、石菖蒲等配伍。

(1) Seminal emission, spontaneous seminal emission, enuresis, frequent urination, white and turbid urine　With the nature of sweet, salty, astringent and acting on the kidney meridian, it can not only consolidate essence and reduce urination, but also nourish the kidney yang and is especially good at treating the former. It is often used to treat enuresis, frequent urination, seminal emission and spontaneous seminal emission due to kidney deficiency. To treat enuresis in children, it is often used alone with the powder form together with rice-water; to treat seminal emission and spontaneous seminal emission due to kidney deficiency, it is often combined with *lóng gǔ, wǔ wèi zǐ* and *zhì fù zǐ* (Aconiti Lateralis Radix Praeparata); to treat mental trance, enuresis, frequent urination, white and turbid urine, it is often combined with *yuǎn zhì* (Polygalae Radix), *lóng gǔ*, and *shí chāng pú* (Acori Tatarinowii Rhizoma).

2. **阳痿**　本品有一定的温补肾阳作用，治疗肾虚阳痿，常与鹿茸、淫羊藿、巴戟天等同用。

(2) Impotence　It has certain effect of warming and tonifying kidney yang, so it can treat impotence due to kidney deficiency with *lù róng* (Cervi Cornu Pantotrichum), *yín yáng huò* (Epimedii Herba) and *bā jǐ tiān* (Morindae Officinalis Radix).

【用法用量 / Usage and dosage】

煎服，6~10g。

Decoction, 6-10g.

【使用注意 / Precaution】

阴虚火旺，膀胱有热而小便频数者忌用。

It should be contraindicated in patients with frequent urination induced by yin deficiency resulting in vigorous fire and damp-heat in the urinary bladder.

【现代研究 / Modern research】

本品主要含蛋白质、脂肪、粗纤维，尚含铁、钙及胡萝卜素样色素等。具有抗利尿、促性腺发育、抗缺氧、抗疲劳、抗氧化、降血糖、降血脂、抗肿瘤等作用。

It mainly contains protein, fat, thick fiber, iron, calcium, and carotene like pigment. It has the functions of antidiuretic, gonadotropic development, anti hypoxia, anti fatigue, antioxidant, hypoglycemic, hypolipidemic and anti-tumor.

海螵蛸 *Hǎi piāo xiāo* **(Sepiae Endoconcha)**

《神农本草经》

Shen Nong's Classic of the Materia Medica (Shén Nóng Běn Cǎo Jīng)

【来源 / Origin】

为乌贼科动物无针乌贼 *Sepiella maindroni* de Rochebrune 或金乌贼 *Sepia esculenta* Hoyle 的干燥内壳。主产于浙江、江苏、广东等地。收集其骨状内壳洗净，干燥，砸成小块，生用。本品气微腥，味微咸。

Hǎi piāo xiāo is the inner shell of *Sepiella maindroni* de Rochebrune or *Sepia esculenta* Hoyle, pertaining to Sepiidae. It is mainly produced in Zhejiang, Jiangsu, Guangdong and other places in China. After the bony inner shell is collected, it is washed clean, dried, smashed into small pieces, and used raw. It smells slightly fishy and taste salty.

【性味归经 / Medicinal properties】

咸、涩，温。归脾、肾经。

Salty, astringent and warm; act on the spleen and kidney meridians.

【主要功效 / Medicinal efficacies】

固精止带，收敛止血，制酸止痛，收湿敛疮。

Astringe essence to arrest vaginal discharge; astringe blood to stanch bleeding; control acid to arrest pain; astringe dampness to heal sores.

【临床应用 / Clinical application】

1. 遗精，带下　本品温涩收敛，有固精止带之功。用治肾虚遗精、滑精，常与山茱萸、菟丝子等同用。用治肾虚带脉不固之带下清稀量多，常与山药、芡实等同用。用治赤白带下，多配伍白芷、血余炭等。

(1) **Seminal emission and vaginal discharge**　With the nature of warm and astringent, it has the functions of consolidating essence to treat vaginal discharge. To treat seminal emission and spontaneous seminal emission due to kidney deficiency, it is often combined with *shān zhū yú* and *tù sī zǐ* (Cuscutae Semen); to treat clear and thin leukorrhea due to kidney deficiency and insecurity of *dài mài*, it is often combined with *shān yào* and *qiàn shí* (Euryales Semen); to treat red and white leukorrhea, it can be used with *bái zhǐ* and *xuè yú tàn* (Crinis Carbonisatus).

2. 崩漏，吐血，便血及外伤出血　本品能收敛止血。用治崩漏，常与茜草、棕榈炭等同用。用治吐血、便血，常与白及等分为末服。用治外伤出血，可单用研末外敷。

(2) **Metrorrhagia and metrostaxis, hematemesis, bloody stool and traumatic bleeding**　It can astringe blood to stanch bleeding. To treat metrorrhagia and metrostaxis, it is often combined with *qiàn cǎo* (Rubiae Radix et Rhizoma) and *zōng lǘ tàn* (Trachycarpi Petiolus Carbonisatus); to treat hematemesis and bloody stool, it is ground with *bái jí* (Bletillae Rhizoma) in equal dosage into powder for oral administration; to treat traumatic bleeding, it can be ground into powder for topical paste.

3. 胃痛吐酸　本品味咸而涩，能制酸止痛，常用于治疗胃酸过多，胃痛吞酸，多与延胡索、白及、瓦楞子等同用。

(3) **Acid regurgitation and stomachache**　With the nature of salty and astringent, it can control acid and relieve pain. It is often used to treat excessive stomach acid, stomachache and acid regurgitation

combined with *yán hú suǒ*, *bái jí* and *wǎ léng zǐ* (Arcae Concha).

4. 湿疮，湿疹，溃疡不敛　本品外用能收湿敛疮。用治湿疮、湿疹，可与黄柏、青黛、煅石膏等研末外敷。用治溃疡多脓，久不愈合，可单用研末外敷，或配伍煅石膏、枯矾、冰片等共研细末，撒敷患处。

(4) Eczema, sore and unclosed ulcer　It can astringe dampness to heal sores. To treat eczema, it can be ground into powder with *huáng bó*, *qīng dài* (Indigo Naturalis) and *duàn shí gāo* (Gypsum Fibrosum Praeparatum) for topical paste; to treat prolonged and unclosed ulcer with profuse pus, it can be used alone or with *duàn shí gāo*, *kū fán* (Dehydratum Alumen) and *bīng piàn*.

【用法用量 / Usage and dosage】
煎服，5~10g。外用适量，研末撒患处。
Decoction, 5-10g. Proper amount for external application with ground powder.

【现代研究 / Modern research】
本品主要含碳酸钙、壳角质、黏液质，尚含多种微量元素，其中含大量的钙，少量的钠、锶、镁、铁以及微量的硅、铝、钛、锰、钡、铜等。具有中和胃酸、保护胃黏膜、抗消化性溃疡、抗肿瘤、抗辐射及接骨等作用。

It mainly contains calcium carbonate, cuticle, mucilaginous, and a variety of trace elements, including a large amount of calcium, a small amount of sodium, strontium, magnesium, iron, and a small amount of silicon, aluminum, titanium, manganese, barium, copper, etc. It has the functions of neutralizing gastric acid, protecting gastric mucosa, resisting peptic ulcer, anti-tumor, anti radiation and bone grafting.

其他收涩药功用介绍见表23-1。

The efficacies of other astringent medicinals are shown in table 23-1.

表23-1　其他收涩药功用介绍

分类	药物	药性	功效	应用	用法用量
固表止汗药	浮小麦	甘，凉。归心经	固表止汗，益气，除热	自汗，盗汗，阴虚发热，骨蒸劳热	煎服，6~12g
	糯稻根	甘，平。归心、肝、肺经	固表止汗，益胃生津，退虚热	自汗，盗汗，骨蒸潮热	煎服，15~30g
敛肺涩肠药	罂粟壳	酸、涩，平；有毒。归肺、大肠、肾经	敛肺，涩肠，止痛	肺虚久咳，久泻久痢，脘腹疼痛，筋骨疼痛	煎服，3~6g。止咳宜蜜炙用，止泻、止痛宜醋炒用
	赤石脂	甘、涩，温。归大肠、胃经	涩肠止泻，收敛止血，敛疮生肌	久泻久痢；崩漏，便血；疮疡久溃，湿疮流水	煎服，9~12g，先煎。外用适量
	石榴皮	酸、涩，温。归大肠经	涩肠止泻，止血，驱虫	久泻久痢，脱肛，便血，崩漏，带下，虫积腹痛	煎服，3~9g。止血多炒炭用
	五倍子	酸、涩，寒。归肺、大肠、肾经	敛肺降火，涩肠止泻，敛汗，固精止遗，止血，收湿敛疮	肺虚久咳，肺热痰咳，久泻久痢，自汗盗汗，遗精滑精，崩漏便血，外伤出血，痈肿疮毒皮肤湿烂	煎服，3~6g

续表

分类	药物	药性	功效	应用	用法用量
固精缩尿止带药	覆盆子	甘、酸，温。归肝、肾、膀胱经	益肾固精缩尿，养肝明目	肾虚不固，遗精滑精，阳痿早泄，肝肾不足，目暗昏花	煎服，6~12g
	莲子	甘、涩，平。归脾、肾、心经	补脾止泻，止带，益肾涩精，养心安神	脾虚泄泻，带下，肾虚遗精滑精，遗尿尿频；心悸失眠	煎服，6~15g
	芡实	甘、涩，平。归脾、肾经	益肾固精，补脾止泻，除湿止带	肾虚遗精滑精，遗尿尿频，脾虚久泻，白浊带下	煎服，9~15g
	金樱子	酸、甘、涩，平。归肾、膀胱、大肠经	固精缩尿，固崩止带，涩肠止泻	遗精滑精，遗尿尿频，崩漏带下，久泻久痢	煎服，6~12g
	椿皮	苦、涩，寒。归大肠、肝经	清热燥湿，收涩止带，止泻，止血	湿热泻痢，久泻久痢；赤白带下，崩漏，便血	煎服，6~9g。外用适量

（高　峰）

题库

第二十四章 涌 吐 药
Chapter 24　Emetic medicinals

PPT

学习目标 | Learning goals

1. **掌握** 涌吐药在性能、功效、主治及使用注意方面的共性。

2. **了解** 涌吐药以及相关功效术语的含义；常山、甜瓜蒂、藜芦的功效以及特殊的用法用量和特殊的使用注意。

1. Master the commonness of emetic medicinals in property, efficacy, indications and cautions.

2. Understand the definitions of emetic medicinals and related terms; the efficacy, special usage and dosage and special precautions of *cháng shān*, *tián guā dì* and *lí lú*.

凡以促使呕吐为主要功效，常用以治疗毒物、宿食、痰涎等停滞胃脘或胸膈以上所致病证的药物，称为涌吐药，又称催吐药。

Medicinals that are used to treat the diseases caused by stagnation in the stomach or above the chest septum of poisons, retained food, phlegm and saliva, with the main effect of inducing vomiting are called emetic medicinals.

涌吐药味多酸、苦，性偏寒凉，归胃经，均具有涌吐功效，通过诱发呕吐，使毒物、宿食、痰涎等迅速排出，以达到治疗疾病的目的。适用于误食毒物，停留胃中，未被吸收；或宿食停滞不化，尚未入肠，胃脘胀痛；或痰涎壅盛，阻于胸膈或咽喉，呼吸喘促；痰浊上蒙清窍所致的癫痫发狂等。

Emetic medicinals are mostly sour and bitter in taste, cold and cool in nature, and has the effect of inducing vomiting through which the poison, retained food, phlegm and saliva can be rapidly discharged, so as to achieve the purpose of disease treatment. It is suitable for ingesting poisons by mistake, which is still in the stomach and not being absorbed; or stagnant food with distending pain in abdomen, or excessive phlegm and saliva obstructed in the throat; or epilepsy and mania caused by clouding of resuscitation by phlegm turbidity.

涌吐药作用强烈，均有毒性，易伤胃气，故只适用于体壮邪实之证。凡体虚之人，或老人、小儿、妇女胎前产后，以及素患失血、头晕、心悸、劳嗽喘咳者等，均应忌用。

Emetic medicinals are toxic and violent in action, and easy to hurt stomach qi, so they are only suitable for the strong body with excess pathogen. It is contraindicated in the cases of the weak, or the elderly, children, the pregnant, women just post-partum, as well as those suffering from blood loss, dizziness, palpitation, pulmonary tuberculosis, or chronic cough, etc.

使用涌吐药时，应注意用量用法。宜从少量渐增，以防中毒或涌吐太过；服药后宜多饮开水以助药力，或用翎毛探喉以助涌吐；如呕吐不止，当采取措施及时解救。

Attention should be paid to the dosage and usage when using the emetics. Generally, the application of emetic medicinals should be increased from small dosage to prevent poisoning or excessive emesis; in order to accelerate vomiting, warm boiled water should be drunk a lot after administration, or use the feather to depress the throat to help emesis; persistent vomiting requires timely measures to rescue.

涌吐药只宜暂用，中病即止，不可连服、久服。吐后当休息，不宜立即进食，待胃肠功能恢复后，再进食流质或易消化的食物，以养胃气。

The emetic medicinals should only be used temporarily, and stopped timely once the pathogens are drained. It should not be taken successively or for a long time. Patients should have a rest after vomiting and not take food immediately. After gastrointestinal function recovers, liquid diet or digestible food should be taken to nourish stomach qi.

因本类药物作用峻猛，药后患者反应强烈、痛苦，故涌吐法现今临床已很少应用。

Because of the violent action and the strong and painful reaction of the patients after administration, the emetics are rarely used in clinic now.

常山　*Cháng shān* (Dichroae Radix)
《神农本草经》
Shen Nong's Classic of the Materia Medica (Shén Nóng Běn Cǎo Jīng)

【来源 / Origin】

为虎耳草科植物常山 *Dichroa febrifuga* Lour. 的干燥根。主产于四川、贵州、湖南等地。秋季采挖，晒干，切片，生用或酒炒用。本品气微，味苦。

Cháng shān is the dry root of *Dichroa febrifuga* Lour., pertaining to Saxifragaceae, mainly produced in Sichuan, Guizhou and Hunan Province, collected in autumn, dried in the sun, sliced, and used raw or stir-fried with wine. It has a slight odor and a bitter taste.

【性味归经 / Medicinal properties】

苦、辛，寒；有毒。归肺、肝、心经。

Bitter, acrid and cold; act on lung, liver and heart meridians.

【主要功效 / Medicinal efficacies】

涌吐痰涎，截疟。

Induce vomiting, and prevent attack of malaria.

【临床应用 / Clinical application】

1. 痰饮停聚，胸膈痞塞　本品生用性善上行，具有较强的催吐作用，能涌吐胸中痰涎。用治胸中痰饮停聚，胸膈痞塞，欲吐不能，常与甘草、白蜜水煎温服。

(1) **Phlegm-fluid retention, stuffiness and fullness in chest and diaphragm**　*Cháng shān* is ascending in nature when it is used in raw form and has a strong action of inducing vomiting and vomiting phlegm-fluid in chest. It treats phlegm-fluid retention, stuffiness and fullness in chest and diaphragm, and nauseous inability in combination with *gān cǎo* (Glycyrrhizae Radix et Rhizoma) decocted with white honey.

2. 疟疾　本品善祛痰而截疟，为治疟之要药。适用于各种疟疾，尤以间日疟和三日疟为佳，可单用浸酒或煎服，或配伍厚朴、槟榔、草豆蔻等。

(2) **Malaria**　*Cháng shān* is good at expelling phlegm and prevent attack of malaria and is an essential medicinal for malaria treatment. It is suitable for all kinds of malaria, especially tertian malaria

and quartan malaria. It can be used only in liquor or decoction, or in combination with *hòu pò* (Magnoliae Officinalis Cortex), *bīng láng* (Arecae Semen) and *cǎo dòu kòu* (Alpiniae Katsumadai Semen).

【用法用量 / Usage and dosage】

煎服，5~9g。入丸、散酌减。涌吐宜生用，截疟宜酒制用。治疟疾宜在寒热发作前半天或2小时服用。

Decoction, 5-9g. It is appropriately reduced in pills or powder. Raw material is used for inducing vomiting while the one stir-fried with alcohol is for checking malaria. Malaria treatment should be taken half a day or two hours before the onset of cold and heat.

【使用注意 / Precaution】

用量不宜过大。孕妇及体虚者不宜用。

The dosage should not be too large. It should not be used by pregnant women or the weak people.

【现代研究 / Modern research】

本品主要含常山碱甲、常山碱乙、常山碱丙、常山次碱、4-喹唑酮、常山素 A、常山素 B 等。具有催吐、抗疟、降压、抗流感病毒、抗阿米巴原虫等作用。

Cháng shān mainly contains dichroine A, B, C, Changshan sub alkali, 4-quinazolone, dichrin A and B. It has the functions of emetic, antimalarial, antihypertensive, anti influenza virus and anti amoeba.

甜瓜蒂 *Tián guā dì* (Pedicellus Melo)
《神农本草经》
Shen Nong's Classic of the Materia Medica (*Shén Nóng Běn Cǎo Jīng*)

【来源 / Origin】

为葫芦科植物甜瓜 *Cucumis melo* L. 的干燥果蒂。全国各地均产。夏、秋二季采收成熟果实，切取果蒂，阴干或晒干，生用或炒用。本品味苦。

Tián guā dì is the dry fruit base of *Cucumis melo* L., pertaining to Cucurbitaceae, produced all over China, collected in summer and autumn, the fruit base cut off, dried in the shade or in the sun, and used raw or stir-fried. It tastes bitter.

【性味归经 / Medicinal properties】

苦、寒；有毒。归胃、胆经。

Bitter, cold and toxic; act on stomach and gallbladder meridians.

【主要功效 / Medicinal efficacies】

涌吐痰食，祛湿退黄。

Induce vomiting, eliminate dampness to remove jaundice.

【临床应用 / Clinical application】

1. **喉痹，癫痫，宿食停滞，食物中毒** 本品味极苦，涌泄之力较强，具有涌吐痰涎、宿食、毒物之功。凡痰涎瘀结胸中所致的癫痫发狂、喉痹喘息，以及宿食停滞胃脘而致胸脘胀痛，或误食毒物不久，尚停留于胃者，可单用本品研末服，或与赤小豆、香豉同用。

(1) **Pharyngitis, epilepsy, stagnation of retained food, food poisoning** *Tián guā dì* is extremely bitter and violent in discharging. It has the action to vomit phlegm and saliva, retained food and poisons. For those who suffer from epilepsy, mania, and pharyngitis caused by phlegm and saliva stagnated in chest, and those with abdominal distending pain caused by retained food in the stomach, or those who are still in the stomach shortly after ingestion of poisons by mistake, it can be used alone and ground into powder for administration, or in combination with *chì xiǎo dòu* (Phaseoli Semen) and *xiāng chǐ* (Sojae

Semen Praeparatum).

2. 湿热黄疸 本品有祛湿退黄的作用。用治湿热黄疸，多单用本品研末吹鼻，令鼻中黄水流出，以引去湿热之邪；或单用本品煎汤内服；或研末送服等，均可收退黄之功。

(2) Dampness-heat jaundice *Tián guā dì* has the action to eliminate dampness and remove jaundice. It treats dampness-heat jaundice alone when it is ground into powder and puffed in nose till some yellow-discharge flows out, so as to remove dampness-heat pathogen; or it is decocted alone for oral taking; or it is ground into powder for administration, all to remove jaundice.

【用法用量 / Usage and dosage】

煎服，2.5~5g；入丸、散服，每次 0.3~1g。外用适量，研末吹鼻，待鼻中流出黄水即停药。

Decoction, 2.5-5g; 0.3-1g for pill or powder. An appropriate dosage for external use, puff through nose till yellow water flows out.

【使用注意 / Precaution】

体虚、胃弱、吐血、咯血、心脏病、上部无实邪者及孕妇忌用。

It is contraindicated in patients with a weak constitution, weakness of stomach, hematemesis, hemoptysis, heart disease, or no pathogenic excess in the upper part, and in pregnant women.

【现代研究 / Modern research】

本品主要含葫芦素 B、葫芦素 D、葫芦素 E（即甜瓜素或甜瓜毒素）、异葫芦素 B 及葫芦素 B 苷，尚含皂苷、氨基酸等。具有催吐、抗肝损伤、降压、抑制心肌收缩力、减慢心率、退黄疸、治疗慢性乙型肝炎及肝硬化等作用。

Tián guā dì mainly contains cucurbitacin B, D, E (i.e., cucurbitacin or melon toxin), isocucurbitacin B and cucurbitacin B glycosides, saponins, and amino acids, etc. It has the functions of emetic, anti liver injury, depressurization, inhibiting myocardial contractility, slowing down of heart rate, removing jaundice, treating chronic hepatitis B and cirrhosis.

其他涌吐药功用介绍见表 24-1。

The efficacies of other emetic medicinals are shown in table 24-1.

表 24-1 其他涌吐药功用介绍

分类	药物	药性	功效	应用	用法用量
涌吐药	藜芦	苦、辛，寒；有毒。归肺、肝、胃经	涌吐风痰，杀虫	中风，癫痫，喉痹，误食毒物；疥癣、白秃，头虱，体虱	入丸、散服，0.3~0.6g，温水送服。外用适量
	胆矾	酸、辛，寒；有毒。归肝、胆经	涌吐痰涎，解毒收湿，祛腐蚀疮	喉痹，癫痫，误食毒物；风眼赤烂，口疮，牙疳；胬肉，疮疡不溃	温水化服，0.3~0.6g。外用适量

（全素安）

第二十五章 攻毒杀虫止痒药

Chapter 25 Medicinals of toxin-eliminating and worms-killing to relieve itching

PPT

学习目标┊ Learning goals

1. **掌握** 攻毒杀虫止痒药在性能、功效、主治、配伍及使用注意方面的共性；硫黄、雄黄、蛇床子的性能、功效、应用以及特殊的用法用量和特殊的使用注意。

2. **了解** 攻毒杀虫止痒药的含义；土荆皮、蜂房、白矾、蟾蜍、大蒜的功效、主治以及特殊的用法用量和特殊的使用注意。

1. Master the commonness on medicinals of toxin-eliminating and worms-killing to relieve itching in efficacy, indications, property, compatibility and cautions; as well as the property, efficacy, application, special usage and dosage and special precautions of *liú huáng*, *xióng huáng* and *shé chuáng zǐ*.

2. Understand the definitions of medicinals of toxin-eliminating and worms-killing to relieve itching; and the efficacy, indications, special usage and dosage and special precautions of *tǔ jīng pí*, *fēng fáng*, *bái fán*, *chán chú* and *dà suàn*.

凡以攻毒疗疮、杀虫止痒为主要功效，常用于治疗疮疡、湿疹、疥癣等病证的药物，称为攻毒杀虫止痒药。本类药物大多有毒，以外用为主，兼可内服，具有攻毒疗疮、杀虫止痒等功效，主治疮痈疔毒、疥癣、湿疹湿疮、蛇虫咬伤等。本类药物外用时，具体方法因病而异，如研末外撒，或煎汤洗渍及热敷、浴泡、含漱，或用油脂及水调敷，或制成软膏涂抹，或制成药捻、栓剂塞于患处，或煎汤熏洗患处等。本类药物内服时，宜作丸、散剂，使其缓慢溶解吸收，且便于掌握剂量。本类药物多具有不同程度的毒性，无论外用或内服，均应严格掌握剂量及疗程，不可过量或持续使用，以防产生毒性和副作用。制剂时应严格遵守炮制和制剂法度，以降低毒性，确保用药安全。

Medicinals with the efficacies of eliminating toxin to heal sore, killing worms to relieve itching and indications of sore, eczema and scabies are known as toxin-eliminating and worms-killing to relieve itching medicinals. Most of them are toxic, so they are mostly applied externally and some can be taken orally. They can be applied in the diseases and syndromes of Surgery, Dermatology and Otorhinolaryngology, such as sores, carbuncles, deep-rooted boils, eczema, and insect or snake bite. These medicinals are mainly for external use, and the specific methods vary according to the diseases, such as grinding into powder and spreading out, or decocting for washing, hot compressing, bathing, gargling, or applying with oil and water, or making into ointment or medicated threads and suppository

医药大学堂
www.yiyaodxt.com

put in the affected area, or washed the affected area with decoction. When this kind of medicinal is taken orally, it should be used as pill or powder for slowly dissolving and absorbing. Because of its toxicity, no matter for external use or internal use, the dosage and courses of treatment should be strictly controlled. Do not overdose or continue to use it to prevent toxic and side effects. In order to reduce the toxicity and ensure the safety of usage, the processing and preparation methods should be strictly followed.

硫黄 *Liú huáng* (Sulfur)
《神农本草经》
Shen Nong's Classic of the Materia Medica (Shén Nóng Běn Cǎo Jīng)

【来源 / Origin】

为自然元素类矿物硫族自然硫。主产于山西、山东、陕西等地。随时采挖，采挖后加热熔化，除去杂质，或用含硫矿物经加工制得。生硫黄只作外用，内服常与豆腐同煮后阴干用。本品有特异的臭气，味淡。《中国药典》规定，含硫（S）不得少于 98.5%。

Liú huáng is the natural ore Sulphur of sulphide mineral and mainly produced in Shanxi, Shandong and Shaanxi Province. It can be collected at any time, heated and melted after mined to remove impurity, or processed with sulfur-containing minerals. Raw one is only for external use; after being boiled with bean curd and dried in shade, it can be taken orally. It has distinctive stink and slight taste. According to *Chinese Pharmacopoeia*, the content of sulfur (S) should be no less than 98.5%.

【性味归经 / Medicinal properties】

酸，温；有毒。归肾、大肠经。

Sour, warm and toxic; act on the kidney and large intestine meridians.

【主要功效 / Medicinal efficacies】

外用解毒疗疮，杀虫止痒；内服补火助阳通便。

External use for resolving toxin and killing worms to relieve itching; internal use for nourishing fire and assisting yang to promote defecation.

【临床应用 / Clinical application】

1. 疥癣，湿疹，阴疽疔疮　本品外用解毒疗疮，杀虫止痒，为治疗疥疮之要药。用治疥疮，可单用研末，麻油调涂。用治湿疹，可单用麻油调涂，或配伍风化石灰、铅丹、轻粉研末，猪油调涂。用治阴痒，可单用，或配伍蛇床子、枯矾等。用治痈疽疮疡，可与雄黄、白矾等研末，外敷患处。

(1) **Acariasis, bald-scalp sore, eczema and scabies**　The external use of *liú huáng* is detoxification to treat scabies, and kill worms to relieve itching, especially to treat scabies. To treat scabies, it can be used alone for grinding and applying with *má yóu*. To treat eczema, it can be used alone or with *má yóu*, or combined with the grinding form of weathered lime, *qiān dān* (Minium) and *qīng fěn* (Calomelas); to treat pruritus vulvae, it can be used alone or combined with *shé chuáng zǐ* (Cnidii Fructus) and *kū fán* (Dehydratum Alumen); to treat eczema and scabies, it is often combined with *xióng huáng* and *bái fán* (Alumen) and ground to powder for applying on the affected area.

2. 阳痿，虚喘冷哮，虚寒便秘　本品内服能补火壮阳通便。用治肾阳不足，阳痿足冷，可与鹿茸、补骨脂、蛇床子等同用。用治肾不纳气之虚寒哮喘，可配伍附子、肉桂、沉香等。用治虚寒便秘，常与半夏同用。

(2) **Impotence, deficiency-type panting and cold asthma, constipation due to deficiency-cold**　*Liú huáng* can replenish fire, invigorate yang and relieve constipation. To treat impotence and

cold foot due to deficiency of kidney yang, it is often combined with *lù róng* (Cervi Cornu Pantotrichum, *bǔ gǔ zhī* (Psoraleae Fructus) and *shé chuáng zǐ* (Cnidii Fructus); to treat deficiency cold asthma due to kidney not holding qi, often combined with *fù zǐ* (Aconiti Lateralis Radix Praeparata), *ròu guì* (Cinnamomi Cortex) and *chén xiāng* (Aquilariae Resinatum Lignum); to treat constipation due to cold of insufficiency, it is often combined with *bàn xià* (Pinelliae Rhizoma).

【用法用量 / Usage and dosage】

外用适量，研末敷或加油调敷患处。内服 1.5~3g，炮制后入丸、散服。

Appropriate amount for external use, apply with the form of grinding or mixing with oil to adjust the affected area; 1.5-3g for internal use in the form of pill or powder after processing and preparation.

【使用注意 / Precaution】

阴虚火旺者及孕妇忌用。不宜与芒硝、玄明粉同用。

It is not suitable for those suffering deficiency of yin and hyperactivity of fire and pregnant women; not suitable to be applied together with *máng xiāo* (Natrii Sulfas) and *xuán míng fěn* (Natrii Sulfas Exsiccatus).

【现代研究 / Modern research】

本品主要含硫，尚含少量砷、硒、铁等。具有杀疥虫、抗细菌和真菌感染、镇咳、抗炎、缓泻等作用。

Liú huáng mainly contains sulfur and a small amount of arsenic, selenium and iron. It has the functions of killing scabies, resisting bacterial and fungal infection, antitussive, anti-inflammatory and diarrhea.

雄黄 *Xióng huáng* (Realgar)
《神农本草经》
Shen Nong's Classic of the Materia Medica (Shén Nóng Běn Cǎo Jīng)

【来源 / Origin】

为硫化物类矿物雄黄族矿石，主含二硫化二砷（As₂S₂）。主产于湖北、湖南、贵州等地。随时采挖，除去杂质，研细粉或水飞，生用。本品有特异的臭气，味淡。《中国药典》规定，含砷量以二硫化二砷计，不得少于 90.0%。

Xióng huáng is the ore of sulphide mineral realgar, and its main ingredient is arsenic disulfide (As_2S_2). It mainly produced in Hubei, Hunan, Guizhou and other places in China. It can be collected at any time and removed impurity, ground into fine powder or refined with water. It has unique odor and light taste. According to *Chinese Pharmacopoeia*, the content of arsenic disulfide should be no less than 90.0%.

【性味归经 / Medicinal properties】

辛，温；有毒。归肝、大肠经。

Acrid, warm and toxic; act on the liver and large intestine meridians.

【主要功效 / Medicinal efficacies】

解毒杀虫，燥湿祛痰，截疟。

Resolve toxin and kill worms; eliminate dampness and phlegm, stop malaria.

【临床应用 / Clinical application】

1. **痈肿疔疮，蛇虫咬伤** 本品有毒，能以毒攻毒，外用、内服均有良好的解毒杀虫作用。用治痈肿疔毒，可单用或入复方，常与白矾等分研末外用。用治痈疽硬肿疼痛，常配伍乳香、没药、麝香等为丸内服。用治蛇虫咬伤，可单用本品粉末，香油调涂患处或用黄酒冲服。

(1) Carbuncle, swollen sore, deep-rooted boil and ulcers, eczema and acariasis, as well as insect or snake bite *Xióng huáng* is toxic and can attack with poison. It has good effects of detoxification and killing worms for external and internal use. It can be used alone or in compound prescription or together with *bái fán* (Alumen); to treat swelling and pain of carbuncle and sore, it is often combined with *rǔ xiāng, mò yào* and *shè xiāng* (Moschus) in pills for oral usage; to treat snake or insect bite, it can be applied to the affected area in the form of powder with oil or prepared with rice wine.

2. 湿疹疥癣 本品有燥湿杀虫止痒之功。用治头癣、体癣、牛皮癣、干癣等多种癣疾，常与全蝎、轻粉、斑蝥等同用。用治热疖、痱、痤、疥、疹、风湿痒疮，常与白矾共为末外用。

(2) Acariasis, bald-scalp sore and eczema It has the function of drying dampness, killing worms and dissolving itching. To treat tinea capitis, tinea corporis, psoriasis, and chronic eczema, it is often combined with *quán xiē, qīng fěn* and *bān máo* (Mylabris); to treat hot boils, acne, scabies, rash, and rheumatic, it is often ground with *bái fán* into powder for external use.

3. 虫积腹痛，惊痫，疟疾 本品内服能杀虫、燥湿祛痰、截疟。传统用治虫积腹痛，惊痫，疟疾等，但现今临床用之甚少。

(3) Abdominal pain due to parasites, epilepsy, malaria *Xióng huáng* can kill worms, eliminate dampness and phlegm and prevent malaria when taken orally. Traditionally, it was used to treat abdominal pain due to parasites, epilepsy, malaria, but now is seldom used.

【用法用量 / Usage and dosage】

外用适量，研末撒敷，或以香油、醋调敷。内服入丸、散，0.05~0.1g。

Appropriate amount for external use, ground into powder or mixed with sesame oil and vinegar. Take in the form of pill or powder internally, 0.05~0.1g.

【使用注意 / Precaution】

内服宜慎，不可久服。外用不宜大面积涂搽及长期使用。孕妇忌用。忌火煅。

It should be used with caution internally and can not be used for a long time. For external use, it is not suitable to apply to large area for a long time. Pregnant women should not use it. Do not calcine it with fire.

【现代研究 / Modern research】

本品主要含二硫化二砷，还有少量有毒成分三氧化二砷，并含少量硅、铅、铁、钙、镁等杂质。具有抑菌、抗肿瘤、抗血吸虫及疟原虫等作用。

Xióng huáng mainly contains arsenic disulfide, and with component of trioxide, and a small amount of silicon, lead, iron, calcium, magnesium and other impurities. It has the functions of bacteriostasis, anti-tumor, anti haemophilus and plasmodium.

蛇床子　*Shé chuáng zǐ* (Cnidii Fructus)
《神农本草经》
Shen Nong's Classic of the Materia Medica (Shén Nóng Běn Cǎo Jīng)

【来源 / Origin】

为伞形科植物蛇床 *Cnidium monnieri*（L.）Cuss. 的干燥成熟果实。全国大部分地区均产。夏、秋二季采收，晒干，生用。本品气香，味辛凉，有麻舌感。《中国药典》规定，含蛇床子素（$C_{15}H_{16}O_3$）不得少于 1.0%。

Shé chuáng zǐ is the mature dry fruit of *Cnidium monieri* (L.) Cuss., pertaining to Umbelliferae. It is produced in most parts of China and collected in summer and autumn when the fruit is ripe and dried in the sun and used raw. It is fragrant in smell, acrid and cool in flavor with a tingling feeling. According to *Chinese Pharmacopoeia*, osthole ($C_{15}H_{16}O_3$) should not be less than 1.0%.

【性味归经 / Medicinal properties】

辛、苦，温；有小毒。归肾经。

Acrid, bitter, warm and slightly toxic; act on the spleen meridian.

【主要功效 / Medicinal efficacies】

杀虫止痒，燥湿祛风，温肾壮阳。

Kill worms and relieve itching; dry dampness and dispel wind; warm the kidney and strengthen yang.

【临床应用 / Clinical application】

1. 阴痒，湿疹，疥癣　本品苦温性燥，外用有燥湿杀虫止痒之功，为治疗瘙痒性皮肤病的常用药。用治妇女阴痒带下，常与白矾共煎汤外洗。现代临床多用治滴虫性阴道炎。用治湿疹瘙痒，可与苦参、黄柏等同用。用治疥癣瘙痒，可单用本品研末，猪脂调之外涂。

(1) Pudendum itching, eczema and pruritus, as well as acariasis　It is bitter, warm and dry and can be used externally to kill worms and dry dampness to relieve itching. It is a commonly used medicinal for pruritus skin diseases. To treat pruritus vulvae andmorbid leucorrhea, it is often decocted with *bái fán* for washing and for modern clinical treatment of trichomonal vaginitis; to treat eczema and pruritus, it is often combined with *kǔ shēn* (Sophorae Flavescentis Radix) and *huáng bó* (Phellodendri Chinensis Cortex); to treat scabies and pruritus, it can be used alone externally in the grinding form with lard oil.

2. 肾虚阳痿，宫冷不孕　本品内服有温肾壮阳、暖宫起痿之功。用治肾阳不足，男子阳痿不育，女子宫冷不孕，常与鹿茸、肉苁蓉、淫羊藿等同用。

(2) Impotence due to kidney deficiency and sterility due to uterus-cold　It has strong function of warming the kidney and uterus and strengthening yang. To treat impotence due to kidney deficiency and sterility due to uterus-cold, it is often combined with *lù róng* (Cervi Cornu Pantotrichum), *ròu cōng róng* (Cistanches Herba) and *yín yáng huò* (Epimedii Herba).

3. 寒湿带下，湿痹腰痛　本品辛散苦燥，性温祛寒，有温阳散寒、燥湿祛风之效。用治寒湿带下，可与山茱萸、鹿茸、海螵蛸等同用。用治湿痹腰痛兼肾阳不足或有寒，常与桑寄生、杜仲、秦艽等同用。

(3) Leukorrhea due to cold damp, and lumbago caused by damp-*bì* syndrome　It has the functions of assisting yang and dissipating cold, drying dampness and dispelling wind. To treat leukorrhea due to cold damp, it is often used with *shān zhū yú* (Corni Fructus), *lù róng* and *hǎi piāo xiāo* (Sepiae Endoconcha); to treat lumbago caused by damp-*bì* syndrome, especially cold-dampness with kidney yang deficiency, it is often combined with *sāng jì shēng* (Taxilli Herba), *dù zhòng* (Eucommiae Cortex) and *qín jiāo* (Gentianae Macrophyllae Radix).

【用法用量 / Usage and dosage】

煎服，3~10g。外用适量，水煎熏洗或研末调敷。

Decoction, 3-10g. Appropriate amount for external use, it is usually decocted to steam and wash or is ground to powder and mixed with water for external application.

【使用注意 / Precaution】

阴虚火旺或下焦有湿热者不宜内服。

It is not advisable to be taken orally for those with fire excess from yin deficiency or those with dampness and heat in the Lower jiao.

【现代研究 / Modern research 】

本品主要含蛇床子素、异虎耳草素、蒎烯、莰烯、异戊酸龙脑酯、异龙脑、甲氧基欧芹酚、佛手柑内酯、二氢山芹醇、当归酸酯等。具有抗炎、杀灭阴道滴虫、抑菌、抗真菌、抗过敏、镇痛、祛痰平喘、降血压、抗骨质疏松等作用。

It mainly contains osthole, iso saxifrage, pinene, camphene, isopentenyl isovalerate, isoborneol, methoxyparshinol, bergamot lactone, dihydrosansyl alcohol and angelic acid ester. It has the functions of anti-inflammatory, killing trichomonas vaginalis, bacteriostatic, anti-fungal, anti-allergic, analgesic, expectorant and antiasthmatic, lowering blood pressure, and resisting osteoporosis.

其他攻毒杀虫止痒药功用介绍见表 25-1。

The efficacies of other medicinals of toxin-eliminating and worms-killing to relieve itching are shown in table 25-1.

表 25-1　其他攻毒杀虫止痒药功用介绍

分类	药物	药性	功效	应用	用法用量
攻毒 杀虫 止痒药	土荆皮	辛，温；有毒。归肺、脾经	杀虫，疗癣，止痒	体癣，头癣，手足癣，疥疮，湿疹，皮炎，皮肤瘙痒	外用适量，醋或酒浸涂，或研末调涂患处
	蜂房	甘，平。归胃经	攻毒杀虫，祛风止痛	疮疡肿痛，乳痈，瘰疬，顽癣瘙痒，鹅掌风，牙痛，风湿痹痛	煎服，3~5g。外服适量，研末油调敷患处，或煎水漱口，或洗患处
	白矾	酸、涩，寒。归肺、脾、肝、大肠经	外用解毒杀虫，燥湿止痒；内服止血止泻，祛除风痰	湿疹，疥癣，痔疮，疮疡，聍耳流脓，便血，吐衄，崩漏，久泻久痢，癫痫发狂	内服，0.6~1.5g，入丸、散剂。外用适量，研末敷或化水洗患处
	蟾蜍	辛，温；有毒。归心经	解毒，止痛，开窍醒神	痈疽疔疮，瘰疬，咽喉肿痛，牙痛，中暑神昏，痧胀腹痛	内服，0.015~0.03g，多入丸、散。外用适量
	大蒜	辛、温。归脾、肺、胃经	解毒杀虫，消肿，止痢	痈肿疮疡，疥癣，肺痨，顿咳，痢疾，泄泻，钩虫病，蛲虫病	煎服，9~15g。外用适量，捣烂外敷，或切片外搽

题库

（叶耀辉）

第二十六章 拔毒化腐生肌药

Chapter 26 Medicinals for removing toxin, resolving putridity and promoting granulation

PPT

学习目标 | Learning goals

1. 掌握 拔毒化腐生肌药在性能、功效、主治及使用注意方面的共性；红粉的性能、功效、应用以及特殊的用法用量和特殊的使用注意。

2. 熟悉 轻粉、砒石、炉甘石、硼砂的功效、主治以及特殊的用法用量和特殊的使用注意。

3. 了解 拔毒化腐生肌药及相关功效术语的含义；铅丹的功效以及特殊的用法用量和特殊的使用注意。

1. Master the commonness of medicinals for removing toxin, resolving putridity and promoting granulation in property, efficacy, indications and cautions; the property, efficacy, application, special usage and dosage and special precautions of *shēng yào*.

2. Familiar with the efficacy, indications, special usage and dosage and special precautions of *qīng fěn, pī shí, lú gān shí* and *péng shā*.

3. Understand the definitions of medicinals for removing toxin, resolving putridity and promoting granulation and related terms; the efficacy, special usage and dosage and special precautions of *qiān dān*.

凡以拔毒祛腐，生肌敛疮为主要功效，常用以治疗痈疽疮疡溃后脓出不畅或久溃不敛等病证的药物，称为拔毒化腐生肌药。

Medicinal with the main effect of removing toxins and resolving putridity, promoting granulation and healing up sores, commonly used to treat pus failing to be expelled after the ulceration of carbuncle sores, or prolonged ulcers, are known as medicinals for removing toxin, resolving putridity and promoting granulation.

拔毒化腐生肌药多为矿石类药物或其加工制品，多有剧毒，以外用为主，具有拔毒化腐、生肌敛疮的功效，主要用于痈疽疮疡溃后脓出不畅或溃后腐肉不去、伤口难以生肌愈合等，也可用于治疗癌肿、梅毒、湿疹、疥癣瘙痒、咽喉肿痛、口舌生疮、目赤翳障、耳疮等。

Most of them are mineral drugs or their processed products, which are highly toxic, mainly for external use with the functions of removing toxin, resolving putridity, promoting granulation and healing up sores. They are mainly used for the treatment of pus failing to be expelled after the ulceration of carbuncle sores, or putrefaction after ulceration, or wounds that are difficult to heal. It can also be used to

467

treat cancer, syphilis, eczema, scabies and pruritus, sore throat, sores in mouth and tongue, red eye with nebula, and ear sores, etc.

本类药物以局部外用为主，方法因病而异，常用方法有研末外撒，或研末加油、加水调敷，或制成软膏药敷贴，或制成药捻外用，或点眼、吹喉、滴耳等。

This type of medicine is mainly for topical external use, and the method varies depending on the disease. Commonly used external methods include powdering and spreading, or powdering and applying oil and water, or making an ointment, or making a medicated thread for external use, or eye dropping, throat blowing, ear dropping, etc.

本类药物多有剧毒和较强的刺激性，为保证用药安全，使用时应严格控制剂量和用法。即使外用亦不宜过量或持续使用，以防中毒。特别是含砷、汞、铅类的药物毒性和副作用尤甚，用药时更应注意安全。

This type of medicine is highly toxic and highly irritating. In order to ensure the safety of medication, the dosage and usage should be strictly controlled. Even for external use, it should not be used excessively or continuously to prevent poisoning. The toxic and side effects of arsenic, mercury, and lead-containing drugs are especially serious, and more attention should be paid to keep safety.

红粉 *Shēng yào* (Hydrargyri Oxydum Rubrum)
《外科大成》
The Great Compendium of External Medicine (Wài Kē Dà Chéng)

【 来源 / Origin 】

由水银、火硝、白矾混合升华而成的红色升华物，又称升药、三仙丹、升丹、小升丹、红升。全国各地均产，以河北、湖北、湖南等地产量较大。研细末入药。本品气微。《中国药典》规定，含氧化汞（HgO）不得少于99%。

Hóng fěn is a red sublimate sublimated by mixture of mercury, saltpeter and alum, also known as *shēng yào, sān xiān dān, shēng dān, xiǎo shēng dān, hóng shēng*. It is produced in all parts of the country, with large output in Hebei, Hubei, and Hunan and ground into fine powder as medicine. It has a slight odor. According to *Chinese Pharmacopoeia*, mercury oxide (HgO) should be no less than 99%.

【 性味归经 / Medicinal properties 】

辛，热；有大毒。归肺、脾经。

Acrid, heat and highly toxic; act on lung and spleen meridians.

【 主要功效 / Medicinal efficacies 】

拔毒，除脓，祛腐，生肌。

Remove toxin, expel pus, resolve putridity, and promote granulation.

【 临床应用 / Clinical application 】

痈疽溃后，脓出不畅，或腐肉不去，新肉不生　本品有大毒，具有良好的拔毒除脓、祛腐生肌作用，为只供外用的外科常用药之一。常与煅石膏研末同用，或撒于患处，或制成药捻填入脓腔，或用药捻插入瘘管中。随病情不同，调整煅石膏与本品的配伍比例，如煅石膏与红粉的用量比为9∶1者，称九一丹，拔毒之力较轻而收敛生肌力较强；用量比为8∶2者，称八二丹，以此类推，可分别配制成七三丹、六四丹、五五丹等。红粉与煅石膏之比为9∶1者，称九转丹，拔毒化腐排脓效力最强。

Poor discharge of pus after ulceration, or deep-rooted carbuncle making new tissue difficult to grow　*Hóng fěn* is highly toxic and has a good effect of removing toxin, expelling pus, resolving putridity, and promoting granulation, and is one of the common surgical drugs for external use. It is often used together with *duàn shí gāo* (Gypsum Fibrosum Praeparatum) ground into powder, or sprinkled on the affected area, or made into a medication thread and inserted into the purulent cavity or into the fistula. The compatibility ratio of the two drugs is usually adjusted according to the different conditions. For example, the dosage ratio of *duàn shí gāo* and *shēng yào* is nine to one which is a formula named *Jiǔ Yī Dān* (Nine-to-one Elixir) with a milder effect of removing toxin and stronger effect of astringing dampness and promoting granulation; if the ratio is eight to two, it is named *Bā Èr Dān* (Eight-to-two Elixir), and so on. It can be made into *Qī Sān Dān* (Seven-to-three Elixir), *Liù Sì Dān* (Six-to-four Elixir), *Wǔ Wǔ Dān* (Five-to-five Elixir), respectively. If the proportion of *hóng fěn* to *duàn shí gāo* is nine to one, it is called *Jiǔ Zhuǎn Dān* which has the strongest action of removing toxin and expelling pus.

此外，本品还可用治湿疹、黄水疮、顽癣、梅毒等。

In addition, *hóng fěn* can also be indicated externally for eczema, yellow water sore, stubborn tinea and syphilis.

【用法用量 / Usage and dosage】

外用适量。本品只供外用，不能内服，且不用纯品，多配伍煅石膏。用时研极细粉干掺或调敷，或以药捻沾药粉使用。

An appropriate amount for external use. *Shēng yào* is for external use only, not for internal use. What's more, pure products can not be applied, mostly used with *duàn shí gāo*. If used, it should be ground into fine powder, dried or mixed with liquid, or dipped with medicated threads.

【使用注意 / Precaution】

本品有大毒，外用亦不可过量或持续使用。外疡腐肉已去或脓水已尽者不宜用。孕妇禁用。

Hóng fěn is highly toxic, and should not be used in excess or continuously. It should not be used when the carrion has been removed or the pus has been used up and forbidden for pregnant women.

【现代研究 / Modern research】

本品主要含氧化汞（HgO），另含少量硝酸汞 [Hg(NO$_3$)$_2$] 等。具有抗菌、促进创口愈合等作用。

Hóng fěn mainly contains mercury oxide (HgO) and a small amount of mercury nitrate [Hg(NO$_3$)$_2$], etc. It has the functions of antibacterial and promoting the healing of wounds.

轻粉 *Qīng fěn* (Calomelas)
《本草拾遗》
Supplement to the Materia Medica (Běn Cǎo Shí Yí)

【来源 / Origin】

为水银、白矾（或胆矾）、食盐等用升华法炼制而成的氯化亚汞（Hg$_2$Cl$_2$），又称汞粉、水银粉。主产于湖北、湖南、云南等地。避光保存，研细末用。本品气微。《中国药典》规定，含氯化亚汞不得少于 99.0%。

Qīng fěn is mercuric chloride (Hg$_2$Cl$_2$) crystalline powder refined by sublimation method such as mercury, alum (or chalcanthite), salt and so on, mainly produced in Hubei, Hunan, and Yunnan Province, kept away from light for storage and ground into powder for use. It has a slight odor. According to *Chinese Pharmacopoeia*, mercuric chloride must not be less than 99.0%.

【性味归经 / Medicinal properties】

辛，寒；有毒。归大肠、小肠经。

Acrid, cold and toxic; act on large intestine and small intestine meridians.

【主要功效 / Medicinal efficacies】

外用杀虫，攻毒，敛疮；内服祛痰消积，逐水通便。

External use: exterminate insects, remove toxin and heal up sores. Internal administration: dispel phlegm and eliminate accumulation, expel retained water and relax the bowels.

【临床应用 / Clinical application】

1. 疮疡溃烂，疥癣，臁疮，湿疹，酒渣鼻，梅毒　本品外用具有较强的攻毒杀虫止痒和生肌敛疮作用。用治疮疡溃烂，久不收口，多与血竭、当归、紫草等制膏贴敷。用治疥疮，常与吴茱萸、硫黄等同用。用治干、湿癣，可与风化石灰、铅丹、硫黄等同用。用治臁疮不合，配伍黄连末、猪胆汁调涂。用治黄水疮、湿疹痒痛，可与黄柏、煅石膏、蛤粉共为细末，凉水或麻油调涂。用治酒渣鼻、痤疮，可配伍大黄、硫黄加凉水调涂。用治梅毒，可与大风子捣烂外涂。

(1) **Sores and ulcers, tinea, chronic shank ulcer, eczema, rosacea, syphilis**　*Qīng fěn* for external use has a strong effect of removing toxin, killing insects, relieving itching, healing up sores and promoting granulation. It is often made into ointment with *xuè jié* (Draconis Sanguis), *dāng guī* (Angelicae Sinensis Radix) and *zǐ cǎo* (Arnebiae Radix) to treat persisting sores and ulcers. For scabies, it is often used in combination with *wú zhū yú* (Evodiae Fructus) and *liú huáng* (Sulphur). For ringworm due to dryness and dampness, it is used with weathered lime, *qiān dān* (Minium) and *liú huáng*. For unhealed chronic shank ulcer, it is combined with powder of *huáng lián* (Coptidis Rhizoma) and pig bile for external paste. For yellow-water sores and eczema itching and painful, it is used with *huáng bó* (Phellodendri Chinensis Cortex), *duàn shí gāo* (Gypsum Fibrosum Praeparatum) and clam powder, ground into powder and mixed with water or sesame oil for external paste. It treats rosacea and acne in combination with *dà huáng* (Rhei Radix et Rhizoma) and *liú huáng* (Sulphur), mixed with cold water for external paste. For syphilis, it can be mashed with *dà fēng zǐ* (Hydnocarpi Semen) for external paste.

2. 痰涎积滞，水肿鼓胀，二便不利　本品内服能通利二便，逐水退肿。用治痰涎喘逆气急，不得平卧，可用本品与鸡蛋清调匀，蒸熟食用。用治水肿鼓胀，二便不通，可配伍大黄、甘遂、大戟等。

(2) **Phlegm and saliva retention, edema, tympanites, difficulty in urination and defecation**　*Qīng fěn* can relax the bowels and expel retained water to alleviate edema for internal application. For phlegm and saliva retention and asthma, it can be mixed with egg white and steamed, and the patient is not allowed to lie flat. For edema, tympanites, and difficulty in urination and defecation, it is combined with *dà huáng* (Rhei Radix et Rhizoma), *gān suí* (Kansui Radix) and *dà jǐ* (Euphorbiae Pekinensis Radix).

【用法用量 / Usage and dosage】

外用适量，研末调涂或干掺，或制膏外贴。内服每次 0.1~0.2 g，每日 1~2 次，多入丸、散或装胶囊内服。

An appropriate amount for external use, grind it into powder for mixing and pasting, or make into ointment for external application. Take orally 0.1-0.2g every time, 1-2 times a day, mostly in pills, powder or capsules.

【使用注意 / Precaution】

内服宜慎，不可过量使用，且服后应漱口。体虚者及孕妇忌服。

It is advisable to use with caution when taking orally, not to overdose, and rinse mouth after taking it. It is contraindicated in weak people and pregnant women.

【现代研究 / Modern research】

本品主要含氯化亚汞。具有泻下、利尿、抗真菌等作用。

Qīng fěn mainly contains mercuric chloride. It has the functions of purgation, diuretic and antifungal.

砒石 *Pī shí* (Arsenolite Ore)
《日华子本草》
Ri Huazi's Materia Medica (Rì Huá Zǐ Běn Cǎo)

【来源 / Origin】

为天然砷华矿石，或毒砂、雄黄等含砷矿物的加工品，又称信石、人言。主产于江西、湖南、广东等地。药材分白砒（白信石）与红砒（红信石），二者三氧化二砷（As_2O_3）的含量均在96% 以上，但前者更纯，后者尚含少量硫化砷等红色矿物质。药用以红砒为主，砒石升华的精制品即砒霜。本品气无，烧之有蒜样臭气。

Pī shí is a natural arsenic ore or a processed product of arsenic-containing minerals of arsenopyrite and realgar, mainly produce in Jiangxi, Hunan and Guangdong Province, also known as *xìn shí*, *rén yán*. The medicinal materials are divided into white arsenic (*bái xìn shí*) and red arsenic (*hóng xìn shí*). The content of arsenic trioxide (As_2O_3) is more than 96%, but the former is more pure, while the latter contains a small amount of red minerals such as arsenic sulfide. Red arsenic is mainly for medicinals, and the refined product of arsenic sublimation is *pī shuāng*. It has no odor and smells like garlic when burned.

【性味归经 / Medicinal properties】

辛，大热；有大毒。归肺、脾、肝经。

Acrid, highly hot and highly toxic; act on lung, spleen and liver meridians.

【主要功效 / Medicinal efficacies】

外用攻毒杀虫，蚀疮祛腐；内服劫痰平喘，截疟。

External use: remove toxin, exterminate insects, erode sores and resolve putridity. Internal administration: dispel phlegm and relieve dyspnea, and prevent attack of malaria.

【临床应用 / Clinical application】

1. 恶疮，瘰疬，顽癣，牙疳，痔疮　本品毒性剧烈，腐蚀性强，外用具有攻毒杀虫、蚀疮祛腐之功，为治疗恶疮、顽癣、瘰疬之要药。虽可单用贴敷，但易引起中毒而导致剧烈疼痛，故多配伍其他药物以缓其毒。用治恶疮日久，可配伍附子、硫黄、苦参等调油为膏，柳枝煎汤洗疮后外涂。用治瘰疬、顽癣、疔疮、牙疳，可与明矾、雄黄、乳香为细末外用。用治痔疮，可配伍白矾、雄黄等。

(1) **Sores, scrofula, stubborn ringworm, ulcerative gingivitis, and hemorrhoids** *Pī shí* is highly toxic and corrosive. It has the functions of attacking poisons and killing insects, eroding sores and resolving putridity, and is an important medicinal for the treatment of sores, stubborn ringworm and scrofula. Although it can be applied alone, it may cause severe pain due to poisoning, so other drugs are used to alleviate its toxicity. It treats persistent sores in combination with *fù zǐ* (Aconiti Lateralis Radix Praeparata), *liú huáng* (Sulphur) and *kǔ shēn* (Sophorae Flavescentis Radix) by mixing with oil as ointment to paste after washing the sores with decoction with willow branch. For scrofula, stubborn ringworm, whitlow, and ulcerative gingivitis, it can be used with *míng fán* (Alumen), *xióng huáng* (Realgar) and *rǔ xiāng* (Olibanum) ground into powder. For hemorrhoids, it can be combined with *bái fán* (Alumen) and *xióng huáng* (Realgar).

2. 寒痰哮喘 本品入肺经，内服能祛寒痰、平喘息。用治寒痰哮喘，久治不愈，可与淡豆豉为丸服。

(2) Cold phlegm and asthma *Pī shí* enters lung meridian, and can dispel cold phlegm and relieve dyspnea. It treats persistent cold phlegm and asthma in combination with *dàn dòu chǐ* (Sojae Semen Praeparatum) in pills.

此外，本品还能攻毒抑癌，用于多种癌肿。古人曾用砒石治疗疟疾，但现已少用。

In addition, *pī shí* can also attack and inhibit cancer, and be used for a variety of cancers. The ancients used to treat malaria with it, but now it is rarely used.

【用法用量 / Usage and dosage】

外用适量，研末撒敷，宜作复方散剂或入膏药、药捻用。内服每次 0.002~0.004g，入丸、散服。

Appropriate amount for external use, spread after grinding into powder. It is suitable for compound powder or into plaster, medicated threads. Take 0.002-0.004g each time for internal use in pill or powder.

【使用注意 / Precaution】

内服宜慎，外用不宜过量，以防局部吸收中毒。不能作酒剂服。孕妇忌用。不宜与水银同用。

It is advisable to use with caution when taking orally, not to overdose it for external use, to prevent local absorption and poisoning. It cannot be used as wine preparation. Pregnant women avoid using it. Not suitable for use with mercury.

【现代研究 / Modern research】

本品主要含三氧化二砷，并有残存的雌黄（As_2S_3）、雄黄（As_2S_2）等原生矿物及云母、石英等矿物。具有杀菌、杀虫、抗癌、抗组胺及平喘等作用。

Pī shí mainly contains arsenic trioxide, residual primary minerals such as orpiment (As_2S_3), realgar (As_2S_2), mica, quartz and so on. It has bactericidal, insecticidal, anticancer, antihistamine and antiasthmatic effects.

其他拔毒化腐生肌药功用介绍见表 26-1。

The efficacies of other medicinals for removing toxin, resolving putridity and promoting granulation are shown in table 26-1.

表 26-1 其他拔毒化腐生肌药功用介绍

分类	药物	药性	功效	应用	用法用量
拔毒化腐生肌药	铅丹	辛，微寒；有毒。归心、肝经	外用拔毒生肌，杀虫止痒；内服坠痰镇惊	疮疡溃烂，湿疹瘙痒；疥癣；惊痫癫狂，心神不宁	外用适量，研末撒布或熬膏贴敷。内服多入丸、散，0.3~0.6g
	炉甘石	甘，平。归肝、脾经	解毒明目退翳，收湿止痒敛疮	目赤翳障，眼睑溃烂；溃疡不敛，湿疮湿疹	外服适量，研末撒布或调敷，水飞点眼、吹喉
	硼砂	甘、咸，凉。归肺、胃经	外用清热解毒；内服清肺化痰	咽喉肿痛，口舌生疮，目赤翳障，痰热咳嗽	外用适量，研极细末干撒或调敷患处。内服1.5~3g，入丸、散

（叶耀辉）

题库

医药大学堂
WWW.YIYAODXT.COM

药名拼音索引
Pinyin index of medicinals

参考文献
Reference

［1］国家中医药管理局，《中华本草》编委会.中华本草［M］.上海：上海科学技术出版社，1999.

［2］南京中医药大学.中药大辞典［M］.2版.上海：上海科学技术出版社，2006.

［3］高学敏，钟赣生.中医药学高级丛书·中药学［M］.2版.北京：人民卫生出版社，2013.

［4］雷载权，张廷模.中华临床中药学［M］.北京：人民卫生出版社，1998.

［5］张廷模.临床中药学［M］.上海：上海科学技术出版社，2012.

［6］钟赣生.中药学［M］.北京：中国中医药出版社，2016.

［7］高晓山.中药药性论［M］.北京：人民卫生出版社，1992.

［8］尚志钧.中国本草要籍考［M］.合肥：安徽科学技术出版社，2009.

［9］唐德才，吴庆光.中药学［M］.3版.北京：人民卫生出版社，2016.

［10］张廷模.中药功效学［M］.北京：人民卫生出版社，2013.

［11］周祯祥.临床中药研究心得［M］.北京：中国医药科技出版社，2005.

［12］王建，张冰.临床中药学［M］.2版.北京：人民卫生出版社，2016.

［13］周凤梧.中药学［M］.山东：山东科学技术出版社，1981.

［14］高晓山.本草文献学纲要［M］.北京：人民军医出版社，2009.

［15］赵军宁，叶祖光.中药毒性理论与安全性评价［M］.北京：人民卫生出版社，2012.

［16］尚志钧，林乾良，郑金生.历代中药文献精华［M］.北京：科学技术文献出版社，1989.

［17］龚千锋.中药炮制学［M］.北京：中国中医药出版社，2016.

［18］滕佳林.中药学［M］.北京：人民卫生出版社，2019.

［19］彭康，张一昕.中药学［M］.北京：科学出版社，2013.